What a gem! The *Lifestyle Medicine Handbook* is ⟨...⟩ as thoroughly referenced. Full of prac⟨...⟩ fect place to start your journey into lifes⟨...⟩ dify and expand your knowledge. This ⟨...⟩ ion for anyone joining the lifestyle med⟨...⟩ ent overview of the field. Congratulations ⟨...⟩ producing such a valuable text!

Wayne S. Dysinger, MD, MPH, FACLM
CEO, Lifestyle and Preventive Medicine, Lifestyle Medicine Solutions

The *Lifestyle Medicine Handbook* is based on state-of-the-art research and best practices, and it is a wonderful guide filled with tips, strategies, tools, and more.

Julie K. Silver, MD
Associate Professor and Associate Chair,
Department of Physical Medicine and Rehabilitation, Harvard Medical School
Author of *Before and After Cancer Treatment: Heal Faster, Better, Stronger*

A remarkable book, full of great tips, but it is especially notable for the human moment that Dr. Frates creates for us by taking us with her as she engages her patients in her "Live and Learn With Dr. Beth Frates" vignettes, which make it easy to read and a friendly powerful way to learn. The style is engaging and the tips are practical and evidence-based. What a great way to introduce the new field.

John Ratey, MD
Associate Clinical Professor of Psychiatry, Harvard Medical School
Author of *Spark: The Revolutionary New Science of Exercise and the Brain*

Since the publication of the first edition of my academic textbook in 1999 which named and framed this discipline, the field of lifestyle medicine has continued to grow and thrive. The *Lifestyle Medicine Handbook* is a welcome new addition to this effort. The handbook is well researched, practical, and inspirational. It draws on the abundant clinical experience and insights of Dr. Frates and her co-authors. This handbook will introduce students and practitioners at all levels to the power and importance of daily habits and actions on health and quality of life. I highly recommend it!

James M. Rippe, MD
Founder and Director, Rippe Lifestyle Institute
Author of *Lifestyle Medicine*

Lifestyle Medicine Handbook
An Introduction to the Power of Healthy Habits

In collaboration with

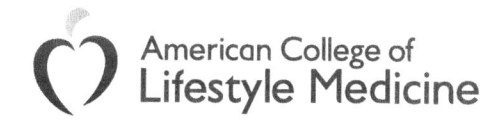

American College of Lifestyle Medicine

Beth Frates, MD
Jonathan P. Bonnet, MD
Richard Joseph, MD
James A. Peterson, PhD

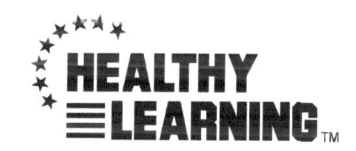

HEALTHY LEARNING

© 2019 Healthy Learning. All rights reserved. Printed in the United States.

No part of this book may be reproduced, stored in a retrieval system or transmitted, in any form or by any means, electronic, mechanical, photocopying, recording, or otherwise, without the prior permission of Healthy Learning.

ISBN: 978-1-60679-413-5
Library of Congress Control Number: 2017956953
Book layout: Cheery Sugabo
Cover design: Becky Hansen
Cover photos: (front, left to right) serezniy/iStock/Thinkstock; iStock.com/oonal; monkeybusinessimages/iStock/Thinkstock; (back, left to right) antoniodiaz/Shutterstock.com; Gettyimages.com; Gettyimages.com

Healthy Learning
P.O. Box 1828
Monterey, CA 93942
www.healthylearning.com

About ACLM

Vision:

A world in which all physicians and allied health professionals
have been trained and certified in evidence-based lifestyle medicine,
integrating healthful behaviors into their own lives,
while incorporating a lifestyle medicine-first approach to
treating root causes of lifestyle-related diseases into their clinical practices.

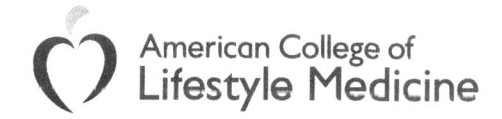

American College of Lifestyle Medicine

The American College of Lifestyle Medicine (ACLM) is the medical professional association for those dedicated to the advancement and clinical practice of Lifestyle Medicine as the foundation of a transformed and sustainable system of health care delivery. More than a professional association, ACLM is a galvanized force for change. ACLM addresses the need for quality education and certification, supporting its members in their individual practices and in their collective mission to domestically and globally promote Lifestyle Medicine as the first treatment option, as opposed to a first option of treating symptoms and consequences with expensive, ever-increasing quantities of pills and procedures. ACLM members are united in their desire to identify and eradicate the cause of disease, striving for sustainable health, sustainable health care and a sustainable world—as all are inextricably connected. For more information, visit www.lifestylemedicine.org. For information about certification in the field of Lifestyle Medicine, please visit www.ablm.co.

Dedication

This book is dedicated to all the lifestyle medicine professionals, patients, researchers, and students who have helped us to realize the power of healthy habits, like routine exercise, nutritious and delicious foods, restful sleep, stress resiliency, mindfulness, meditation, a growth mindset, and so much more. We are grateful to Healthy Learning and the American College of Lifestyle Medicine for their partnership in getting this handbook completed.

Acknowledgments

I was approached about creating a lifestyle medicine handbook in 2014, and it is finally happening. We want to thank Susan Benigas for her support of the handbook. We are also grateful to David Ferriss and Amanda McKinney, two board members of the ACLM, who reviewed the contents of the book, and provided feedback. Specifically for the nutrition chapter, we want to thank Susan Benigas, Paulina Shetty, Brenda Rea, George Guthrie, Cate Collings, and Kayli Dice for helping to make the chapter an accurate reflection of the ACLM's position stand on nutrition. In addition, I would like to acknowledge the students in my Harvard Extension School class. If not for them, this book would not have come to fruition. They asked for the book and many helped get it going. Specifically, thank you Kate Simeon, Yasamina McBride, Irena Matanovic, and Merl Coriolan for your initial edits and help with formulation.

—Beth Frates

Foreword

The Lifestyle Medicine Revolution

Beth Frates has written one of the most comprehensive and useful books about the power of lifestyle medicine. I feel honored to write the foreword to it and highly recommend it. She has also been an important leader in advancing this field.

This is the era of lifestyle medicine: that is, using simple yet powerful lifestyle changes not only to prevent but also to treat and often to reverse the progression of the most common chronic diseases as well as to help prevent them.

Our bodies often have a remarkable capacity to begin healing, and much more quickly than we had once believed, when we work at this causal level: the lifestyle changes choices we make each day. These include what we eat, how we respond to stress, how much exercise we get, and how much love and support we have.

Lifestyle medicine is the most exciting movement today in health and healing—a revolutionary tidal wave that hasn't yet even begun to crest.

There is a convergence of forces and a growing recognition of the importance and power of lifestyle medicine that finally make this the right idea at the right time. These include an increasing body of scientific evidence documenting the limitations of high-tech medicine at the same time that there is a growing recognition of the power of lifestyle medicine to reverse and prevent a wide variety of chronic diseases. This is why Medicare and many insurance companies are now covering our lifestyle medicine program for reversing heart disease.

For example, the latest studies are showing that lifestyle changes are not only as good as drugs and surgery but in some cases even better in treating and actually reversing many of the most prevalent chronic diseases. Here are two examples:

1. *Coronary heart disease:* A review of all eight randomized controlled trials concluded that stents don't prevent heart attacks, don't reduce the need for bypass surgery, don't reduce angina (chest pain), and don't prolong life in most patients with stable coronary heart disease.[1, 2, 3]

---

1. Stergiopoulos K, Brown DL. Initial coronary stent implantation with medical therapy vs medical therapy alone for stable coronary artery disease: meta-analysis of randomized controlled trials. *Archives of Internal Medicine.* February 27 2012;172(4):312-319.
2. Boden WE, O'Rourke RA, Teo KK, et al. COURAGE Trial Research Group. Optimal medical therapy with or without PCI for stable coronary disease. *New England Journal of Medicine.* 2007;356(15):1503-1516.
3. Al-Lamee R, Thompson D, Dehbi H M, et al. Percutaneous coronary intervention in stable angina (ORBITA): a double-blind, randomized controlled trial. *Lancet.* 2017; published online Nov 2. http://dx.doi org/10.1016/S0140-6736(17)32714-9.

In contrast, my colleagues and I conducted the first randomized controlled trials showing that lifestyle medicine can reverse the progression of even severe coronary heart disease in most patients, without drugs or surgery. There was even more reversal after five years than after one year and 2.5 times fewer cardiac events, and there was a 91 percent reduction in the frequency of angina.[4] PET scans revealed that blood to the heart was 400 percent higher in the group that went on this lifestyle medicine program when compared to the randomized control group.[5]

Stents can be lifesaving in someone who is having a heart attack or is unstable. But most patients who have undergone these procedures are stable.

Recently, several patients with such bad heart disease that they were told they needed a heart transplant went through our lifestyle medicine program and improved so much in only nine weeks that they no longer needed a heart transplant! In addition to saving over $1 million per patient and avoiding a lifetime of immunosuppressive medications, these improvements graphically show how powerful and meaningful lifestyle medicine can be. What's the more radical intervention—lifestyle changes or a heart transplant?

2. *Early-stage prostate cancer:* Two randomized controlled trials in *The New England Journal of Medicine* documented that surgery and radiation do not prolong life after 10 years in men with early-stage prostate cancer.

In contrast, my colleagues and I conducted the first randomized controlled trial (in collaboration with the chairs of urology at Memorial Sloan-Kettering Cancer Center and at UCSF) showing that lifestyle medicine may slow, stop, or even reverse the progression of early-stage prostate cancer, without drugs or surgery.[6]

There is a relatively small subset of men—approximately one out of 50—who have especially aggressive forms of prostate cancer and may benefit from surgery or radiation. Dr. Carroll has developed algorithms to help identify these patients. Most men are much more likely to die *with* prostate cancer than *from* prostate cancer.

Also, surgery and radiation can maim men in the most personal ways by often causing impotence and incontinence. Most men with diagnosed prostate cancer want to *do something,* not just "watchful waiting," even if the results of conventional treatments of surgery and radiation are often worse than the disease. Lifestyle medicine provides a third, better alternative for many patients.

---

4. Ornish DM, Scherwitz LW, Doody RS, et al. Effects of stress management training and dietary changes in treating ischemic heart disease. *JAMA.* 1983;249:54-59.
5. Gould KL, Ornish D, Scherwitz L, et al. Changes in myocardial perfusion abnormalities by positron emission tomography after long-term, intense risk factor modification. *JAMA.* 1995;274:894-901.
6. Ornish DM, Weidner G, Fair WR, et al. Intensive lifestyle changes may affect the progression of prostate cancer. *Journal of Urology.* 2005;174:1065-1070.

Of course, there is a time and a place for high-tech medicine. We've all benefited from it. Drugs and surgery can be lifesaving in a crisis. And in the early stages of treating and reversing chronic diseases, drugs may be necessary in addition to intensive lifestyle changes at least at the beginning while your body is healing. And some people may need drugs and/or surgery even when they make comprehensive lifestyle changes. Even then, though, we need to address the underlying causes—which are usually lifestyle related and often treatable and even reversible with lifestyle medicine.

Also, more than 86 percent of the $3.2 trillion in annual U.S. healthcare costs go toward treating chronic diseases, which can often be prevented and sometimes even reversed by making comprehensive lifestyle changes, at a fraction of the cost. Lifestyle medicine can make better care available to more people at lower costs—and the only side effects are good ones.

Dean Ornish, MD
Founder and President, Preventive Medicine Research Institute
Clinical Professor of Medicine, University of California, San Francisco
www.ornish.com

Contents

About ACLM 5
Dedication 6
Acknowledgments 7
Foreword (Dean Ornish) 9
Preface 14

Chapter 1: Understanding Lifestyle Medicine 17
Chapter 2: Empowering People to Change 43
Chapter 3: Collaborating, Motivating, Goal-Setting, and Tracking 89
Chapter 4: Improving Health Through Exercise 119
Chapter 5: The Nutrition-Health Connection 167
Chapter 6: Sleep Matters 242
Chapter 7: Stress and Resilience 273
Chapter 8: Peace of Mind With Meditation, Mindfulness, and Relaxation 297
Chapter 9: The Power of Connection 328
Chapter 10: Positively Positive 350
Chapter 11: Substance Abuse 377
Chapter 12: Staying the Course 411

Appendix A: A Weekly Health Prescription 437
About the Authors 440

Preface

This book is for anyone who wants to learn the key factors involved in lifestyle medicine. It is designed as an introductory book that will explore the history of lifestyle medicine, as well as its six pillars, including nutrition, exercise, sleep, stress resiliency, addiction, and social connection. The research, guidelines, clinical cases, and prescriptions for each of the pillars are addressed. In addition, this book details the importance of collaborating with the patient and using a coach approach when counseling people about adopting and sustaining healthy habits. Furthermore, the text reviews the important role of the stages of behavior change, motivational interviewing, appreciative inquiry, positivity, a strengths-based approach, a growth mindset, and other evidence-based models for change.

One of the reasons that this book is unique is because each chapter provides updated medical information and cutting-edge research on the topic addressed. It also features a series of "Live and Learns" as a way to share best practices in lifestyle medicine. Similar to "M&M" or "Morbidity and Mortality" conferences in general medicine, in lifestyle medicine, we offer "L&L" or "Live and Learns" as a viable means to focus on different strategies to empower people and guide them on the path to optimal health and wellness.

On occasion, what we try does not work. In these instances, we share our missteps with others, in the hope that we can learn from each other. The underlying goal is to build on each other's experiences as practitioners. This book emphasizes a growth mindset, targeting the fact that every misstep is an opportunity to learn and grow. In other words, together everyone achieves more (T.E.A.M.).

This handbook is an attempt to introduce basic lifestyle medicine principles and to create a team of like-minded practitioners who will continue to collaborate with the goal of transforming healthcare and reducing the burden of lifestyle-related diseases on the individual level, as well as on the population and global levels. As such, this book is designed to get the basic information related to lifestyle medicine into the hands of as many people as possible.

The material in this handbook is based on information and insights derived from more than 30 years of studying and practicing lifestyle medicine principles. My father had a heart attack and subsequent stroke, when he was 52 and I was 18, which is when my journey into healthy habits started. Subsequently, I was researching and learning about heart health to help my father live a longer and healthier life. Then, I began to practice the principles attendant to a healthy lifestyle for myself. This effort transformed into my life's passion—to help other people reach their optimal state of well-being in body, mind, and spirit.

Through research for my senior thesis in college, I studied the effect of mental stress on the function of the heart. Later, in medical school, I investigated the impact of a diet rich in nitric oxide on the arterial walls, as well as the build-up of plaque. During my residency in physiatry, I researched the habits of physicians, with regard to exercise. In the process, it became apparent to me that physicians who exercise tend to counsel on exercise. As such, if physicians engaged in strength training, they counseled on strength training. If they did not strength train, they did not counsel on it. The same factor was true for aerobic exercise.

During residency, I examined the general knowledge of stroke survivors (and their caregivers) about their condition. For example, did they know what kind of stroke they had? Were they aware of what medications they were taking? Were they familiar with the steps they could take to prevent a second stroke? And so on. I was surprised to discover that less than half of stroke survivors and caregivers could answer these questions correctly. In my mind, this situation called out for a book about stroke prevention. I attempted to fill this gap in the literature by working with colleagues in the Harvard Department of Physical Medicine and Rehabilitation on a book entitled *Life After Stroke: The Guide to Recovering Your Health and Preventing Another Stroke*.

It was then that I dove deep into the medical literature on exercise, nutrition, and stress resiliency. After that, I was determined to help everyone I could to lead healthy lives, prior to experiencing a health setback, such as a stroke. This mindset led me to join the lifestyle medicine movement in 2008 at Harvard Medical School (HMS), with Dr. Edward Phillips at the Institute of Lifestyle Medicine. We co-created CME courses, live and online, and developed the institute together. In addition, I started the Lifestyle Medicine Interest Group at HMS, which has been operating, at this point, for over 10 years.

In 2014, I was invited to teach a college-level course on lifestyle medicine at Harvard Extension School. It was at this time that I put together a full lifestyle medicine syllabus, which is now shared with the American College of Lifestyle Medicine (www.lifestylemedicine.org). After teaching the course for three years, I finally decided to proceed with writing a handbook on lifestyle medicine that could accompany the syllabus. The students in the course at the Harvard Extension School kept asking for a book. At this point, no basic handbook was yet available at the introductory level for college students, pre-medical students, first- and second-year medical students, nurses, physical therapists, nutritionists, health coaches, psychologists, and social workers, as well as other healthcare providers. This handbook is designed to help fill that void.

In 2015, I attended my first national meeting of the American College of Lifestyle Medicine (ACLM) and, at that time, became part of the national and global movement. In 2016, I was honored to be elected to the board of directors for ACLM and have been actively involved with the education and publication committees ever since. It is through a close collaboration with ACLM that we have been able to complete this handbook. My co-authors include Jon Bonnet, a sports and obesity medicine physician, who was a teaching assistant in my Harvard Extension School course; Richard Joseph, a medical resident at the Brigham and Women's Hospital and a mentee of Dr. David Katz, while he was at Yale; and Dr. Jim Peterson, a sports medicine consultant and a fellow of ACSM.

In collaboration with my three co-authors, I wrote this book to both inform and inspire individuals about the extensive array of benefits that are attendant to adhering to healthy habits. If this book helps a single reader to prevent or reverse a chronic health disease, then the effort to put it together will have been more than worthwhile. Enjoy!

—Beth Frates

CHAPTER 1

UNDERSTANDING LIFESTYLE MEDICINE

"The part can never be well unless the whole is well."

—Plato
Classical Greek Philosopher
428 to 348 BCE

❏ Chapter Goals:

- Introduce the field of lifestyle medicine.
- Encourage readers to consider their own healthy habits.
- Provide a roadmap for the remainder of the book.

❏ Learning Objectives:

- To understand what lifestyle medicine is and what it means to be evidence-based
- To understand why lifestyle medicine is important for individuals, society, and healthcare
- To be aware of the history, economics, and competencies attendant to lifestyle medicine

❏ Guiding Questions:

- What are some of the lifestyle-related problems that patients, providers, and healthcare systems are currently facing?
- How is lifestyle medicine meeting the needs of patients, providers, and healthcare systems in the 21st century?
- How can patients and providers acquire the necessary knowledge, skills, and tools required to prevent, treat, and reverse lifestyle-related diseases, such as diabetes, obesity, cardiac disease, stroke, and metabolic syndrome?
- What is the evidence supporting lifestyle medicine?

❏ Important Terms:

- *Lifestyle medicine:* The use of evidence-based lifestyle therapeutic approaches, such as a predominantly whole food, plant-based diet, regular physical activity, adequate sleep, stress management, avoidance of risky substance use, and other non-drug modalities to treat, oftentimes, reverse and prevent the lifestyle-related, chronic disease that's all too prevalent

- *Quality of life:* The patient's ability to enjoy normal life activities
- *Evidence-based:* In medicine, pertaining to the conscientious, explicit, and judicious use of current best evidence in making decisions about the care of individual patients

The material in this chapter provides a framework from which to build a healthy lifestyle. Starting from 600 BC with the wisdom of Hippocrates, there have been many important leaders and forefathers of lifestyle medicine. In addition to various individuals, there are critical historical events that have contributed to the development of this burgeoning field of medicine. Exploring how vaccines and antibiotics changed the landscape of medicine and how the Industrial Revolution played a part in the spread of lifestyle-related diseases provides perspective on how the worldwide epidemic of obesity and diabetes started. In addition, the economics of lifestyle medicine are important, given the cost and burden of chronic diseases, such as diabetes, obesity, and cardiac disease. This chapter provides an introduction to lifestyle medicine in a way that is meant to inspire, unnerve, and motivate readers.

THE PAST

The history of lifestyle medicine is intricately tied to the history of the mankind. Humans were hunters and gatherers for the majority of their existence. Then came farming and agriculture. Families and workers would toil all day in the fields, and, only after hours of hard labor, did they sit down for a home-cooked meal, derived from the crops and animals on their farms. Relatively speaking, they had to engage in a great deal of work to consume a small amount of food each day. During the farming era, people spent most of their time outside in nature, and they were moving. Today, people do the exact opposite. Most individuals spend little time moving, little time outdoors, and little time preparing food—and hence, the emergence of the term "fast food."

Movement is a critical component of a healthy lifestyle. It is rumored that Albert Einstein's breakthrough insights in his general theory of relativity came not while he was diligently working at a desk, but rather during one of his breaks, while he was riding a bicycle outside! He looked at some clocks while riding, and, suddenly, everything in his lab made sense.

It is important to note that experiencing a creativity breakthrough with exercise is not just for famous inventors. Routine exercisers often experience a similar surge of inspiration (albeit not at the same scope of importance as Einstein's). After a run, a bicycle ride, or even a walk in the woods, many exercisers often have a 'creativity moment,' one in which the solution to a particular problem or novel idea pops into their head. After exercise, like a walk in the woods or a yoga class, the brain waves enter an alpha state, which is associated with a reflective, clearheaded state of mind, ripe for new ideas. In such an instance, that particular bout of exercise can be a game changer.

THE CURRENT STATE OF HEALTH

What does the present state of health look like for people in the United States? People are sitting, people are eating fast food and processed food, people are watching TV, and people are walking their dogs, on occasion, while they themselves drive a car. This latter snapshot is, in fact, *true*. It has been documented on the Internet and witnessed by credible observers that some people walk their dogs, while sitting in a car, one hand on the wheel and one hand on a leash, hanging out the driver's window.

Technology has afforded many advances to Americans. Without question, the U.S. is a productive society. A wide variety of advances have occurred since 1760 and the Industrial Revolution, including the steam engine, car engine, telegraph, sewing machine, telephone, light bulb, and then, of course, the computer and the digital revolution.

This plethora of inventions has changed societal norms in a number of ways. In fact, the three big Ts—transportation, television, and technology—have made a significant impact on the lifestyles of most individuals:

- *Transportation:* In 1908, the invention of the Ford Model T changed human existence for good, moving the nation from a physically active society to a more-sedentary driving society.
- *Television:* All factors considered, TV is great for spreading information and news and for providing some comic relief (which can be very positive, since it's well-known that laughing half an hour a day promotes good health). Conversely, sitting in front of a TV for hours each day, as many people do, is also correlated with weight gain and disease.
- *Technology:* Humans can have a face-to-face meeting with other people hundreds of miles away, with the click of a button on a phone or computer. This interaction can be very time-efficient and useful for cultivating and retaining relationships, both personal and professional. The problem is that replacing in-person meetings with virtual meetings can lead an individual to miss some of the essential features and joys of being human, including touch experienced with a handshake, a high-five, a hug, or a tap on the back. As such, the health value of human touch is well-established. For example, the feel-good hormone oxytocin, known as the "cuddle hormone" or the "love hormone," is released from the pituitary gland when people connect physically with other humans.

THE TIMES THEY ARE CHANGING

Over the past hundred years or so, not only have huge gains been undertaken in industry that have made life easier, less strenuous, and more productive (e.g., resulting in more food being available for everyone), but great advances in healthcare settings have also been achieved. For example, vaccinations for measles and other diseases that extended the lifespans of Americans have been developed; surgical anesthesia has been devised; efforts to clean water and improve sanitation have been undertaken; and antibiotics, such as penicillin (one of the most important discoveries ever in medicine) have been unearthed.

In fact, any listing of the medical breakthroughs that have occurred would be extensive and would include such items as the birth control pill, open-heart surgery, randomized controlled clinical trials, radiologic imaging, early and improved diagnostic tests for cancer detection, advances in childbirth (resulting in fewer deaths) and enhancements in organ transplantation. Because of those advances, the health of individuals has improved dramatically, along with their lifespan.

❑ Health and Life Expectancy

At the present time, the average life expectancy in the United States is 77.9. As a rule, 66.2 of those years tend to be healthy, unimpaired ones. In other words, most people will face 11.7 *impaired, unhealthy* years of life. In that regard, lifestyle medicine can not only help to increase the number of healthy years, it can also help to decrease the number of impaired years of life that a person experiences. This factor enables most humans to enjoy a relatively high quality of life right up to the end of their life. Living until 80 years old is a step in the right direction—particularly if the 80-year-old is able to converse with loved ones, laugh, eat the food they want, move freely and without pain, and be productive and independent.

The primary causes of death in the United States have also evolved considerably in the past century. Figure 1-1 shows the leading and actual causes of death in the United States in 2000. Actual causes of death are defined as lifestyle and behavioral factors, such as smoking and physical inactivity, that contribute to this nation's leading killers

Leading Causes of Death*
United States, 2000

- Heart disease
- Cancer
- Stroke
- Chronic lower respiratory disease
- Unintentional injuries
- Diabetes
- Pneumonia/influenza
- Alzheimer's disease
- Kidney disease

Percentage (of all deaths): 0, 5, 10, 15, 20, 25, 30, 35

Actual Causes of Death†
United States, 2000

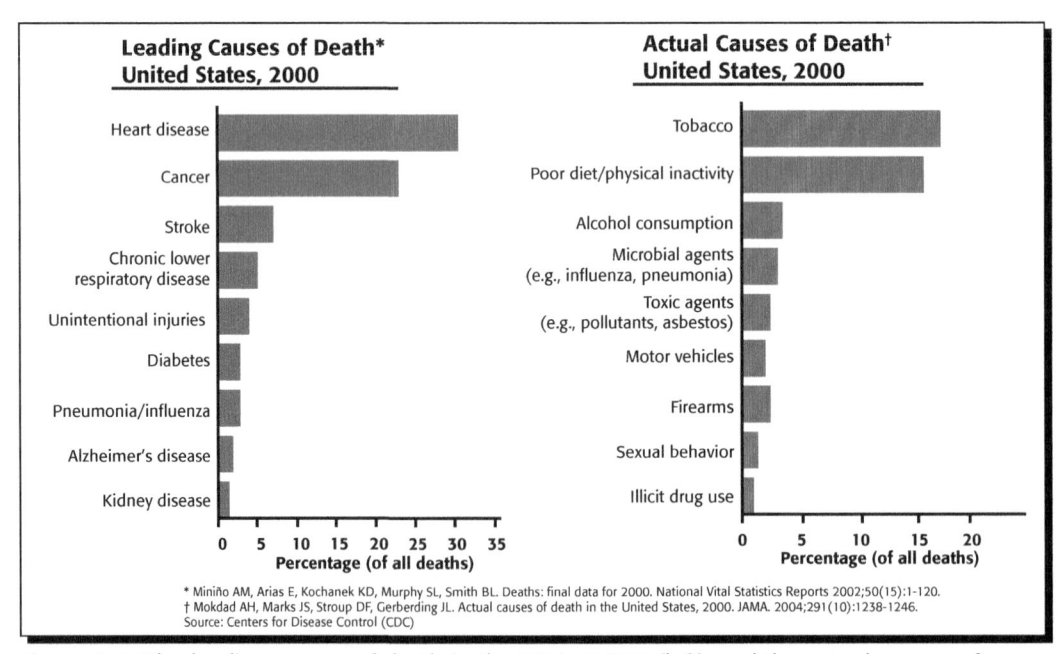

- Tobacco
- Poor diet/physical inactivity
- Alcohol consumption
- Microbial agents (e.g., influenza, pneumonia)
- Toxic agents (e.g., pollutants, asbestos)
- Motor vehicles
- Firearms
- Sexual behavior
- Illicit drug use

Percentage (of all deaths): 0, 5, 10, 15, 20

* Miniño AM, Arias E, Kochanek KD, Murphy SL, Smith BL. Deaths: final data for 2000. National Vital Statistics Reports 2002;50(15):1-120.
† Mokdad AH, Marks JS, Stroup DF, Gerberding JL. Actual causes of death in the United States, 2000. JAMA. 2004;291(10):1238-1246.
Source: Centers for Disease Control (CDC)

Figure 1-1. The leading causes of death in the US in 2000 (left) and the actual causes of death in the US in 2000 (right)

including heart disease, cancer, and stroke. It is important to note that the top three causes of death (and arguably a few of the other factors) are all related to lifestyle choices. Collectively, the lifestyle-related factors account for an astonishing 80 percent of the attributable premature deaths in the country.

A snapshot of the American healthcare scene presents a mixed message. On one hand, some medical conditions have experienced tremendous progress (e.g., infectious disease). On the other hand, some have unfortunately regressed (e.g., heart disease and obesity).

• *Infectious disease.* One of the areas in which healthcare innovations and advances have had a conspicuous impact on health is in a marked reduction in the death rate for infectious disease in the United States. For example, during the period 1918-1920, an influenza pandemic occurred that resulted in an estimated 20-40 million deaths. With the invention of the first vaccination for the flu in the late 1930s, however, influenza was no longer the devastating health threat that it once was. Subsequently, penicillin was developed—a miracle drug designed to treat bacterial infections that would previously have been life-threatening.

In 1900, most Americans died by 50 years of age. As previously noted, the average age of death today is closer to 80 years old. This number could arguably be even higher were it not for the counterproductive impact that lifestyle-related decisions have on various medical conditions. Perhaps, the most calamitous conditions that are impacted by lifestyle are heart disease, obesity, and diabetes.

• *Heart disease.* Despite noteworthy medical advances in recent years, heart disease (also referred to as cardiovascular disease), which includes atherosclerotic coronary heart disease (i.e., partially or completely obstructed coronary arteries), stroke, angina pectoris (i.e., chest pain/pressure), and congestive heart failure (the heart's inability to pump effectively, which causes a reduced level of blood flow to the tissues of the body), remains the leading cause of death in most developed countries, including the United States.

Heart disease causes approximately one out of every four U.S. deaths each year. Quantitatively, that disturbing statistic translates to nearly 2,300 American deaths a day (e.g., one death every 37 seconds). In addition, heart disease and stroke also have an economic downside, costing the nation an estimated $318 billion in healthcare expenditures and lost productivity. As subsequent chapters in this book will clearly point out, most of those deaths could and would be prevented if individuals adhered to sound lifestyle choices.

• *Obesity.* As recently as 2000, obesity (body mass index of 30+) was not recognized by the public as a significant health problem. It wasn't until 2013 that the American Medical Association declared that obesity was a disease. Until that time, physicians, other healthcare providers, insurance agencies, and the general public typically did not take obesity seriously enough. By 2000, however, obesity had reached epidemic proportions in the United States. It was clear that something needed to be done to address this serious health-related crisis. For example, considerable evidence has been found that obesity increases a person's risk for contracting a variety of chronic medical conditions, including heart disease, type 2 diabetes, high cholesterol, high blood pressure, stroke, obstructive sleep disorders, and fatty liver. Furthermore, the estimated annual healthcare costs of obesity-related illness are over $190 billion, including $14 billion alone in direct medical costs for childhood obesity.

Appropriately so, it has been recognized that medical professionals will need lifestyle tools and strategies to help their patients undertake and sustain behavioral changes that will enable them to successfully manage their weight. One of the key focal points of this book is to detail those resources.

- *Diabetes.* According to the Centers for Disease Control and Prevention, more than 29 million Americans have diabetes (a group of metabolic disorders in which high blood sugar levels are present in the body over a prolonged period). Almost equally disturbing is the fact that the total annual cost of diabetes exceeds $245 billion, including $176 billion in direct medical costs and $69 billion in reduced productivity. Furthermore, estimates indicate that an additional 86 million individuals in the U.S. have prediabetes (elevated blood sugar levels that will lead to diabetes if not corrected). Shockingly, the results of some investigations suggest that *one in three* American adults could have diabetes by the year 2050.

This group of metabolic diseases (type 1 and type 2 diabetes) results in a person having abnormally high blood glucose levels (blood sugar), either because insulin production is inadequate (type 1 diabetes), or because the body's cells do not respond properly to insulin (type 2 diabetes), or both. Over time, having too much glucose in the blood can lead to serious medical problems, including heart disease and damage to a person's eyes, kidneys, and nerves. Fortunately, individuals can take a number of lifestyle-related steps that can significantly lower (if not eliminate) their risk of contracting type 2 diabetes.

THE LIFESTYLE MEDICINE IMPERATIVE

Without question, the United States is in the midst of a healthcare crisis. The number of Americans suffering from at least one chronic medical condition is rising. The corresponding cost of healthcare is exceptionally high, and essentially unsustainable on the current path. The trend is alarming, and presents a call-to-action for those individuals who are ready to take up the challenge.

The renowned French writer Victor Hugo, author of the acclaimed novel *Les Misérables*, once remarked that "Nothing is as powerful as an idea whose time has come." With regard to healthcare, that idea is both compelling and straightforward—a strategy must be adopted that results in people making essential changes in their lifestyle. Without an appropriate shift in how people live their lives and how they view their health, the perilous course on which the American healthcare system is headed will continue unabated.

Given the situation, at least two basic questions arise. First, what can be done to help address the current state of affairs of healthcare in the United States? Second, who are the change agents who must help lead the way to implement the proposed solutions? All factors considered, the answer to the first query is to get individuals to subscribe to the six pillars of lifestyle medicine. This situation will likely include public health efforts to help make these individual lifestyle choices the default choices. The response to the second issue is to put physicians and allied health professionals at the forefront of the effort. The fundamental centerpiece in both instances is understanding, advocating, and abiding by the core tenets of lifestyle medicine.

The official definition of lifestyle medicine from the American College of Lifestyle Medicine (www.lifestylemedicine.org) is that it is the use of evidence-based lifestyle therapeutic approaches, such as a predominantly whole food, plant-based diet, regular physical activity, adequate sleep, stress management, avoidance of risky substance use, and other non-drug modalities to treat, oftentimes, reverse and prevent the lifestyle-related, chronic disease that's all too prevalent. This definition harkens back to the concept of healthy life years, previously discussed in this chapter, in which the basic objective is to increase the number of healthy life years that people live. This subtlety is important, given that the underlying objective of lifestyle medicine is not to simply add years to life (though it will do this), but to add life to those years (the real prize).

The underlying blueprint for achieving the aforementioned goal entails adhering to the six pillars of lifestyle medicine: exercise, nutrition, sleep, smoking cessation, social connection, and mind-body health. As such, the focus is to help individuals become more physically active, improve their diet, enhance the quantity and quality of their sleep, eliminate their use of tobacco, strengthen their relationships with the people around them, and lessen the physical and emotional effects that they may face from the pressures of everyday life. All of these elements are vital aspects of lifestyle medicine. The power of lifestyle medicine lies in the combination of these pillars.

Lifestyle medicine acknowledges the link between lifestyle and health outcomes. Lifestyle medicine also recognizes the science behind health behavior change. The importance of providing tailored nutrition and exercise prescriptions and recognizing the value of a multi-disciplinary approach is foundational to lifestyle medicine. Lifestyle medicine emphasizes the value of a team approach and the need for support of a qualified healthcare team to get the prescriptions written and filled. Physicians can't do it all on their own. Lifestyle medicine is a team specialty, similar in scope to any team sport, e.g., football, basketball, soccer, etc. In order for the team to be successful, each member of the team must bring their own unique skillset to help patients make sustainable lifestyle changes.

Lifestyle medicine practitioners need to be knowledgeable in a variety of areas, including lifestyle assessments, effective relationships, collaborating with patients, working with a team of caregivers, making referrals, utilizing medical information technology, and promoting healthy habits as a foundation for health. Another core competency involves the need for and value of the personal practice of a healthy lifestyle (i.e., practice what they preach). Taking self-care seriously is not selfish. That is an important lesson for the lifestyle medicine practitioner to practice and to preach.

THE FOREFATHERS OF LIFESTYLE MEDICINE

While there are many extraordinary individuals who have helped grow the lifestyle medicine field, several individuals have had a particularly noteworthy impact on the field, including the following:

❑ *Nathan Pritikin:* Pritikin was a renowned author, a well-respected nutritionist, and a longevity researcher. Pritikin conceived the underlying concepts for lifestyle medicine, long before the emergence of the data reviewed in this chapter. Nathan Pritikin was brilliant—an inventor, but also a chemist, physicist, and a nutritionist.

What propelled Pritikin? Certainly, his heart attack in 1950 played a key role. (It should be noted that an interesting story can almost always be found behind the people in the field of lifestyle medicine.) He tried to heal himself with diet and exercise, and it worked. Subsequently, he started the widely successful Pritikin Longevity Centers.

Eventually, he began giving lectures to internal medicine physicians and cardiologists about the diet he had created that was comprised of whole foods, with little to no sugar (which was being consumed to excess at that time, just as it is now) and moderate to low levels of fat. Pritikin Centers currently operate in locations around the U.S. While they are keeping pace with the updated theories and documented evidence about lifestyle medicine, the diet they advocate remains very similar to the whole-foods diet that Pritikin recommended in the 1970s.

Over time, Pritikin conducted several clinical trials on the efficacy of his theories and convictions. He published papers in 1983 and 1985 on his intensive in-house program (an undertaking in which my father actually participated). He found that of the patients who stayed with the program through 26 in-patient days, 77 percent were able to go off their diabetes medication, while 25 percent had a reduction in their total cholesterol level.

Other studies on the "Pritikin" diet have determined that positive changes in BMI, blood sugars, and LDLs occur—changes that moderate the effects of metabolic syndrome, a disease complex that includes diabetes, hypertension, and coronary artery disease.

❑ *Caldwell Esselstyn, Jr., MD:* Dr. Esselstyn is a former surgeon, who is currently a clinician and researcher at the Cleveland Clinic. Since 1985, he has conducted research on whole foods and plant-based nutritional therapy to reverse coronary artery disease. An author, as well as a former Olympic rowing champion, he has written a best-selling book on preventing and reversing heart disease, in which he advocates consuming a low-fat, whole foods, plant-based diet that avoids all animal products.

During his career, Esselstyn has also published several important papers in his area of expertise. In his publications, Esselstyn reported on three people who had been treated with traditional medicine and then came to him for lifestyle medicine. His data demonstrated drastic improvements in these patients' cardiovascular health after following his regimen. He has also performed trials utilizing his dietary approach and followed patients for four years. His research found out that of 198 patients with cardiovascular disease, 177 were adherent to his diet and only 0.6 percent of those individuals had a recurrent coronary vascular disease event. In contrast, the people who were not adherent to his plan had a 62 percent recurrence rate.

❏ *Dean Ornish, MD:* Dr. Ornish studied internal medicine at Baylor College of Medicine, did his residency at Massachusetts General Hospital, and completed a fellowship at Harvard Medical School. His work in this area began in 1978 when he completed a pilot study demonstrating improved blood flow to the heart after 30 days of his lifestyle program. He performed this study while still in medical school and cleverly figured out a way to study lifestyle factors when there was not much support or belief in this area of medicine. In fact, without his own medical facility where patients could stay to receive treatment and be monitored, he cleverly arranged for his patients to stay at a near by hotel. Since that time, Dr. Ornish has completed several randomized controlled studies that demonstrated the power of lifestyle medicine to not only reverse severe cases of heart disease but to also help with early stage prostate cancer. His studies have revealed the impact of lifestyle changes on genes and chromosomes. He found that lifestyle changes could alter how 500 different genes were expressed, turning on health promoting genes and turning off genes that promote heart disease and some cancers including prostate, breast, and colon. In addition, one of his studies showed that telomere length increased with lifestyle medicine interventions. The telomeres are found at the end of chromosomes and they protect the chromosome from damage and deterioration. Thus, longer telomeres have been correlated with longer life spans.

Dr. Ornish is currently the president and founder of the nonprofit Preventive Medicine Research Institute in Sausalito, California, as well as a clinical professor at the University of California, San Francisco. He is also heavily involved in the American College of Lifestyle Medicine. His outpatient intensive, integrative lifestyle medicine program Undoit with Ornish is currently reimbursed by insurance agencies, which is a feat in and of itself. Dr. Ornish's research and his clinical work developing an effective outpatient lifestyle medicine program were pivotal for the field and part of the reason he won the Lifetime Achievement Award at the annual meeting for the American College of Lifestyle Medicine.

❏ *David L. Katz, MD, MPH:* Dr. Katz is a board-certified specialist in both internal medicine and preventive medicine/public health. Currently an associate adjunct professor in public health practice at the Yale University School of Medicine, he is also a well respected author, who has written several well-received books on a variety of health-related topics. Dr. Katz is a prolific writer and has written many substantial and influential articles for LinkedIn, Huffington Post and other platforms that have helped to put lifestyle medicine on the map for the public.

In 2015, Dr. Katz established the True Health Initiative to help convert what is known about lifestyle medicine into what can be done about it. A recognized authority on lifestyle as a powerful tool for the prevention of chronic health-related conditions, he is a past-president of the American College of Lifestyle Medicine, as well as the co-founding director of the CDC-funded Yale-Griffin Prevention Research Center.

Dr. Katz is widely regarded as an eloquent advocate for lifestyle medicine. Among his more acclaimed quotes is the following: "We have not yet done nearly a good enough job empowering people to make them feel like they really can get to the prize, the prize being sustainable weight loss, their weight controlled without being hungry [and] miserable for the rest of their lives."

❏ *James Rippe, MD:* Dr. Rippe is a cardiologist who was trained at Harvard University. He left cardiology after becoming frustrated with what was happening in the field with the misguided, often singular focus on interventions and medications. Currently, he is the founder and director of the Rippe Lifestyle Institute, which conducts numerous studies every year on a variety of lifestyle-related topics, including physical activity and healthy weight management.

Dr. Rippe is a prolific author, having written over 400 publications on issues in medicine, health and fitness, and weight management. He has also written 50 books, including 32 medical textbooks and 18 well-received books on health and fitness that were targeted at the general public. He authored the first book (*Lifestyle Medicine*, currently in its 2nd edition) that was designed to help guide physicians in the diverse aspects of how to incorporate lifestyle issues into the practice of modern medicine. His textbook is considered the main source of academic information in the field, as it has 1568 pages and thousands of references. In terms of articles in lifestyle medicine, Dr. Rippe is the Editor-in-Chief of the American Journal of Lifestyle Medicine, which is the official Journal of the American College of Lifestyle Medicine. Dr. Rippe continues to propel the field forward with his publishing, writing and editing.

❏ *Garry Egger, MPH, PhD:* Dr. Egger is a pioneer of lifestyle medicine in Australia and a professor of health and human sciences at Southern Cross University in East Lismore, Australia. He is the author of 30 books, including the landmark text, *Lifestyle Medicine: Managing Diseases of Lifestyle in the 21st Century*. Considered one of Australia's leading authorities on lifestyle medicine and chronic disease, he has worked in public, corporate, and clinical health for over four decades. Among his professional undertakings is conducting training programs in lifestyle medicine and chronic disease management for over 7,000 Australian clinicians and allied healthcare professionals. In recent years, he has resumed being involved in both clinical and community research.

A ROADMAP FOR SUCCESS

The cost of healthcare will soon approach 20 percent of the GDP ... in other words $1 out of every $5 spent in America will be spent on healthcare. Such a situation is simply not sustainable. America needs to move from the current, reactive "sick care system," to a proactive healthcare model—one that prevents chronic disease, which is responsible for the largest proportion of healthcare expenditures. This dire financial situation has neither shown signs of abating, nor produced meaningful results with regard to preventing or treating a wide variety of chronic health problems.

Attempts to identify the factors that have been major contributors to this epidemic of medical issues have produced an array of probable etiologies ... poor eating habits, a sedentary lifestyle, stress, smoking, etc. Concurrently, numerous attempts have been undertaken to identify what—if anything—can be done to diminish the number and/or severity of the medical problems affecting the public. These efforts have provided considerable evidence that adhering to the fundamental tenets of lifestyle medicine can result in substantial medicinal benefits for individuals of all ages.

In a number of ways, the aforementioned industrialization has hindered the efforts of the U.S. to enhance the health of its citizens. One of the major drawbacks of transforming from an agrarian to an industrial society entails "quality-of-life" issues. In contrast to an agrarian lifestyle, urbanization has often resulted in longer working hours and an enhanced level of stress, which has led to the exact issues highlighted by the previously noted six pillars of lifestyle medicine.

Dr. David Katz, past president of the American College of Lifestyle Medicine, articulates a phrase that aptly summarizes the compelling need for lifestyle medicine—"The Three Fs" (feet, forks, and fingers). In other words, "How often do people move their feet each day? How do people use their forks each day? Are people using their fingers to smoke?"

Although the three Fs seem somewhat mundane, these daily lifestyle choices matter far more than most people realize. The top three actual causes of death (i.e., smoking, poor diet/physical activity, alcohol consumption) are modifiable lifestyle behaviors that also have the power to prevent, treat, and, in some cases, reverse chronic disease.

In a relatively large study by Ford et al. in Potsdam, Germany, it was estimated that approximately 80 percent of chronic diseases could be prevented by adhering to four healthy lifestyle factors: never smoking, maintaining a body mass index lower than 30, being physically active for greater than 3.5 hours per week, and adhering to a healthy diet, consisting of high intake of fruits, vegetables, whole-grain bread, and low meat consumption.

While prevention is ideal, intensive lifestyle treatment can also be used to minister to and reverse chronic disease. Though not always emphasized by physicians, lifestyle behaviors are typically first-line treatment for many chronic diseases, including diabetes, hypertension (high blood pressure), hypercholesterolemia (high cholesterol), and hypertriglyceridemia (high triglycerides), to name a few. In a landmark study published in *The New England Journal of Medicine*, 3,234 subjects with elevated blood sugar levels (early stages of developing diabetes) were randomized to three different treatment groups: placebo; a medication called metformin (the first line pharmaceutical treatment for type 2 diabetes); and a lifestyle-modification program.

This nearly three-year study found a surprising difference among these three groups *in favor of lifestyle intervention*. Compared to the placebo group, the people in the metformin group had a 31 percent lower incidence of diabetes, while the people in the lifestyle intervention group had a 58 percent lower incidence of diabetes. In other words, changing a person's lifestyle was more effective than placebo and more effective than metformin.

This study was disruptive, because in the 2000s, most experts firmly believed that medication was necessary to treat diabetes. In fact, very few people believed that lifestyle could have a significant impact on the body's ability to control diabetes or to handle high blood glucose levels. This study helped to put lifestyle medicine on the map in mainstream medicine as a powerful treatment tool.

Finally, lifestyle medicine has been shown to reverse cardiac disease. Although there are many medications that help treat and control risk factors for heart disease, there are *no medications* that have been shown to actually reverse this onerous cause of death. The groundbreaking Lifestyle Heart Trial, conducted by Dean Ornish, MD in 1990, revealed that a lifestyle intervention, consisting of a low-fat vegetarian diet, smoking cessation, stress management training, and moderate exercise, was able to reverse coronary artery stenosis in 82 percent of patients in the intervention group, without the use of cholesterol lowering drugs.

A follow-up study, published in 1998 involving the same population, demonstrated additional coronary atherosclerosis regression after five years of the dietary intervention. Concerningly, it also showed that the coronary atherosclerosis in the control group (non-lifestyle intervention group) continued to worsen and that these subjects experienced more than twice as many cardiac events as the intervention group.

While questions remain concerning how beneficial lifestyle medicine interventions can be for a variety of other disease, the aforementioned examples highlight a few of the powerful outcomes that have been published. In addition to the potential superiority of lifestyle medicine compared to medications, it is a fraction of the cost of expensive pharmaceutical drugs. Furthermore, it has almost no negative side effects. Quite simply, lifestyle medicine is some of the best medicine that individuals have.

LIVE AND LEARN WITH DR. BETH FRATES

Consider this common story of a middle-aged man. When he was 52, he was an overworked, overweight, overstressed, New York City businessman. His diet consisted almost exclusively of steak, potatoes, chocolate chip cookies, chocolate cake, and hard candies that he stored in the middle drawer of his desk at work. Despite the fact that he had been an excellent high school and college athlete, playing baseball, basketball, and soccer, at this time in his life, he was sedentary. He was running his own business in New York City, and his only form of physical activity was an occasional sprint from Park Avenue to Grand Central Station to catch the last train home at 11:07 p.m. If he didn't catch that train, he would have to stay overnight in his office on a cot, which he did on occasion. To avoid the cot, however, he would sprint as fast as he could in an attempt to catch the train.

On one of these mad dashes at 11:07 at night, this gentleman felt a little pressure, a little pain in his chest. Because "no pain, no gain" was one of his mantras, though, he forged forward and made that train. About a half an hour later, he felt as if there were an elephant accompanying him on the train ride, sitting on his chest. The pain was severe. He also experienced numbness and tingling down his left arm. He was sweating and very short of breath. His wife dutifully picked him up at 11:33 p.m. at the home station, as she had done countless times before.

His wife was a school teacher with no medical training, whatsoever. But she took one look at him and declared, "This is not right." Immediately, she rushed him to the local emergency room, where he suffered a massive myocardial infarction and a right middle cerebral artery infarction that left him paralyzed on his left side. This scenario all occurred in one evening.

This chronicle is the story of many Americans—middle-aged, younger, and older. These individuals are living life on a work treadmill—not literally on a treadmill exercising, but on the work bandwagon. They're not caring for themselves. They're eating poor diets, consisting of the easiest, quickest meals they can find. The story is one that has propelled me in my work every day since I was 18 years old. The man in the story was my dad.

Fortunately, my father made a full recovery after a year of hard work, with physical therapy, occupational therapy, and routine walking. His only residual deficit was in the fine motor movement in his left hand. I watched his recovery and transformation in amazement. My father was the type of person to research topics and to do what he could to create his own destiny. When he discovered he had heart disease, he found the top programs in the country that could help people reverse their disease through diet and exercise.

At that time, in the 1980s, because Nathan Pritikin and Dr. Julian Whitaker had successful intensive lifestyle medicine programs, my dad traveled across the country to participate in these residential programs. He started a whole new life, and my mother was with him every step of the way. She acted as his personal health and wellness coach, although she had no training in healthcare or coaching. Yet, my mother was a compassionate, supportive, and smart woman, who knew that my dad needed to make big changes in his life in order to prevent another health setback.

My father started eating salads, vegetables, complex carbohydrates, and fish. He avoided desserts. He had fruit instead. The hard candies disappeared, as did his supply of Oreo cookies. In addition, my dad bought an exercise bike, which he religiously rode five days a week for one half hour, while listening to the financial news on the radio or TV. In terms of work, my dad found more balance. He worked from 10 a.m. to 2 p.m. which also allowed him to sleep the recommended 7-8 hours a night, instead of the 3-4 he used to get. With those changes, the stress in his life was significantly reduced. Another change happened in his social life. Dad spent more time with family and friends. He always had a good sense of humor, but he used it more frequently after his health setback. Also, for the first time in my life, I saw him kiss my mom in front of me. It was a little peck on the cheek, but it was a big change and an important rearranging of his priorities. I saw that my dad was a loving person, someone who was able to express his love for my mom in front of others. Their relationship really blossomed after his heart attack and stroke.

My father would always say that his heart attack and stroke were a blessing in disguise. He felt that he started to truly live life to its fullest and actually reached optimal health and wellness after his health setback. He lived another 27 more years, and he lived life to its fullest until he died.

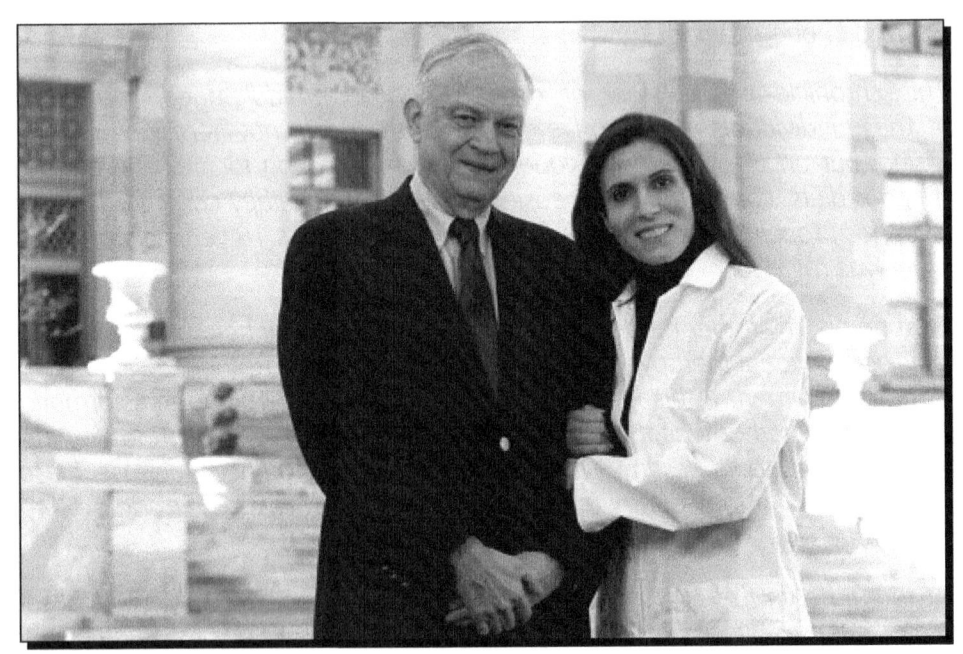

Dr. Beth Frates and her father, Donald Pegg

My father passed away a few years ago, but I still have all of his books from the Pritikin program, as well as his exercise bike. His story is one that resonates with many people. They may know someone like my dad, or feel they are just like my dad themselves. My father's stroke was the inspiration for my book, Life After Stroke: The Guide to Recovering Your Health and Preventing Another Stroke. *After witnessing his recovery, my goal was to empower stroke survivors to make the lifestyle changes they needed to make so that they could live their best years after their stroke. Now, I run lifestyle medicine wellness groups for stroke survivors and their loved ones at Spaulding Rehabilitation Hospital as part of the Stroke Institute for Research and Recovery. My dad's health setback set me on this lifestyle medicine journey, back when I was 18. Good things can come out of challenging situations.*

INFORMATION MAY NOT BE ENOUGH

Francis Bacon's expression that "Knowledge is power" is often quoted. After I had written my stroke book, I thought, "That's it, that's enough." Subsequently, I started talking to anyone and everyone who would listen to me. I wanted to tell them all about the warning signs for stroke. I created a whole mnemonic: FALLING, which stands for "face, arm, leg, language, I-eyesight, nasty headache, and gait (walking instability)." If someone is FALLING off of their baseline, then they might be having a stroke.

I wanted everyone to know the facts, the risk factors, and the guidelines for exercise and diet. I lectured at public libraries—in reality, anywhere I could. Then, one day I wondered, "Are these lectures empowering people to change? Are people listening to my lectures and then making lifestyle changes?" I considered doing a research project to determine if people who read my book or listened to my lecture actually changed their behaviors.

A mentor of mine advised me that this type of research study would not be a useful endeavor, given that most people will not change their behavior simply by increasing their knowledge. He suggested that only about 10 percent of people would change. Instead of doing a research study, he recommended that I learn more about the *process* of behavior change. So, I did.

In 2008, I became certified in health and wellness coaching. At that time, there were only a handful of physicians who were certified in coaching. Fortunately, there are now many more. I have completed four different coaching programs, including the Diabetes Prevention Program lifestyle coach training, as well as a certificate course in motivational interviewing course from the University of Massachusetts. Other trainings that have influenced my practice of lifestyle medicine include Herbert Benson's Mind Body Medicine Training, Jon Kabat-Zinn's Mindfulness Stress Reduction, nutrition courses, and yoga classes.

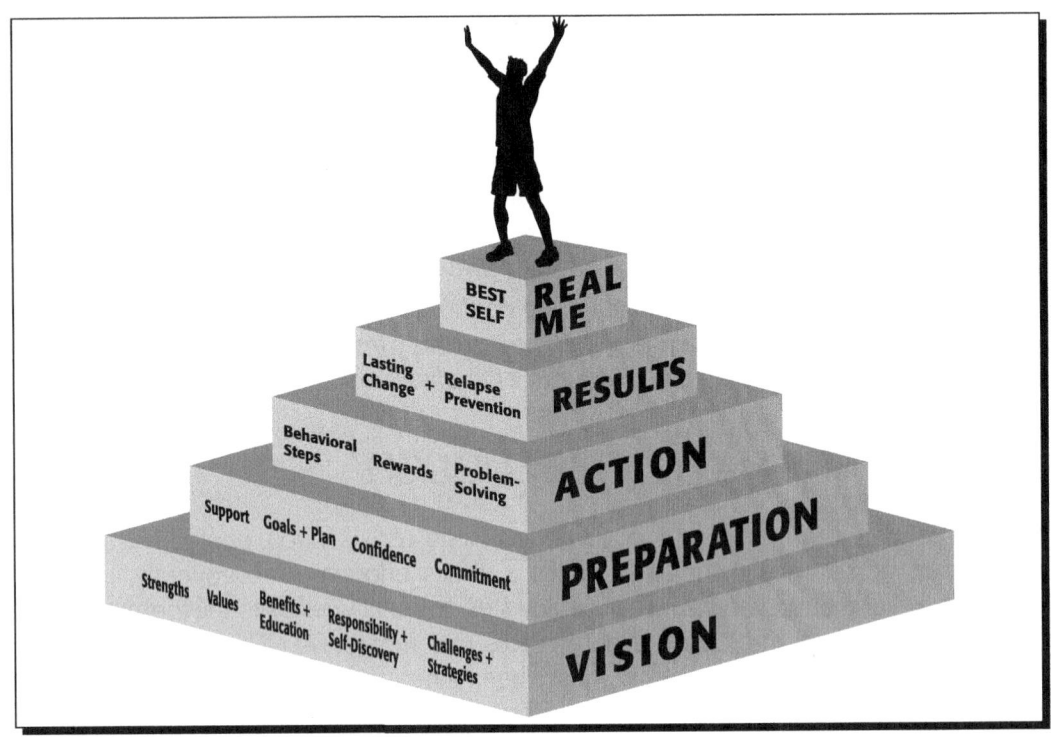

Figure 1-2. Behavior change pyramid. Adapted with permission from the book, *Coaching Psychology Manual*, 1E.

    I am constantly trying to learn how to empower others so that they will make and sustain healthy changes. Yes, knowledge is important, and that is what reading books and taking classes provides. Getting people to change their behavior, however, entails more than knowledge. For physicians and allied health practitioners to be successful at helping people make changes, they need practice. They also need to work on their own personal behavior changes in the areas of diet, exercise, stress management, sleep, social connection, attitude, and positivity.

    During one of the coaching courses I completed, we learned about a behavior change pyramid. There were many steps or blocks in this pyramid of behavior change (Figure 1-2). It should be noted that only one of the 15 blocks in this pyramid addresses education. The others covered a variety of elements, including obstacles, strategies, values, strengths, responsibility, goals, planning, commitment, self-efficacy, problem-solving, and relapse prevention.

    Personally, I have been trying to learn about behavior change for over 30 years. My goal is to help people get to be their best selves. Just like my mom was a powerhouse coach for my father after his stroke, I want to be a powerhouse coach for other people. In this handbook, I am sharing my life's work, as well as my life's passion with the readers of the book, so that they too, can benefit from the journey into lifestyle medicine.

KEY POINTS/TAKEAWAYS FOR CHAPTER 1

❏ Chapter Review:

- Overall goal: Define evidence-based lifestyle medicine.
- Application goal: Understand how lifestyle medicine can positively impact the your own health and the health of those around you.

❏ Discussion Questions:

- What is an example of at least one major advancement or change in society that has occurred in the last century and how it has affected health?
- What makes lifestyle medicine an appealing approach to improving healthcare and bringing down costs?
- What are your current thoughts about healthy lifestyles?
- Where did you gain this knowledge?
- How do you find evidence-based information on lifestyle?
- What do you hope to get out of this book?

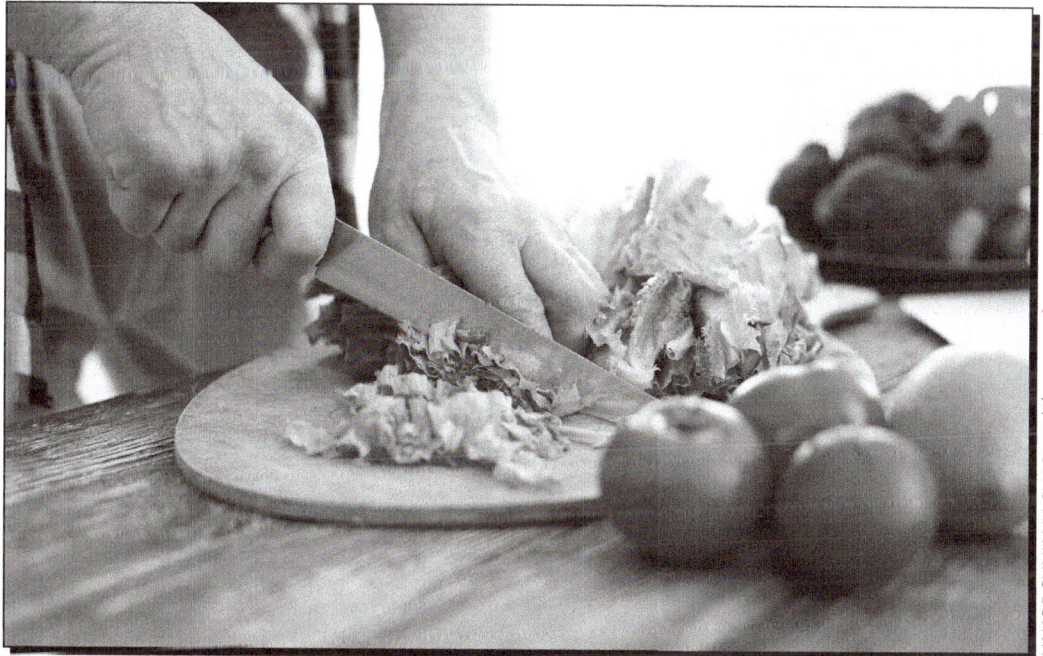

The official definition of lifestyle medicine from the American College of Lifestyle Medicine (www.lifestylemedicine.org) is that it is the use of evidence-based lifestyle therapeutic approaches, such as a predominantly whole food, plant-based diet, regular physical activity, adequate sleep, stress management, avoidance of risky substance use, and other non-drug modalities to treat, oftentimes, reverse and prevent the lifestyle-related, chronic disease that's all too prevalent.

	TITLE	AUTHORS	JOURNAL	YEAR	KEY FINDINGS
General Lifestyle Medicine					
1	Actual causes of death in the United States	McGinnis JM, Foege WH	JAMA	1993	This landmark study revealed that tobacco use, diet/physical activity patterns, and alcohol were the actual leading causes of death, accounting for approximately 80% of premature deaths in the U.S.
2	Actual causes of death in the United States, 2000	Mokdad AH, et al.	JAMA	2000	Smoking remained the leading cause of mortality. However, evidence suggested that "poor diet and physical inactivity may soon overtake tobacco as the leading cause of death. These findings, along with escalating health care costs and aging population, argue persuasively that the need to establish a more preventive orientation in the US health care and public health systems has become more urgent."
3	Healthy living is the best revenge: findings from the European Prospective Investigation Into Cancer and Nutrition—Potsdam study	Ford ES, et al.	Archives of Internal Medicine	2009	In Potsdam, Germany researchers found that an estimated 80% of chronic diseases could be prevented by four healthy lifestyle factors: never smoking, maintaining a body mass index lower than 30, being physically active for greater than 3.5 hours per week, and adhering to a healthy diet consisting of high intake of fruits, vegetables, whole-grain bread, and low meat consumption.
4	Influence of individual and combined health behaviors on total and cause-specific mortality in men and women: the United Kingdom health and lifestyle survey	Kvaavik E, et al.	Archives of Internal Medicine	2010	A prospective cohort study done in the United Kingdom that examined the effect that physical activity, diet, smoking, and alcohol had on all-cause mortality. Having all four poor health behaviors resulted in an estimated chronological age of being 12 years older.
5	Healthy lifestyle habits and mortality in overweight and obese individuals	Matheson EM, King DE, Everett CJ	Journal of American Board Family Medicine	2012	This study looked at healthy behaviors and mortality in normal weight, overweight, and obese individuals. It found that practicing healthy lifestyle habits was "associated with a significant decrease in mortality regardless of baseline body mass index."
6	Can we say what diet is best for health?	Katz DL, Meller S	Annual Review of Public Health	2014	This systematic review examined all mainstream dietary approaches and the published evidence pertaining to their impact on health. It found that "the fundamentals of virtually all eating patterns associated with meaningful evidence of health benefit overlap substantially." Furthermore, "A diet of minimally processed foods close to nature, predominantly plants, is decisively associated with health promotion and disease prevention and is consistent with the salient components of seemingly distinct dietary approaches."

Figure 1-3. Lifestyle medicine landmark studies

	TITLE	AUTHORS	JOURNAL	YEAR	KEY FINDINGS
General Lifestyle Medicine (cont.)					
7	A systems medicine approach: translating emerging science into individualized wellness	Bland JS, Minich DM, Eck BM	*Advances in Medicine*	2017	A discussion of the increasingly important role that personalized lifestyle medicine will have in treating lifestyle-related noncommunicable diseases. Remarks on the numerous technical and logistical changes of translating "big data" into actionable and clinically relevant solutions and advocates for healthcare practitioners and all related stakeholders to work together to solve the non-communicable disease epidemic that we face.
8	Lifestyle medicine: A brief review of its dramatic impact on health and survival	Bodai BI, et al.	*Permanente Journal*	2017	This article describes the effect of lifestyle medicine on chronic disease and its' impact on the Kaiser Permanente health system. The authors conclude that "we believe that lifestyle medicine should become the primary approach to the management of chronic conditions and, more importantly, their prevention."
Cardiovascular Disease					
9	Low-risk diet and lifestyle habits in the primary prevention of myocardial infarction in men: a population-based prospective cohort study	Akesson A, et al.	*Journal of the American College of Cardiology*	2014	In Sweden, this study showed that 79% of myocardial infarctions could be prevented through healthy lifestyle choices ["a healthy diet (top quintile of Recommended Food Score), moderate alcohol consumption (10 to 30 g/day), no smoking, being physically active (walking/bicycling >/=40 min/day and exercising >/=1 h/week), and having no abdominal adiposity (waist circumference <95 cm)"].
10	Can lifestyle changes reverse coronary heart disease? The Lifestyle Heart Trial	Ornish D, et al.	*Lancet*	1990	Ornish and colleagues showed that "comprehensive lifestyle changes may be able to bring about regression of even severe coronary atherosclerosis after only 1 year, without use of lipid-lowering drugs."
11	Comprehensive lifestyle changes may be able to bring about regression of even severe coronary atherosclerosis after only 1 year, without use of lipid-lowering drugs	Ornish D, et al.	*JAMA*	1998	This study was a continuation of the prior trial that demonstrated that coronary atherosclerosis continued to regress in patients who continued the program, compared to the control group, which had progression of their coronary atherosclerosis.
12	Lifestyle medicine and the management of cardiovascular disease	Doughty KN, et al.	*Current Cardiology Reports*	2017	A review of the effects of lifestyle interventions in individuals with established cardiovascular disease. "Findings were mixed, but most interventions improved at least some markers of cardiovascular risk…The benefits of lifestyle change for cardiovascular disease patients have been established by decades of evidence. However, further research is needed to determine the optimal intensity, duration, and mode of delivery for interventions."

Figure 13. Lifestyle medicine landmark studies (cont.)

	TITLE	AUTHORS	JOURNAL	YEAR	KEY FINDINGS
Cardiovascular Disease (cont.)					
13	Lifestyle interventions to prevent cardiovascular events after stroke and transient ischemic attack	Deijle IA, et al.	*Stroke*	2017	This meta-analysis of 22 randomized controlled trials evaluated the effectiveness of lifestyle interventions in preventing recurrent cardiovascular events, reducing mortality, and improving cardiovascular disease risk factors in patients who had a stroke. They found that lifestyle interventions were effective in lowering systolic blood pressure (mean difference 3.6 mm Hg) but found no effect of lifestyle interventions on cardiovascular event rate mortality, diastolic blood pressure, or total cholesterol.
14	Healthy lifestyle medicine in the traditional healthcare environment—primary care and cardiac rehabilitation	Williams MA, Kaminsky LA	*Progress in Cardiovascular Diseases*	2017	Reviews the literature and discusses value and limitations of implementing healthy lifestyle medicine into traditional models of healthcare. "One opportunity which should be considered is expanding access to currently available options, such as cardiac rehabilitation programs and worksite wellness programs." They also emphasize focusing on community-based centers development utilizing specialists, such as counselors, exercise physiologists, dietitians, and physical therapists.
15	Primary prevention and risk factor reduction in coronary heart disease mortality among working aged men and women in eastern Finland over 40 years: population based observational study	Jousilahti P, et al.	*BMJ*	2016	This study came out of Finland's North Karelia Project, which was started in 1972. It is a large, population-based project that utilized a multilevel approach that focused on reducing sodium intake and replacing saturated fat with unsaturated fat on a population level targeted at the public at large. Data from this population 40 years later reveal a persistent 82% and 84% reduction in coronary heart disease mortality in men and women, respectively.
Diabetes/Metabolic Syndrome					
16	Reduction in the incidence of type 2 diabetes with lifestyle intervention or metformin	Knowler WC, et al.	*New England Journal of Medicine*	2002	This landmark study compared lifestyle intervention to the diabetes drug metformin. It found that both "lifestyle changes and treatment with metformin both reduced the incidence of diabetes in persons at high risk. The lifestyle intervention was more effective than metformin." Lifestyle medicine has the power to outperform some of the best medications for chronic conditions.
17	Beneficial effects of high dietary fiber intake in patients with type 2 diabetes mellitus	Chandalia M, et al.	*New England Journal of Medicine*	2000	This trial showed the concurrent benefits that adopting a healthy diet can have on diabetes treatment. It found that "a high intake of dietary fiber, particularly of the soluble type, above the level recommended by the ADA, improves glycemic control, decreases hyperinsulinemia, and lowers plasma lipid concentrations in patients with type 2 diabetes."

Figure 1-3. Lifestyle medicine landmark studies (cont.)

	TITLE	AUTHORS	JOURNAL	YEAR	KEY FINDINGS
Diabetes/Metabolic Syndrome (cont.)					
18	Association of an intensive lifestyle intervention with remission of type 2 diabetes	Gregg EW, et al.	*JAMA*	2012	A study done involving overweight adults that demonstrated that "intensive lifestyle intervention was associated with a greater likelihood of partial remission of type 2 diabetes compared with diabetes support and education."
Stroke/Dementia					
19	Lifestyle and stroke risk: a review	Galimanis A, et al.	*Current Opinion Neurology*	2009	"Stroke can be substantially reduced by an active lifestyle, cessation of smoking and a healthy diet. Both public and professional education should promote the awareness that a healthy lifestyle and nutrition have the potential to reduce the burden of stroke."
20	Prevention of age-related cognitive decline: which strategies, when, and for whom?	Shatenstein B, Barberger-Gateau P, Mecocci P	*Journal of Alzheimer's Disease*	2015	This paper reviewed evidence-based strategies to enhance cognition and prevent cognitive decline. Their findings "imply that we can target modifiable environmental, lifestyle, and health risk factors to modify the trajectory of cognitive decline before the onset of irreversible dementia. Because building cognitive reserve and prevention of cognitive decline are of critical importance, interventions are needed at every stage of the life course to foster cognitive stimulation, and enable healthy eating habits and physical activity throughout the lifespan."
21	Primary prevention of stroke by healthy lifestyle	Chiuve SE, et al.	*Circulation*	2008	A large prospective study that examined the impact that lifestyle factors had on stroke. They specifically defined a low-risk lifestyle as "not smoking, a body mass index <25 kg/m(2), >or=30 min/d of moderate activity, modest alcohol consumption (men, 5 to 30 g/d; women, 5 to 15 g/d), and scoring within the top 40% of a healthy diet score." They found that 47% of total and 54% of ischemic stroke cases were attributable to lack of adherence to a low-risk lifestyle; among the men, 35% of total and 52% of ischemic stroke may have been prevented" with better lifestyle choices.
22	Secondary prevention of new vascular events with lifestyle intervention in patients with noncardioembolic mild ischemic stroke: a single-center randomized controlled trial	Kono Y, et al.	*Cerebrovascular Disease*	2013	This randomized controlled trial investigated the role of lifestyle intervention on secondary stroke prevention. In patients with prior ischemic stroke, lifestyle intervention, in addition to medication, resulted in fewer vascular events and improved vascular risk factors as compared to the control group.

Figure 1-3 Lifestyle medicine landmark studies (cont.)

#	TITLE	AUTHORS	JOURNAL	YEAR	KEY FINDINGS
Stroke/Dementia (cont.)					
23	Mediterranean diet, cognitive function, and dementia: a systematic review	Lourida I, et al.	*Epidemiology*	2013	A systematic review that concluded that "greater adherence to Mediterranean diet is associated with slower cognitive decline and lower risk of developing Alzheimer disease."
Cancer					
24	Combined impact of healthy lifestyle factors on colorectal cancer: a large European cohort study	Aleksandrova K, et al.	*BMC Medicine*	2014	The authors sought to develop a healthy lifestyle index, consisting of five modifiable lifestyle factors—healthy weight, physical activity, not smoking, limited alcohol consumption and a healthy diet, and relate it to colorectal cancer risk. The study found that 16% of new colorectal cancer cases were attributable to not adhering to the healthy lifestyle index behaviors.
25	Proportion and number of cancer cases and deaths attributable to potentially modifiable risk factors in the United States	Islami F, et al.	*CA: A Cancer Journal for Clinicians*	2017	This article sought to estimate the proportion of cancer cases and deaths that were attributable to modifiable risk factors (i.e., cigarette smoking, secondhand smoke, excess body weight, alcohol intake, consumption of red and processed meat, low consumption of fruits/vegetables, dietary fiber, dietary calcium, physical inactivity, ultraviolet radiation, and six cancer-associated infections). They estimated that 42% of all incident cancers and 45.1% of cancer deaths were attributable to the aforementioned risk factors. Cigarette smoking accounted for the highest proportion of cancer cases (19%) and deaths (28%), followed by excess body weight (7.8% and 6.5%, respectively) and alcohol intake (5.6% and 4%, respectively).
26	Changes in prostate gene expression in men undergoing an intensive nutrition and lifestyle intervention	Ornish D, et al.	*Proceedings of the National Academy of Sciences of the United States of America*	2008	This pilot study found evidence that a three-month intensive nutrition and lifestyle intervention could positively modulate prostate gene expression in patients with prostate cancer.
Genetics					
27	The effect of a short-term hypocaloric diet on liver gene expression and metabolic risk factors in obese women	Hietaniemi M, et al.	*Nutrition, Metabolism, and Cardiovascular Diseases*	2009	Researchers demonstrated that eight weeks of a hypocaloric diet in women with obesity resulted in down-regulation of 142 hepatic genes.

Figure 1-3. Lifestyle medicine landmark studies (cont.)

	TITLE	AUTHORS	JOURNAL	YEAR	KEY FINDINGS
Genetics (cont.)					
28	Lifestyle intervention up-regulates gene and protein levels of molecules involved in insulin signaling in the endometrium of overweight/obese women with polycystic ovary syndrome	Ujvari D, et al.	*Human Reproduction*	2014	This study of overweight/obese women with polycystic ovarian syndrome showed that lifestyle intervention up-regulated endometrial genes with subsequent improvement in glucose control and endometrium function.

References

1. McGinnis JM, Foege WH. Actual causes of death in the United States. *JAMA*. 1993;270:2207-2212.
2. Mokdad AH, Marks JS, Stroup DF, et al. Actual causes of death in the United States, 2000. *JAMA*. 2004;291:1238-1245.
3. Ford ES, Bergmann MM, Kroger J, et al. Healthy living is the best revenge: findings from the European Prospective Investigation Into Cancer and Nutrition—Potsdam study. *Archives of Internal Medicine*. 2009;169:1355-1362.
4. Kvaavik E, Batty GD, Ursin G, et al. Influence of individual and combined health behaviors on total and cause-specific mortality in men and women: the United Kingdom health and lifestyle survey. *Archives of Internal Medicine*. 2010;170:711-718.
5. Matheson EM, King DE, Everett CJ. Healthy lifestyle habits and mortality in overweight and obese individuals. *Journal of the American Board of Family Medicine*. 2012;25:9-15.
6. Katz DL, Meller S. Can we say what diet is best for health? *Annual Review of Public Health*. 2014;35:83-103.
7. Bland JS, Minich DM, Eck BM. A systems medicine approach: translating emerging science into individualized wellness. *Advances in Medicine*. 2017:1718957. doi:10.1155/2017/1718957.
8. Bodai BI, Nakata TE, Wong WT, et al. Lifestyle medicine: a brief review of its dramatic impact on health and survival. *Permanente Journal*. 2017;22. doi: 10.7812/TPP/17-025.
9. Akesson A, Larsson SC, Discacciati A, et al. Low-risk diet and lifestyle habits in the primary prevention of myocardial infarction in men: a population-based prospective cohort study. *Journal of the American College of Cardiology*. 2014;64:1299-1306.
10. Ornish D, Brown SE, Scherwitz LW, et al. Can lifestyle changes reverse coronary heart disease? The Lifestyle Heart Trial. *Lancet*. 1990;336:129-133.
11. Ornish D, Scherwitz LW, Billings JH, et al. Intensive lifestyle changes for reversal of coronary heart disease. *JAMA*. 1998;280:2001-2007.
12. Doughty KN, Del Pilar NX, Audette A, et al. Lifestyle medicine and the management of cardiovascular disease. *Current Cardiology Reports*. 2017;19(11):116. doi: 10.1007/s11886-017-0925-z.
13. Deijle IA, Van Schaik SM, Van Wegen EEH, et al. Lifestyle interventions to prevent cardiovascular events after stroke and transient ischemic attack. *Stroke*. 2017;48:174-179.
14. Williams MA, Kaminsky LA. Healthy lifestyle medicine in the traditional healthcare environment—primary care and cardiac rehabilitation. *Progress in Cardiovascular Diseases*. 2017;59(5):448-454. doi: 10.1016/j.pcad.2017.01.008.
15. Jousilahti P, Laatikainen T, Peltonen M, et al. Primary prevention and risk factor reduction in coronary heart disease mortality among working aged men and women in eastern Finland over 40 years: population based observational study. *BMJ*. 2016;352:i721.
16. Knowler WC, Barrett-Connor E, Fowler SE, et al. Reduction in the incidence of type 2 diabetes with lifestyle intervention or metformin. *New England Journal of Medicine*. 2002;346:393-403.
17. Chandalia M, Garg A, Lutjohann D, et al. Beneficial effects of high dietary fiber intake in patients with type 2 diabetes mellitus. *New England Journal of Medicine*. 2000;342:1392-1398.
18. Gregg EW, Chen H, Wagenknecht LE, et al. Association of an intensive lifestyle intervention with remission of type 2 diabetes. *JAMA*. 2012;308:2489-2496.
19. Galimanis A, Mono ML, Arnold M, et al. Lifestyle and stroke risk: a review. *Current Opinion in Neurology*. 2009;22:60-68.
20. Shatenstein B, Barberger-Gateau P, Mecocci P. Prevention of age-related cognitive decline: which strategies, when, and for whom? *Journal of Alzheimer's Disease*. 2015;48:35-53.
21. Chiuve SE, Rexrode KM, Spiegelman D, et al. Primary prevention of stroke by healthy lifestyle. *Circulation*. 2008;118:947-954.
22. Kono Y, Yamada S, Yamaguchi J, et al. Secondary prevention of new vascular events with lifestyle intervention in patients with noncardioembolic mild ischemic stroke: a single-center randomized controlled trial. *Cerebrovascular Disease*. 2013;36:88-97.
23. Lourida I, Soni M, Thompson-Coon J, et al. Mediterranean diet, cognitive function, and dementia: a systematic review. *Epidemiology*. 2013;24:479-489.
24. Aleksandrova K, Pischon T, Jenab M, et al. Combined impact of healthy lifestyle factors on colorectal cancer: a large European cohort study. *BMC Medicine*. 2014;12:168.
25. Islami F, Goding Sauer A, Miller KD, et al. Proportion and number of cancer cases and deaths attributable to potentially modifiable risk factors in the United States. *CA: A Cancer Journal for Clinicians*. November 21, 2017. doi.org/10.3322/caac.21440.
26. Ornish D, Magbanua MJ, Weidner G, et al. Changes in prostate gene expression in men undergoing an intensive nutrition and lifestyle intervention. *Proceedings of the National Academy of Sciences of the United States of America*. 2008;105:8369-8374.
27. Hietaniemi M, Jokela M, Rantala M, et al. The effect of a short-term hypocaloric diet on liver gene expression and metabolic risk factors in obese women. *Nutrition, Metabolism, and Cardiovascular Diseases*. 2009;19:177-183.
28. Ujvari D, Hulchiy M, Calaby A, et al. Lifestyle intervention up-regulates gene and protein levels of molecules involved in insulin signaling in the endometrium of overweight/obese women with polycystic ovary syndrome. *Human Reproduction*. 2014;29:1526-1535.

Figure 1-3. Lifestyle medicine landmark studies (cont.)

REFERENCES

- Abramson S, Stein J, Schaufele M, Frates EP, Rogan S. Personal exercise habits and counseling practices of primary care physicians: a national survey. *Clinical Journal of Sports Medicine.* 2000;10(1):40-48.
- AHA Policy Statement. Forecasting the Future of Cardiovascular Disease in the United States. Available at: http://circ.ahajournals.org/content/123/8/933. Accessed November 2016.
- American College of Lifestyle Medicine. Core Competencies. Available at: http://www.lifestylemedicine.org/Core-Competencies. Accessed November 2016.
- American Heart Association—Statistical Update. Heart Disease and Stroke Statistics—2011 Update. Available at: http://circ.ahajournals.org/content/123/4/e18.full.pdf+html. Accessed November 2016.
- American Public Health Association. Healthy Outlook: Public Health Resources for Systems Transformation. Available at: http://www.apha.org/~/media/files/pdf/topics/aca/tranformation/healthyoutlookcomplete.ashx. Accessed November 2016.
- Barnard RJ, Massey MR, Cherny S, O'Brien LT, Pritikin N. Long-term use of a high-complex-carbohydrate, high-fiber, low-fat diet and exercise in the treatment of NIDDM patients. *Diabetes Care.* May-June 1983;6(3):268-273.
- Boyle D. Watch: Cardiff Driver Hunted After 'Walking' Dog From Moving Car's Window. Available at: http://www.telegraph.co.uk/news/uknews/crime/11942307/Cardiff-driver-walks-dog-from-moving-car-South-Wales-Police.html. Accessed November 2016.
- Burke JE, Hultgren BP. Will physicians of the future be able to prescribe exercise? *Academic Medicine.* 1975;50(6):624-626.
- Centers for Disease Control and Prevention (CDC). Achievements in public health, 1900–1999. *Morbidity and Mortality Weekly Report.* July 1999;29:621-647.
- Centers for Disease Control and Prevention (CDC). Behavioral Risk Factor Surveillance System (BRFSS). Available at: http://www.cdc.gov/brfss/. Accessed November 2016.
- Centers for Disease Control and Prevention (CDC). Diabetes Report Card 2012. Available at: www.cdc.gov/diabetes/pubs/pdf/DiabetesReportCard.pdf. Accessed November 2016.
- Centers for Disease Control and Prevention (CDC). October 6, 2000 Press Release. Available at: https://www.cdc.gov/media/pressrel/r2k1006a.htm. Accessed November 2016.
- Centers for Medicare and Medicate Services. National Health Expenditures 2014 Highlights. Available at: https://www.cms.gov/research-statistics-data-and-systems/statistics-trends-and-reports/nationalhealthexpenddata/downloads/highlights.pdf. Accessed November 2016.
- Childs D, Kansagra S. 10 Health Advances That Changed the World. ABC News. September 20, 2007. Available at: http://abcnews.go.com/Health/TenWays/story?id=3605442&page=3. Accessed November 2016.

- Connaughton AV, RM RMW, Connaughton D. Graduating medical students' exercise prescription competence as perceived by deans and directors of medical education in the United States: implications for Healthy People 2010. *Public Health Reports*. 2011;116:226-234.
- Diabetes Prevention Program Research Group. Reduction in the incidence of type 2 diabetes with lifestyle intervention or metformin. *New England Journal of Medicine*. 2002;346:393-403. Available at: http://www.nejm.org/doi/pdf/10.1056/NEJMoa012512. Accessed September 2017.
- Dictionary.com. Evidence-based. Available at: http://www.dictionary.com/browse/evidence-based. Accessed November 2016.
- Dysinger W. Lifestyle medicine competencies for primary care physicians. *Virtual Mentor*. 2013;15(4):306-310.
- Egger G, Binns A, Rossner S. *Lifestyle Medicine: Managing Diseases of Lifestyle in the 21st Century*. North Ryde, N.S.W.: McGraw-Hill; 2010.
- Esselstyn C, Golubic M. The nutritional reversal of cardiovascular disease—fact or fiction? three case reports. *Clinical Cardiology*. 2014;20(7):1901-1908.
- Esselstyn CB, Gendy G, Doyle J, Golubic M, Roizen MF. Way to reverse CAD? *The Journal of Family Practice*. 2014;63(7):356-364.
- Exercise is Medicine. Available at: http://www.exerciseismedicine.org/. Accessed November 2016.
- Fahey TD, Insel PM, Roth WT. *Fit and Well: Core Concepts and Labs in Physical Fitness and Wellness*. Mountain View, CA: Mayfield Pub. Co.; 1994.
- Forman D, Bulwer BE. Cardiovascular disease: optimal approaches to risk factor modifications of diet and lifestyle. *Current Treatment Options in Cardiovascular Medicine*. 2006;8:47-57.
- Frank E, Breyan J, Elon L. Physician disclosure of healthy personal behaviors improves credibility and ability to motivate. *Archives of Family Medicine*. 2000;9:287-290.
- Frates EP, Moore M, Lopez CN, McMahon GT. Coaching for behavior change in physiatry. *American Journal of Physical Medicine & Rehabilitation*. December 2011;90(12).
- Garry JP, Diamond JJ, Whitley TW. Physical activity curricula in medical schools. *Academic Medicine*. 2002;77:818-820.
- Halm J, Amoako E. Physical activity recommendation for hypertension management: does healthcare provider advice make a difference? *Ethnicity and Disease*. Summer 2008;18(3):278-282.
- Katz D. Lifestyle is medicine. *Virtual Mentor*. 2013;15(4):286-292.
- Katz D. What Really Kills Us Huffington Post Online Edition. November 11, 2013. Available at: http://www.huffingtonpost.com/david-katz-md/chronic-disease_b_4250092.html. Accessed November 2016.
- MedicineNet.com. Definition of Quality of Life. MedTerms. Available at: http://www.medicinenet.com/script/main/art.asp?articlekey=11815. Accessed November 2016.

- Mokdad AH, Marks JS, Stroup DF, Gerberding JL. Actual causes of death in the United States, 2000. *Journal of the American Medical Association.* 2004;291(10):1238-1245.
- Moore M, Tschannen-Moran B. *Coaching Psychology Manual.* New York: Lippincott Williams & Wilkins; 2010.
- Peek ME, Tang H, Alexander GC, Chin MH. National prevalence of lifestyle counseling or referral among African-Americans and whites with diabetes. *Journal of General Internal Medicine.* November 2008;23(11):1858-1864.
- Pritikin N. *The Pritikin Program for Diet and Exercise.* New York: Random House Publishing Group; 1979.
- Rosenthal MB, Barnard RJ, Rose DP, Inkeles S, Hall J, Pritikin N. Effects of a high-complex-carbohydrate, low-fat, low-cholesterol diet on levels of serum lipids and estradiol. *American Journal of Medicine.* January 1985;78(1):23-27.
- Stein J, Silver J, Frates EP. *The Guide to Recovering Your Health and Preventing Another Stroke.* Baltimore, MD: Johns Hopkins University Press; 2006.
- Sullivan S, Samuel S. Effect of short-term Pritikin diet therapy on the metabolic syndrome. *Journal of Cardiometabolic Syndrome.* 2006;1(5):308-312.
- U.S. Preventive Services Task Force. Behavioral Counseling Interventions to Promote a Healthful Diet and Physical Activity for Cardiovascular Disease Prevention in Adults: U.S. Preventive Services Task Force Recommendation Statement. September 4, 2012. Available at: https://www.uspreventiveservicestaskforce.org/Home/GetFile/1/1721/physrs/pdf. Accessed November 2016.

CHAPTER 2

EMPOWERING PEOPLE TO CHANGE

"The secret of change is focusing all of your energy, not on fighting the old, but on building the new."

—Socrates
One of the Founders of Western
Philosophy
470 to 399 BCE

❏ Chapter Goals:

- Challenge readers to think differently about how to empower people to change.
- Invite readers to consider the pros and cons of direct advice versus negotiation in the area of behavior change.
- Consider the role of education in behavior change.
- Demonstrate how to be a coach by highlighting the "being" and "doing" characteristics/attributes of a coach through patient examples and case studies.
- Explain the five As of behavior change counseling.
- Introduce the Transtheoretical Model of Change.

❏ Learning Objectives:

- To examine health and wellness coaching strategies
- To explore the differences between the coach-like approach and the expert-like approach
- To know when to use the expert-like approach and when to use the coach-like approach
- To be aware of the essential elements of being a coach
- To grasp the five As of behavior change counseling
- To recognize the six stages of change in the Transtheoretical Model of Change
- To understand the concept of the Frates COACH™ Approach

❏ Guiding Questions:

- What are the attributes of an effective health and wellness coach?
- How does the coach-like approach differ from the expert-like approach?
- What is the Frates COACH Approach?

- How can the Transtheoretical Model of Change benefit both patients and providers?
- How can a clinical environment be created that facilitates lasting behavior change?
- What are the key factors involved in behavior change counseling?

❑ Important Terms:

- *Lifestyle medicine:* The use of evidence-based lifestyle therapeutic approaches, such as a predominantly whole food, plant-based diet, regular physical activity, adequate sleep, stress management, avoidance of risky substance use, and other non-drug modalities to treat, oftentimes, reverse and prevent the lifestyle-related, chronic disease that's all too prevalent.
- *Quality of life:* The culmination of objective indicators of physical, mental, emotional, and social health with subjective interpretation of the quality of those factors for a unique individual, based on the person's personal goals and values
- *Transtheoretical Model of Change:* A psychological theory that encompasses a cycle of mental stages that individuals progress (and regress) through as they engage in behavior modification
- *Vision:* A vivid aspirational picture of future accomplishment or state of being, which can be clearly articulated and used to determine and plan courses of action
- *Wellness:* The state of being in good health based on a holistic interpretation of health that includes emotional, physical, mental, spiritual, and social health

Coaching is *the* key verb in lifestyle medicine. It is the way to evoke behavior change. There are distinct differences between being a coach and being an expert, which this chapter explores in depth. The chapter examines both the being and doing skills involved in coaching.

As such, coaches have many tools in their toolbox. They use a whole different approach to the patient. This chapter introduces some of the most important tools that empower the "doing" aspects of coaching. The theory, evidence, and practice of health and wellness coaching are covered in this chapter, as well. The "being" aspects of the coach-like approach are exemplified in the Frates COACH Approach, with an emphasis on curiosity, openness, appreciation, compassion, and honesty. To fully appreciate the value of using coaching skills in the behavior change process, examples of trying the expert-like approach with a patient who has congestive heart failure and a poor diet and the coach-like approach with an 84-year-old patient who wanted to begin jumping rope will be discussed. As you will see, using coaching strategies helps not only with patient interactions but also with communications with colleagues, family, and friends.

Before discussing behavior change and how to apply coaching strategies, it is important to understand that the underlying focus of lifestyle medicine practitioners is to help individuals and families adopt and sustain healthy behaviors that affect their health and quality of life. What is quality of life? In that regard, one commonly accepted definition of this subjective factor is that it is the patient's ability to enjoy normal, routine, everyday activities. In a coaching relationship, the goal is to empower people to make changes that lead them to their optimal level of health and wellness.

Wellness, in turn, considers the whole person and the individual's feeling of balance, energy, peace, and productivity. Wellness pioneer John Travis, MD, MPH, defines wellness as "a way of life—a lifestyle that you design to achieve your highest potential for well-being" and also "a process—a developing awareness that there is no end point, but that health and happiness are possible in each moment, here and now." Gerhard William Hettler, III, one of the co-founders of the National Wellness Institute, detailed an even more comprehensive overview of wellness, outlining the six different dimensions of wellness, including emotional, physical, intellectual, social, occupational, and spiritual.

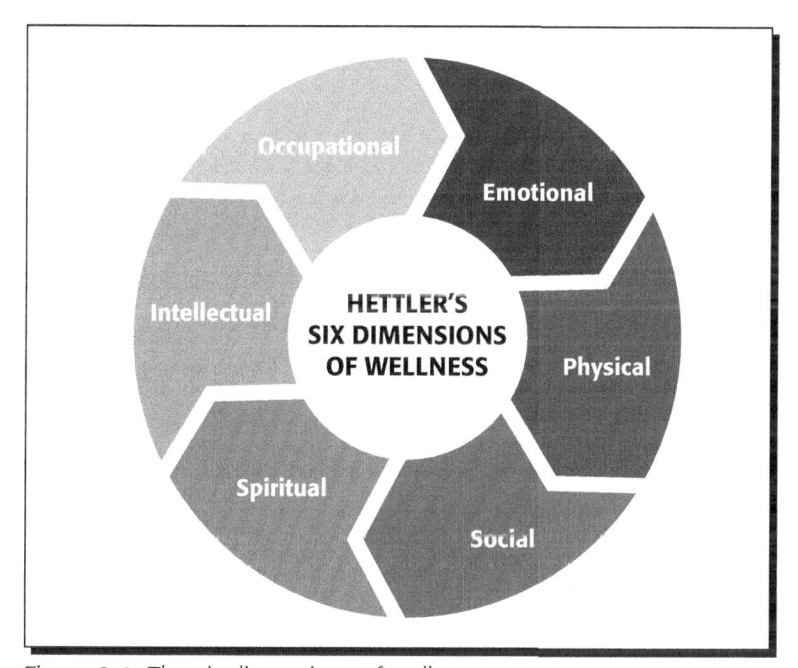

Figure 2-1. The six dimensions of wellness

A fundamental characteristic of lifestyle medicine is that it is an *evidence-based* area of medicine. What does evidence-based mean? David Sachet, one of the forefathers of the evidence-based approach to medicine, argues that evidence-based medicine is "the conscientious, explicit, and judicious use of current best evidence in making decisions about the care of the individual patient. It means integrating individual clinical expertise with the best available external clinical evidence from systematic research."

It should be noted that it wasn't until after 1990 that the term "evidence-based" became mainstream in medicine. At the present time, medical textbooks with the tagline "evidence-based" on their cover exist in almost every field of medicine. In fact, a textbook that specifically addressed the issue, *Evidence-Based Coaching*, was published in 2006.

Evidence exists concerning how patients can be empowered to make behavior changes. This data raises two important questions. First, how do lifestyle medicine practitioners use their words and their body language to develop rapport and connect with patients? (The underlying goal is that by the end of a coaching session, the patient feels capable of making a specific behavior change.) Second, how do practitioners increase patient self-efficacy, so that individuals are confident in their ability to complete a certain target task?

Clinical evidence provides some of the answers to these questions. Some of the attendant issues, however, remain unanswered and, as such, are active areas of research. Although medicine and behavioral change are based on research findings, they are also inextricably an art. While science informs that art, creativity, emotional intelligence, and instincts allow the art and the respective fields to flourish.

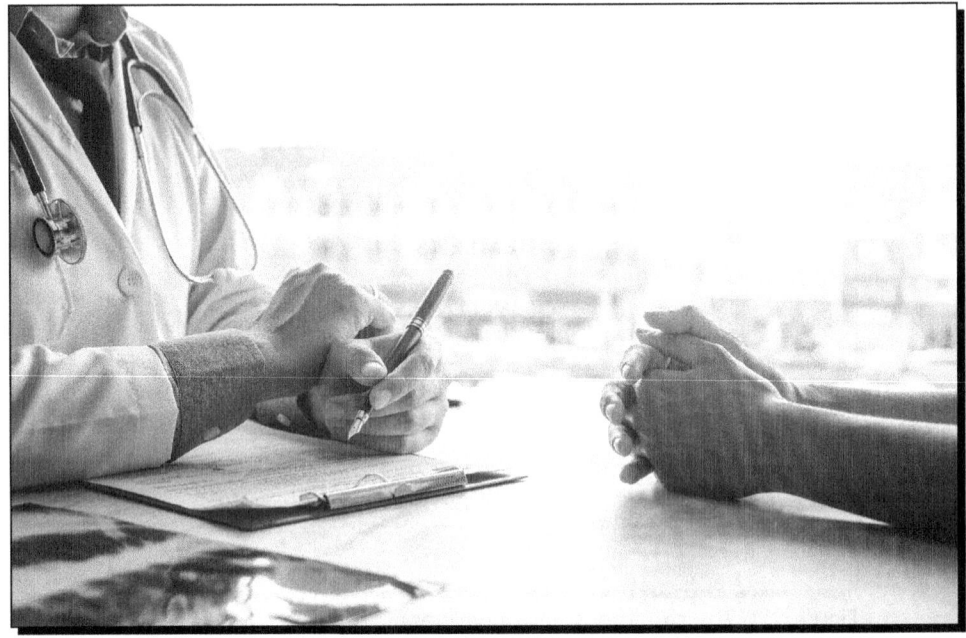

Coaching is the key verb in lifestyle medicine.

LIFESTYLE MEDICINE VS. TRADITIONAL MEDICINE

A difference exists between *traditional medicine* and lifestyle medicine. In traditional medicine, practitioners treat individual risk factors. Patients are passive recipients of care. They come into the office, and they expect a cure—usually in the form of a pill or procedure.

In this scenario, patients are not required to make big changes. Doctors just give them the solution (advice, medicine, or an intervention), and they take it. Adherence to a medication regimen, in most cases, is the behavioral change that is prescribed and the treatment is often short-term. In this instance, responsibility primarily lies with the clinician to diagnose the problem appropriately and to treat it with the right intervention, such as the correct antibiotic for an infection or the optimal antihypertensive medication that will bring the patient's blood pressure down.

In contrast to traditional medicine, lifestyle medicine practitioners look carefully at the lifestyle-related causes of disease. They look at the whole patient. They examine what the patients do on a daily basis with regard to selected lifestyle-related factors, such as their exercise, nutrition, social connections, sleep, and stress management, etc. Patients are active partners in the lifestyle medicine process, and practitioners frequently ask or invite patients to make big changes in their daily routines—altering habits that may have been ingrained for years or even decades. The key question in this process is how do lifestyle medicine practitioners engage their patients as active partners, when so many of these individuals are conditioned to be passive recipients of care?

The lifestyle medicine treatment is generally long-term. The process includes having patients forecast and *backcast* their goals by asking them where they want to be in five years, one year, six months, three months, one month, and then in one week. This method takes the long-range vision approach, creating an image of what patients see for themselves in the distant future. Subsequently, after creating this distant vision, the lifestyle practitioner works with the patient to craft visions of themselves for the near future. When creating a vision, it is best to make an attempt to use all the senses and try to have the patients craft clear images of themselves in 20 years, 10 years, or 5 years. Ask them how they imagine themselves feeling, walking, and talking? Next comes goal-setting. Goal-setting is completed for each month and week, with detailed specifics concerning days and times for particular activities.

Lifestyle medicine practitioners are not against medications. There are certain times when medication is advised, such as for extremely high cholesterol levels, high blood pressure, or poor glucose control with diabetes. Especially in the beginning of the lifestyle medicine journey, patients might make one of their goals to reach a point where they require a smaller and smaller dose of a specific medication. As such, any decision to prescribe medication should be based on the signs and symptoms of the patient, as well as the lab results for that individual. In the case of depression, anxiety, or other psychiatric issues, the prescription and ingestion of medicine depends on the severity of the patient's symptoms. The process is a personalized one, and treatments or interventions are as unique as the people are.

LIFESTYLE MEDICINE AND PREVENTION

Health and wellness coaching and the coach-like approach emphasize motivation and collaboration. With this style of counseling, patients and providers work together on disease management, reversal or prevention. In terms of prevention, there is primary, secondary, and tertiary prevention. *Primary prevention* involves individuals who are very healthy and want to stay that way. *Secondary prevention* is used when people who have risk factors for a disease, and want to avoid receiving a diagnosis for that disease. In contrast, *tertiary prevention* is needed with patients who have already suffered an event, such as a stroke, or already have a diagnosis like heart disease, and they are trying to prevent any consequences of the disease, with the hopes of attenuating the disease process or even reversing it.

LIFESTYLE MEDICINE AS A COLLABORATIVE PRACTICE

Traditional medicine has typically been an individual "sport" or a solitary specialty. Patients may go to a general practitioner (GP) for overall healthcare and minor health concerns, but they will be referred to specialists for specific problems. For example, patients will go to a cardiovascular specialist, if they have heart disease; a pulmonary specialist, if they suffer from asthma; a nephrologist or renal physician for kidney problems; or an endocrinologist for diabetes and hormone disorders. These specialists typically work in their own silos and operate independently on a one-on-one basis with their patients. They rarely interact with the GP, apart from perhaps sending a progress note. If patients have more than one problem, they might visit multiple specialists—and these specialists might not communicate with one another or the GP. As a result, they could develop different plans for addressing a specific patient's needs and interests. This situation is clearly not ideal. Fortunately, a number of people are working to change the system. Coordinated care is the goal for many medical practices now.

While traditional medicine has adopted more of a team approach in recent years, lifestyle medicine has been team-based since its inception. It involves a group of medical professionals, such as nurses, therapists, psychologists, health and wellness coaches, nutritionists, fitness professionals, case managers, social workers, etc. Collectively, these individuals must all communicate and work together to help patients make and sustain behavioral changes. In addition, a lifestyle medicine practitioner will work with a patient's primary care doctor and the other specialists who are involved with the patient. This undertaking requires a great deal of communicating, in person, via email, and through the individual's medical record.

Physiatry—physical medicine and rehabilitation—is a unique medical specialty that utilizes such a team approach. When working with a stroke patient, for example, the physiatrists interacts closely with a variety of other practitioners, such as a physical therapist, occupational therapist, speech therapist, recreational therapist, vocational therapist, nutritionist, psychologist, social worker, nurse, and nurse's aide. There are team meetings with all of these health professionals in the room. In addition, family members are part of the team.

In lifestyle medicine, practitioners are increasingly calling upon allied health professionals to utilize their skills, talents, and time to assist patients. As such, in lifestyle medicine, the physician is just one member of the team.

COACHING CONVERSATIONS IN LIFESTYLE MEDICINE

The differences between the *expert-like approach* and the *coach-like approach* are detailed in Figure 2-2. It can also be helpful to consider how traditional medicine compares with the expert-like approach. There are many similarities between the traditional medicine approach described earlier in this chapter and the expert-like approach. Traditionally, trained physicians treat and educate each of their patients, while relying on their own skills and knowledge. As the expert, they strive to have all the answers. As such, the letters of the word EXPERT can sometimes stand for examine, x-ray, plan, explain, repeat, and tell, - an acronym that, on occasion, is referred to as the "sell-and-tell" approach (Figure 2-3).

Medical training generally favors the expert-like approach. Healthcare professionals read countless volumes of textbooks and numerous work-related materials throughout their careers. As a result, they feel the need to not only utilize all of that information, but share as much of it as possible with their patients. Acquiring knowledge and sharing it are useful and important goals, but not everyone is ready and willing to hear the information that the medical expert wants to share.

Expert-Like Approach	**Coach-Like Approach**
Treats patients.	Helps patients help themselves.
Educates.	Builds motivation, confidence and engagement.
Relies on skills and knowledge of expert.	Relies on patient self-awareness and insights.
Strives to have all the answers.	Strives to help patients find their own answers.
Focuses on the problem.	Focuses on what is working well.
Advises.	Collaborates.

Figure 2-2. The differences between the expert-like approach and the coach-like approach

EXPERT

E = Examine

X = X-ray

P = Plan

E = Explain

R = Repeat

T = Tell

Figure 2-3. The "EXPERT" acronym created by Dr. Beth Frates

The expert focuses on the problem. For example, an expert may ask themselves, "What is the problem? It's my responsibility with all my knowledge, training, and skills to fix this problem." After finding the answer to the problem, the expert then follows a pattern of advising and directing. The patient often has little say in this situation. The conversation is mostly one-way. Satisfaction is also often felt predominately by the physician expert, who is excited to have solved the mystery. Patients, however, may still feel alone, confused, and in the dark about their particular condition.

When dealing with life-threatening situations, such as in an emergency room, the expert-like approach is invaluable and necessary. This one-sided approach, however, is rarely effective in producing behavior change. There is an important art to affecting behavior change, given that the issues addressed are often neither straightforward nor are they completely evident to the physician or patient. For example, "What will it take for you to quit smoking?"

In contrast, using the coach-like approach enables the practitioner to approach patients in a way that empowers them to find their own ideal solutions to their lifestyle problems and unhealthy habits. As a coach, the objective is to build motivation, confidence, and engagement in the process of lifestyle change. Coaches rely on patient self-awareness and insights, viewing the patient as the expert on their own lifestyle and their own life. To embody the being skills underlying the Frates COACH Approach, an individual must rely on curiosity, openness, appreciation, compassion, and honesty (refer to Figure 2-4).

The coach strives to help patients find their own answers. The focus is on a *strengths-based approach*, or what is working for patients. The coach starts with the positive. What is going well in the patient's lifestyle at this point in the person's life? This strategy is all about *appreciative inquiry*, and how that theory plays into lifestyle medicine consulting. After all, what individuals appreciate, appreciates. Thus, appreciating the positive is a great way to start a coaching conversation. Coaching is a

> **COACH**
>
> **C** = Curiosity
>
> **O** = Openness
>
> **A** = Appreciation
>
> **C** = Compassion
>
> **H** = Honesty

Figure 2-4. The Frates COACH Approach acronym

real example of a collaborative process. The underlying goal is to cultivate a high quality connection with the patient by listening, questioning, negotiating, and co-creating.

A 2008 study yielded a startling statistic about hypertensive patients, finding that only one-third of them received counseling to engage in physical activity as a way to manage their hypertension. This situation occurred, despite the fact that research has repeatedly indicated that having patients exercise decreases their blood pressure. Studies show that physicians who lack training or time do not necessarily counsel their patients to engage in physical activity. This situation occurred despite the fact that when patients were counseled to exercise, 71 percent of them followed the recommendations. It also suggests that routine physician counseling alone may not be sufficient for nearly 30 percent of patients. This research was a wake-up call to physicians, years ago.

Patients can struggle to follow prescriptions for exercise; they do the same with written prescriptions, and they do so at about the same rate. For example, approximately one-third of the prescriptions that physicians write never get filled. In these situations, the physicians invest significant amounts of time and use their expert skills and knowledge, in order to find the right medication—for instance, an antibiotic to combat a particular type of bacterial infection. Then, they write out the prescription, and the patient may say to themselves, "I don't need this. I'm just going to take Vitamin C."

After that, patients may throw the prescription in the trash, figuratively and literally. Some patients do what they want to do, especially if they do not understand the rationale for the prescription, as it was written or for a recommendation that was made. Perhaps, the prescription was not explained well, or a connection was not made between the prescription and the patient's health. Perhaps there was no connection between the patient and the physician. If so, there may have been no trust.

The underlying concept in lifestyle medicine is that writing a prescription for exercise, nutrition, stress management, or sleep is only the first step. The real challenge lies in working diligently with the patient to ensure that the prescription actually gets filled.

This factor raises several other important questions that research has worked to address. For example, how is this effective communication accomplished? How can lifestyle medicine practitioners use words to negotiate and communicate with a patient in such a way that the patients walk away and actually feel motivated to make the desired change?

One strategy is *self-disclosure*—physicians sharing what works for them in their medical practices. Dr. Erika Frank has conducted research to help us to appreciate this technique. An example of applying this technique might sound like: "I actually know it's really hard to exercise. I bike to work. It's also hard to have healthy snacks. I eat an apple." This approach goes against the routine practice and the training that many practicing physicians received during medical school. Usually, it is best to focus only on the patient. Research in lifestyle medicine, however, reveals that demonstrating that the physician is taking healthy habits seriously and trying to sustain them for themselves can be motivating to their patients. The physician does not need to be perfect to be motivating. In fact, they just need to be real and actually trying to eat healthy foods, exercise regularly, sleep seven to eight hours, and follow the other evidence-based lifestyle medicine recommendations. It's not about perfection. It's about progress and staying on the healthy lifestyle journey.

RESEARCH SPOTLIGHT

In most instances, advising people to engage in more exercise is simply ineffective. This point was proven in a randomized, controlled trial of physical activity promotion in primary care that looked at physician styles of counseling. Titled "Advising People to Take More Exercise Is Ineffective," the study involved three groups. One group offered direct advice, one group focused on negotiation, and the third group served as the control. In the control group, the primary care physicians treated the patients in their usual manner.

A physician giving direct advice in the first group in the study might sound like this: "You need to exercise more. Exercise is good for you. It helps our heart, your lungs, your brain. It helps everything. You need to make it a priority and just do it!"

Meanwhile, the negotiating physicians in the aforementioned research project were told to ask questions, in particular, open-ended questions. Their basic goal was to find out a little bit about the patient and their current actions. The negotiating physician may sound like this: "How are you doing with exercise?" As such, the client might respond that they do not exercise at all. The negotiating physician would then respond, "Oh really? What's getting in your way?" At that point, they talk about the barriers. Then, the physician might say, "Oh, so you have diabetes. Do you know how exercise can help you manage your diabetes? Do you know what exercise you would do to help you manage your diabetes?"

In both groups, whether giving direct advice or negotiating, the physician and patients talked for a half hour. All patients in the experimental groups, either through direct advice or negotiation, were counseled to increase their level of physical activity engagement.

The final group was the control. The physicians in this group did not change the way they treated their patients. They also did not specifically counsel the patient about their activity level. In addition, they were told not to spend more than a half hour or any extra time with the patient.

When the study concluded, the patients were asked follow-up questions about their level of physical activity since their clinic visit. The results revealed that the patients in the negotiation group significantly increased their minutes of physical activity over those in the control group. The direct advice approach, however, was no more likely to spur patients to exercise than the routine approach (control group). This study suggests that if a physician is going to take the time to address lifestyle behaviors, then the negotiation approach is best.

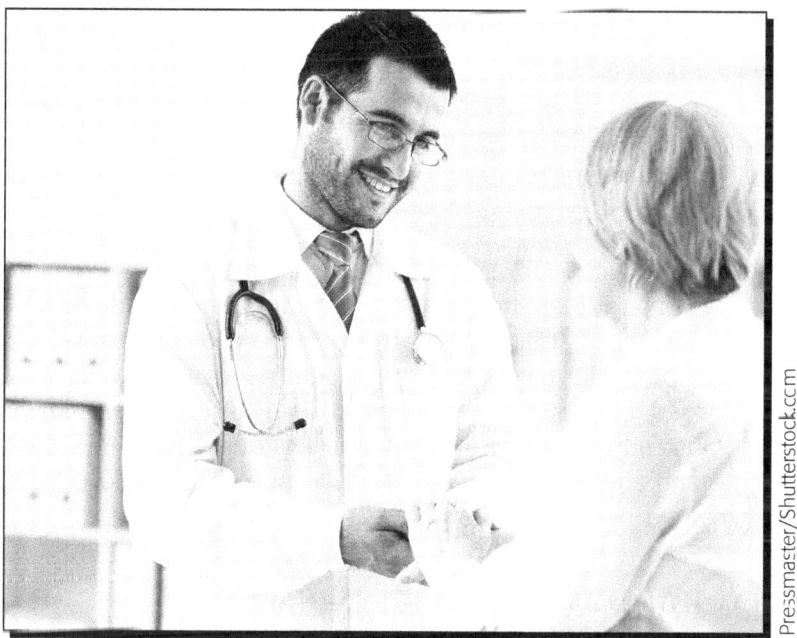

The first step in using the coach-like approach involves engaging and learning.

SWITCHING FROM THE EXPERT-LIKE APPROACH TO THE COACH-LIKE APPROACH

How does a practitioner, after years of training, start using a more collaborative coach-like approach? Many healthcare professionals have been trained to be experts and to have all the answers. The expert wants to provide knowledge and employs a directive style—tell/sell, teach as much as possible, and inform the patient.

The first step in using the coach-like approach involves engaging and learning. It begins with being curious about the patient or client. Instead of assuming that the patient needs the information, the lifestyle medicine practitioner starts with a question. This method is similar to the negotiation arena mentioned in the study, "Advising People to Take More Exercise Is Ineffective." For example, the practitioner will inquire of the patient, "What do you know about stroke?" or "What do you already know about diabetes?"

The practitioner will check to see what the patient's understanding of the topic is and what the individual is interested in learning. "Oh, would you like to know how diet could affect your chance of stroke?" a practitioner might ask. "No, not really, because you know what, I have a nutritionist, and she went over all that for me," could be the response of the patient. "Okay, great," replies the practitioner, understanding that the patient does not need another lecture, because the individual has already heard it before. At that point, the practitioner might ask, "How do you feel about what you are eating?" or "How is your diet going?"

Another option might be to ask, "What do you understand about how your diet can help you prevent another stroke?" If the patient answers and shares a great deal of information, then the practitioner can move on to a different topic. This way, the practitioner can supply information that the patient needs and wants. As a result, the practitioner provides what is referred to as "just in time information," which saves everyone time. Instead of the practitioners wasting their time with lectures, they can focus their time and attention on areas that have not yet been covered and thus still "need" to be covered.

LIVE AND LEARN WITH DR. BETH FRATES

I'd like to share my personal experience as a patient, going in for an annual visit, a few years ago.

In all honesty, I was hoping to talk with my physician about exercise. I enjoy exercise, and I had been faithful to a routine exercise schedule for many years. At this time in my life, however, I had kids and was writing a book chapter. There seemed to be countless obstacles standing in my way to get out and run. I am used to being the person helping others and negotiating with others to empower them to lead healthy lives and exercise regularly. Now, it was my turn to be the patient, and I was looking forward to it.

My physician entered the room in a rush. He was a little late, but I did not mind that at all. He also seemed quite frazzled. Actually, he said, "Oh. I am so glad it is you, because I am running so late today. I need to make up some time. You are an easy one!" When he asked me about physical activity, it was in a general way; he didn't give me much leeway to respond. For years, I have answered this question the same way, by replying, "I usually jog five days a week for about a half an hour, and I also practice yoga one to two times a week." I started with this standard answer, hoping to clarify my response, since these were not the current facts.

But my physician interjected, "So, you're still exercising? You're still exercising five days a week? You're still doing that? Right?" What's more, while he said this, he was looking at the computer screen, facing the wall with his back to me, trying to type and fill in my electronic medical record during the interview. Behind his back, I replied, "Yeah, I'm still exercising. Yeah, I mean I'm exercising."

Quickly, he quipped, "Okay, so you're still exercising regularly." Feeling like a liar, I tried to explain, "Yeah, but—yeah." However, he had already moved on to the next question in the electronic medical record. "Alright. And, so, let's see, looks like your weight, and your blood pressure are the same." He then just went on and on. Okay, well alright. "I guess I missed my chance," is the thought that entered my mind. I also felt badly for him, because he had already confided to me that he was running late. So, I did not want to take up his time. I figured I would have to figure out my exercise issues on my own.

At that point, with his eyes still glued to the computer, checking my data, he said, "Oh, I see you need a mammogram this year." To which, I simply stated, "Oh, I thought I had one last year. Does that mean I need one this year?" In reality, I just wanted a "yes" or "no" from him. If he said, "Yes, you need it this year," I was going to be perfectly fine with that. If he said, "Oh, no, you're right, I didn't realize you had one last year," I would have been fine to just move on to the next part of the exam. It did not go like that.

Instead, he took his eyes away from the computer and looked at me. He then started to deliver an unexpected and unwanted lecture by commenting, "Oh, haven't you seen the latest research? Let me tell you about it. So, there is data to support women undergoing mammograms every year."

Quite frankly, I don't know what else he said, because I was looking at him and thinking to myself, "Oh my gosh, this is how patients feel when practitioners go on and on, counseling them on topics that are of no interest to them." I remember feeling strange and thinking, "I see his mouth moving, but I am not hearing her or making sense of her words." It seemed to me as if everything was in slow motion.

Finally, he concluded with, "Isn't that interesting?" At that point, all I said was, "So, do I need a mammogram this year?" "Yes," was his reply.

On occasion, physicians need to use the expert-like approach during their clinical encounters. If a patient is suffering a heart attack, for example, the expert-like approach is the way to handle the situation. With acute care issues or urgent care, the patients need to see their physicians to take charge and help them. A heart attack, stroke, anaphylaxis, or sepsis are not times for negotiating.

It would be absurd for an emergency room physician to ask a heart attack victim, "How are you feeling? Do you want to take the nitroglycerin (a medicine that helps open up blood vessels) and put it under your tongue? Would you like one or two? Would you like to hear more about it before you consider taking it?"

In this situation, the physician needs to take the expert-like approach and inform the patient that they are having a heart attack and that these little white pills, called nitroglycerin, will help their heart. Without question, an important role exists for the expert-like approach in medicine.

Experts, like healthcare providers, often rely on their cognitive listening skills. As such, they search for the facts. They can listen carefully to the patient's stories, picking up red flags and symptoms that can help to solve the individual's mystery and explain what is going on with the person. They can listen to the beating of the heart, percuss the liver to discern its size, and listen for carotid bruits in the neck. Healthcare providers have a lot of great listening skills, and they utilize them for diagnosis and treatment in an acute care setting. This skillset is very important.

In the coach-like approach, practitioners also need to use well-developed listening skills—just different ones. As a coach, the goal is to build rapport and connect to the patient to develop a therapeutic relationship. With the coach-like approach, the practitioners utilize themselves as healing agents, hoping that their presence and their interaction will soothe, inspire, and motivate the patient. In lifestyle medicine and coaching, practitioners can employ the Frates invitation-to-learn, a technique that is also known as live and learn or simply L & L.

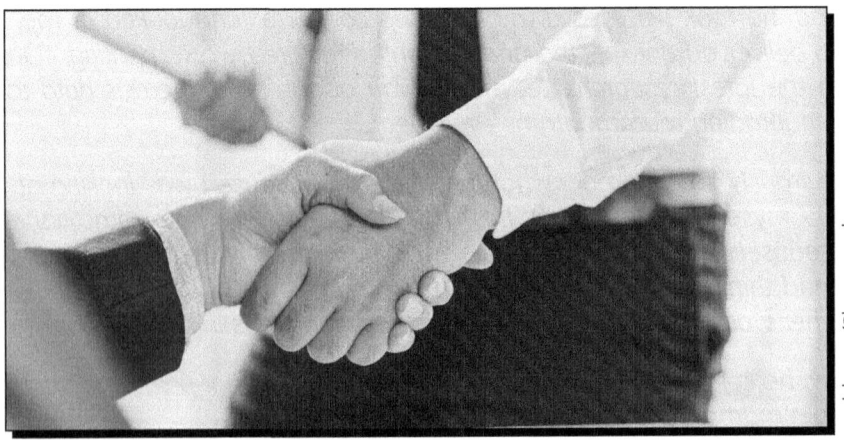

As a coach, the goal is to build rapport and connect to the patient to develop a therapeutic relationship.

LIVE AND LEARN WITH DR. BETH FRATES

Years ago, after I had become a licensed coach, I went back to Spaulding Rehabilitation Hospital, where I had worked with stroke patients during my residency. After my coach training, I started a wellness group for stroke patients and their caregivers. It was really exciting. It was wonderful, and I loved it.

For my first wellness group, I started with a roundtable discussion—with all of the stroke survivors and caregivers positioned around a large, wooden, oval table. During the first session, people were invited to tell their stories, for which they had an allotted period of time.

For this introductory activity, I really looked forward to listening, really listening, to the patients undistracted—no writing, no wriggling, just holding eye contact with my hands on the table. I did not even take notes, which felt a little uncomfortable to me. I was accustomed to listening, while writing and filling out paperwork, which is what I had done to stay on top of my work and remain productive.

On occasion, I would even talk to the patient, while I examined them. I recall times when I was flying around the room, pretending to listen and pay attention, when all the while, I was desperately trying to multitask. Mindfulness had not entered my vocabulary.

This instance was the first time I remember saying to myself, "I'm just sitting here and listening. That's it. I'm going to just listen to the real story behind everyone's stroke, what happened to them and why." Mostly, I listened intently, because I wanted to be able to help them, by teaching them important information relevant to them and their particular situations. From my previous research, I knew that many stroke survivors and caregivers didn't know their risk factors, their type of stroke, or their medications. Accordingly, I wanted to listen carefully to each person. But, I learned an unexpected lesson that day.

It was great. I am proud to say that I did listen intently, with my hands folded and my eyes on the person talking the entire time. Nothing else was on my mind, except each person's story, all of which were fascinating. Previously, with stroke patients, I would access their medical record ahead of time so that I knew the important details about each patient and did not even really need to interview the individual once they arrived to the rehabilitation hospital.

Basically, I knew the punch line—the type of stroke and how it happened, because it's documented. Unless you're an ER doctor, who otherwise translates it for all of us, this information is provided to us through the medical record. In this instance, however, I knew nothing. I was just meeting these patients for the first time, and they were an empty slate to me. After hearing their stories, I did give a little lecture about stroke basics (risk factors, warning signs, types of strokes, and medications) and then answered a few questions they had about strokes.

As I do with any coaching session, at the end of it, I asked, "What was helpful to you during our time together?" Subsequently, when this coaching session was done, I asked the same question. The responses varied. Some people said the best part was hearing about warning signs. Most people said hearing other people tell their stories was the most helpful. I will never forget what the last gentleman said. He sat there, with tears in his blue eyes and looked at me. Softly, he said, "You know, you're the very first doctor who has listened, really listened to my story. You cared about my story. No one else listened." And then, he broke down into tears.

At that point, of course, the rest of the group cried, and I almost cried. I wanted to cry, not only because he was crying, but because I had actually never listened to a patient's stroke story before in that same powerful therapeutic way. I was always rushing around. In hindsight, I feel sorry both for the patients whom I interviewed and for myself. As such, I missed a number of great opportunities to be a healer. That experience taught me how important it is to listen wholeheartedly, affectively, and fully to the words, the body language, the patient's eyes, the tone of voice, speed of speech, pitch, and velocity.

In reality, there is so much to listen to with each patient. The power of listening has long been appreciated and written about. For example, Zeno Citium, an ancient Greek philosopher, once remarked, "We have two ears and one mouth, so we should listen more than we say." The importance of listening is not new information, but emphasizing its power in the clinical setting is a good reminder for everyone.

DEVELOPING A QUESTIONING ATTITUDE

Another challenge the practitioner faces, when using the traditional expert-like approach, is the rigid reliance on a specific questioning format, such as the review of systems. This undertaking entails a series of closed-ended questions developed to identify any problems in the multiple organs and systems in the body. These questions require a "yes" or "no" answer, and run along the lines of inquiries, such as, "Are you having pain on urination? Are you coughing? Are you short of breath? Are you having chest pains?" These questions are designed to help practitioners in an acute care setting and are focused on the expert's agenda.

Normally, practitioners follow their own agenda in an acute care visit. When employing the traditional expert-like approach, the expert's agenda is the focus.

In situations involving the coach-like approach, such as visits for chronic health problems that would benefit from behavioral change, lifestyle medicine practitioners use open-ended questions and follow the patient's agenda. Why? They are curious about what the patient is thinking and what makes that individual feel unhealthy, stressed, tired, anxious, or unwell.

How do practitioners elicit that information? Their basic strategy is to allow patients to talk and to focus on listening to them. Lifestyle medicine practitioners ask, "How would your life be different if you were exercising now?", rather than, "Why aren't you exercising when you, know it is good for your health?" Furthermore, they ask, "What things are preventing you from exercising?", instead of, "You are following my recommendations to exercise five days a week, aren't you?"

Coaching-type questions open up conversation and allow for the process of discovery. Examples of other open-ended questions include the following:
- How are you feeling about your exercise routine now?
- What would life be like if you quit smoking?
- What has to happen in order for you to consider drinking less?
- Tell me more about your relationship with alcohol.
- Talk to me about …

The essential point to remember is that letting the patients talk and share their thoughts plays a key role in lifestyle medicine counseling. As such, it is helpful to keep in mind that patients are the experts in their own life.

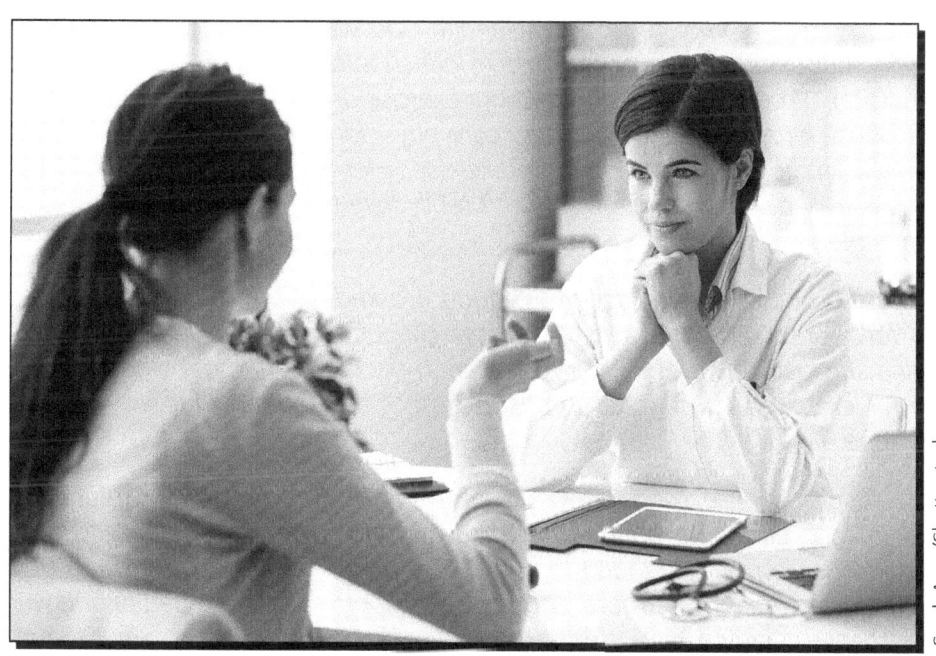

The essential point to remember is that letting the patients talk and share their thoughts plays a key role in lifestyle medicine counseling.

LIVE AND LEARN WITH DR. BETH FRATES

I once had a client, an 82-year-old woman who was about 100 pounds, 5'2", fit, doing well, and walking 20 minutes a day twice a week with her husband. One day, she walked into my office with a smile on her face and declared, "Well, I am here today, because I want to do more exercise. I mean I have osteoporosis. I know it's good for me, so I want to do more exercise."

Her attitude perplexed me. I kept thinking that she is exercising for 20 minutes two times a week by walking with her husband. She enjoys that. Why not walk for 20 minutes another day or extend the walks to 30 minutes? The solution seemed too easy.

I also got sidetracked, because I heard her brief statement about having osteoporosis. Somewhat serendipitously, I had just given a lecture at the Medical School on this topic. In the process, I had created this wonderful diagram about how vitamin D works with sunshine to help bones. I was very excited to share this new diagram with her. Inherently, I very much wanted to say, "Oh, let me share this with you. I just shared this helpful diagram with the medical students, and I know you will love it too."

I had recently completed my first health and wellness coach training program when this happened, however, so I didn't launch into lecture mode. Instead, I asked the question, "Would you like to hear about exercise and osteoporosis?" To my dismay, her response was, "No, no. My primary care physician already told me all about that. That's why I'm here. I want to do more exercise." Her response saved both of us time, but it was truly disappointing, given that I really love to lecture, and that the diagram was intricate yet simple to understand. .

Focusing back onto her agenda though, I asked, "What are you thinking about doing for more exercise?" I was genuinely curious. I kept thinking to myself, "Why wouldn't she just walk more"? Her response to my question about what do you want to do for exercise was a great surprise to me. She reported that she wanted to... "jump rope."

My initial response (again) was to jump into lecture mode—emergency lecture mode, in fact, given the dangers—with an emphasis on threatening, scaring, and preventing her from doing that. I thought, "No. What? That's crazy. You are 82 years old, skinny, and frail. Furthermore, you have osteoporosis." Before health and wellness coach training, I would have started shouting, "At your age, you cannot jump rope, that is one of the best ways I know to fracture your hip. At your age, hip fracture means hospitalization, which then that leads to pneumonia, and finally the proverbial old man's friend—death."

Such thoughts were racing through my mind, and my lips were practically moving, before I stopped and took a breath. You cannot predict the answers inside the patient's head. That's why it is good to be curious. So, instead, I said, "What makes you say that?"

She responded with, "My sister and I used to do double-dutch jump rope when we were little. We used to sing songs and jump rope for hours, and I was thinking about that. My sister passed away from pancreatic cancer two months ago. That's why I really want to jump rope and sing our songs. Somehow, I want to feel closer to her."

Well, her response changed everything for me. Her feelings were interesting, and I wondered to myself, "Is there a way she can jump rope safely? Can I clear a space? Can I talk with her about how to do this? Would this be possible?"

Accordingly, I asked another question. "Do you have a jump rope?" You need to know how serious the person is about the intended activity. She was serious. Earlier in the week, she had purchased a jump rope.

Arguably, she was likely going to jump rope, regardless of what I said. Her jumping rope was what the whole visit was about. On the other hand, I did point out, "Okay, let's talk about this. It can be very unsafe. Are you familiar with hip fractures?"

I asked if she wanted to understand and know more about the dangers of hip fractures. I also inquired if she would like to talk about a safe way to jump rope, perhaps make it more of a walking-rope or even use an imaginary rope. In addition, I queried if she wanted any additional support to help with her sadness about her sister passing away. Who could have guessed that an 82-year-old would want to jump rope? The point is that you will not know if you don't ask.

PROBLEM-SOLVING AS A COACH

Experts love to solve problems. That is why many physicians go into medicine. Solving problems and finding solutions can be enjoyable and rewarding, especially if it saves someone's life or helps them to heal.

When using the coach-like approach, the mystery is also compelling. Coaches, however, do not have a microscope or lab values to help them find the solution to the problem with which they are concerned. Instead, they must rely on information given to them by their patients, as well as rely on their own patience to draw it out of them.

Instead of diving in and trying to solve the problem, as if it were an emergency, the coach has to work with the patient by asking open-ended questions, listening, and discovering the solution. For example, if a problem exists with someone not exercising, that person might come by to visit and say, "You know what, I wanted to exercise five days a week, but I only exercised one. I mean I put my sneakers on other days, but I just couldn't get out the door."

Coaches do not have to interrogate patients about every detail to try and solve the problem like Sherlock Holmes. In fact, interrogating patients can lead to discomfort and resistance. Asking an open-ended question, however, such as, "What were the circumstances when you could not get out the door?" can be helpful. As a rule, in such a situation, the patient is likely to give great insight concerning the event. For example, a patient might say, "One time, I got a phone call and needed to stay at home to talk to my friend, because she was going through a divorce, you know." Hearing feedback can help the practitioner to better understand how to help the patient.

After listening to the patient talk about a particular problem, it can be tempting to spew out solutions that may work for the practitioners, such as, "The next time that happens, if you get a phone call, and you're ready to go for a walk, use your cell phone. You can walk and talk at the same time with your cell phone." Now, that suggestion might work. It might resonate with that particular patient. However, it could also be off-putting or alienating, especially if the person does not have a cell phone.

Another technique that is in alignment with the coach-like approach might be to ask another question that calls upon the wisdom inside the patient. "Hmm, what could you do, if next time you're going for a walk, you've got your shoes on, and your phone rings? What do you think you could do differently?" In this instance, the solution a patient might give is, "Tell my friend I will call her back, when I am done walking, invite my friend to come over and walk with me, or take a walk to my friend's house." Arguably, those are great solutions, too. In reality, people are more likely to stick with a solution that they created or that they selected from a series of options. Brainstorming ideas together and asking the patient to think about solutions, along with you, can work well, too. In the end, the patient needs to select the solution they like best and the one they think will work best for them. The point is that it is essential to honor the autonomy of the patient, instead of the practitioner imposing their own solution on that individual.

LIVE AND LEARN WITH DR. BETH FRATES

I once had a patient who came to me one day and said, "You know, I'm doing really well with the exercise. I've lost 10 pounds, but I can't get over this plateau. And, I'm a night eater. After 9:00 p.m., I watch television, and, I eat. I eat potato chips. I eat cookies. I sit. I watch, and I eat. Actually, one of my favorite treats is those little pastries that I keep in the refrigerator. They've got cream, and they're really good. During the commercials, I go into my refrigerator, and I get them. Truth be known, I just really enjoy eating at night, but, then, I feel really bad about my actions the next morning."

Before my health and wellness coach training, I would have said, "Look, what we're going to do is we're going to lock you out of the kitchen. Just lock the door to the kitchen at 9:00 p.m. Someone else will take the key, and you won't be able to go in again until the next day. Or, you could lock the cabinets up somehow, put padlocks on them perhaps." If that did not work, I would have recommended that she just sip water after 9 p.m. All factors considered, restricting the ingestion of foods and fluids to water was a good solution that could be useful, given that I had other clients who only drank water after dinner and that worked wonders for them.

I stopped, however, before I started to speak. I thought to myself, "What does this patient know that I don't know? What has she considered doing to stop her nighttime eating binges? I bet she has thought about the just-sip-water option." So, I asked, "Well, what do you think would work for you to—would you want to stop that? You're telling me about it as if it's something you're unhappy with." She replied, "Yeah, I don't want to do it anymore." I then inquired, "Well, so what do you think can help?"

She responded, "Well, I don't know. My nighttime eating is an addiction. I have to stop it, but I don't know how. What do you think? What should I do?"

This situation was an exceptional opportunity for the coaching strategy referred to as brainstorming. If the patient reports that they can't think of any solutions, then brainstorming can be a great way to invite creativity into the problem-solving session. For example, you can say to the patient, "Let's brainstorm together. You think of an idea that might work, and I"ll think of other ideas. We keep taking turns, suggesting different solutions, until you hear some ideas you like. Some of my ideas might be funny, crazy, and outside-the-box, but who knows? They might just work for you. How does that sound?"

My brainstorming session with this client was memorable. She wanted me to start. "What about a padlock on your refrigerator?" I asked, and she burst out laughing. Then, for her turn at brainstorming, she said, "You know what, I have an exercise ball in my TV room that has been sitting in the corner for months. I look at it as I'm on my recliner getting a massage and having my pastry. I look at it, and I say hmm, it would be good to use that. You know what I think I should do? Get rid of the recliner, put the recliner in the corner, and get the exercise ball out. If I sit and bounce on the exercise ball throughout the show I can't actually be eating my pastries."

My response to her idea was simply, "Brilliant." I then gave another potential solution of sipping water after 9 p.m., which she quickly stated would not work. She thought of not watching TV, but dismissed it immediately. In the end, she settled on using the exercise ball when watching TV, and she loved it. I have actually used her solution with other clients in other brainstorming sessions. That give-and-take session yielded an example of a solution that I would not have thought of on my own. I am not the expert of her house or her habits. I had no idea that she had an exercise ball in her TV room. As such, her expertise was needed to find the ideal solution for her.

TAKING RESPONSIBILITY AND CARING FOR PATIENTS

Physicians who are on call overnight at the hospital can feel alone and stressed, thinking that they are primarily responsible for the health and safety of several patients who are very ill. On-call physicians have to address every problem, and it's a heavy weight when they are using the "expert-like approach" all night at the hospital. It can be difficult to handle all that responsibility.

When someone needs a coach, however, they usually are not in the hospital, and they are not acutely ill. Most patients with chronic diseases due to unhealthy behaviors, such as smoking, are not in an emergency situation, requiring a medical expert when they come to see the health and wellness coach. At that point, they need someone who can engage and empower them, someone who can talk to them, and someone to help find out what is actually going on.

It is not practical for health and wellness coaches to take responsibility to go to the houses of patients, wake them up early, put on their sneakers, tie the laces of their shoes, and go for a walk with them. One coach cannot do all of these tasks with multiple patients. In this instance, the coach would be taking on too much responsibility for the behavior of patients. In reality, patients need to take responsibility for their own actions and behaviors.

Behavior change is a journey. It is not a quick fix. All patients are on their own wellness journeys, on which they will experience many successes and setbacks. Coaches are there to provide support, regardless of circumstances. Coaches, like experts, want to help a patient find health and wellness. The expert does this through testing, treatment, and procedures. In contrast, the coach helps by promoting *self-efficacy* in patients—the belief in one's ability to accomplish certain tasks or achieve particular goals. Through the coaching relationship, the patients gain confidence in themselves. This confidence helps patients sustain their positive lifestyle-related actions and continue on their wellness journey.

LIVE AND LEARN WITH DR. BETH FRATES

The following is a really difficult anecdote for me to share, because it is a situation in which I feel like I failed. I am sharing it so others can learn and grow from my mistakes, just as I did. This patient example highlights five different approaches of experts versus coaches: sharing knowledge, listening, asking open-ended questions, finding solutions, and taking responsibility.

Years ago, I was working in the emergency room (ER) as an intern. It was notorious for being a place of controlled chaos one moment, to a peaceful, quiet place the next.

One night, around midnight, it got quiet. On this particular night, I went into our call room. We were all resting, when suddenly the alarm went off, and the ambulance driver called in a patient case. We heard, "Frank D. is coming in, and he can't breathe. He is short of breath. He looks blue. We have got him on oxygen."

All of a sudden, the nurses, the doctors, therapists, everyone there, expressed similar sentiments, "Are you kidding me? Not Frank again. He is a frequent flyer in this place. I am telling you, we almost got shuteye." I was a new intern and not yet jaded, so I was thinking, "The man can't breathe. Did anyone hear that part of the report? He is really suffering. I'm sorry, the man can't breathe. It's our job to help him. We shouldn't be mad at him."

Frank came in and was diagnosed with congestive heart failure (CHF). CHF is often scary for patients because they feel like they are drowning. Frank could not even breathe without the help of an oxygen mask, which is a horrible feeling. I haven't felt it myself, but I have taken care of many patients who had CHF. In essence, they are at risk for having excess water accumulation in their lungs because the heart can't pump it out. This situation results in the sensation of drowning.

In the ER, we took the expert-like approach with Frank, which was appropriate and expected. Immediately, we administered IV Lasix to help his kidneys eliminate the excess fluid from his body. Once we got enough fluid out of his system, he could breathe again. At that point, the attending physician wrote a prescription to increase the dose of his diuretic to help him eliminate fluid on a daily basis. The hope being that he would not be back to see us again next week. When she saw the prescription, one of the nurses said, "We did that before, but we'll increase it now, again."

This word again caught my attention. I felt that we clearly needed a new approach. So, I went into Frank's room with my Netter anatomy textbook to educate him about CHF. I said to myself, "Oh, this is great, because he is stable." Things are again quiet, so I can take this time to fortify Frank with knowledge and power.

I then got my Netter out and showed him the diagram of the kidney. Subsequently, I said, "Frank, you have congestive heart failure. The basic problem is that your heart is not pumping well. If you can't pump your blood through your system well, then it can get backed up in your body, your legs, and your lungs. You might not realize this point, but your kidneys are really important for you to eliminate excess fluid. This is really cool, actually."

I lectured excitedly and enthusiastically. With a huge smile on my face, I explained to him about the renal tubules. I explained how the kidney creates homeostasis in the body, and why salt (NaCl) is an important compound. In fact, I took him all the way through a tour of the loop of Henle to explain ATP pumps and potassium pumps. It was fun for me!

At that point, I asked Frank a question—closed-ended—'Do you eat anything with salt?" With a bewildered look on his face, he responded, "I don't know. What do you mean?" I went back into lecture mode, "Well, soup is the number one culprit for packing in extra salt." His eyes lit up, "Yes. I eat soup."

'Bingo," I thought. I nailed it. Frank eats a ton of soup. That is the problem. So, I shared some more information, "Frank, if you consume a lot of salt, and you have congestive heart failure, you will go into a crisis like this."

Boy, was I ever so proud of myself. I was telling myself, "No one else saw it. I found it with my Netter book and my examples. I solved this. I saved the day and, certainly, the quality of his life. This is great. Furthermore, he is not going to come in again, which is good."

At that point, I then talked to Frank some more, my volume rising with my excitement, "Okay, look, you eat soup now, but from now on—NO SOUP FOR YOU!" With a fearful look, he nodded at me. I don't even know what his body language was saying to me, because I wasn't in tune with his feelings at all. Frankly, I didn't care, because I was so busy with my Netter, my renal tubules, and my own self-congratulations.

What happened next? One week later, I'm was in the ER again, and we get the very same call about Frank, again. We were all ready to go for our rest around midnight, and everyone is mad again, including me. I'm mad because I'm thinking, "He better not have eaten soup. I told him not to have any soup." My mindset is embarrassing, but true. That's the live-and-learn aspect of medical practice. At this point, Frank was wheeled in on a gurney, panting and panicked. We proceeded in a similar manner as before—IV Lasix and oxygen by a mask.

Once he was stabilized, I pounced, "Hi, Frank. How are you doing?" Without waiting for an answer, I asked THE question, "Did you have soup?" Sheepishly, he quietly mutters, "Yes." With fire in my eyes and smoke coming out of my ears, I demanded, "Why did you have soup? The soup has the salt. Remember the renal tubules and the loop of Henle?" Looking confused, "Not really," he admits. "So, you said no soup, but I have about 50 cans of soup at home. So, I thought I would just get rid of them. I would just eat them and be done with them. Then, I wouldn't ever buy more soup. Quite frankly, I could not waste the soup or the money. But, then, when it was gone… no soup, no soup for me."

All of the anger drained from my body, as I thought, "Oh dear. Who would have thought? Who would have thought that would be the solution, to just eat all your soup? I didn't know. Oh no. Okay." Then, I explored other salt-containing foods to try to better understand his home situation, asking, "Do you have crackers? Do you have any other packaged goods? What else do you have to eat at home?" From these open-ended questions, I discovered that Frank had chips, crackers, boxed macaroni and cheese, and lots of other packaged food, all with tons of salt. As such, it wasn't just the soup that was the problem.

So what did I learn from my experience with Frank? I had taken a directive approach with Frank in an attempt to get him to change his eating habits, and it didn't work. I could have taken the Frates COACH Approach, and asked if he even wanted to learn about the loop of Henle and the renal tubules. Furthermore, I could have inquired as to whether or not he wanted to know more about the impact of salt on his health. I could have asked open-ended questions, such as, "Do you know any foods that are full of salt?"

I also could have listened to his answers to these questions, paid attention to his body language, and invited him to take responsibility for the change in his diet by asking him how he could decrease the amount of salt he was consuming.

If I could go back in time, I would have asked, "Would you like to hear about CHF, including what causes it? Do you know about the connection between salt and CHF? Do you want to take a look at my anatomy textbook and see the renal tubules?" Surely, he would have said "no" to looking at Netter. I get that now. Back then, however, I thought it was a great idea.

Other great questions I wish that I had asked included, "What does your cupboard look like? How often do you have soup? What could you do to reduce your intake of salt? Tell me what you want to do." If he responded, "I have a lot of soup, and I'm going to just eat it all this week and then, never eat it again," I could have brainstormed other effective solutions to the salt problem. In situations like this, it is not as simple as advising, "No soup for you!"

THE POINT OF THE LIVE AND LEARNS IN THIS HANDBOOK

The key point of this live and learn example, as well as the other live and learn examples detailed in this chapter, is to demonstrate how the coach-like approach relates to real-life situations. These stories draw attention to the inherent value of this approach. To embrace this approach, practitioners should focus on using the Frates COACH Approach—employing its "being" skills: Curiosity, Openness, Appreciation, Compassion, and Honesty—the key components of being a change agent.

In the coaching world, there is a common analogy that coaching is like dancing with a client, while the expert-like approach of advising and directing is like wrestling a client down. Of note, health and wellness coaches refer to those with whom they work as clients. They are cognizant that the person is paying for their services and that the coach is there to serve them, as a customer. With dancing, two people are aware of the other person, paying attention to body language, negotiating, collaborating, and working together. With wrestling, the people involved are fighting, twisting each other's arms and legs, bending over backwards to win the argument, and trying to overpower the other person to ultimately win a battle.

Lifestyle medicine practitioners do not need to train in health and wellness coaching or become certified coaches, but it might help many of them to be able to counsel effectively, if they hone the "doing" and "being" skills of the coach-like approach.

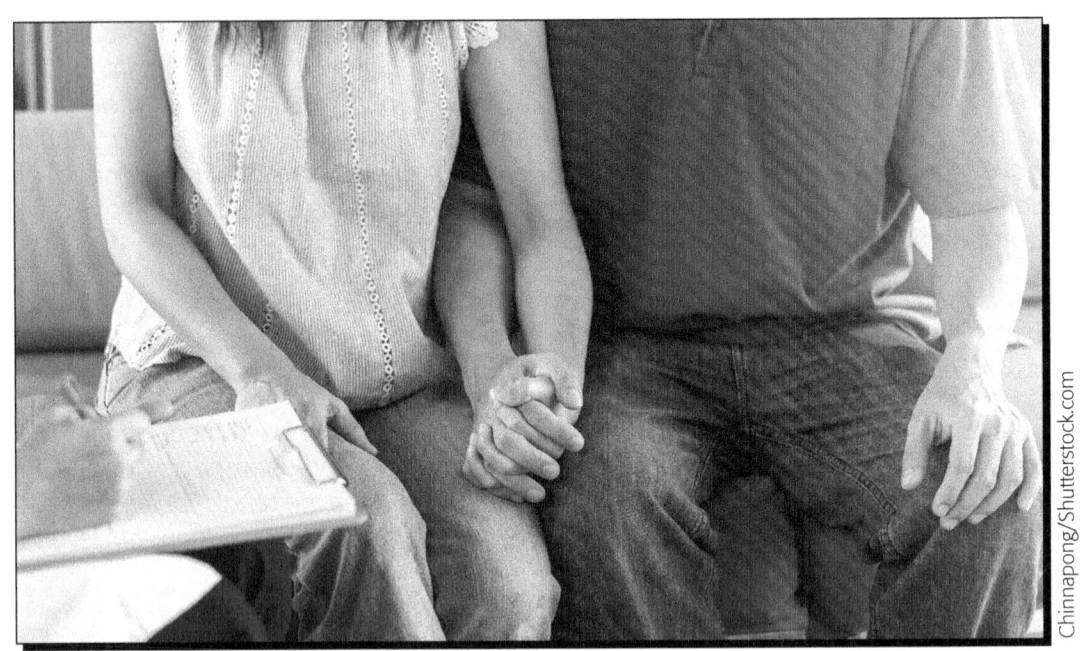

    Practitioners who commit to the coach-like approach are much more likely to dance with their patients. In addition, it's a lot more fun than just being the boss all of the time. Lifestyle medicine practitioners do not need to train in health and wellness coaching or become certified coaches, but it might help many of them to be able to counsel effectively, if they hone the "doing" and "being" skills of the coach-like approach. It will take learning and practicing. Trying to think about lecturing less and listening more; educating the patient on relevant information that they don't already know when they are receptive to it; asking more open ended questions; trying to listen to the body language of the patients; and empowering the patient to take responsibility for change will help lifestyle medicine practitioners to use their time efficiently and effectively, when they're counseling patients on adopting healthy habits. This method might take more time and practice for some practitioners who are entrenched in the expert mode and less time for others who are practicing medicine in a collaborative, non-authoritarian style already. Mindfully expressing the Frates COACH Approach on a daily basis (focusing on curiosity, openness, appreciation, compassion and honesty) will serve all healers well by creating the space for a therapeutic relationship.

EVIDENCE BASE FOR HEALTH AND WELLNESS COACHING

Although health and wellness coaching is relatively new, a significant amount of evidence exists that supports the efficacy of type of coaching. Life coaching and executive coaching have been around for years and the International Coach Federation is the governing body for his group. Health and Wellness Coaching also has a National Certification procedure that have come together recently after years of groundwork. In that regard, randomized controlled trials, the gold standard of medical studies, have been conducted in the area of health and wellness coaching. These studies have investigated the effects of health and wellness coaching on health outcomes. Among the key questions to ask when reviewing these studies are:
- What type of study is it?
- How many patients were in it?
- What interventions were used?
- What coaching techniques were used?
- How were the coaches trained?
- What were the lengths of the coaching sessions?
- What was the frequency of the coaching sessions?

As such, all of this information matters. A more in-depth look at these factors is offered in "Coaching for Behavioral Change in Physiatry," an article that appeared in the *American Journal of Physical Medicine and Rehabilitation*.

In 2008, research into health and wellness coaching was still in its beginning stage. In fact, there were only about 13 randomized controlled trials, one non-randomized trial, four qualitative reports, one case study, one project demonstration, and numerous descriptive articles on the topic. In addition, there were also two articles that specifically examined the use of health and wellness coaching in medical education. In one, medical students used health coaching techniques to counsel patients in a primary care clinic. Examining the results of the randomly controlled trials (RCTs) is particularly important for healthcare practitioners, given the fact that this type of research yields the most unbiased and most useful data.

RESEARCH SPOTLIGHT

In 2003, Vale and colleagues examined the effect of coaching on 792 cardiac patients. The study included a coach-like approach group and a control group. In the coach-like approach group, the cholesterol level of the subjects dropped 21 milligrams versus seven milligrams for individuals in the control group. In another study, Kenneth R. Whittemore, MD, looked at 53 women with diabetes and found qualitative data that supported the premise that coaching resulted in a better diet, and that self-management led to less diabetes related to stress, distress, and a higher satisfaction with care.

In medicine, most practitioners are very interested in numbers. It is equally important, however, to think about the patient's experience and how it is altered with the interventions imposed by physicians. In that regard, health psychologist, Ruth Wolever, PhD, conducted considerable research on health and wellness coaching and published it while she was at Duke University, prior to her move to Vanderbilt. One of her investigative efforts included 56 patients with type 2 diabetes. In this particular study, Wolever and her colleagues found significant reduction in hemoglobin A1c levels (hemoglobin A1c is a marker for average blood glucose levels over a 90-day period) in subjects who were coached, as compared to subjects who received the usual counseling and care.

In another study, Fisher and colleagues looked at the effect of coaching on children with asthma. When the children and their parents were coached about how to manage asthma, there was a decreased re-hospitalization rate, compared to the participants who were in the control group. This decrease in hospitalizations also translated into a significant amount of cost savings.

In yet another investigation, Oliver and colleagues utilized a pre-visit coaching session with 67 cancer pain patients. Amazingly, the single, 30-minute coaching intervention decreased their level of pain severity compared to members of the control group. This single coaching intervention included questions, such as, "What is going on with your pain? Do you know how to manage your pain? What are you using to manage your pain? What are you going to speak to the physician about? And what does pain mean to you?" Their decrease in pain severity, which was noted during a follow up visit, was achieved by simply coaching and listening for 30 minutes.

The aforementioned studies represent some of the initial research into coaching and its potential application. There are also a number of issues attendant to this research. For example, they involve a relatively small number of subjects, which makes them not all generalizable to all populations. In addition, there is a lack of consistency with the coaching specifics, such as who performed the coaching, the techniques used, the number and duration of coaching sessions, the duration of the study, and the length of the follow-up.

In the area of coaching, large studies are needed—studies that involve thousands of patients. Longer follow-ups, for example, ideally out to 10 years, would also be helpful. Research is ongoing in the field and with time, more powerful studies will be reported in the literature. At the present time, however, a limited amount of documented evidence shows that there are improved outcomes after coaching, among patients with cardiovascular disease, diabetes, cancer pain, and asthma. It should also be noted that there are several common threads in these studies, such as a one-to-one relationship, the use of collaboration and negotiation, goal-setting, accountability, and an educational component.

In a large, systematic review conducted by Ruth Wolever, PhD, and her colleagues in 2013, the group of researchers examined more than 1,000 abstracts and full-text articles on health and wellness coaching. Research from the full-text articles revealed the following:

- Fully or partially patient-centered care was a common feature in 86 percent of these studies.
- The patient determined the goals 71 percent of the time.
- Self-discovery and the active learning process were present in 63 percent of the settings.
- Accountability for behavior (i.e., someone was checking in on them) occurred in 86 percent of the studies.
- Some kind of education was provided in 91 percent of these coach interventions.
- A relationship with a trained coach (e.g., a one-on-one relationship) existed in 78 percent of the patients.

Advances in the area of health and wellness coaching continue to be made. A large review of 150 studies in health and wellness coaching was compiled and published in the *American Journal of Lifestyle Medicine* in 2017 (http://journals.sagepub.com/doi/full/10.1177/1559827617708562). This compendium evaluated randomized studies, as well as longitudinal and qualitative research in the areas of heart disease, hypertension, high cholesterol, cancer, diabetes, obesity, and wellness. The compendium authors concluded that health and wellness coaching was worthy of consideration for patients with heart disease, cancer and diabetes, which confirms prior studies. They also found that there was evidence that patients with hypertension, obesity, and high cholesterol could possibly benefit from health and wellness coaching.

Since there were no nationally recognized standard guidelines for coach training programs or for health and wellness practice for many years, the research is confounded by a variety of coaches having been trained a variety of ways and using a variety of different techniques. In reality, there are several coaching training organizations with excellent programs and coaching companies, such as Mentor Coach, Bark Coaching Institute, Real Balance Coaching, Wellcoaches, Wellness Inventory, and Functional Medicine Coaching Academy, among others. In addition, there are several academic institutions that are involved with health and wellness coach training, including Duke University, Vanderbilt University, and University of Minnesota, which has a Masters Degree in the area. Recently, the International Consortium for Health and Wellness Coaching created a national exam and a national certification process is in place, which is designed to help to standardize the training and the practice of health and wellness coaching moving forward.

COACHING FOR BEHAVIOR CHANGE

Research in the United States on behavior change has focused on five As: *assess, advise, agree, assist,* and *arrange*. The all-important step of agreeing is included in the five As. The patient needs to agree with the treatment plan and the plan for behavior change if the plan has any chance of working and being implemented.

❏ Assess

Lifestyle medicine practitioners need to assess the patient on multiple levels. Knowing what is going on inside the body by checking blood tests is often helpful. Lab tests, including fasting cholesterol, LDL cholesterol, HDL cholesterol, C-Reactive Protein, iron, hemoglobin A1c (for glucose control), fasting glucose, thyroid function tests, Vitamin D levels, Vitamin B12 levels, and other blood chemistries, can help the practitioners assess the patient.

Assessing the patient's readiness to change is another important factor, one that is discussed in the section of this chapter on the Transtheoretical Model of Change (TTM). Inquiring about the patient's understanding of their disease process or risk for disease can help the practitioner learn about the patient's level of knowledge. In turn, it can also help inform the practitioner about what education might be useful to the patient. For example, what are the patient's motivators for change, both intrinsic (internal like wanting to feel more energetic) and extrinsic (wanting to lose weight to fit into a bathing suit)? Other valuable questions include, "Where are you now in terms of your lifestyle? Or, "What information are you seeking today?"

The answers to such questions can help the practitioner to better understand the patient. How confident is the patient in change? How important is the change to the patient? What obstacles are in the way? What are the patient's strengths? Where does the patient see themselves in 10 years? What is the difference between where they are now and where they want to be? Assessing the patient by asking these questions will help the practitioner better serve the patient and co-create a plan that has meaning for that patient.

❏ Advise

Lifestyle medicine practitioners will need to give their opinions and advise the patient on the best way forward. For example, after noting that a patient is obese by BMI, the practitioner will need to share that information in a non-judgmental and open minded way with language such as "According to your BMI, you fall into the obese category. What do you think about that?" If the patient says "It's no big deal. I have always been like this, and my family is like this," then the practitioner can advise the patient with, "There has been a lot of research on the role of obesity on developing different disease, and reaching a healthy BMI is important for your body." A follow-up question, such as "What do you think you can do to reach a healthy BMI?" will help keep the consultation a conversation rather than a lecture. If a patient is smoking, a lifestyle medicine practitioner will need to advise that patient, "One of the best things you could do for your health is to quit smoking." Following up with a question such as "How are you feeling about your smoking?" will engage the patient to transition the advice into conversation. The goal of advice-giving is to lay out the medical facts and to open the door for a conversation about them.

☐ Agree

This A is probably the most important A in the five As. The patient needs to agree with a plan for change. After the assessment, advice, and discussion, the practitioner and patient work to co-create a plan for moving forward. This is a co-creation because the patient needs buy in and needs to feel some responsibility for taking action steps to make a change. By using the coach-like approach, the lifestyle medicine practitioner will be collaborative, when dealing with the patient. This step will occur naturally.

☐ Assist

The lifestyle medicine practitioner assists the patient in order to help make the co-created plan a reality. The assistance can come in the form of setting a SMART goal, helping to make sure that the goal is specific, measurable, action oriented, realistic, and time-sensitive. The practitioner could also help the patient to find resources that might be helpful to them, for example, local YMCAs, community classes, Farmer's Markets, or online stress management classes that might be of value.

☐ Arrange

The lifestyle medicine practitioner needs to arrange for a follow-up with the patient. If plans are co-created, and there is no follow-up, then, the patient could forget about the plan and, thus, no progress will be made. By arranging follow up, the practitioner is signaling to the patient that they will be held accountable for the plan, and there will be a check-in. It also tells the patient that someone cares. Someone will be asking about the plan, the goals, and the progress. This approach is a way of making the patient feel important and valued.

THE TRANSTHEORETICAL MODEL OF CHANGE (TTM)

Renowned University of Rhode Island psychologist Dr. James Prochaska has been studying behavior change since the 1980s. His father, who was an alcoholic, died of complications of the disease. After that, Dr. Prochaska was determined to understand alcoholism and addiction so that he could help others avoid the suffering that his father and family experienced. Dr. Prochaska, working hard to try to solve the mystery of addiction, made tremendous progress in this area.

After studying addiction for more than three decades, Prochaska and his colleagues created the stages of change model known as the Transtheoretical Model of Change (TTM). This model has enabled healthcare providers to be more effective in their behavior-change counseling of patients who suffer with addiction, as well as those individuals seeking to change their unhealthy behaviors. The model allows practitioners to identify a patient's current stage of change and then target the consultation and counseling to that person with stage-appropriate processes. As a result, the practitioner is able to meet the patient where they are during the consultation. Rather than talk at them, they can talk with them.

❑ Stages of Change

There are six stages of change: *pre-contemplation, contemplation, preparation, action, maintenance,* and *termination*, which are discussed at length in Prochaska's book, *Changing for Good*. The authors have suggested specific interventions that have been found to be effective for the various stages. While the interventions or processes can be employed at many different stages, ideally, practitioners should try experiential and cognitive processes with those individuals who are in the early stages of change (pre-contemplators and contemplators) and behavior processes for those patients in later stages (preparation, action, maintenance, and termination).

STAGES OF CHANGE

PROCESSES	Pre-Contemplation	Contemplation	Preparation	Action	Maintenance
	Consciousness raising →				
	Environmental re-evaluation →				
	Dramatic relief →				
	Social liberation →				
		Self-reevaluation →			
			Self-liberation →		
			Helping relationships →		
			Counterconditioning →		
				Reinforcement management →	
				Stimulus control →	

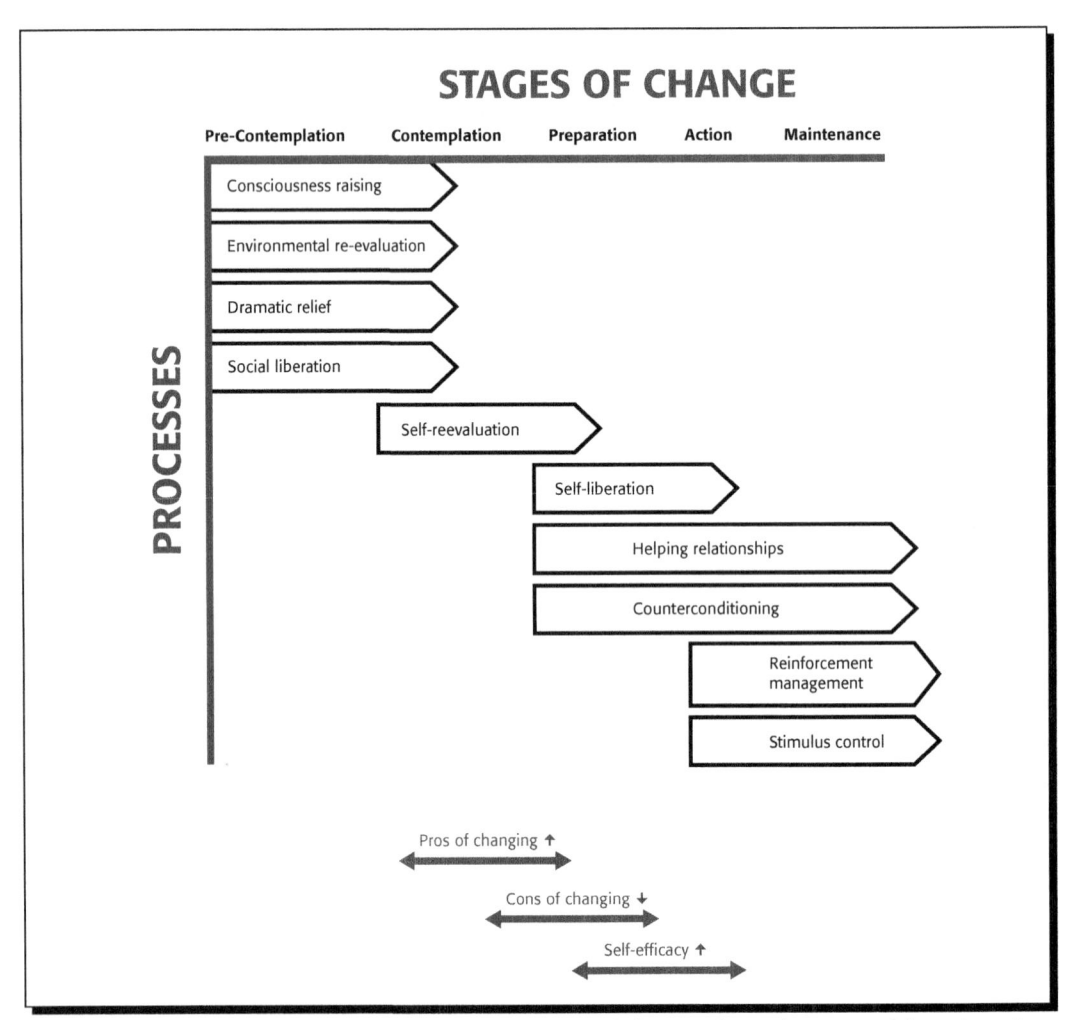

Pros of changing ↑
Cons of changing ↓
Self-efficacy ↑

Figure 2-5. Processes emphasized in different stages of change (based on an article written by James Prochaska and Wayne Velicer)

USING TTM INTERVENTIONS

❏ The Transtheoretical Model of Change—Pre-Contemplation Stage

Pre-contemplators are those individuals who are resistant to change. As such, they are not intending to take any action in the foreseeable future. They may be either uninformed or under-informed about the specific behavior. The interventions and processes suggested for patients in this stage are experiential and cognitive. For example, a pre-contemplator might make statements, such as "I'm not going to do it." "I can't exercise. I have absolutely no time. I mean, you don't understand my schedule. It's crazy. I couldn't possibly exercise." Or, "I refuse to quit smoking."

How does a practitioner work with someone who is in the pre-contemplation stage? In medical school in the '90s, students were taught to manage smokers with a standard response. So, when someone says, "I'm not going to quit smoking. I smoke. I'm not going to talk about it," the physician would respond with something like, "Smoking is really dangerous for your health. You need to quit. You have to set a quit date. When's it going to be?"

According to this practice, the physician should then direct the patient into quitting and get them to sign a quit-date declaration right on the spot. Today, the situation is different, and there are many techniques, skills, and strategies that are well-accepted methods of managing and helping patients who are smoking and refusing to quit (i.e., pre-contemplators). An example of one such tool is motivational interviewing, which is discussed in Chapter 3.

For individuals who are pre-contemplative, practitioners can use *consciousness-raising* efforts. For example, they could be asked, "Are you familiar with the risks of smoking? Specifically, did you know it was connected to erectile dysfunction?" Patients might say "yes," they might say "no." The key is to make the information personally relatable and relevant. If the patient responds with, "Well no, what do you mean?", for instance, the practitioner can share knowledge about that particular topic. As a rule, after agreeing or granting permission to the practitioner to explain the facts further, the patient will likely be more receptive to education and counseling.

The next step may be to suggest how the issue may impact others—*environmental reevaluation*. For example, practitioners might inquire if patients notice the effect of smoking on others—children, colleagues, elderly parents—living with them and if they have considered the issue of secondhand smoke. Another example might involve a pre-contemplator who is unwilling to change their eating habits. For example, if the patient is a mom who eats a lot of junk food and keeps it in the kitchen cabinets at home, the practitioner might ask, "What effect does your eating have on your immediate family?" In turn, if the patient is a doctor who eats lots of sweets and brings leftover cookies and treats to the office for both the patients and the staff, the question could be asked, "What is the health effect of this behavior on those individuals in the office?"

Another TTM technique is *dramatic relief*, which involves paying attention to feelings. This stage involves inviting the pre-contemplator to feel something emotionally about the unhealthy actions they are taking. For example, sharing stories of patients who actually quit smoking and what happened when they quit. Explaining how the lives of those patients changed is one way to help a patient visualize a role model and feel the rewards of quitting—before actually quitting. An opposite approach to this technique would be to describe the ill effects of continuing to smoke, perhaps by showing photos of cancer survivors or sharing a comparative model of the lungs of smokers versus the lungs of nonsmokers. The underlying premise of this method is to evoke emotion—e.g., fear, sadness, excitement, surprise, disgust, or anger—and invite the patient to pay close attention to these feelings. Having patients identify their feelings, explain why they feel that way, and what they could do to feel differently is a useful strategy with pre-contemplators.

It is also helpful when counseling pre-contemplators to acknowledge social trends. This step elicits the *social liberation process* in the TTM. This process brings in the outside forces that influence the patient in their strategy for pre-contemplators.

No person is completely free of influence. There are immediate family members, work environments and colleagues, extended family and friends, neighborhood rituals, city laws, state laws, and national guidelines that influence individuals. For example, if a person works at a college campus that is smoke-free, then that individual needs to make accommodations to explore alternate, often inconvenient, areas in which to smoke during the workday. Constant reminders that smoking is bad for a person's health are all around the employee, such as "SMOKE-FREE ZONE" signs, which may influence that person's behavior. These are examples of social liberation.

Social trends are well-known to affect the individuals living in certain environments and cultures. For example, states where marijuana is legal to use have different social norms than do states in which marijuana is illegal. As such, individuals who live in the former states will feel different pressures than those individuals who live in the latter states. It should be noted that the practitioners can try to make connections between the unhealthy behaviors of their patients and the negative outcomes that are likely to occur. Alternately, it can be highly effective if the practitioner encourages the patients to make the connections themselves.

❑ The Transtheoretical Model of Change—Contemplation

The next TTM stage is the contemplation stage. Patients in this stage may be thinking, "Hmm, I've been thinking about changing, but I just don't know. I don't think I can do it. I'm not sure. I mean I want to do it, but then again I don't want to do it."

This stage is marked by ambivalence. This is another stage in which *motivational interviewing* is an appropriate tool to use. People can also be in a state of what is called *chronic contemplation*. For example, they may proclaim (for years, sometimes), "I know I should exercise regularly. I know it's really good for me. I just can't get started."

The key feature of contemplation is that the patients are actually thinking about their situation. Whereas, in pre-contemplation, patients are saying, "No way!" contemplators are saying, "I'm thinking about making a change." For contemplators, the pros of change often equal the cons of change, or the pros may be less than the cons the way they are viewing it. That is what may make it difficult for them to decide to change.

Similar to the pre-contemplative stage, the processes suggested for contemplators are experiential and cognitive. They may include the same techniques used with pre-contemplators, such as consciousness raising, environmental reevaluation, dramatic relief, and social liberation (social trends). In addition, the cognitive process of *self-reevaluation* is a suggested strategy to use with contemplators. Self-reevaluation helps patients create a new self-image. For example, the practitioner might ask, "Imagine you were free from smoking. How would you feel about yourself? How would you feel each day? How would that change the way you feel in the morning? How would it change your life?"

Asking such questions, with an intention of connecting the answers to the core values of the patients, can be incredibly motivating. It allows the patient to see how a new self-image or a reevaluation of themselves, without the unhealthy behaviors, will enable them to be their authentic selves. For example, if they are contemplating change, a practitioner can say, "Well, I know that your family is really, really important to you. Tell me about how changing this behavior would affect your feelings about how you care for your family."

On occasion, contemplators just need a cognitive "kaizen" step. Kaizen is a Japanese business management concept that has been adopted into psychological counseling and coaching. It is actually "a way of life philosophy that assumes that every aspect of our life deserves to be constantly improved. One of the most notable features of kaizen is that big results come from many small changes accumulated over time."

Imagine the following scenario: the patient has a treadmill in their basement, which has become a clothing rack for clothes that are now too small. The patient is contemplating starting to exercise. Consider what would happen if the practitioner says, "Just do it. Just get off your butt and exercise. Get those clothes off the treadmill. Start jogging on it five days a week and aim for 30 minutes to reach the suggested exercise guidelines."

Chances are that this approach is not going to work, because it does not involve internal motivation. A different approach to the contemplator might be to invite them to take a cognitive kaizen step or baby-step for self-improvement. For example, the practitioner might ask, "What needs to be in place for you to start using the treadmill?" The patient might answer, "Well, first all that stuff needs to be put away and that is overwhelming." The practitioner might then say, "What would you think about going down to the basement with your coffee one morning and simply looking at the treadmill? And then, after a minute or two, perhaps you might consider taking one article of clothing off of it?"

With this approach, the patient does not feel intimidated or afraid. It is a small step and finding success with this step is relatively easy. From there, success breeds success. There is a good chance that if the individual goes down to look at the treadmill and considers taking one piece of clothing off of it, they will either clear it all off or decide that the treadmill is not an option. Either way, they have completed the small step of looking at the treadmill.

❏ The Transtheoretical Model of Change—Preparation

The next stage in the TTM is preparation. Patients in this stage say, "I want to do this. I'm going to do this. I am planning to do this soon." It is almost like they are saying, "I just need a good plan. I just need confidence." As such, the people in the preparation stage of change are intending to take action within the next month.

For these people, Prochaska and his colleagues recommend moving into the behavioral steps. *Self-liberation*, a recommended process for this stage, involves making a commitment to change. If a patient tells a friend, "I'm going to start ... exercising this week," that friend is likely going to ask about it the following week. By committing to change verbally or writing it down, patients make the behavior or goal real for themselves, as well as for other individuals hearing or reading the commitment. This is liberating because the desire and intention is no longer bottled up inside the patient. Rather, it is expressed and freed from the confinements of the patient's mind. A statement of self-liberation sounds like, "I'm going to start on this walking program at the YMCA on Tuesday at 10 a.m." The statement is specific concerning when, where, and how the behavior is going to be accomplished.

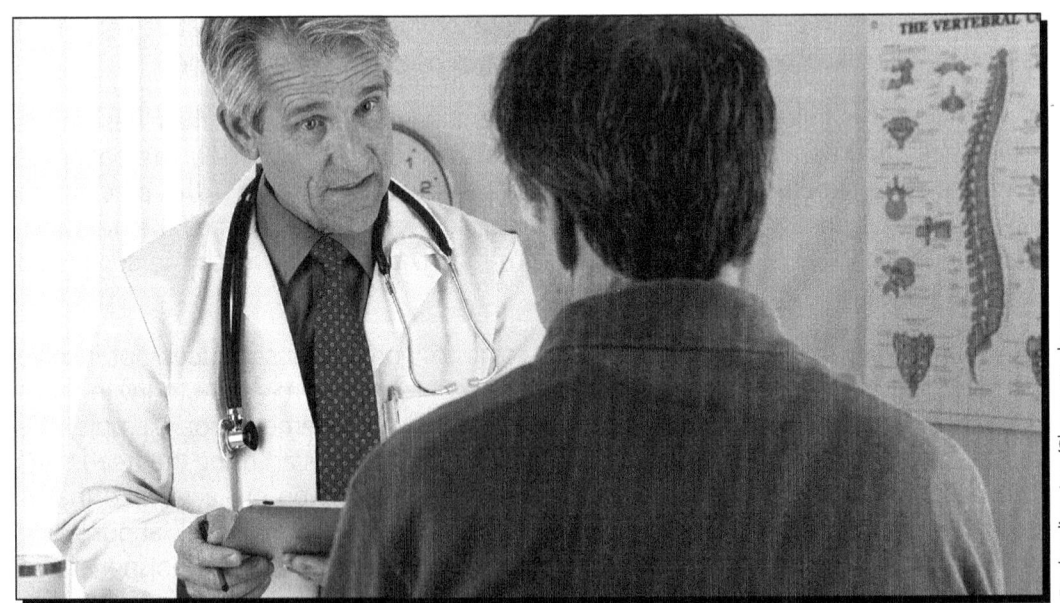

Asking questions, with an intention of connecting the answers to the core values of the patients, can be incredibly motivating.

In the preparation stage, *helping relationships* are useful. Since the patient is ready and willing to change, identifying supportive people and relationships can be the difference between remaining in the preparation stage and moving into the action stage. For example, if the patient has friends who also want to change their eating patterns and adopt a whole-food, plant-based diet, then connecting with those friends and creating a plan together will increase the chances of success. Not only will the patient have partners who are just as interested in the process as the patient, they will also have built-in accountability. The partners can talk about recipes together, grocery shop with each other, and, perhaps, share meals together.

Counter-conditioning (or substitutions) represents a third important process for people in the preparation stage. If patients are used to going to a fast-food restaurant after work each night, and they want to adopt a whole-food, plant-based diet, there are several options for counter-conditioning available in such a scenario. One might be able to substitute the burger for a salad at the fast-food chain. Another option might be to consider a fast food chain that has a vegetable burrito bowl or a healthier version of fast food as a substitution to start. There are chains that cater to people with allergies and food sensitivities, as well as to vegetarians and vegans. These chains offer several whole food, plant-based options.

Being realistic about the substitutions is important. How likely is the patient to order a salad instead of a burger at their favorite fast food chain. The smell of the burger and fries may be too hard to resist, and going to the same location might just bring the patient into the old habit. So, mapping out a different way home, one that avoids that fast-food chain and leads the patient to a farmer's market or other healthy option would be helpful. The farmer's market may have premade healthy options that are whole foods and plant-based, which might be a good substitute to begin the change process. Another alternative might be to buy veggie burgers or bean burgers at the grocery store, instead of ordering hamburgers at a fast-food chain. In addition, buying sweet potato fries from the grocery store, in place of buying the french fries sold at the fast-food chain, would certainly be a healthier option. In all of these possibilities, the key point is that the preparation stage is a process that will take time to navigate through and will require many small steps.

❏ The Transtheoretical Model of Change—Action

Patients in the action stage of change have actually been engaging in the healthy behavior for several weeks. However, just because these patients are undertaking the intended action does not mean the practitioner should ignore them. Importantly, these patients need specific counseling, as well, in order to encourage them to continue on to the maintenance phase of the TTM, because patients in the action stage can relapse and go right back into chronic contemplation. TTM is not a stepwise model for change, but rather, more similar to a spiral model (Figure 2-6).

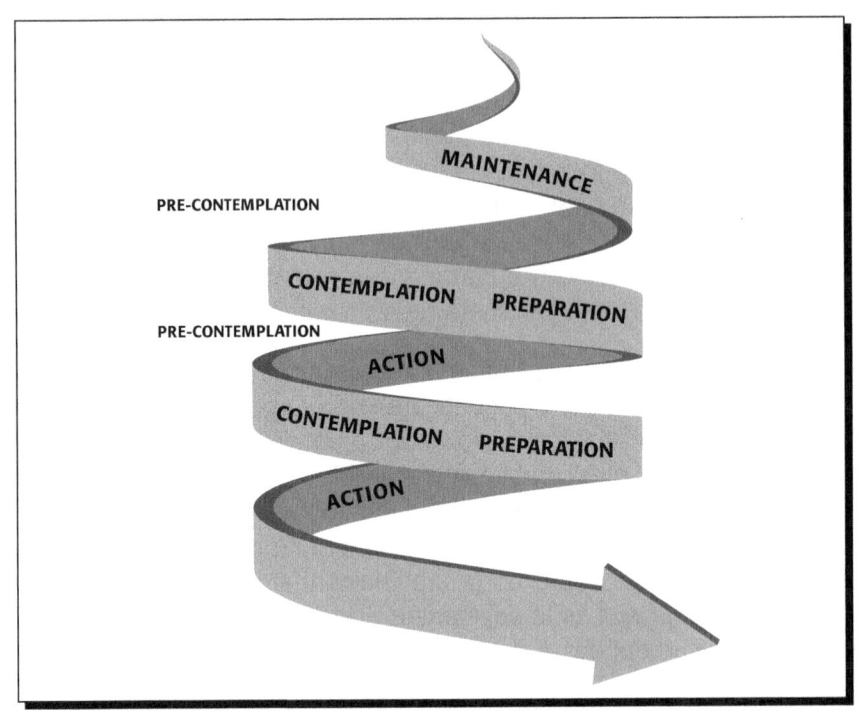

Figure 2-6. James Prochaska's depiction of the spiral model of the TMC

In the action stage, the practitioner can use the techniques of helping relationships and counter-conditioning, when counseling the patient to encourage them to continue on with the healthy behavior, in the same way these processes were used in the preparation stage. Additional processes that are recommended for those individuals in the action stage include *reinforcement management* and *stimulus control*.

Reinforcement management involves using rewards to reinforce the positive behavior. A practitioner can invite the patients to acknowledge the benefits of the newly adopted healthy behavior by asking, "Now that you have been exercising for a couple of weeks, what have you noticed that is different?" Allowing the patients to express the changes that they notice in themselves gives them the opportunity to reflect on these changes and to appreciate them. Patients can then realize, "Wow I'm doing this. And I feel more energized, more focused at work, and I am sleeping better too."

If the duration has been sufficiently (approximately a month or more), the practitioner can also point out any physical or lab changes, such as changes in body weight, waist circumference, blood pressure, or cholesterol levels. By acknowledging the health benefits, the patient receives an added incentive to continue the healthy behavior.

Stimulus control is another important process in the action stage. Using the social ecological model of change, the practitioner can help the patient recognize the events, the people, the places, and the objects that encourage the newly adopted behavior. Conversely, the practitioner can help the patient understand and appreciate the factors that tempt them to return to old unhealthy behaviors. Appreciating these various stimuli is critical to this stage of change.

To control the stimulus, patients must first recognize the triggers or cues that encourage the healthy habit, as well as those factors that encourage the unhealthy habit. After identifying the stimulus of the undesired behavior, patients can create a plan to increase exposure to people, places, and events that encourage the new target behavior. Patients can also avoid or rid themselves from the cues, triggers, and experiences that sabotage the efforts to change. For example, a patient who quit smoking might get rid of all ashtrays and rearrange the living room so that their favorite smoking chair is in a different place or even a different room. Altering the routine and taking away the 'comfort zone" for the unhealthy behavior will help to keep it at bay.

❑ The Transtheoretical Model of Change—Maintenance

In the maintenance stage of TTM, patients have been in action for at least six months. On occasion, practitioners may be tempted to ignore these patients and assume that they do not need further assistance. The image of the spiral stairway, however, is a constant reminder to practitioners that the process of change includes slips, lapses, and relapses. It is therefore recommended that practitioners ask patients in the maintenance stage about the desired healthy habit. For someone who is a jogger, for example, the conversation might involve the following: "How is the jogging going? Remind me what you are going to do in the winter, when the snow starts to fall."

In this example, the practitioner is looking ahead at the potential barriers and obstacles confronting the patient, as well as helping the patient to strategize solutions that address those challenges. Asking the patient to share their motivation for continuing to jog will remind both the patient and the practitioner of the importance of this activity to the patient. For example, the practitioner might say, "What is motivating you to keep on going? Wow, you've been doing this for a long time. Congratulations! I'd love to hear more about how you do this." The patient may then respond that their motivator is stress relief right now. Motivators change, however, and tapping into the patient's current motivators can be illuminating.

Reviewing the benefits of the new behavior, such as jogging, as well as the physical and lab changes that occur as a result of engaging in the action stage, can also be used in maintenance. Furthermore, stimulus control can be useful in this stage as well.

❑ The Transtheoretical Model of Change—Termination

Termination is the sixth step. In the termination stage, patients have no temptation to return to the old unhealthy habit. According to Prochaska and his colleagues, "The termination stage is the ultimate goal for all changers … your behavior will never return …" Over the years, the thoughts and ideas about this stage have evolved. Not everyone discusses or works with this stage. Many individuals feel that smokers are in the maintenance stage forever, as are people who start exercising. In reality, it seems that most behavior change requires some sort of maintenance. More often than not, it is something that the patients are going to continue striving to do for the rest of their lives.

BASIC TTM AXIOMS

- You cannot get people to change unless they truly want to change.
- You cannot force people to listen to you, if they do not want to listen.
- If you get resistance from a patient, you should let them know you are here for them when they are ready.
- The best first step is to listen to your patient. Not only will you build rapport, but you will be better able to understand where they actually are in the process of change.
- You are a facilitator to the patients' own discoveries. While suggestions, knowledge, and prompts may be very helpful to expand the conversation, patients are the experts in themselves and will be able to tell you what their goals are and what they will be capable of doing.
- Though patients may turn to you for motivation, true motivation comes from their desire to make the change for themselves. While you can provide accountability, expertise, and observations (both concerning the positive effects of the change and the negative barriers they may be experiencing), the underlying goal is to help them find their intrinsic motivators.

KEY POINTS/TAKEAWAYS FOR CHAPTER 2

❑ Chapter Review:

- Overall goal: Review the factors that affect the ability of a person to change.
- Application goal: Understand the differences between the expert-like approach and the coach-like approach when dealing with patients who need to change their behavior.

❑ Discussion Questions:

- What are the necessary ingredients for the behavior change process?
- What are the necessary ingredients or "being skills" to be a coach or change agent?
- How does an individual create lasting behavior change?
- How can a healthcare provider hinder the behavior change process?
- What evidence exists that the coach-like approach leads to better health outcomes?

	TITLE	AUTHORS	JOURNAL	YEAR	KEY FINDINGS
1	Personal exercise habits and counseling practices of primary care physicians: a national survey	Abramson S, et al.	*Clinical Journal of Sports Medicine*	2000	The authors demonstrated that physicians who exercise were more likely to counsel their patients to exercise. Physicians that do aerobic training counsel on aerobic training, and those that do strength training counsel on strength training. The main barriers that physicians faced preventing them from counseling on exercise were: inadequate time, lack of knowledge/experience with exercise counseling.
2	Physician disclosure of healthy personal behaviors improves credibility and ability to motivate	Frank E, Breyan J, Elon L	*Archives of Family Medicine*	2000	This study compared the effect that two different educational videos had on physicians' abilities to motivate patients to adopt healthy habits. It found that subjects viewed the video in which the physician discussed their own personal health habits with subtle supporting cues (i.e., apple on the desk, bike helmet in view) to be more believable and motivating regarding exercise and diet.
3	A randomized controlled evaluation of the effect of community health workers on hospitalization for asthma: the asthma coach	Fisher EB, et al.	*Archives of Pediatrics & Adolescent Medicine*	2009	A population-based study of 191 African-American children who were hospitalized for asthma. The intervention tested to see if community health workers could reach low-income parents and reinforce basic asthma education and key management behaviors through home visits and phone calls. They found a significant decrease in children rehospitalized for asthma where both the parents and children received coaching. They found a significant decrease in rehospitalization rate for the intervention subjects (35.6%) as compared to controls (59.1%).
4	Coaching for behavior change in physiatry	Frates EP, et al.	*American Journal of Physical Medicine & Rehabilitation*	2011	Discusses the coach approach and how it differs from the expert approach. Focuses on importance of collaborating with patients by being empathetic, aligning motivation, building confidence, setting SMART goals, and setting accountability. It also reviews many of the randomized controlled trials of health and wellness coaching. It found preliminary evidence to suggest that health and wellness coaching is an important useful adjunct to usual care for managing hyperlipidemia, diabetes, cancer pain, cancer survival, asthma, weight loss, and increasing physical activity.
5	Physical activity recommendation for hypertension management: does healthcare provider advice make a difference?	Halm J, Amoako E	*Ethnicity & Disease*	2008	Revealed that only one-third of hypertensive patients received counseling to engage in physical activity to manage their hypertension. However, of those that were counseled, 71% who followed the recommendations to exercise were able to reduce their blood pressure by 3.1 mm Hg on average.

Figure 2-7. How to evoke behavior change for yourself and those you care for personally and professionally evidence

	TITLE	AUTHORS	JOURNAL	YEAR	KEY FINDINGS
6	Advising people to take more exercise is ineffective: a randomized controlled trial of physical activity promotion in primary care	Hollisdon M, et al.	International Journal of Epidemiology	2002	Demonstrated that brief negotiation, as compared to direct advice and control, was significantly better at increasing the minutes of physical activity per week.
7	Running as a key lifestyle medicine for longevity	Lee DC, et al.	Progress in Cardiovascular Disease	2017	"This review details the findings surrounding the impact of running on various health outcomes and premature mortality, highlights plausible underlying mechanisms linking running with chronic disease prevention and longevity, identifies the estimated additional life expectancy among runners and other active individuals, and discusses whether there is adequate evidence to suggest that longevity benefits are attenuated with higher doses of running."
8	Individualized patient education and coaching to improve pain control among cancer outpatients	Oliver JW, et al.	Journal of Clinical Oncology	2001	A small study of 67 patients with cancer pain that demonstrated that a brief education and coaching intervention was associated with improved average pain levels.
9	The transtheoretical model of health behavior change	Prochaska JO, Velicer WF	American Journal of Health Promotion	1997	A discussion of the transtheoretical model of health behavior change, including the 10 processes of change that had been identified for producing progress, decisional balance, self-efficacy, and temptations. It suggested that for at-risk populations, roughly 40% of people are in the pre-contemplation, 40% are in the contemplation, and 20% are in the preparation stage of change.
10	Compendium of the health and wellness coaching literature	Sforzo GA, et al.	American Journal of Lifestyle Medicine	2017	A comprehensive systematic review on health and wellness coaching for lifestyle behavior change. They concluded that the literature "generally reveals health and wellness coaching as a promising intervention for chronic diseases though further research is needed in most categories."
11	Coaching patients on achieving cardiovascular health (COACH): a multicenter randomized trial in patients with coronary heart disease	Vale MJ, et al.	Archives of Internal Medicine	2003	This study examined the effect of the COACH Program on the cholesterol levels of 792 patients with cardiac disease. The results found a cholesterol drop of 21 mg/dL in the coaching group vs. 7 mg/dL in the usual care group.

Figure 2-7. How to evoke behavior change for yourself and those you care for personally and professionally evidence (cont.)

	TITLE	AUTHORS	JOURNAL	YEAR	KEY FINDINGS
12	A nurse coaching intervention for women with type 2 diabetes	Whittemore R, et al.	Diabetes Educator	2004	In a six-month study of 53 women with diabetes, this study found that coaching, as compared to usual care, resulted in better diet self-management, less diabetes-related distress, and higher satisfaction with care.
13	Integrative health coaching for patients with type 2 diabetes: a randomized clinical trial	Wolever RQ, et al.	Diabetes Educator	2010	"Fifty-six patients with type 2 diabetes were randomized to either 6 months of integrative health coaching or usual care (control group)." The researchers found a significant reduction in hemoglobin A1c among subjects with baseline ≥7.
14	A systematic review of the literature on health and wellness coaching: defining a key behavioral intervention in healthcare	Wolever RQ, et al.	Global Advances in Health and Medicine	2013	A systematic review of health and wellness coaching in the literature that sought to identify the common features of coaching in the health literature. They found that most approaches were fully or partially patient-centered (86%), have patient-determined goals (71%), involve self-discovery and active learning processes (63%), create accountability for behaviors (86%), provide some type of education (91%), and entail a relationship with a trained coach (78%).

References

1. Abramson S, Stein J, Schaufele M, et al. Personal exercise habits and counseling practices of primary care physicians: a national survey. *Clinical Journal of Sports Medicine.* 2000;10(1):40-48.
2. Frank E, Breyan J, Elon L. Physician disclosure of healthy personal behaviors improves credibility and ability to motivate. *Archives of Family Medicine.* 2000;9:287-290.
3. Fisher EB, Strunk RC, Highstein GR, et al. A randomized controlled evaluation of the effect of community health workers on hospitalization for asthma: the asthma coach. *Archives of Pediatrics & Adolescent Medicine.* 2009;163(3):225-232. doi:10.1001/archpediatrics.2008.577
4. Frates EP, Moore MA, Lopez CN, et al. Coaching for behavior change in physiatry. *American Journal of Physical Medicine & Rehabilitation.* December 2011;90(12):1074-1082. Available at: http://www.wellcoaches.com/images/pdf/Coaching-Am-Journal-Physical-Medicine-Dec-2011.pdf. Accessed September 2017.
5. Halm J, Amoako E. Physical activity recommendation for hypertension management: does healthcare provider advice make a difference? *Ethnicity & Disease.* 2008;18(3):178-182.
6. Hollisdon M, Thorogood M, White I, et al. Advising people to take more exercise is ineffective: a randomized controlled trial of physical activity promotion in primary care. *International Journal of Epidemiology.* 2002;31:808-815.
7. Lee DC, Brellenthin AG, Thompson PD, et al. Running as a key lifestyle medicine for longevity. *Progress in Cardiovascular Disease.* 2017;60(1):45-55. doi:10.1016/j.pcad.2017.03.005.
8. Oliver JW, Kravitz RL, Kaplan SH, et al. Individualized patient education and coaching to improve pain control among cancer outpatients. *Journal of Clinical Oncology.* 2001;19(8):2206-2212.
9. Prochaska JO, Velicer WF. The transtheoretical model of health behavior change. *American Journal of Health Promotion.* September 1997;12(1):38-48.
10. Sforzo GA, Kaye MP, Todorova I, et al. Compendium of the health and wellness coaching literature. *American Journal of Lifestyle Medicine.* 2017. doi:10.1177/1559827617708562.
11. Vale MJ, Jelinek MV, Best JD, et al. Coaching patients on achieving cardiovascular health (COACH): a multicenter randomized trial in patients with coronary heart disease. *Archives of Internal Medicine.* 2003;163(22):2775-2783.
12. Whittemore R, Melkus GD, Sullivan A, et al. A nurse coaching intervention for women with type 2 diabetes. *Diabetes Educator.* September-October 2004;30(5):795-804.
13. Wolever RQ, Dreusicke M, Fikkan J, et al. Integrative health coaching for patients with type 2 diabetes: a randomized clinical trial. *Diabetes Educator.* July-August 2010;36(4):629-639.
14. Wolever RQ, Simmons LA, Sforzo GA, et al. A systematic review of the literature on health and wellness coaching: defining a key behavioral intervention in healthcare. *Global Advances in Health and Medicine.* July 2013;2(4):38-57.

Figure 2-7. How to evoke behavior change for yourself and those you care for personally and professionally evidence (cont.)

REFERENCES

- American College of Lifestyle Medicine. What Is Lifestyle Medicine. Available at: http://lifestylemedicine.org/What-is-Lifestyle-Medicine. Accessed September 2016.
- Centers for Disease Control and Prevention (CDC). Health Effects of Cigarette Smoking. Available at: https://www.cdc.gov/tobacco/data_statistics/fact_sheets/health_effects/effects_cig_smoking/. Accessed September 2016.
- Centers for Disease Control and Prevention (CDC). The Social-Ecological Model: A Framework for Prevention. Available at: http://www.cdc.gov/violenceprevention/overview/social-ecologicalmodel.html. Accessed September 2016.
- Cooperrider DL, Whitney D, Cady S. Appreciative inquiry: a positive revolution in change. In: Holman P, Devane T, Cady S, eds. *The Change Handbook.* San Francisco: Berrett-Koehler Publishers Inc.; 2007.
- Covey SR. *The 7 Habits of Highly Effective People.* Revised edition. New York: Free Press; 2004.
- Egger G, Binns A, Rossner S. *Lifestyle Medicine: Managing Diseases of Lifestyle in the 21st Century.* North Ryde, N.S.W.: McGraw-Hill; 2010.
- Fernandez A, Goldberg E. Chapter 4. *The Sharpbrains Guide to Brain Fitness: How to Optimize Brain Health and Performance at Any Age.* New and expanded 2nd ed. San Francisco: Sharpbrains, Inc.;2013.
- Fisher EB, Strunk RC, Highstein GR, et al. A randomized controlled evaluation of the effect of community health workers on hospitalization for asthma. *Archives of Pediatrics and Adolescent Medicine.* March 2009;163(3):225-232.
- Frank E, Breyan J, Elon L. Physician disclosure of healthy personal behaviors improves credibility and ability to motivate. *Archives of Family Medicine.* 2000;9:287-290.
- Frates EP, Moore MA, Lopez CN, McMahon GT. Coaching for behavior change in physiatry. *American Journal of Physical Medicine & Rehabilitation.* December 2011;90(12):1074-1082. Available at: http://www.wellcoaches.com/images/pdf/Coaching-Am-Journal-Physical-Medicine-Dec-2011.pdf. Accessed September 2017.
- Ghorob A, Willard-Grace R, Bodenheimer T. Health coaching. *Virtual Mentor.* 2013;15(4): 319-326.
- Halm J, Amoako E. Physical activity recommendation for hypertension management: does healthcare provider advice make a difference? *Ethnicity and Disease.* Summer 2008;18(3):178-82.
- Hollisdon M, Thorogood M, White I, Foste C. Advising people to take more exercise is ineffective: a randomized controlled trial of physical activity promotion in primary care. *International Journal of Epidemiology.* 2002;31:808-815.

- Jordan M, Wolever RQ, Lawson K, Moore M. National training and education standards for health and wellness coaching: the path to national certification. *Global Advances in Health and Medicine*. May 2015;4(3):46-56.
- Kaizen Institute. What Is Kaizen?. Available at: https://www.kaizen.com/about-us/definition-of-kaizen.html. Accessed September 2016.
- Moore M, Tschannen-Moran B. *Coaching Psychology Manual*. New York: Lippincott Williams & Wilkins; 2010.
- National Wellness Institute. The Six Dimensions of Wellness Model. Available at: http://c.ymcdn.com/sites/www.nationalwellness.org/resource/resmgr/docs/sixdimensionsfactsheet.pdf. Accessed September 2016.
- Oliver JW, Kravitz RL, Kaplan SH, Meyers FJ. Individualized patient education and coaching to improve pain control among cancer outpatients. *Journal of Clinical Oncology*. 2001;19(8):2206-2212.
- Prochaska JO, Diclemente CC, Norcross JC. In search of how people change. *American Psychologist*. September 1992;27(9):1102-1114.
- Prochaska JO, Norcross IC, DiClemente CC. *Changing for Good*. New York: William Morrow Paperbacks; 2007.
- Prochaska JO, Velicer WF. The transtheoretical model of health behavior change. *American Journal of Health Promotion*. September 1997;12(1):38-48.
- Rippe IM. Chapter 27. *Lifestyle Medicine*. 2nd ed. Hoboken, NJ: CRC Press; 2013.
- Sackett DL, Rosenberg WMC, Gray JAM, Haynes RB, Richardson WS. Evidence based medicine: what it is and what it isn't. *British Medical Journal*. 1996;312:71-72.
- Sackett DL, Strauss SE, Richardson WS, Rosenberg W, Haynes RB. *Evidence-Based Medicine: How to Practice and Teach EBM*. London: Churchill-Livingstone; 2000.
- Sforzo GA, Kaye MP, Todorova I, et al. Compendium of the health and wellness coaching literature. *American Journal of Lifestyle Medicine*. 2017. doi: 10.1177/1559827617708562.
- Tamblyn R, Eguale T, Huang A, Winslade N, Doran P. The incidence and determinants of primary nonadherence with prescribed medication in primary care: a cohort study. *Annals of Internal Medicine*. 2014;160(7):441-450.
- Travis JW. *The Wellness Workbook: How to Achieve Enduring Health and Vitality*. 3rd ed. New York: Celestial Arts; 2004.
- Vale MJ, Jelinek MV, Best JD, et al. Coaching patients on achieving cardiovascular health (COACH): a multicenter randomized trial in patients with coronary heart disease. *Archives of Internal Medicine*. 2003;163(22):2775-2783.
- Value Based Management.net. Kaizen Philosophy/Kaizen Method. Available at: http://www.valuebasedmanagement.net/methods_kaizen.html. Accessed September 2016.

- Whittemore R, Melkus GD, Sullivan A, Grey M. A nurse coaching intervention for women with type 2 diabetes. *Diabetes Educator*. September-October 2004;30(5):795-804.
- Wolever RQ, Dreusicke M, Fikkan J, et al. Integrative health coaching for patients with type 2 diabetes: a randomized clinical trial. *Diabetes Educator*. July-August 2010;36(4):629-639.
- Wolever RQ, Simmons LA, Sforzo GA, et al. A systematic review of the literature on health and wellness coaching: defining a key behavioral intervention in healthcare. *Global Advances in Health and Medicine*. July 2013;2(4):38-57.

CHAPTER 3

COLLABORATING, MOTIVATING, GOAL-SETTING, AND TRACKING

"The good physician treats the disease; the great physician treats the patient who has the disease."

–William Osler, MD
Professor of Clinical Medicine
Co-founder of Johns Hopkins Hospital

❏ Chapter Goals:

- Introduce techniques that practitioners can use to empower patients, including change talk with *motivational interviewing* and finding the positives by using the *appreciative inquiry model*.
- Provide a history of goal-setting in relation to organizational behavior.
- Review the *5-step model* for creating a collaborative coach-patient relationship.

❏ Learning Objectives:

- To review goal-setting theory
- To introduce *motivational interviewing, appreciative inquiry,* and the *social-ecological model of change* into practice
- To describe SMART goals
- To understand the *5-step model* for collaboration and coaching conversations
- To demonstrate collaboration as the key piece of goal-setting
- To appreciate the importance of respecting autonomy when setting goals
- To review strategies for accountability and monitoring

❏ Guiding Questions:

- Why does it matter whether or not a healthcare provider sets goals with patients?
- What is the difference between a healthcare provider setting a goal for a patient and a healthcare provider co-creating a goal with a patient?
- What types of goals motivate people?
- What is the difference between setting a goal and holding a person responsible for a goal?
- How does tracking progress add value to the behavior-change process?

❑ Important Terms:

- *5-step coaching cycle model:* A model for collaborative coaching-patient relationships to promote behavior change created by Dr. Beth Frates and her colleagues
- *Appreciative inquiry model:* A systematic line of questioning advocated by Case Western Reserve University Professor David Cooperrider that searches for the best in people, organizations, and environments
- *Emotional intelligence (EI):* The concept of recognizing your own emotions, as well as those of other individuals, introduced by psychologist Dr. Daniel Goleman in his landmark book *Emotional Intelligence*
- *Goal-setting theory:* A theory introduced by Edwin A. Locke that describes the relationship between goal-setting, working toward those goals, motivation, and performance. In essence, this theory states that working toward a goal provides a major source of motivation to actually reach that goal, which, in turn, improves performance
- *Motivational interviewing (MI):* A style of communication, developed by psychologists William R. Miller and Stephen Rollnick, utilized in healthcare settings that is focused on setting personalized goals and strengthening the motivation of patients to change to healthy behaviors
- *Social-ecological model of change:* A model that describes interrelations among environmental conditions and human behavior and well-being. It is based on the premise that both individual and social-environmental factors play a role in human behavior
- *SMART goals:* Goals set in a specific way to enhance the likelihood that the task (e.g., the healthy new behavior) will be successfully achieved. The acronym SMART stands for: S = specific; M = measurable; A = action-oriented; R = realistic; T = time-sensitive

Lifestyle medicine practitioners use and acknowledge the patient's expertise (their habits, their desires, their feelings, their dreams, their motivators, their obstacles, their strengths, their creativity, their solutions, and their goals). To practice lifestyle medicine, a collaborative approach must be employed, with a focus on uncovering the patient's intrinsic motivators. Intrinsic motivators bring internal rewards, such as experiencing a runner's high after a run, the feeling of being energized after a walk, the feeling of satisfaction after a healthy meal, the feeling of having a sense of calm after meditation, or the feeling of being well rested after seven hours of sleep. While extrinsic motivators, such as receiving a prize at work for the most steps taken in a week, might be effective when initiating a new healthy behavior, for lasting change, however, a powerful intrinsic motivator must be found.

Furthermore, a practitioner must be able to help patients to set goals that are not only suitable to the needs and interests of the particular patient, they also need to be appropriate for the patient's stage of change for a given targeted behavior. It is important to note that patients can be in different stages of change for different behaviors. As such, the behavior-related goals will be different. A patient might be in preparation for dietary changes but in pre-contemplation for smoking cessation.

Building self-efficacy—confidence that a person can complete a task—is critical in lifestyle medicine. Co-creating SMART goals that are specific, measurable, action-oriented, realistic, and time-sensitive is also essential so that patients can experience at least relatively small successes, as well as be motivated to continue their lifestyle changes. It is important to appreciate the fact that the best goals are the ones that patients perceive as important and believe that they can complete. Caregivers might feel that their patients should complete goals that they (the caregivers) believe are very important. On the other hand if the patients don't view those particular goals as worthy, important, or interesting, then they are not going to work toward them.

Setting goals is just one piece of the puzzle—keeping patients accountable for those goals is another factor. If no one is checking on patients, then they may forget or just ignore the goals they have set. Accordingly, being able to develop and implement effective strategies for keeping patients accountable for their goals is another powerful skill for lifestyle medicine practitioners to practice.

MASTERING MOTIVATIONAL INTERVIEWING

Motivational Interviewing (MI) is a critical technique that lifestyle medicine practitioners need to master. In general, MI is defined as a collaborative conversation style for strengthening an individual's motivation and commitment to change. It was developed by psychologists Stephen Rollnick and William R. Miller, authors of *Motivational Interviewing in Health Care*.

Miller and Rollnick describe MI as a person-centered counseling style for addressing the common problem of ambivalence about change. The underlying premise is that while people want to change, they also want to stay the same, because it is easier and requires less effort. MI is designed to strengthen an individual's motivation for, and commitment to, achieving a specific goal. It fosters this situation by using techniques that focus on listening and exploring a person's reasons for change within an atmosphere of acceptance and compassion. One of the main objectives of MI is to elicit change talk, to have the patients state the reasons that it is good for them to change so that they end up convincing themselves of the need to change.

Inviting patients to list the pros and cons of a behavior is a constructive way for them to weigh their options concerning whether or not to change. This process is referred to as creating decisional balance and is often very enlightening for patients. For example, one MI tactic that sometimes startles smokers is for practitioners to ask, "Tell me all the pros about smoking." While this effort may not elicit change talk, it helps patients to evaluate their thoughts and feelings about smoking.

By listening to the pros about smoking, practitioners can learn what their patients will need to replace. For example, a number of smokers report that they like the stress relief they experience while smoking. Many of them also admit that they like leaving work and going outside for a break. On occasion, they socialize with other smokers on their smoke breaks, which is enjoyable to them as well.

Understanding the patient's underlying motivations can help the practitioner to come up with healthy substitutions that will allow a patient to get a break, relieve stress, and connect with fellow co-workers, in place of smoking. This approach is the counter-conditioning technique, which was addressed in the previous chapter.

For example, exercise, such as a five-minute walk, which can reduce a person's state of anxiety, could be a substitute for having a smoke. Walking with friends could add the social element. In addition, asking patients, "What else could you do for stress relief?" opens the opportunity for them to share some of the ideas that they may have been considering or even some they have already tried.

The next phase in the process, in this hypothetical example, involves moving from listing the pros to detailing the cons of smoking. As a rule, this stage evokes some level of change talk from the patients. Often, smokers report similar cons for smoking, for example, "It's so expensive. Oh gosh, and you know what, I smell. Also, I have a baby, and I have to change my clothes every time I go out for a butt and come back. It's really draining. And you know what, it's embarrassing, because in restaurants I have to go outside, and we can't stay in certain hotel rooms. Sometimes, all of the smoking rooms are booked or the hotels don't even have smoking rooms. Then, we are out of luck and have no place to stay." The cons just keep coming. For example, "And besides which, I'm having trouble breathing now."

Once a patient reviews their pros and cons of smoking, and they feel the pros of changing outweigh the cons of changing, they are ready to actually consider the importance of making a healthy behavioral change. Using a simple Likert (importance) scale will help patients to rate the importance level of making the change. Likert scales can be graded from 0 to 10, with 10 being most important and 0 being not important at all. For example, if a patient verbalizes that quitting smoking is an 8 on the Likert scale, the practitioner will know that the patient feels strongly about quitting.

The next area to check is the confidence level of the patients, again using a Likert scale from 0 to 10. For example, the practitioner can ask "How confident are you in your ability to quit smoking?" If the patient answers with the number 4, then the practitioner can ask "Why did you say a 4 and not a 1?" With this technique, patients are invited to list all of the reasons why they feel confident that they can quit. Subsequently, they may realize that they have more reasons to be confident than the number 4 represents. As a result, patients may begin to convince themselves that they can actually quit smoking.

MI focuses on evoking change talk, encouraging the patient to talk about change and seeks to help patients convince themselves that they would benefit from changing.

In MI, the practitioner is not meant to lecture or threaten the patient. In MI, the key is to encourage the patient to lecture themselves. For example, a good question that encourages smokers to lecture themselves to stop smoking is, "Why don't you smoke more?" What follows is change talk, such as, "Well, I don't smoke more because it's too expensive. It smells. I mean, if I smoke more, I will be like a chimney, and I will never get married. My girlfriend broke up with me, because she cannot stand the smoke! I'm ruining my life. I cannot smoke more."

The RULE mnemonic. In their book, Miller and Rollnick share a useful MI guiding-principle mnemonic they refer to as RULE:
- **R** = resist the righting reflex. In the Live and Learn section in the previous chapter, I explained how I couldn't resist the righting reflex in telling the gentleman, who was struggling with congestive heart failure in the ER, that he could not eat soup. "No soup for you!" I exclaimed. The urge to set this gentleman on the right path took over. Resisting the righting reflex means resisting the need to be the expert, to lecture, and to find all of the solutions.
- **U** = understand the patient's motivation. This factor reinforces the importance of listening and empathy. The expression, "No one cares what you have to say until they know how much you care," says it all. As such, a practitioner needs to understand a patient's motivation, spend time connecting with the patient, so that the patient feels that the practitioner cares about them and for them.
- **L** = listen. This point may sound simple, but it requires energy and mindfulness.
- **E** = empower your patient. Using MI tools and skills, as well as evoking change talk by utilizing decisional balance, importance scales, and confidence scales, will help practitioners empower their patients.

❏ *Four ways of being with patients.* The underlying spirit of MI embodies four ways of being with patients:
- Collaboration
- Acceptance
- Evocation
- Compassion

Collaboration refers to the notion that practitioners are creating a partnership, conducive to change with their patients. They do not act in a coercive or overbearing manner with their patients.

Acceptance refers to honoring each person's own worth, internal perspective, and right of self-direction and autonomy. Acceptance also entails uncovering the strengths of each patient and affirming them. In that regard, a practitioner can identify a patient's strengths, while listening to the individual, and then use reflections to point them out to him.

Evoking what is already present, as opposed to installing what is missing, is another pillar of MI. MI practitioners take the view that patients have what they need to make a change, and that by partnering together they can find it. Patients are seen as whole. MI practitioners help draw out the knowledge, skills, and tools that patients need to change their behavior.

Finally, compassion requires that practitioners actively promote the welfare of others to give priority to their needs. In other words, practitioners actively think of the patient first, not how much the practitioner might want to give the osteoporosis lecture (as was described in the previous chapter) to an 80-year-old woman with osteopenia, who wants to jump rope. Reflecting back on the Live and Learn by Beth Frates in Chapter 2, Dr. Frates did not want her patient to break a hip, so her focus was going to be on making sure that the patient knew about bone health. The patient, however, wanted to jump rope to feel closer to her sister, who had died of pancreatic cancer. As such, she kept thinking of the fond memories of them jumping double Dutch together as kids.

Although Dr. Frates reported that she really wanted to give one of her mini-lectures, as it turned out, the patient had already heard the osteoporosis lecture and did not need the information. The only way Dr. Frates could have known that would have been to ask the patient if she wanted to hear about osteoporosis. By inquiring about it, Dr. Frates learned that the patient actually wanted to know more about how to fit more exercise into her life. Specifically, she wanted to talk about jumping rope. If Dr. Frates had not asked the question, "What makes you say that?" when the patient told her that she wanted to jump rope, Dr. Frates would not have heard the story of her sister and felt the compassion she needed to feel in order to patiently work through how that patient could safely satisfy her desire to jump rope.

❑ *MI counseling continuum.* There is a continuum of counseling in MI, moving from directing to guiding and then to following. With guiding, the practitioner uses questions and reflections to evoke change talk. Subsequently, with directing, the MI practitioner makes sure that the conversation is focusing on the unhealthy behavior. For example, the practitioner might look at their watch, notice the time, and make a statement, such as, "Okay, in our last few minutes, let's think about a goal. What have you learned in this session and how do you want to move forward?" The term "following" means just listening. As such, the practitioner might not even make any statements, but rather just quietly listen to the patient. While an MI interview is composed of a mix of all three styles, the predominant counseling style is guiding.

❑ *OARS.* Miller and Rollnick teach four basic skills of MI, which they call OARS:
- O = open-ended questions
- A = affirmations
- R = reflections
- S = summaries

One of the mainstays of MI is asking open-ended questions, as opposed to the closed yes/no or one-word answer questions. This strategy provides patients with the opportunity to speak and share their wisdom. In general, closed-ended questions are conversation stoppers, while open-ended questions are idea generators.

Affirming change talk and encouraging patients to take positive steps toward their health goals are crucial elements in promoting lifestyle change. Recognizing patient strengths and calling attention to them is another way to affirm patients. When a patient says, "You know, I lost 20 pounds, but I just can't quit smoking," an MI practitioner might respond with, "Wow, you lost 20 pounds! That is hard to do, and you did it!" That statement is both a reflection and an affirmation.

A follow-up, open-ended question might be, "How do you feel about that?" The patient might then answer, "Well, I feel good. I worked really hard. I exercised. I watched my diet. And, I did it!"

In turn, the practitioner could respond with, "So, with a structured program, you were able to reach your goal." That feedback affirms the patient's strategy of hard work and planning. Another patient might share, "I just got a promotion at work. Wow, I worked hard. I just can't get exercise in, but I worked hard on my project. I had goals, and I hit them. I got the promotion that I have been wanting for a year now."

The practitioner could respond to this reply with, "It sounds like when you're goal-directed, you are successful. You hit the mark in work. How do you think you can translate that type of goal-setting and planning into your health goals as well?"

Reflections demonstrate to patients that practitioners are listening intently. In order to do this successfully, practitioners are called upon to be mindful when interviewing a patient, so that they can repeat the main concepts that the patients just shared. This strategy is a great way to build rapport and show compassion. It takes interest and energy to follow the thought process of another person. By reflecting sentences and sentiments expressed by patients, practitioners help patients feel heard, understood, and cared for.

There are two basic types of reflections: simple and complex. A simple reflection might sound like, "I hear you. You're not ready to quit smoking." There are also complex reflections, amplified reflections, and double-sided reflections in MI. In reality, when practitioners first start employing simple reflections, it may feel funny to repeat what patients say. For example, a patient might say, "Yeah, I don't have time to exercise. Just no way." "So, it sounds like what you're saying is you don't have time to exercise." Then, the patient repeats, "Right. I have no time to exercise."

The practitioner could repeat again, "You said you have no time to exercise." The patient might then say "It feels like you are repeating what I am saying." If the practitioner then states, "It feels to you that I am repeating what you are saying," that might indicate trouble, in that the practitioner is using too many simple reflections.

Instead, the practitioner could use an amplified reflection, such as, "There is absolutely no way you could possibly exercise any day this week or next week or any week in the near future." The patient could respond to this with, "I did not say that! I just said that I don't have time to exercise. I might in have time in a week or two." At that point, the patient is explaining how they might actually have time to exercise. Reflecting not only shows patients that practitioners are listening, it also allows for an opportunity to evoke change talk. Choosing to reflect statements that have a lot of energy behind them is particularly effective.

Another MI technique is called "summarizing." This approach is designed to demonstrate that practitioners have been listening for the entire interview. After one 15- or 20-minute consultation, if practitioners are able to put pieces of the story together and share it with their patients in the form of a summary, patients may then see their problem in a new light and develop insight into it. In addition, the patient will be impressed that the practitioner was paying attention so carefully that they could assimilate the information and pull it together in a concise statement at the end of the consultation.

For example, at the end of an interview a practitioner might say, "So, you're overweight now. You just gained 20 pounds. It sounds like you added the weight over the course of two months, a fact which seems to be really disturbing you. Yet, you feel very frustrated, because you don't have the time or the resources right now to tackle your weight gain. You have twins at home and a new baby. It sounds like it's been a real struggle these past few weeks. Furthermore, you felt like you were reaching the end of your rope. Now, you want to work on finding help so that you can take naps during the afternoon, which you believe will energize you. Do I have that right?" By checking to make sure the practitioner understood the patient correctly, the practitioner acknowledges the patient is the only one that knows the real story and is the expert in their life. The power is with the patient.

Scientific Evidence for MI

There is a great deal of evidence underlying MI, including its effectiveness in producing behavioral change. A really interesting one was published in 2010, involved 40 primary care physicians who were counseling 461 overweight or obese patients. The researchers evaluated each physician during their consultations to check for MI-consistent behavior, including collaborating, reflections, asking open-ended questions, affirmations, summaries, and signs of listening (basic OARS). They also listened for MI-inconsistent behaviors, such as coercing, directing, threatening, and arguing. The results showed that the patients of MI-consistent physicians had lost weight over the study period, as opposed to the patients of the MI-inconsistent physicians, who actually gained or maintained their weight over the course of the study.

In another study by Watkins, Wathan, and Leathley, titled, The 12-month effects of early motivational interviewing after acute stroke: a randomized controlled trial, published in the journal *Stroke*, in 2011, the intervention was simply four weekly sessions of MI for post-stroke patients. At 12 months, the patients in the MI group were found to have achieved improvements in mood, as well as had a reduced mortality rate (death rate), when compared to the control group, which received usual care for stroke survivors.

APPRECIATIVE INQUIRY MODEL

Another interviewing style employed in behavior change counseling is appreciative inquiry (AI). AI entails a systematic line of questioning that searches for the best in people, organizations, and environments.

Dr. David Cooperrider is the Case Western Reserve University psychologist and professor who originally described AI with colleagues in 1987 and created much of the foundational theoretical work for AI. In *The Change Handbook: The Definitive Resource on Today's Best Methods for Engaging Whole Systems*, he describes the AI model as a "cooperative search for the best in people, their organizations, and the world around them. It involves systematic discovery of what gives a system 'life,' when it is most effective and capable in economic, ecological, and human terms. AI involves the art and practice of asking questions that strengthen a system's capacity to heighten positive potential. It mobilizes inquiry through crafting an 'unconditional positive question,' often involving hundreds or sometimes thousands of people."

AI is different from problem-solving. With problem-solving, there is some ideal way for things to be done, and the goal is to find that ideal solution. In AI, things are socially constructed by the attendant system, and the goal is to find a way to change them. In the problem-solving mode, if a situation is not as people would like it to be, then it's a problem to be solved. With AI, in any situation, there are seeds of excellence upon which to build. As such, the goal is to search for the good in whatever is happening.

In the problem-solving mode, the way to be successful is to break the problem into parts and then analyze them. In AI, the way to be successful is to seek out examples of excellence and share stories of exceptional performance throughout the system being studied. After locating excellence, the goal is to bring it to the forefront and to replicate the good.

Dr. David Cooperrider contends that the concept of the AI spiral entails five steps in the spiral—defining, discovering, dreaming, designing, and delivering (Figure 3-1). This technique is being utilized in healthcare settings for institutions (hospitals), as well as with patients. Each of the five stages has its own unique intent, for example:

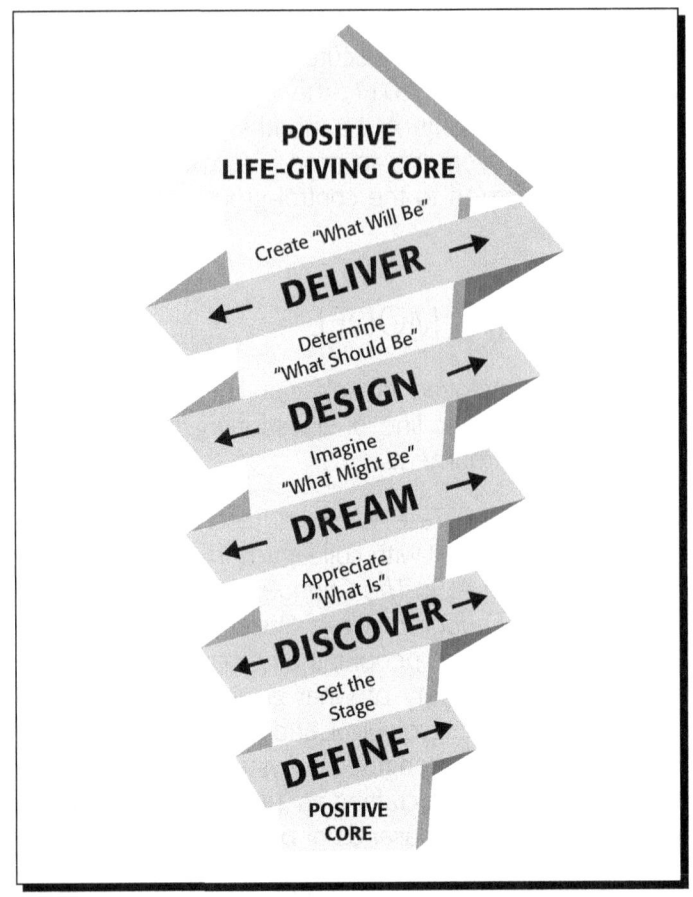

Figure 3-1. The 5D AI spiral model of development

❑ *Defining:* In the first step, the focus is to understand the patient, to the degree possible, in order to help clarify where the patient is in the process. For instance, when working with a patient, the practitioner might state, "Define where you are right now. What is happening in your life? Let's get clarity on what brings you here."

❑ *Discovery:* The second phase of inquiry explores what gives life to this patient, to this organization, to a group of physicians who are struggling? What is good? What can you appreciate? Because what you appreciate, appreciates. The underlying concept is to discover the good and replicate it.

❑ *Dream:* The third stage focuses on envisioning what might be. For example, the practitioner might ask the patient, "What would your life be like if you were exercising five days a week?" or "What would your life be like if you quit smoking?" The practitioner and the patient dream for a little while together, and then create a vision that can draw them toward goals. By developing a specific vision that utilizes all five senses (sight, sound, smell, taste, and touch), a greater feeling of connection and hope is created concerning where the patient wants their life to go.

❏ *Designing:* In the fourth stage, the patient and the practitioner co-construct a process for changing individual behaviors. The process is similar to developing architectural plans for a house. For example, there are specific goals to be accomplished at different stages of the building project. The goals are meant to be specific, as well as easy-to-follow.

❏ *Delivery/Destiny:* During the final step, the practitioner and patient see what is happening and what has occurred with the co-constructed plan. Where did the patient end up? How did it go? More than likely, some progress was made. At this point, the practitioner and patient might need to return to the first step to further define the problem or area of focus. The AI methodology can then begin again, traversing through discovery, dreaming, designing, and delivery/destiny.

The following principles serve as the underlying foundation for the 5D AI spiral model:
- First, the constructionist principle, which entails what people believe to be true will affect the way they act and the way they approach change
- Second, the simultaneity principle, which states that the initial questions asked set the stage for what is found and discovered. Accordingly, with AI, a practitioner and patient start with what is working well. (Similarly, in coaching interactions for behavior change, the coach will start each session with what went well during the past week.) Beginning on a positive note sets the stage for subsequent positive interactions and energy.
- Third, the poetic principle, which suggests that the past, present, and future are endless sources of learning, inspiration, and interpretation. In other words, people are constantly learning and evolving.
- Fourth, the anticipatory principle, which is based on the concept that a person's behavior in the present is influenced by the future they anticipate. That's why practitioners utilize AI. They're dreaming. They're anticipating. They're creating the vision.
- Fifth, the positive principle, which stipulates that the more positive the questions used to guide the change process, the more long-lasting and effective the change will ultimately be.

THE SOCIAL-ECOLOGICAL MODEL OF CHANGE

The social-ecological model of change takes into account the individual, that person's immediate relationships, the surrounding community, and the larger society as a whole, when contemplating behavior change (Figure 3-2). This model states that in order to create successful behavior change, a practitioner or a program cannot just target the unhealthy habits of the individual. The practitioner must look into a patient's relationships, the people closest to that person, the individual's neighbors, community, societal norms, including understood rules and regulations governing that person's behavior, and what official state or federal laws are in place that may influence that individual's behaviors. Results from the famous Framingham Heart Study, published in *The New England Journal of Medicine* in 2007, which found that people who had obese friends, siblings, or spouses were more likely to become obese themselves, validate this model of change.

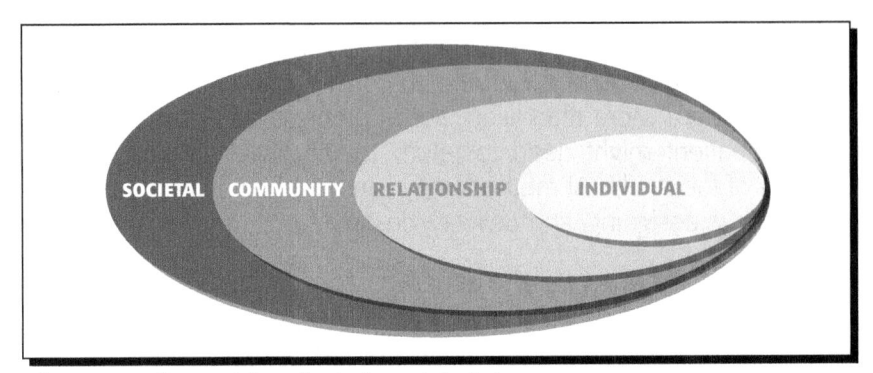

Figure 3-2. The social-ecological model of change

Keeping the social-ecological model of change in mind when practicing lifestyle medicine is important, if the ultimate goal is a culture change. Helping patients achieve lasting change involves altering their environments to make them conducive to exercise, as well as amenable to eating healthy, nutritious foods. When people are surrounded by several different healthy options, making a single healthy choice is easier.

The definition of ecology is the study of the relationship between organisms and their environment. A real connection exists between people and their environments. The interrelationships among environmental conditions and human behavior and their well-being are strong influencers that lifestyle practitioners need to address. For example, to achieve better diets for kids, school administrators and superintendents can change school lunch menus and vending machine snacks. They can also require recess five days a week and include physical education classes in elementary school, middle school, and high school to help kids stay active.

Communities and organizations can change the current system and make it healthier by developing and promoting programs that focus on the concept "move to improve." For example, local YMCAs already offer health-oriented programs for people of all ages. Most towns host 5K road races for various charities. These events can serve as the spark that gets people moving and engaged with other community members.

Finding and creating opportunities for people to congregate, connect, and share healthy behaviors in a fun and exciting way is one strategy to cultivate a culture of healthy living. Encouraging people to buy produce at farmers' markets is also a viable option to support and encourage a whole-foods, plant-based diet that is relatively widely known to provide health benefits. Planting fruits and vegetables at local community gardens is yet another way to make healthy living an integral part of life, as well as provide a great opportunity for patients to connect with fellow community members. Furthermore, some restaurants are helping to promote local farms by buying their produce locally and advertising this aspect of their business on their menus. Many restaurants also provide guidelines on healthy meal options by indicating which meals are heart healthy, which often are both vegan and gluten-free. By creating social norms, all of these community programs and influencers can help to shape the behavior of individuals who live together in specific geographic areas.

THE 5-STEP COACHING MODEL FOR CREATING A COLLABORATIVE COACH-CLIENT RELATIONSHIP

About a decade ago, I developed a 5-step coaching cycle model (Figure 3-3) that works really well to build a strong relationship between a lifestyle practitioner and a patient. The model, which was published in the *American Journal of Physical Medicine and Rehabilitation* in 2011, is still relevant and useful today. It focuses on the basics of being empathetic, aligning motivation, building confidence, setting SMART goals, and creating a mechanism for accountability. The model features the following five steps, which are designed to help practitioners negotiate and collaborate with their patients:

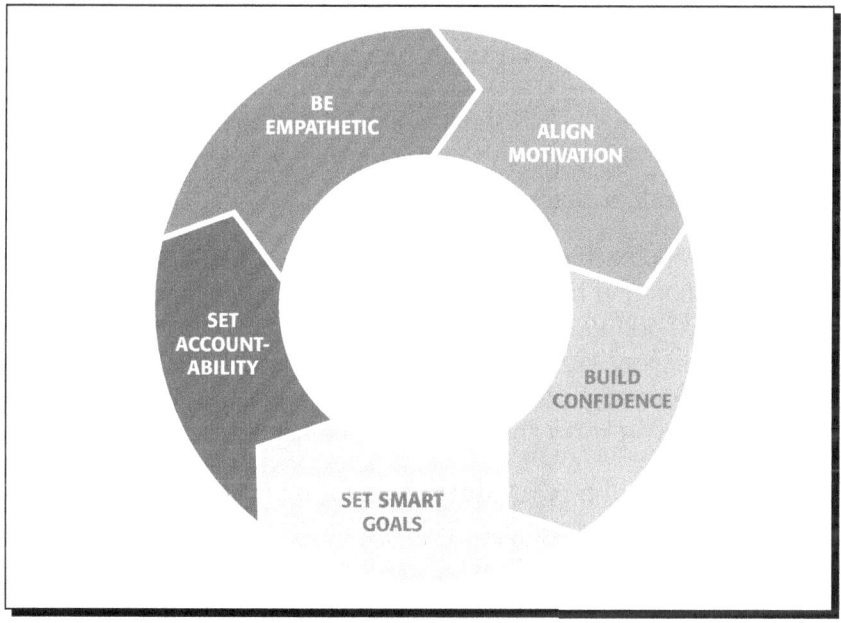

Figure 3-3. The 5-step coaching cycle model

Step #1 Be Empathetic

Empathy begins and ends (or rather, restarts) the 5-step coaching cycle. Empathy is the fuel that propels the cycle around. It is also the keystone for building a relationship with a patient.

What is empathy? *The American Heritage Dictionary* defines the term as "identification with and understanding of another individual's situation, feelings, and motives." The concept that underlies this step builds on several of the points of emphasis that have been addressed thus far in this chapter: sitting with patients, eye-to-eye, at their level, undistracted, while being mindful. Empathy requires that the practitioner be fully present and engaged with the patient. Among the key features of being empathetic are sharing a caring relationship, being trustworthy, listening and demonstrating attention with reflections, being nonjudgmental, being respectful, being supportive, and being genuinely curious about the patient.

When practitioners are using the Frates COACH Approach (curiosity, openness, appreciation, compassion, and honesty), they are able to easily express empathy. For the Frates COACH Approach to work, there needs to be honesty. The practitioner must be comfortable with knowing and sharing the truth. For example, if the patient has a BMI that puts him in the obese category, the practitioner must convey this information in a straightforward way, but face to face. One patient told me that he received his blood test results in the mail with a note from his physician saying, "You are obese. Your BMI is 31. You need to lose weight."

Such feedback was the truth, and the physician was being honest. By communicating this information through a written, mailed document, however, the physician wasn't able to gauge the response to the message or react in a supportive manner to the patient's reaction. In fact, the patient who received this letter became angry. He did not like either hearing the truth or how it was communicated to him. In fact, this patient wanted to change providers after receiving this note.

A Frates COACH Approach strategy to relaying the fact that a patient is obese is one that fosters collaboration and honesty. For example, a coach might say, "Joe, I see here that your weight is 200 pounds. For your height of 5'8", that gives you a BMI of 31, which falls into the obese category. Were you aware of this?" Depending on the way the patient responds, the practitioner might continue with the following feedback, "So, it sounds like this is news to you. Do you know about the risks of a high BMI and obesity?"

If the patient says no, the practitioner can educate him. If the patient responds in the affirmative, the practitioner can ask, "Is there anything you want to do about it?" It is important for the practitioner to remain both curious and non-judgmental. For example, the patient might respond with, "Well, I will keep doing what I am doing because it is working. I have lost 30 pounds in a year."

At this point, the practitioner can express appreciation for the patient's success by congratulating him and asking how he lost the weight. If the strategy involved increased physical activity and adopting healthy eating habits, then the conversation would progress one way. On the other hand, if the patient's strategy for losing weight was to forgo eating for days at a time and take "special supplements," the conversation would go another way.

By asking open-ended questions in a non-judgmental way, the practitioner maximizes the opportunity to create a bond with the patient and to use the therapeutic relationship to help the patients forge forward on their journeys to change their behaviors. In sum, if the objective is to support and empower the patient, then focusing on curiosity, openness, appreciation, compassion, and honesty with the Frates COACH Approach will help the practitioner meet the goal.

❑ *Emotional Intelligence (EI) and Empathy:* Using the Frates COACH Approach invites practitioners to call upon their *emotional intelligence*, a concept that was discussed previously in this chapter. EI (sometimes referred to as emotional IQ or EQ) has been recognized to be as important, or perhaps more important, than IQ in predicting success in employment and social relationships. As a result of Dr. Daniel Goleman's efforts in this area, the social brain has become a topic of conversation for educators, leaders, and healthcare practitioners.

One key aspect of EI is empathy. In his book on the subject, Goleman describes several different types of empathy, including the following:

- *Cognitive empathy.* This form of empathy refers to the practice of striving to understand what the speaker is saying—listening to the words and making sense of the intended message. Cognitively, the person understands the language and expressions of the other individual and can repeat parts of the story back to the speaker.
- *Emotional empathy.* When practicing emotional empathy, a person attempts to feel what the speaker is feeling. The listener understands not just the words, but also the emotions expressed by the speaker by paying attention to body language, facial expressions, tone of voice, pitch, volume, and cadence of speech. This type of empathy is the basis of a therapeutic relationship, when the listener can walk with the speaker and "be in his shoes."
- *Empathic need.* In this form of empathy, a person strives to sense the needs of the speaker before the speaker even expresses them. The listener uses all of the senses to understand the speaker—the "vibes" in the air, the tension in the room, the intangibles, the unspeakables, and the feelings bottled up in the patient awaiting expression. For example, when a person begins to use a slightly shaky voice, look down at the floor, and a tear begins to well up in his eyes, providing a box of tissues before the speaker even appears to need one means the listener is meeting the empathic need of the speaker. Working at the level of empathic need allows practitioners to fully connect with patients and build strong alliances.

If empathy is that important, should medical schools be training medical students in empathy? Can someone learn to be empathetic? Medical educators have been pondering these issues and studying empathy for decades. A few years ago, Thomas Jefferson University Medical School piloted a program to teach empathy to medical students. They conducted a course titled "The Art of Attending," which included workshops in art and theater. In this course, the medical students were asked to look at pictures and describe what they saw. The course tried to push students beyond their comfort zones by not just asking them to state what images were in the painting, but also to use different senses and describe the textures of the work and the emotion conveyed by the work. The course invited medical students to use their social brain and call upon their EI to interpret and analyze a painting. The desired outcome was that this exercise would help train the students in being empathetic.

This pilot program was designed to harken back to ancient times and use art as a way of expressing emotion. For example, in the days of the Greek empire, theater was a way for people to cope with the realities of war and loss. The plays written and produced at the time reflected what was going on in the world around the Greeks.

Watching theater performances was a way for people to manage the difficult times of men lost in battle or at sea. These productions played out the lives of people in the audience, and the theater gave the people in the audience a place to weep, cry, and mourn their losses. For those individuals who had not experienced those losses directly, it was a way for them to empathize with the process in front of them that the actors were portraying. As such, theater was a way of having an empathic experience.

Another resident training program, this one conducted at the University of Washington, called "Improving Clinical Management of Stillbirth," also sought to develop empathy in health practitioners. Developed by Dr. Maureen Kelly, an associate professor at UW in the Department of Pediatrics and Bioethics, the goal of the program was to help medical students deal with the emotional repercussions of handling patients who have stillbirths—not just the medical aspect of having a stillbirth and being involved with a stillbirth, but getting to the emotional impact for both the physician and the patient.

In this program, patients shared their personal stories in front of the physicians who were in training, expressing their fears, tears, and sorrows openly. After listening to the patients, the physicians were encouraged to ask questions and to interact with the patients. The underlying goal of the program was that when faced with a stillbirth in the delivery room, the medical students would have the coping skills and experience to deal empathically with the patient and the emotional process.

A third empathy-oriented medical education training program was designed by Dr. Helen Reese at Massachusetts General Hospital (MGH) in Boston. Dr. Reese, Director of the Empathy and Relational Science program, developed three 60-minute modules that were targeted at increasing empathy in residents. A pilot study revealed that residents who completed these modules improved their ability to express empathy—a fact that was noted by patients, who rated these residents more empathetic than residents who had not completed the modules. In addition, residents responded positively to the program, reporting that the modules helped them get back in touch with their own sense of empathy, as well as enhanced their ability to express empathy.

One of the physicians who went through the program at MGH was deeply touched by his experience with these empathy modules. He reported that, for many years, he had basically just been running in and out of patients' rooms and taking care of urgent business. One day after completing the modules, however, when the physician was doing his inpatient rounds, he noted that a patient's neck was tilted awkwardly, while she laid in bed. Because the patient looked really uncomfortable, he reflexively reached over and fluffed up her pillow, which brought a smile to her face.

This gesture is an example of expressing the third type of empathy (empathic need) described by Dr. Daniel Goleman. The physician remembered this act as a transformative moment for him. Furthermore, he felt a profound effect by performing that one small act of kindness. No words were spoken. He just looked at the patient, sensed her pain, and relieved her discomfort. It is not difficult to imagine the patient perceiving this feat as, "You understood that I was in pain, and you responded, without my even saying anything. You are a compassionate physician."

A study conducted at Northwestern University School of Medicine by Enid Montague and her colleagues reported on the benefits of expressing empathy through nonverbal communication, such as the scenario involving the physician that was described previously. This study concluded that practitioners who made a lot of eye contact were perceived by patients to be more empathetic and more likeable than other physicians, a finding that reinforces the premise that patients know when a doctor is really present with them in the room.

To hold eye contact successfully, physicians need to pay attention and focus on the person in front of them. Patients are put off when a physician rushes through a visit and forces them to stare at the back of the doctor, while the doctor stares at a screen and types into the medical record. Setting up the office visit to encourage level, face-to-face conversation can help to alleviate this alienating way of conducting patient visits.

Step #2. Align Motivation

According to self-determination theory, a foundation for behavior change counseling that was created by Edward Deci, PhD, and Richard M. Ryan, PhD, at the University of Rochester, people experience volitional motivation that helps them persevere with their goals when three specific needs are met: they feel a sense of autonomy; they feel competent to achieve the goal; and they feel a sense of relatedness or connection. The work of these two renowned psychologists separates extrinsic (external) motivation from intrinsic (internal) motivation. Examples of extrinsic motivators include:
- "I'll get paid $10, if I take 10 pounds off."
- "I'll win the prize at work, if I lose 30 pounds."
- "My doctor will be happy and stop harassing me, if I lose some weight by the next visit."

Examples of intrinsic motivators include:
- "I will feel more energized at work in the afternoons, if I walk every day at lunch."
- "I will be able to move around more comfortably, if I lose a few more pounds."
- "My fasting glucose levels will come down to the normal range if I lose weight; as a result, I will be less worried about the consequences of diabetes."

- "I will be more focused at work and get more sleep at night if I exercise regularly."
- "I love the way I feel after a run. There is nothing like a runner's high!"

When patients make changes because they are working toward internal rewards that are important to them, they are more likely to sustain healthy behaviors than when they are working toward external rewards. The key for providers is to be curious about what is important and meaningful to each individual patient.

Consider the following hypothetical example: A smoker of 40 years was finally able to quit when he realized that his smoking was a habit that greatly disturbed his grandchildren. He gleaned this information when he heard them talking about his smoking as they rode in his car. One child said to the other, "Don't worry, it stinks in here, but you will get used to it after a couple of car trips with Papa." Connecting with his grandchildren and not exposing them to a smelly, uncomfortable environment was the only thing that spoke to this smoker. He had heard about cancer, stroke, heart disease, and early death many times, but his grandchildren's words touched him deeply and gave him the intrinsic motivation to change.

Although this man longed for connection with his grandchildren and was now worried that his habit could jeopardize his grandchildren taking rides with him, he wanted to quit smoking, and he wanted to do it his way—he wanted to self-determine the course of his behavior change. It was his choice, not his wife's or his physician's. He felt that going cold turkey was the best method for him, because it had worked in the past, at least temporarily. Furthermore, this time, the intrinsic motivator to connect and spend time with his grandchildren was so powerful that he was able to stay smoke-free.

Step #3. Build Confidence

After cultivating motivation, the 5-step coaching cycle focuses on building confidence. One effective way to accomplish this objective is to talk about a patient's strengths and past successes. Examples of useful questions at this stage of the collaboration include the following:
- What are your strengths?
- Can you tell me about a time when you were successful at work, school, or home?
- What would your friends say are your positive attributes?
- Tell me about a time when you felt like you were at your best. What were you doing?
- What skills were you using? What character strengths were shining bright?

By inquiring about positive experiences and strengths, a physician can find out what is working well. This factor harkens back to Dr. David Cooperrider's appreciative inquiry model. Practitioners can build on the positive by appreciating it.

Several psychological theories support the concept of building confidence to empower lasting change, including social cognitive theory, positive psychology, and hope theory. Each of these approaches has its own set of unique features.

❑ *Social Cognitive Theory:* Dr. Albert Bandura developed this theory, which postulates that self-efficacy is developed from external experiences and self-perception. Interpreting this premise in a clinical context, the practitioner helps the patient to make sense of external experiences and explores the patient's self-perceptions. There is an emphasis on self-talk, as an expression of self-perceptions, given that it is important in the development of self-efficacy. With a close connection to a patient, the practitioner can inquire about self-perceptions and how the patient has experienced various social situations.

❑ *Positive Psychology:* The positive psychology movement was initiated by applied psychologist Dr. Martin Seligman. He advanced the notion that the focus should be on a strengths-based approach to mental health, rather than a deficit approach. Dr. Seligman, who has written several influential books—including *Authentic Happiness* and *Flourish*, teaches a world-renowned course at the University of Pennsylvania. He has an exceptional website (www.authentichappiness.sas.upenn.edu) that is both informative and innovative. Furthermore, several of his graduate students have gone on to do really important work, including Tal Ben-Shahar, PhD, who arguably taught the most popular course at Harvard College (on positive psychology), and has written several books, including *Being Happy, Happier, Even Happier,* and *Choose the Life You Want*, that offer powerful advice on how to be happy and lead a meaningful life.

The underlying focus of positive psychology is to work with strengths and virtues that enable individuals and communities to thrive. Asking patients to take the strengths and virtues quiz available online (at www.viacharacter.org/www/Character-Strengths) is one way to help them to identify their strengths, as well as provide material for conversations with them going forward.

Another positivity researcher is Dr. Barbara Fredrickson, who has developed the broaden and build theory. Her theory is based on her research, which found that positive emotions, such as love, joy, pride, and awe, lead to resiliency, creativity, and life satisfaction. As such, positivity can help patients and providers solve complex problems.

Dr. Fredrickson's research led to the positivity ratio of 3:1, which surmises that three positive emotions are needed for every one negative emotion, in order for a person to remain focused and creative. Subsequently, her statistical methods were called into question. As a result, the ratio of 3:1 might not be as exact as she might have wanted. On the other hand, focusing on appreciating the positive and experiencing positive emotions in a ratio of about 3:1 or greater, but not as much as 11:1, can help people persevere through challenging times, with confidence and resilience. More information on positivity is included in Chapter 12 of this book.

Everyone has negative thoughts. They are a part of life. Psychologists often refer to them as ANTs (automatic negative thoughts). Most people have an inner critic that lives inside their head. This critic finds fault with just about anything and everything, depending on the person. For example, someone might think, "I'll never exercise. I know I should, but I never will. I've never been an exerciser." The concept that Dr. Fredrickson advocates is to balance that negative thought with three positives: "Wait a minute, when I have a goal, and it's meaningful to me, I hit that goal. (One positive thought.) Actually, there was a time in my life I was exercising regularly, and I enjoyed it. (Second positive thought.) Furthermore, I used a pedometer when I did that, and maybe that is a tool I can use. (Third positive thought.)" Adding these positive thoughts to the self-talk mix, as well as recalling occasions when success was achieved, helps people to forge forward in their journey for achieving behavioral change. Even better is to address the inner critic. Some people call it the gremlin. It is possible to fire the gremlin and hire a positivity princess or prince who tries to encourage, support, and build you up. Working with patients on being a self-advocate and using self-compassion is helpful when trying to adopt and sustain lifestyle change.

❑ *The Hope Theory:* The hope theory was developed by Dr. C.R. Snyder and supports confidence building to create hope. His work found that setting inspiring goals enabled people to build confidence and improve outcomes. Identifying pathways to change provides hope that change is possible. This hope can then, in turn, help to increase self-confidence.

LIVE AND LEARN WITH DR. BETH FRATES

The 3:1 ratio of positive to negative emotions was utilized at Harvard Medical School in the 2000s, when I was teaching in the school's tutorial system. We reviewed Dr. Fredrickson's work and used it when we gave constructive criticism to students about their performance. This feedback was essential for students to learn and grow. The recommended methodology was to share two positive performance comments and then one negative comment, revealing an area ripe for improvement and then, end with a final positive comment.

In essence, the process was a positive sandwich. For example, for a student that does well on tests and is very bright, but does not put the effort into daily homework assignments, an instructor might say, "You're really participating in every class. It's great to see you doing that. Your exam scores have been outstanding. You're definitely able to understand the material—you're able to put the information together and make sense of it and then relay it. On the other hand, I also notice that you don't always hand in your homework, and it's not always fully completed when you do. This matter might be an area we can work on in the next two weeks. What could you do differently to allow you to hand in your completed assignments on time?" After a brief discussion, the instructor would end with another positive comment, such as, "Another area where you excel is that you are a great team player during tutorials. You're really good about utilizing the ideas of others and building on them. That is a great skill to continue to use and hone, and it will come in handy on the wards, as well as in your personal life."

The emphasis on positivity gives hope for a bright future—not to mention that hope, in itself, can be therapeutic.

Step #4. Set SMART Goals

Part of building self-confidence is setting goals that are realistic and achievable. This factor leads to the fourth step in the 5-step coaching cycle, setting SMART goals—namely goals that are specific, measurable, action-oriented, realistic, and time-sensitive).

Most business people are familiar with goal-setting. Stephen R. Covey's best-selling book, *The 7 Habits of Highly Effective People: Powerful Lessons in Personal Change*, addressed the subject and listed the following foundations for success:

- Be proactive.
- Begin with the end in mind.
- Put first things first, prioritize.
- Think win/win.
- Seek first to understand, then to be understood.
- Synergize and work with people.
- Sharpen the saw. Always take a break and sharpen the saw. Don't just be cutting down all the trees.

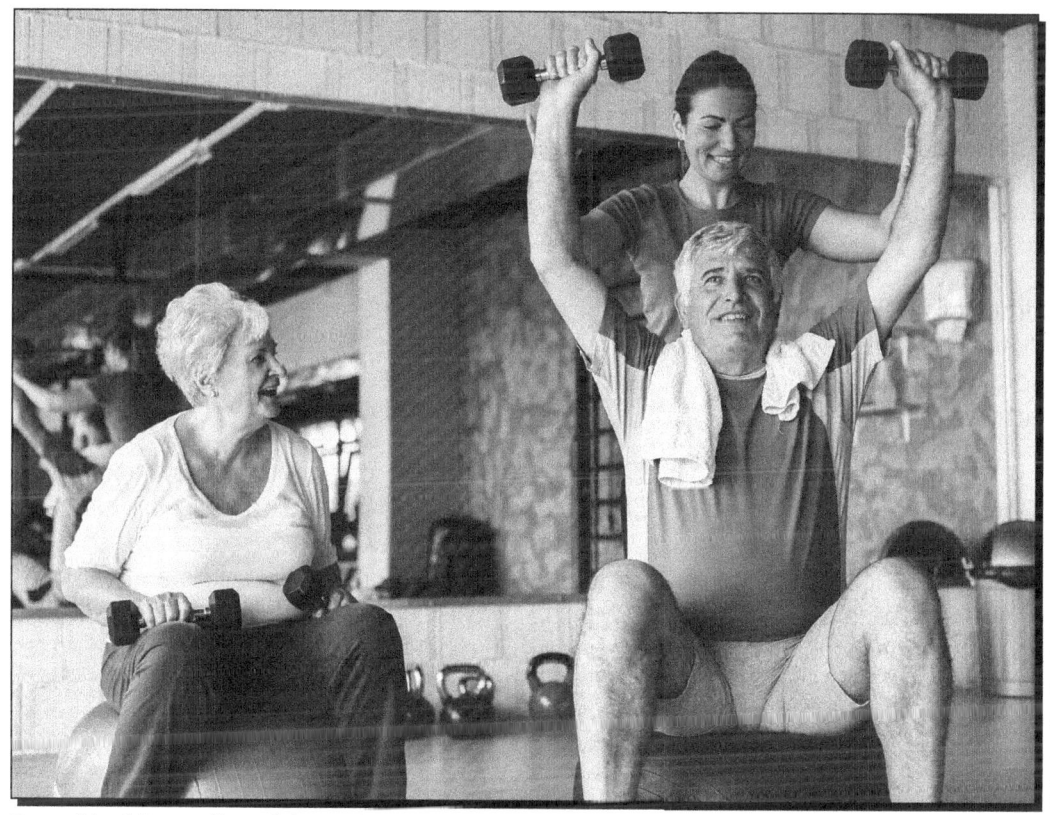

Part of building self-confidence is setting goals, such as exercising on a regular basis, that are realistic and achievable.

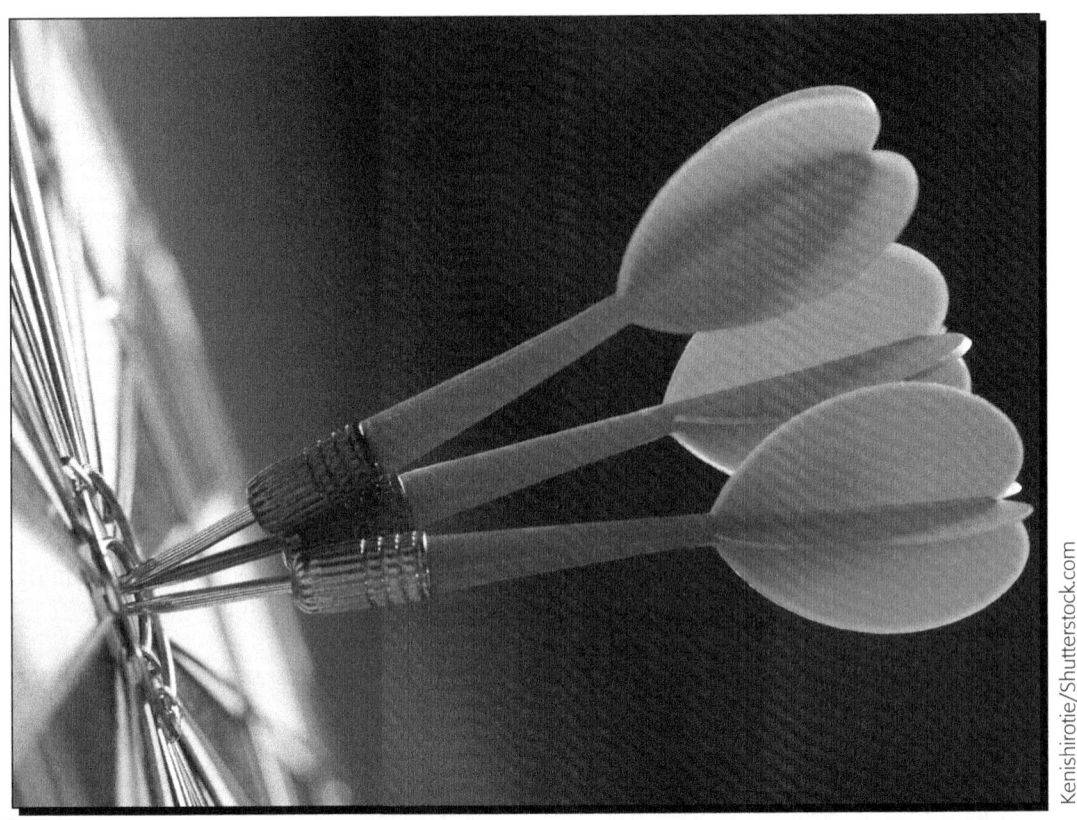

Goals must be clear and present the appropriate level of challenge, neither too difficult nor too easy to achieve.

Diana Scharf Hunt, PhD, an author and researcher who has done a lot of work on time management, advances the notion that "goals are dreams with deadlines." As noted previously, the appreciative inquiry model includes a dreaming step. People like to think big and dream of what can be. They then need to establish specific steps to achieve those dreams.

The goal-setting theory, which was developed by organizational psychologist Dr. Edwin Locke and his colleague, Gary Lathan, is particularly applicable in this situation. This theory surmises that working toward a goal provides a major source of motivation to actually reach that goal, which in turn improves performance. Locke's and Latham's model promotes developing a goal with clarity, challenge, complexity, commitment, and feedback. Subsequently referred to as the 4CF model of goal-setting, the model states that the goal must be clear and must present the appropriate level of challenge, being neither too difficult nor too easy to achieve. It also needs the right amount of complexity, avoiding too many steps or intricacies. In addition, there has to be a commitment to the goal. Finally, there needs to be feedback on the progress toward the goal.

❏ *Adult Learning Theory:* Another important theory related to goal-setting is adult learning theory, which was developed by Malcolm Knowles, PhD. Dr. Knowles' theory has had an impact on how practitioners work with adults on goal-setting. Knowles emphasized that adult learners are different from school-aged learners. He demonstrated that adult learners are full of experience, tend to be autonomous, and are self-directed (consistent with the self-determination theory). They also are relevancy-oriented, practical, and goal-oriented. In order for education in behavior change counseling and setting goals to be effective in adult learners, information must be delivered "just in time," when the learner is in need of the information and ready to receive it.

When setting SMART goals, it is important to begin with the end in mind. In other words, it is essential that practitioners determine their end goal first and foremost. It is often helpful to create a vision of the future. Think about life in the future and how it might be. What do patients want? What are they striving for? What do they want to be like in 10 years, 20 years?

The more specific and creative this vision—including as many senses as possible—the better. Once the vision is set, goal-setting can begin. First, choose some long-term goals: one-year, six-month, three-month, and one-month goals. Then, tackle short-term goals. What can patients accomplish in a week? What will they do on a specific day of the week? Starting with the end in mind, the vision and taking the long-term view can then help with short-term planning, as well as goal-setting.

What type of goal? It is important to be specific with goal-setting strategy. What is the motivation for setting the goal? How does it relate to a patient's purpose, values, and vision? Is this a specific goal? How will it be measured? What actions will the patient take? What is the time frame for completing the goal?

The best way to determine if a goal is realistic is to check on the patient's confidence level about completing the goal. Using a scale of 0 to 10 can be helpful. If patients say that they're at a 10 for confidence, then that is a realistic goal. On the other hand, a 10 rating might also suggest the goal is too easy. Inquiring if they want to increase the challenge is appropriate in this instance, as is allowing the patients to set a simple goal and be successful.

If an individual picks a 6 out of 10 for a confidence level, then the patient and the practitioner need to reconsider that goal. Asking patients how they could adjust the goal so that it is a little easier for them to achieve will help keep them focused and motivated through the behavior change process.

It is important to select goals that are challenging and complex, but not too challenging or complex. If the goals are realistic, then patients can attain them. Success breeds success. Every time a patient achieves a goal, the patient feels a reward. There can be a surge of dopamine released in the brain that increases motivation to keep making goals and achieving them. This process is how small changes bring big rewards.

Step #5. Set Accountability

The last step in the 5-step coaching cycle is setting accountability. While it is critical to set goals, it is just as critical to follow up on them. This stage involves the F for feedback in the Locke and Latham 4CF model. The practitioner needs to check in with the patient. Alternatively, the practitioner and patient can set up a buddy system in which the patient enlists a spouse, friend, coworker, or relative to be their accountability buddy. This person checks in with the patient on a routine basis—at least once a week.

Tracking systems can be helpful for accountability as well. As Peter Drucker, regarded as the father of modern management theory, states, "What gets measured gets managed." While there are currently several options available in the marketplace for wearable devices to track exercise and other metrics, sometimes a simple pedometer or even a pen-and-paper log is the most useful strategy for patients.

SMART Quiz

Review the following scenarios and select yes or no concerning whether they are SMART goals (i.e., specific, measurable, action-oriented, realistic, and time-sensitive):

1. I will lose 10 pounds. Yes No

2. I will eat less processed foods and more vegetables. Yes No

3. This week, I'll exercise three times for 20 minutes each. Monday before work, I'll walk the dog. Wednesday, I'll go to the park with a friend at lunch and walk after we eat. And the third time, on Saturday, I'll ride my bike on the bike path near my house. Yes No

4. I'll call my friend Mary on Tuesday after work, and tell her that I'm making a plan to adopt healthy habits. Yes No

Answer Key:

1. No, this is not a SMART goal. It is specific and measurable, but not action-oriented or time-sensitive. It is hard to tell if it is realistic, because there is no time frame specified.

2. No, this is not a SMART goal. It sounds specific, but is it measurable? What is the person referring to specifically when the individual states, "I will eat less." Less than what? How many? More than how many? Is the goal action-oriented? Yes, the patient is going to do something. Is it realistic? It is hard to know without knowing the patient's current eating habits. Is it time-sensitive? No, it is not.

3. Yes, this is a SMART goal, because it meets all of the criteria for specificity, timeliness, and action.

4. Yes, this is also a SMART goal. It's specific—I'll call my friend. It's action-oriented, and it's got a timeline. Furthermore, it's measurable—the person will either call or won't call her friend.

It all depends on the age and interests of the person. Patients might use journaling, logging, apps, websites, heart-rate monitors, weight, blood tests, or other measures to keep track of their progress. Even a calendar with stars on it for days exercised can provide motivation for adults. It is important to keep in mind that such a simple tool is not just for children.

Competitions with family members or coworkers can also help keep people accountable for the period of time during the competition. A long-term accountability system, however, needs to be put in place. The system could change with time. Making SMART goals and striving toward them with no one watching or checking in can allow for small deviations, which could cause a person to revert back to old habits.

❑ *Finally: Restart Empathy*

After establishing a system for accountability, the 5-step coaching cycle resumes its focus on empathy. Whatever the patient reports back after setting goals and striving toward those goals, the practitioner needs to express empathy for the patient. For example, if patients state that they would walk four days that week, but only walked one, the practitioner can start by asking what happened on the day that they did walk. Inquiring about what went well and what strategies patients employed to complete the walk can help both parties assess what needs to be in place for the individuals to be successful. Listening non-judgmentally to the problems the patient encountered on the other days can help the patient feel understood. Realizing that they can learn and grow from each misstep can help them stay focused and motivated on their journey for behavior change.

KEY POINTS/TAKEAWAYS FOR CHAPTER 3

❑ Chapter Review:

- Overall goal: Review techniques that practitioners can employ with their patients to empower them to change their behavior.
- Application goal: Understand how to create a collaborative coach-patient relationship by using the 5-step model.

❑ Discussion Questions:

- What are SMART goals?
- What is motivational interviewing?
- What is the importance of goal-setting in the practice of lifestyle medicine?
- How does the concept of empathy relate to the practice of lifestyle medicine?
- What are strategies for accountability and monitoring?

	TITLE	AUTHORS	JOURNAL	YEAR	KEY FINDINGS
1	Intrinsic and extrinsic motivation for smoking cessation	Curry S, Wagner EH, Grothaus LC	Journal of Consulting and Clinical Psychology	1990	Examined an intrinsic-extrinsic model of motivation for smoking cessation with two samples of smokers who wanted to quit smoking. "Logistic regression analyses indicated that smokers with higher levels of intrinsic relative to extrinsic motivation were more likely to achieve abstinence from smoking."
2	Reasons for quitting: intrinsic and extrinsic motivation for smoking cessation in a population-based sample of smokers	Curry SJ, Grothaus L, McBride C	Addictive Behaviors	1997	Using the validated questionnaire from the study by Dr. Curry (see #1), researchers sampled 1,137 smokers and found that "higher levels of intrinsic relative to extrinsic motivation were associated with more advanced stages of readiness to quit smoking and successful smoking cessation at a 12-month follow up." Furthermore, "improvement in stage of readiness to quit over time was associated with significant increases in health concerns and self-control motivation."
3	The "what" and "why" of goal pursuits: human needs and the self-determination of behavior	Deci EL, Ryan RM	Psychological Inquiry	2000	A discussion of self-determination theory with attention to how needs specify the necessary conditions for psychological growth, integrity, and well-being. It also describes how psychological needs pertain to cultural values, evolutionary processes, and contemporary motivation theories.
4	The five step collaboration cycle: a tool for the doctor's office	Frates EP	International Journal of School and Cognitive Psychology	2015	Discusses patient and physician collaboration using a Five Step Collaboration Cycle: 1) Communication, 2) Empathy, 3) Respect, 4) Mutual Goals, and 5) Mutual Trust.
5	Physicians' empathy and clinical outcomes for diabetic patients	Hojat M, et al.	Academic Medicine: Journal of the Association of American Medical Colleges	2011	Using the Jefferson Scale of Empathy, this study of 29 family physicians and 891 diabetic patients found that: "Patients of physicians with high empathy scores were significantly more likely to have good control of Hemoglobin A1c (56%) than were patients of physicians with low empathy scores (40%, $p<0.001$). Similarly, the proportion of patients with good LDL-C control was significantly higher for physicians with high empathy score (59%) than physicians with low scores (44%, $p<0.001$)."
6	The ABCDs of lifestyle counseling	Lehr AL, Driver SL, Stone NJ	JAMA Cardiology	2016	An overview of lifestyle counseling that advocates using the following framework when counseling: Assess (A), Barriers (B), Commit (C), Demonstrate (D).
7	Motivational interviewing in medical care settings: a systematic review and meta-analysis of randomized controlled trials	Lundahl B, et al.	Patient Education Counseling	2013	A review including 48 studies that analyzed the efficacy of motivational interviewing (MI) in medical care settings. Found a statistically significant, modest advantage for MI. Areas of promise included HIV viral load, dental outcomes, death rate, body weight, alcohol and tobacco use, sedentary behavior, self-monitoring, confidence in change.

Figure 3-4. Goal setting, accountability, and tracking for lifestyle medicine evidence

	TITLE	AUTHORS	JOURNAL	YEAR	KEY FINDINGS
8	Nonverbal interpersonal interactions in clinical encounters and patient perceptions of empathy	Montague E, et al.	*Journal of Participatory Medicine*	2013	This study analyzed 110 videotaped clinical encounters for clinician and patient nonverbal cues and compared the behaviors to patient-completed questionnaires. It found that the "length of visit and eye contact between clinician and patient were positively related to the patient's assessment of the clinician's empathy. Eye contact and social touch were significantly related to patient perceptions of clinician empathy."
9	Effect of a self-determination theory-based communication skills training program on physiotherapists' psychological support for their patients with chronic low back pain: a randomized controlled trial	Murray A, et al.	*Archives of Physical Medicine and Rehabilitation*	2015	A randomized controlled trial involving 24 physiotherapists and 24 patients with chronic low back pain. Half of the physiotherapists received eight hours of communication skills training focused on supporting patients' psychological needs, while the others served as controls. The physiotherapists who received the training were rated by blinded raters to be significantly more supportive of patients' needs than the control physiotherapists.
10	Goal setting as a strategy for dietary and physical activity behavior change: a review of the literature	Shilts M, Horowitz M, Townsend M	*American Journal of Health Promotion*	2004	A literature review including 28 studies that concluded "goal setting has shown some promise in promoting dietary and physical activity behavior change among adults." However, the study was limited by methodological issues with the studies and lack of reported effectiveness from children and adolescent studies.
11	The 12-month effects of early motivational interviewing after acute stroke: a randomized controlled trial	Watkins CL, et al.	*Stroke*	2011	This randomized controlled trial of 411 stroke patients examined whether motivation interviewing can benefit patients' mood and mortality post-stroke. The intervention group consisted of four individual, weekly sessions of motivational interview. At the 12-month follow-up, it found a significant benefit of motivational interviewing over usual stroke care for mood (OR 1.66, CI 1.08-2.55, p=0.020) and mortality (OR 2.14, CI 1.06-4.38, p=0.035).

Figure 3-4. Goal setting, accountability, and tracking for lifestyle medicine evidence. (cont.)

References

1. Curry S, Wagner EH, Grothaus LC. Intrinsic and extrinsic motivation for smoking cessation. *Journal of Consulting and Clinical Psychology*. 1990;58:310-316.
2. Curry SJ, Grothaus L, McBride C. Reasons for quitting: intrinsic and extrinsic motivation for smoking cessation in a population-based sample of smokers. *Addictive Behaviors*. 1997;22:727-739.
3. Deci EL, Ryan RM. The "what" and "why" of goal pursuits: human needs and the self-determination of behavior. *Psychological Inquiry*. 2000;11:227-268.
4. Frates EP. The five step collaboration cycle: a tool for the doctor's office. *International Journal of School and Cognitive Psychology*. 2015;2:3.
5. Hojat M, Louis DZ, Markham FW, et al. Physicians' empathy and clinical outcomes for diabetic patients. *Academic Medicine: Journal of the Association of American Medical Colleges*. 2011;86:359-364.
6. Lehr AL, Driver SL, Stone NJ. The ABCDs of lifestyle counseling. *JAMA Cardiology*. 2016;1(5):505-506. doi:10.1001/jamacardio.2016.1419
7. Lundahl B, Moleni T, Burke BL, et al. Motivational interviewing in medical care settings: a systematic review and meta-analysis of randomized controlled trials. *Patient Education Counseling*. 2013;93:157-168.
8. Montague E, Chen Py, Xu J, et al. Nonverbal interpersonal interactions in clinical encounters and patient perceptions of empathy. *Journal of Participatory Medicine*. 2013;5.
9. Murray A, Hall AM, Williams GC, et al. Effect of a self-determination theory-based communication skills training program on physiotherapists' psychological support for their patients with chronic low back pain: a randomized controlled trial. *Archives of Physical Medicine and Rehabilitation*. 2015;96:809-816.
10. Shilts M, Horowitz M, Townsend M. Goal setting as a strategy for dietary and physical activity behavior change: a review of the literature. *American Journal of Health Promotion*. 2004;19(2):81-93. Available at: http://www.csus.edu/indiv/s/shiltsm/pdf/Goal%20setting%20review%20PDF.pdf. Accessed September 2017.
11. Watkins CL, Wathan JV, Leathley MJ, et al. The 12-month effects of early motivational interviewing after acute stroke: a randomized controlled trial. *Stroke*. 2011;42:1956-1961.

Figure 3-4. Goal setting, accountability, and tracking for lifestyle medicine evidence (cont.)

REFERENCES

- American Heritage Dictionary. Empathy. Available at: https://ahdictionary.com/word/search.html?q=Empathy. Accessed January 2017.
- Ben-Shahar T. *Being Happy: You Don't Have to Be Perfect to Lead a Richer, Happier Life*. New York: McGraw-Hill Education; 2009.
- Ben-Shahar T. *Choose the Life You Want: 101 Ways to Create Your Own Road to Happiness*. New York: The Experiment; 2012.
- Ben-Shahar T. *Even Happier: A Gratitude Journal for Daily Joy and Lasting Fulfillment*. New York: McGraw-Hill; 2010.
- Ben-Shahar T. *Happier: Learn the Secrets to Daily Joy and Lasting Fulfillment*. New York: McGraw-Hill; 2007.
- Centers for Disease Control and Prevention (CDC). The Social-Ecological Model: A Framework for Prevention. Injury Prevention and Control: Division of Violence Prevention. Available at: https://www.cdc.gov/violenceprevention/overview/social-ecologicalmodel.html. Accessed December 2016.
- Cerasoli CP, Nicklin JM, Ford MT. Intrinsic motivation and extrinsic incentives jointly predict performance: a 40-year meta-analysis. *Psychological Bulletin*. 2014;140:980-1008.
- Cooperrider DL, Whitney D. Appreciative inquiry: a positive revolution in change. In: Holman P, Devane T, Cady S, eds. *The Change Handbook: The Definitive Resource on Today's Best Methods for Engaging Whole Systems*. San Francisco: Berrett-Koehler Publishers, Inc.; 2007.
- Covey SR. *The 7 Habits of Highly Effective People*. Revised edition. New York: Free Press; 2004.

- Curry S, Wagner EH, Grothaus LC. Intrinsic and extrinsic motivation for smoking cessation. *Journal of Consulting and Clinical Psychology.* 1990;58:310-316.
- Curry SJ, Grothaus L, McBride C. Reasons for quitting: intrinsic and extrinsic motivation for smoking cessation in a population-based sample of smokers. *Addictive Behaviors.* 1997;22:727-739.
- Deci EL, Ryan RM. *Intrinsic Motivation and Self-Determination in Human Behavior.* New York: Plenum; 1985.
- Deci EL, Ryan RM. The "what" and "why" of goal pursuits: human needs and the self-determination of behavior. *Psychological Inquiry.* 2000;11:227-268.
- Donnan S. What Is Appreciative Inquiry? Metavolution. Available at: http://www.metavolution.com/rsrc/articles/whatis_ai.htm. Accessed December 2016.
- Fraser GE. Vegetarian diets: what do we know of their effects on common chronic diseases? *American Journal of Clinical Nutrition.* 2009;89(5):1607S–1612S. doi:http://dx.doi.org/10.3945/ajcn.2009.26736K.
- Frates EP, Bonnet J. Collaboration and negotiation: the key to therapeutic lifestyle change. *American Journal of Lifestyle Medicine.* 2016;10(5):302-312. https://doi.org/10.1177/1559827616638013.
- Frates EP, et al. Behavior change and nutrition counseling. In: Rippe JM, ed. *Nutrition in Lifestyle Medicine.* Switzerland: Humana Press; 2017:51-84.
- Frates EP, Moore MA, Lopez CN, McMahon GT. Coaching for behavior change in physiatry. *American Journal of Physical Medicine & Rehabilitation.* December 2011;90(12):1074-1082.
- Frates EP. The five step collaboration cycle: a tool for the doctor's office. *International Journal of School and Cognitive Psychology.* 2015;2:3.
- Fredrickson BL. *Positivity.* New York: Crown Archetype; 2009.
- Knowles M. *The Adult Learner: A Neglected Species.* 3rd ed. Houston, TX: Gulf Publishing; 1984.
- Kong A, Bain CE, Beresford SA, Mctiernan A, Jeffery RW, Xiao L, et al. Self-monitoring and eating-related behaviors are associated with 12-month weight loss in postmenopausal overweight-to-obese women. *Journal of the Academy of Nutrition and Dietetics.* 2012;112(9):1428-1435. Available at: http://www.ncbi.nlm.nih.gov/pmc/articles/PMC3432675. Accessed September 2017.
- Kristakis NA, Fowler JH. The spread of obesity in a large social network over 32 years. *New England Journal of Medicine.* 2007;357:370-379.
- Locke EA, Latham GP. *A Theory of Goal Setting & Task Performance.* Englewood Cliffs, NJ: Prentice-Hall, Inc.; 1990.
- Media Health Leaders. Training Physicians for Empathy. Available at: http://www.healthleadersmedia.com/physician-leaders/training-physicians-empathy#. Accessed January 2017.
- Miller WR, Rollnick S. *Motivational Interviewing: Helping People Change.* 3rd ed. New York: The Guilford Press; 2012.

- Montague E, Chen Py, Xu J, Chewning B, Barrett B. Nonverbal interpersonal interactions in clinical encounters and patient perceptions of empathy. *Journal of Participatory Medicine.* 2013;5.
- Park YH, Chang H. Effect of a health coaching self-management program for older adults with multimorbidity in nursing homes. *Patient Preference and Adherence.* 2014;8: 959-970. Available at: http://www.dovepress.com/effect-of-a-health-coaching-self-management-program-for-older-adults-w-peer-reviewed-article-PPA. Accessed September 2017.
- Pollak KI, Alexander SC, Coffman CJ, et al. Physician communication techniques and weight loss in adults: Project CHAT. *American Journal of Preventive Medicine.* 2010;39(4):321-328.
- Riess H. Teaching empathy can improve patient satisfaction. *Vital Signs.* October 2012;8:6.
- Seligman MEP. *Authentic Happiness: Using the New Positive Psychology to Realize Your Potential for Lasting Fulfillment.* New York: Atria Paperback; 2002.
- Seligman ME. *Flourish: A Visionary New Understanding of Happiness and Well-being.* New York: Free Press; 2011.
- Shilts M, Horowitz M, Townsend M. Goal setting as a strategy for dietary and physical activity behavior change: a review of the literature. *American Journal of Health Promotion, Inc.* 2004;19(2):81-93. Available at: http://www.csus.edu/indiv/s/shiltsm/pdf/Goal%20setting%20review%20PDF.pdf. Accessed September 2017.
- Team FME. Pages 8-29. *Effective Goal Setting: Productivity Skills.* 2013. Available at: http://www.free-management-ebooks.com/dldebk-pdf/fme-effective-goal-setting.pdf. Accessed September 2017.
- The Appreciative Way. Appreciative Inquiry and Churches. Available at: https://www.appreciativeway.com/appreciative-inquiry/appreciative-inquiry-church.cfm. Accessed December 2016.
- Tuso PJ, Ismail MH, Ha BP, Bartolotto C. Nutritional update for physicians: plant-based diets. *The Permanente Journal.* 2013;17(2):61-66. doi:10.7812/TPP/12-085.
- Watkins CL, Wathan JV, Leathley MJ, et al. The 12-month effects of early motivational interviewing after acute stroke: a randomized controlled trial. *Stroke.* 2011;42:1956-1961.

CHAPTER 4

IMPROVING HEALTH THROUGH EXERCISE

"Physical fitness is not only one of the most important keys to a healthy body; it is the basis of dynamic and creative intellectual activity."

–John F. Kennedy
35th President of the United States

❏ Chapter Goals:

- Emphasize the health benefits of physical activity on the body and the brain.
- Review the evidence-based guidelines for physical activity levels.
- Consider ways to present physical activity to patients as both doable and enjoyable.

❏ Learning Objectives:

- To review definitions of exercise
- To provide an overview of physical activity guidelines
- To utilize a framework to make exercise prescriptions
- To discuss the benefits and risks of exercise and review the risk stratification system developed by the American College of Sports Medicine

❏ Guiding Questions:

- What are the primary benefits of exercise?
- What are some less commonly known benefits of exercise?
- How does exercise affect the 11 systems of the body?
- What are the risks of exercise?
- Why don't people exercise?
- How can physical activity become part of daily life in the 21st century?
- What is the evidence that physical activity affects health?

❏ Important Terms:

- *Exercise:* Physical activity that is planned or structured. Exercise involves repetitive bodily movements done to improve or maintain one or more of the components of physical fitness.
- *Exercise prescription:* A descriptive recommendation for exercise, entailing frequency, intensity, time, and type of activity or FITT, as well as volume and progression
- *Physical activity:* Any bodily movement produced by skeletal muscles that results in an expenditure of energy
- *Physical fitness:* A set of attributes that people have or achieve that relates to the ability to perform activities of daily living (e.g., cardiorespiratory fitness, muscular fitness, flexibility, and body composition)

All factors considered, the average person has a better chance of living a longer, healthier life than ever before—but only if they take a proactive approach concerning the key factors involved in achieving such a life. Arguably, one of the most documented and widely accepted aspects in that regard is the need to be physically active on a regular basis.

Young or old, male or female, athletic or not, fit or not, the potential benefits of exercise are extensive and pervasive. In fact, there is virtually no one, including individuals suffering from chronic disease, whose life would not be enhanced by exercising on a regular basis. After all, the human body is designed to move.

Given the positive consequences of being physically active, physicians and allied health professionals face several key issues. For example, how can they make their patients appreciate the exercise-health connection? What can they do to get individuals to resist the tide toward a sedentary lifestyle? What can be done to help ensure that their patients will commit to being totally fit?

In reality, a list of the potential strategies for addressing the aforementioned issues is practically endless. Among the more viable steps are the following:

- Be knowledgeable about how exercise impacts the 11 systems of the body.
- Be aware of the numerous benefits of exercise. In other words, be an articulate spokesperson for the exercise-health connection.
- Be effortlessly conversant in the basic components of total fitness—what they are and how they can be developed.
- Be able to assess the basic components of total fitness and use that information to discuss, design, and prescribe a tailored exercise regimen, appropriate for a specific patient.
- Be able to help patients set realistic, appropriate exercise and fitness goals for themselves.
- Be well-informed about the potential downside of exercising too much.
- Be a good listener and value the patient's expertise—their own past efforts, failures, successes, fears, dreams, obstacles, opportunities, and environments.

THE IMPACT OF EXERCISE ON THE 11 SYSTEMS OF THE BODY

The human body has 11 systems that collectively work together to enable individuals to function. Among the more obvious of those functions are breathing, moving, speaking, and digesting food. While the impact of exercise on each of these systems can be an endless source of debate among members of the medical and allied healthcare communities, depending on the specific system being considered, the following information offers a commonly held viewpoint on the subject:

❑ Circulatory System

- What? The circulatory system consists of the heart and blood vessels. Collectively, these tissues facilitate the circulation of blood and transportation of nutrients (e.g., amino acids and electrolytes), oxygen, carbon dioxide, hormones, and blood cells to and from the cells of the body to provide nourishment and help in fighting diseases, stabilizing temperature and pH, and maintaining homeostasis.
- Impact of exercise? Raises the "good" cholesterol (HDL). Reduces the level of bad cholesterol (LDL). Lowers the heart rate (in the long-term). Reduces the level of blood pressure. Protects against heart attacks, strokes, and diabetes.

❑ Digestive System

- What? The digestive system of the body (e.g., mouth, throat, pharynx, esophagus, stomach, small intestine, large intestine, colon, rectum, and anus), working together with the various digestive organs (e.g., liver, gallbladder, and pancreas), converts food into energy, as well as into basic nutrients, to feed the entire body. The digestive system also packages the residue for waste disposal.
- Impact of exercise? Over the long term, regular exercise can relieve constipation and promote healthy digestion while at rest. Furthermore, regular light-to-moderate-intensity exercise can have a protective effect against diverticular disease and colon cancer. However, depending on how close a person eats to when they exercise and what and how much is consumed, exercise can result in digestive symptoms (e.g., loose stools, nausea, vomiting, abdominal pain and cramping, etc.). Because exercise time does not coincide with digestion time, mixing the two can cause uncomfortable results.

❑ Endocrine System

- What? The endocrine system consists of a series of glands (e.g., pituitary, hypothalamus, thyroid, pineal body, adrenals, parathyroids, and pancreas) that secrete hormones. These hormones help regulate certain bodily functions including growth, sexual development, and metabolism.
- Impact of exercise? In the short-term, physical activity facilitates the production of human growth hormone by the pituitary gland, as well as the secretion of hormones

that facilitate movement (e.g., adrenaline, noradrenaline, erythropoietin, etc.). With regard to the endocrine system, exercise also helps lower blood sugar levels and improve insulin levels.

❑ Immune System

- What? The immune system consists of organs, tissues, proteins, and specialized cells that collectively help protect the body from harmful organisms. This system helps prevent infections and keep the body healthy.
- Impact of exercise? There is evidence that suggests that exercise helps to strengthen the body's immune system. Regular, moderate-intensity exercise has been shown to help protect people against some diseases, particularly those that involve the upper respiratory tract, such as the common cold. However, overtraining or strenuous exercise can temporarily suppress immune function, making an individual more susceptible to infectious illnesses.

❑ Dermatologic System

- What? The dermatologic system consists of the skin, hair, nails, and mucous membranes of the body. Collectively, this system serves several key functions, which include regulating body temperature, protecting the body from damage, absorbing nutrients, and maintaining homeostasis. The skin helps the body get rid of sweat and dead skin cells. This system, in conjunction with the nervous system, also allows individuals to experience the sense of touch.
- Impact of exercise? In the short-term, exercise helps to cool the body by enabling heat to dissipate through the pores of the skin when the blood flow to the skin increases. In the long-term, physical activity helps keep the skin looking more youthful, feeling softer, and being more pliable.

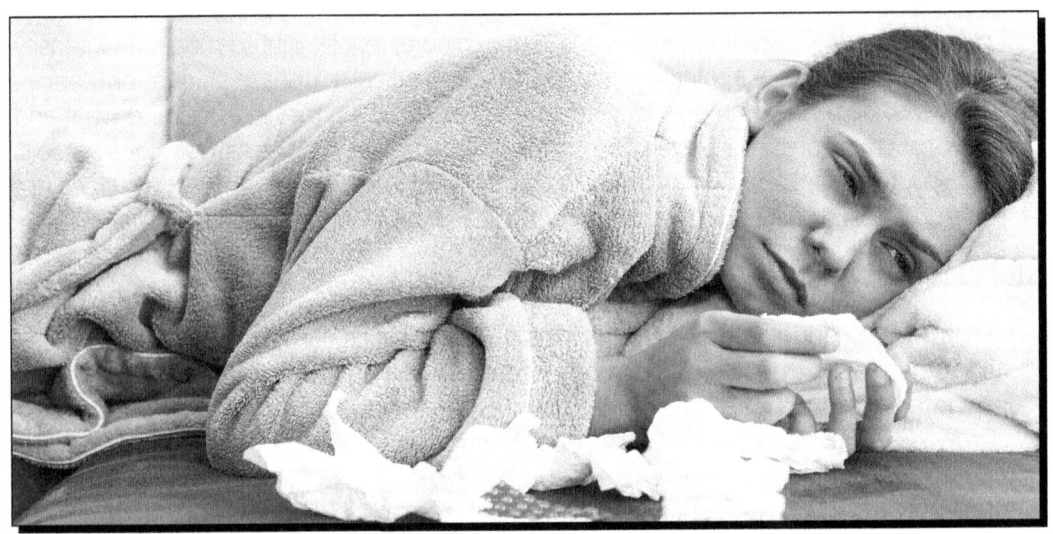

Regular, moderate-intensity exercise has been shown to help protect people against some diseases, particularly those that involve the upper respiratory tract, such as the common cold.

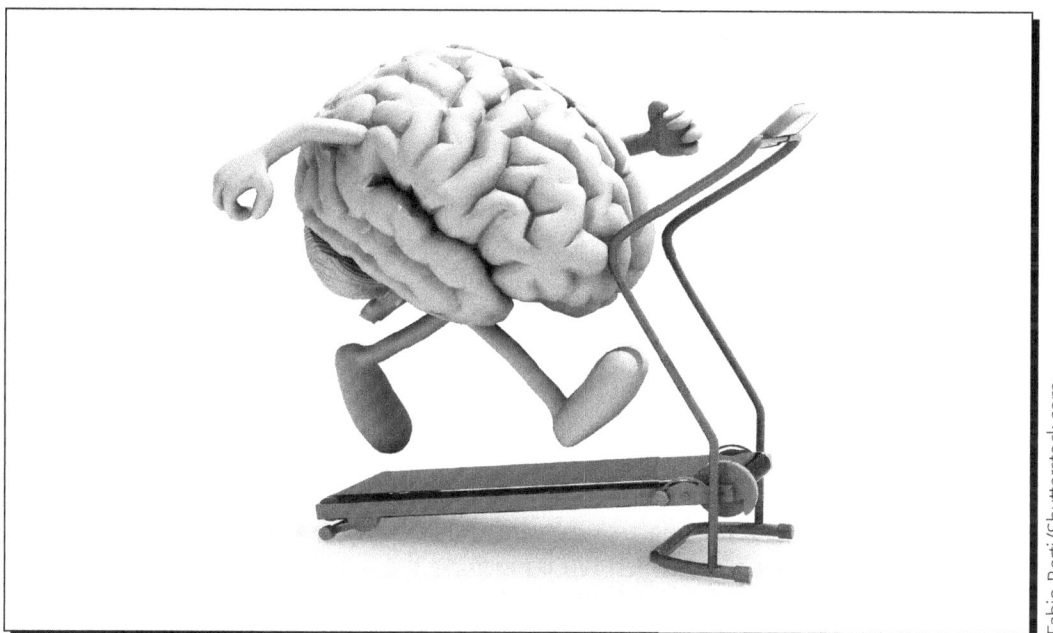

Exercise facilitates the development of new brain cells; increases the number of pathways for oxygen, energy, and the removal of waste products from the brain; improves cognitive function; enhances alertness; and reduces the level of stress

❏ Muscular System

- What? The muscular system consists of three types of muscle: smooth (e.g., pushes food through the digestive tract); cardiac (e.g., helps circulate blood throughout the body by contracting); and skeletal (e.g., supports the body and aids in movement).
- Impact of exercise? In the short-term, the acute stress of exercise coupled with adequate rest, facilitates muscular development and growth. In the long-term, physical activity can strengthen the muscles, as well as develop muscular endurance, depending on the exercise regimen. Exercise can also enhance flexibility when it is performed through a full range of motion. Resistance exercise, along with proper nutrition, can actually increase the size of the body's muscles. Finally, regular exercise can increase the number of mitochondria in the muscle cells of the body. Mitochondria are the powerhouses of the cells that create energy by biochemical processes called cellular respiration. More mitochondria, more energy.

❏ Nervous System

- What? The nervous system of the central nervous system and the peripheral nervous system. The basic role of the central nervous system (brain and spinal cord) is to receive information and transmit instructions. The fundamental job of the peripheral nervous system (the nerves in the body) is to send out messages to other parts of the body.

- Impact of exercise? Helps facilitate the development of new brain cells; increases the number of pathways for oxygen, energy, and the removal of waste products from the brain; improves cognitive function; enhances alertness; and reduces the level of stress.

❑ Reproductive System

- What? The male reproductive system consists of the scrotum, testes, spermatic ducts, sex glands, and penis. Collectively, these male organs work together to produce sperm, the male gamete, and the other components of semen. The female reproductive system consists of ovaries, fallopian tubes, uterus, vagina, vulva, breasts, and mammary glands. Collectively, these female organs are involved in both the production of sex hormones and the transportation of gametes. This system also facilitates the fertilization of ova by sperm, as well as supports the development of the infant during pregnancy and infancy.
- Impact of exercise? Moderate-intensity endurance exercise has been shown to increase sperm quality—speed, shape, and volume. In addition, exercise can work to help dilate blood vessels, which would include those in the penis, which aids with erectile dysfunction. With regard to the female reproductive system, an excessive amount of exercise can lead to a dysfunctional condition referred to as the "female athlete triad," which includes ammenorrhea (not have a period) or oligomenorrhea (few periods), osteopenia (low bone mass) or osteoporosis (extremely low bone density with susceptibility for fractures), and eating disorders (anorexia, low energy availability). On a more constructive note, a moderate level of physical activity has been found to have a positive impact on a woman's reproductive health, including improvements in menstrual cyclicity, ovulation, and fertility.

❑ Respiratory System

- What? The respiratory system consists of the lungs, diaphragm, mouth, trachea, and nose. Collectively, this system controls breathing as a means of transporting oxygen and carbon dioxide in blood in the body to and from muscles and tissues. The lungs expel carbon dioxide and other waste gases.
- Impact of exercise? In the short-term, exercise causes the heart rate to increase. In addition, the rate and depth of breathing are also increased, which helps make certain that more oxygen is absorbed into the blood, as well as that more carbon dioxide is removed from it. Over the long-term, physical activity can also have permanent, positive changes in an exerciser's respiration function, including a slowing of the resting respiration rate, an improved level of air flow volume and lung capacity, and an increased capacity to perform work (e.g., sustained physical activity).

❑ Skeletal System

- What? The skeletal system consists of all of the bones and the network of tissues (ligaments, tendons, and cartilage) that help connect them together. Collectively, the skeletal system performs several essential functions, including supporting the

body, enabling the body to move, protecting the body, producing blood cells, storing calcium, and helping regulate the endocrine system.
- Impact of exercise? In the short-term, exercise increases the amount of an oil-like synovial liquid, which helps to keep the joints healthy, the cartilage from drying out, and the cartilage well-nourished. In the long-term, physical activity can increase the density, size, and weight of bones. This effect not only makes the bones stronger, it also makes them more resistant to injuries and able to recover more quickly after being injured.

❏ Renal/Urinary System

- What? The renal system consists of the kidneys, ureters (tubules from the kidneys to the bladder), bladder and the urethra (tubule from the bladder to excretion). Collectively, these organs work together to rid the body of waste, which is excreted in the form of urine; to help maintain the body's fluid and acid-base balance; to help regulate electrolyte levels in the body; and to secrete several essential hormones. The kidneys remove waste by filtering the blood and expelling waste in the urine.
- Impact of exercise? Exercise affects the urinary system in several important ways, including diminishing the flow of blood to the kidneys (which helps exercisers maintain their level of blood pressure); maintaining fluid balance (which helps the kidneys conserve sodium and reabsorb water, which contributes to a reduction in urine production, stimulating the secretion of the hormones aldosterone and angiotensin II (which are responsible for the restoration of the electrolyte balance in the body following exercise); and helping maintain the appropriate acid-base balance in the body by metabolizing some of the lactic acid that remains in the body following exercise and converting it into glucose (blood sugar). Exercise changes the rate at which the kidneys filter the blood. Exercise also increases sweat levels.

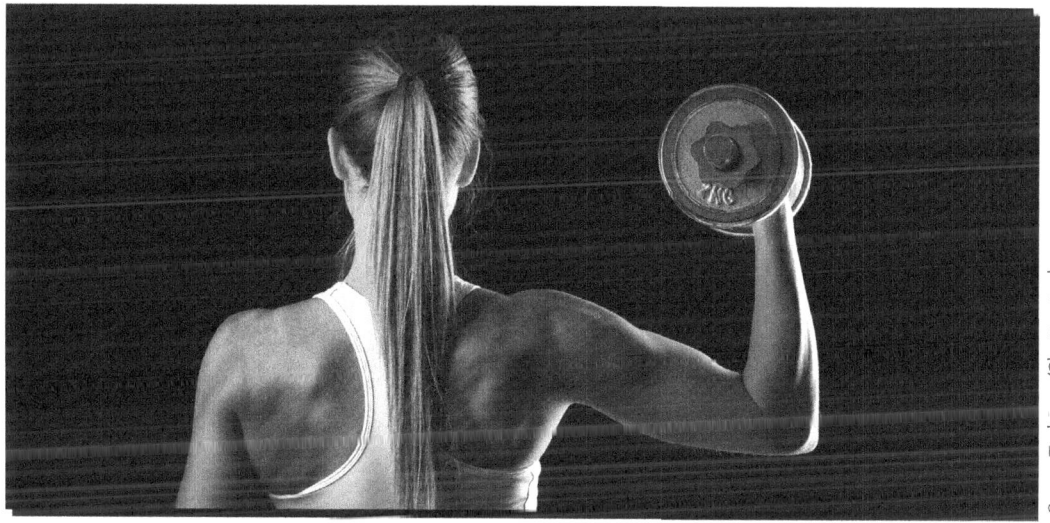

Exercise not only makes the bones stronger, it also makes them more resistant to injuries and able to recover more quickly after being injured.

MORE THAN JUST THE BODY

Most individuals know that exercise is good for the bodily systems, but fewer people appreciate what benefits exercise can have on the mind and psyche. These are the benefits that invite people to really lean in, listen, and learn about the power of exercise, for example, improved sleep, increased interest in sex, relief of stress, better mood, enhanced energy and stamina, reduced tiredness, and more mental alertness.

❑ Depression and Anxiety

There has been a significant amount of research conducted that demonstrates that routine exercise decreases levels of depression and anxiety and also improves quality of life. Studies comparing the use of antidepressants to routine exercise (approximately half an hour a day, five days a week) have shown similar results over the course of six to eight weeks. Both groups experienced a similar increase in serotonin levels (a neurotransmitter that is known to be important in mood balance) and had similar decreases in their depressive symptoms as well. This trial suggests that for some people exercise can be as potent an antidepressant as medication. This scenario sounds familiar.

While the effects of exercise can be quite powerful, it is important to align patient expectations appropriately. For example, an antidepressant typically takes three to four weeks to work. Exercise is similar in that it takes time to fully reap some of the benefits. This factor underscores the importance of sharing this information with patients, so that they understand that a single bout of exercise is not going to change their life, mood, or disease process. It can decrease their state of anxiety after a run or even a walk. One exercise session is a good step in the right direction, but a regular exercise routine is needed to get all of the benefits of physical activity.

❑ BDNF

One mind-exercise benefit that has yet to be well publicized has to do with brain-derived neurotrophic factor (BDNF), a protein produced by the brain. John Ratey, MD, discusses BDNF in his book, *Spark*, and describes it as "Miracle-Gro for the brain," because it combines with hormones to grow brain cells.

A number of years ago, the understanding about the brain was that people were born with a certain number of brain cells, without an ability to gain additional brain cells. Current evidence, however, demonstrates that this situation is not the case, and that people *can* increase their number of brain cells with regular exercise (among other things). Research studies reveal that the hippocampus, a part of the brain involved with consolidating memories and learning, can increase in volume after weeks of regular exercise. This information may be of particular interest to patients, given that many of the older ones are worried about Alzheimer's disease, and the younger ones are concerned about school and work performance. BDNF not only helps generate new brain cells, it also protects and repairs neurons from injury and degeneration.

Numerous studies examining the effect of exercise on cognition show that exercise enhances prefrontal executive functions, such as working memory, spatial awareness, attention, and planning—the higher-level brain processes that make us human. In other words, exercise is essential for optimal brain function throughout a person's lifespan.

❑ Runner's High

A more commonly known exercise benefit is associated with a euphoric type of feeling or what has been termed the "runner's high." Less well known is why this happens. The presumption is that these feelings are related to the endorphins (i.e., feel-good chemicals) that are released during exercise.

Exercise is also associated with the production of alpha waves in the brain, which are linked with a state of relaxation. These alpha waves are often present when people are daydreaming, meditating, practicing mindfulness, or relaxing. Interestingly, alpha waves are also produced after exercise, which may help explain why people report that they feel more creative after a workout.

The brain chemical serotonin is released during exercise, which further enhances mood. In fact, many antidepressants (most notably selective serotonin reuptake inhibitors or SSRIs) work on serotonin receptors to block the re-uptake of serotonin, thereby increasing serotonin levels in the brain.

Antidepressants also work to increase levels of norepinephrine, dopamine, and other natural brain chemicals. Exercise works to increase these brain chemicals as well. By increasing norepinephrine, exercise helps to improve focus and attention. People with ADHD, attention-deficit hyperactivity disorder, often take medications that work, in part, to increase levels of norepinephrine. Thus, exercise acts like another medicine in this capacity.

Finally, dopamine levels are elevated after exercise. Dopamine is associated with reward, motivation, and pleasure. Drugs like cocaine act to increase the release of dopamine, but exercise is a natural way to increase levels of dopamine in the body, and to feel reward, motivation, and pleasure.

Furthermore, exercise is also associated with improved learning and focus. As such, research has found that exercise can have a positive effect on a person's cognitive (brain) function throughout their lifetime. While no one knows for certain why exercise enhances an individual's "brainpower," many professionals believe that this situation is a byproduct of several exercise related factors, including increased circulation in the brain of nutrient-rich blood and the creation of mitochondria—the cellular structures that generate and maintain a person's energy, both in their muscles and in their brain.

UNDERSTANDING THE VALUE OF EXERCISE

❏ A Little Exercise Can and Does Go a Long Way

In reality, deciding whether to start a program of regular exercise is a straightforward decision, if patients are interested in their health, well-being, and appearance. The answers to some simple questions show how relatively easy such a decision should be. Are the benefits of regular exercise worth the time and effort involved? Without question! Can an exercise program be designed that is appropriate to a person's particular interests and needs? Absolutely! How soon will the individual see results? No easy answer to this one. Some bodies respond more quickly than others. The underlying strategy for any exercise regimen should be to design an individualized program, keep track of the exerciser's progress, modify the program to meet the individual's personal needs, and let the body adapt to the exercise the way it has been designed to do for millions of years.

Everyone has seen before-and-after pictures of men and women who turned obese or skinny bodies into healthy, muscular figures. No such changes happen overnight. In reality, a healthy-looking body isn't accomplished merely by thinking, wishing, or praying. It requires that individuals commit to a lifestyle of sound choices regarding their health. It's important to remember that some of the most important outcomes of regular physical activity cannot be seen in the mirror, but rather in how someone feels and functions.

The point to keep in mind is that even small steps can collectively have a major impact on a person's health. Although incremental acts, such as walking during the lunch hour, eating a piece of fruit instead of a candy bar, playing with their kids, etc., can seem inconsequential, eventually, they do make a difference. Accordingly, the sooner an individual gets started on an exercise program, the sooner they will experience the countless benefits of exercising.

As noted previously, regular exercise has been shown to have a positive effect on both the length and the quality of a person's life. In other words, exercising can enable an individual not only to live longer, but live better. The impact of sound exercise on a person's health and sense of well-being is substantial and well documented. For example, exercise can improve an individual's ability to perform activities of daily living, make them think more clearly, improve their ability to maintain their weight at the desired level, improve their mood, and even have a positive impact on their sex life. More importantly, exercise can substantially reduce their risk of contracting certain diseases and medical conditions, all caused by or worsened by being physically inactive.

A report by the United States Department of Health and Human Services, entitled *Physical Activity and Health: A Report of the Surgeon General*, states that "for every hour you exercise, you extend your life by up to two hours." Too many people are simply unaware of the negative consequences of an inactive lifestyle. The value of a sound exercise program goes beyond the fact that it may allow an individual to live longer. In fact, exercise can also affect the quality of a person's life in a number of viable ways.

EXERCISE IS MEDICINE

In 2007, the American Medical Association (AMA) and the American College of Sports Medicine (ACSM) launched the "Exercise is Medicine" campaign. This undertaking was in response to the overwhelming body of evidence that has repeatedly and consistently shown that exercise offers significant mental and physical health benefits. The campaign seeks to encourage healthcare providers to assess the activity level of all patients at every visit, evaluate whether patients are meeting national guidelines for exercise, and briefly counsel patients on exercise. On its website (www.exerciseismedicine.org), the campaign provides tools and protocols that encourage physicians to write exercise prescriptions and counsel patients about exercise. In addition, the website provides stages-of-change protocols that help physicians tailor recommendations to patients' specific stages of change. The Transtheoretical Model of Change (TTM) was reviewed in detail in Chapter 2.

LIVE AND LEARN WITH DR. BETH FRATES

In my practice, I have had a lot of experience working with sedentary patients. I've learned a great deal from these people, and I've also learned that it is effective to counsel patients while we walk, so we both get some exercise.

In particular, I recall an elderly woman who came to see me. During our first walking session, she was aghast when I asked, "What are you doing for exercise these days?" She responded, "Oh, exercise? I don't do that. I was never an athlete. Look at me. This body is not built to exercise. Take a look at this caboose," and she pointed to her derriere. This patient had a sense of humor and was remarkably outgoing.

When I mentioned that walking was indeed exercise, the patient stopped in her tracks. "This is not exercise," she exclaimed. This led us into a conversation about the definitions of exercise and physical activity, as well as the benefits of movement for the body and mind.

By the end of the hour-long walk, the elderly woman said that she could not believe she had walked for an hour. Prior to that visit, the woman had not walked more than five or 10 minutes at a time, and that was only while doing errands in the mall. It wasn't purposeful. The woman reported that she had liked our walk so much that she was going to walk an hour a day, until she saw me again. I immediately recognized that as an overly ambitious goal that was likely to result in failure. I began to negotiate with her to develop a SMART goal that was suitable for her and that she could actually achieve. After negotiation, collaboration, and careful consideration of her schedule, her SMART goal turned out to be walking 30 minutes, three times a week.

MAKING A FIRM COMMITMENT TO TOTAL FITNESS

Obviously, it is not enough merely to be aware of the importance of a physically active lifestyle. In order to receive the vast array of benefits afforded by exercising, a person has to engage in a sound exercise program on a regular basis. In this regard, the essential step that an individual must take is to make a firm commitment to developing "total fitness."

❑ What Is Total Fitness?

Broadly defined, total fitness involves the ability to engage in activities of daily living, without either becoming unduly tired or being injured. If individuals are totally fit, they have the ability to do the necessary and desired activities at work, home, and at play—all without a heightened risk of injury. Collectively, fitness is a by-product of four basic health-related components of fitness—cardiorespiratory fitness, muscular fitness, flexibility, and body composition. In contrast, skill-related components of fitness (i.e., motor skills, such as power, agility, coordination, kinesthetic awareness, balance, quickness, and foot speed) are important for performing athletic-type activities, but have little to do with a person's long-term health (Figure 4-1).

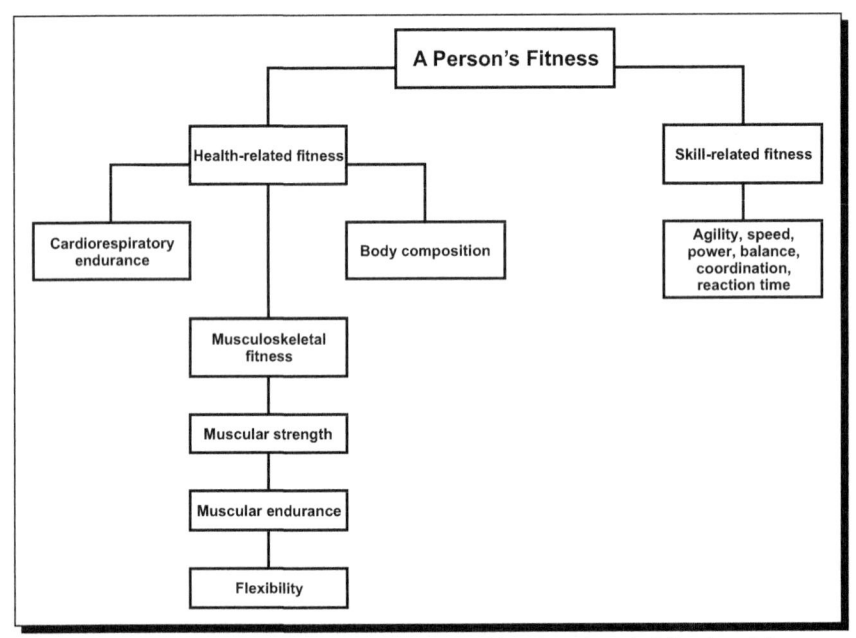

Figure 4-1. "Total fitness" consists of both health-related and skill-related fitness

The health-related components of fitness are those factors that have an impact on an individual's long-term health. Total fitness is attained when all four health components are developed and maintained at an appropriate level. In this regard, the key point to remember is that an individual can be exceptionally fit in three of these components and not be totally fit. Total fitness involves all four fitness elements.

Cardiorespiratory fitness (sometimes referred to as aerobic fitness) is commonly defined as the coordinated ability of the pulmonary system (lungs), cardiovascular system (heart and blood vessels), and metabolic pathways within a person's muscular system to take in, deliver, and utilize oxygen. All factors considered, the more oxygen an individual can take in, deliver, and utilize, the more aerobically fit that person is.

Muscular fitness can best be defined as the ability of the muscles to do what the person wants them to do when they need them to do it. Traditionally, many people view muscular fitness as encompassing two distinct applications of muscular work—muscular strength and muscular endurance. As such, muscular strength is defined as the ability of a muscle or muscle group to exert maximal force. Muscular endurance, on the other hand, can be defined as the ability of a muscle or a muscle group to exert submaximal force for an extended period of time.

Flexibility is generally defined as the ability of a skeletal joint to move through its full range of motion. Range of motion is highly specific to a given joint and is primarily dependent on the musculature that controls the movement of that joint. For example, the ability of a person to be able to scratch the middle of their back is affected by the relative tightness of their shoulder muscles.

The fourth component of total fitness is body composition—a relative indicator of the amount of fat stored in the body. In more specific terms, body composition is defined as the ratio of fat (adipose tissue) to fat-free mass (muscle, bone, water, and protein) in the body. Contrary to what most people believe, it is not how much a person weighs that is important to their health, it's how much fat they have. Considerable evidence shows that in order for a person to be in good health, it is essential that they have an appropriate fat to fat-free mass ratio, since an excessive level of fat has been found to be a significant risk factor for a number of diseases, including coronary heart disease, hypertension, and diabetes. Fat carried in the middle or abdomen is riskier than fat carried in the buttocks. Apple-shaped people are at increased risk for cardiovascular disease compared to pear-shaped people.

While each health component is a distinct entity unto itself, performing activities of daily living usually involves the simultaneous interaction of all four components. As such, a person's life can be viewed as a synergistic environment in which they need each of these components at various times, in varying degrees.

Obviously, how these components interact can vary from task-to-task, individual-to-individual, and situation-to-situation. For example, at a minimum, carrying groceries up several flights of stairs can require both cardiorespiratory fitness and muscular fitness. In turn, putting those groceries away in an overhead cabinet can involve flexibility, as well as muscular fitness.

❏ Making Exercise Work

From a physical and mental health standpoint, a physically active life can easily be distinguished from a sedentary one. Fortunately, a healthier tomorrow is well within an individual's reach. The key is making a commitment to be fit. Such an undertaking can be more easily achieved and maintained, if a person adopts a commonsense approach and starts exercising today (i.e., stop procrastinating); focus on making relatively small changes over time in physical activity patterns; exercise with a partner who can help encourage and provide ongoing support; and make the exercise efforts enjoyable. Exercise does not—should not—have to involve drudgery. In addition, it should be noted that individuals should not punish themselves if they have temporary setbacks in their exercise efforts. Once a person develops an awareness of the need to be totally fit, they will likely find that exercising on a regular basis is one of the best things they've ever done for themselves.

ASSESSING FITNESS

If people want to maximize the body's capacity to withstand the demands imposed upon it by their lifestyle (at work, home, play), they should periodically assess their level of physical fitness. A similar need to assess one's fitness exists for someone who has decided to start exercising.

Although an individual may presuppose a certain level of fitness, a more structured evaluation can offer a quantified basis for deciding whether to take specific steps to remedy a particular functional deficiency. Subsequently, information obtained from such an assessment can also help provide a basis for evaluating how well their conditioning efforts are working.

Medical and allied healthcare professionals should be aware of the fact that it's never too late to test someone. Furthermore, an individual doesn't need to be fit or of a particular age to be tested. If the tests for checking out a patient's level of fitness provide meaningful feedback, that person has everything to gain and nothing to lose.

One of the easiest ways for medical and allied healthcare professionals to set the stage for testing is to ask the individual a series of questions. For example, does the patient have difficulty moving a heavy object from one point to another? Does the patient have the energy to do the things they like to do? Do they have trouble lifting something over their head? Does the patient often suffer from nagging aches and pains? In other words, is the person capable of handling the demands of their lifestyle? To what degree? And based on what assessments and metrics?

Surprisingly enough, the easiest approach to responding to a patient's answers to these questions is relatively straightforward. Once it has been determined how fit a patient is, the medical and allied healthcare professionals can do whatever is necessary, to have that person commit to doing whatever is necessary to improve their level of fitness. Since the methods that can be used to assess an individual's level of fitness vary considerably in their ease of administration, cost, and degree of accuracy, medical and allied healthcare professionals need to carefully consider the testing options they have in their testing toolbox.

❏ What Factors Should Be Tested?

The initial task of medical and allied healthcare professionals should be to determine what factors or measures to test. The most common approach is to separately assess the four basic health-related components of total fitness (cardiorespiratory fitness, muscular fitness, flexibility, and body composition).

❏ Why Should an Individual's Fitness Level Be Assessed?

The results of a patient's fitness assessment efforts can provide medical and allied healthcare professionals with a "sense" of their fitness profile. The test results can also be helpful in other ways. At a minimum, the test scores can be useful in developing a personalized exercise program for the person. Periodic testing can also help the medical or allied healthcare professional to oversee (monitor) the patient's progress in their conditioning regimen and to determine to what degree the patient is achieving their fitness goals. Accordingly, the assessment results can enable the medical or allied healthcare professional to know whether adjustments in the individual's training program need to be made. Patients can also track their progress this way. When they see their fitness level improving, they will likely feel more motivated to continue the program. Finally, the fitness evaluation can provide a patient with a "snapshot" of any fitness-associated issues that they may be facing in later life.

THE KEY TO SUCCESSFUL TESTING

In order to make a person's testing efforts as productive as possible, proven and actionable methods need to be utilized to assess each of the four basic components of total fitness. Then, whatever steps are necessary to ensure that each test is conducted properly need to be followed. It is important to note that if the proper way to perform a specific test is compromised in any way, the usefulness of any information obtained from that test might also be imperiled.

A number of assessment tests and procedures are available to test each component of fitness, some of which include: a submaximal cycle ergometer or treadmill test to evaluate cardiorespiratory fitness; resting and exercise heart rate and blood pressure to ascertain cardiorespiratory fitness; a sit-and-reach test to assess trunk flexibility; tests for both muscular strength (bench press and leg press) and muscular endurance (sit-ups or push-ups); and a body composition evaluation (percentage of body fat and lean muscle mass) by either bioelectrical impedance, skinfold testing, or measuring the circumference of various body areas.

HOW AEROBICALLY FIT IS THE PATIENT?

Cardiorespiratory fitness (commonly referred to as "aerobic fitness") is a reflection of the body's ability to take in, deliver, and utilize oxygen during endurance activities, such as walking, jogging, swimming, and cycling. All factors considered, the better the body's pulmonary system (lungs), cardiovascular system (heart and blood vessels), and metabolic pathways within the body's muscular system accomplish these tasks, the more aerobically fit an individual is.

The most widely accepted measure of aerobic fitness is based on how much physical activity a person can do before they become fatigued. This measure is commonly referred to as an individual's level of maximal oxygen uptake— $\dot{V}O_2$max. Numerous ways exist to determine the $\dot{V}O_2$max, including estimating maximal oxygen uptake, conducting a submaximal test, and predicting maximum from the submaximal data, and measuring the person's maximal performance directly. Typically, $\dot{V}O_2$max testing involves the direct measurement of the gases the individual exhales, while exercising during a submaximal effort. Analyzing the exhaled oxygen and carbon dioxide levels has been shown to provide a very accurate measurement of a person's $\dot{V}O_2$max.

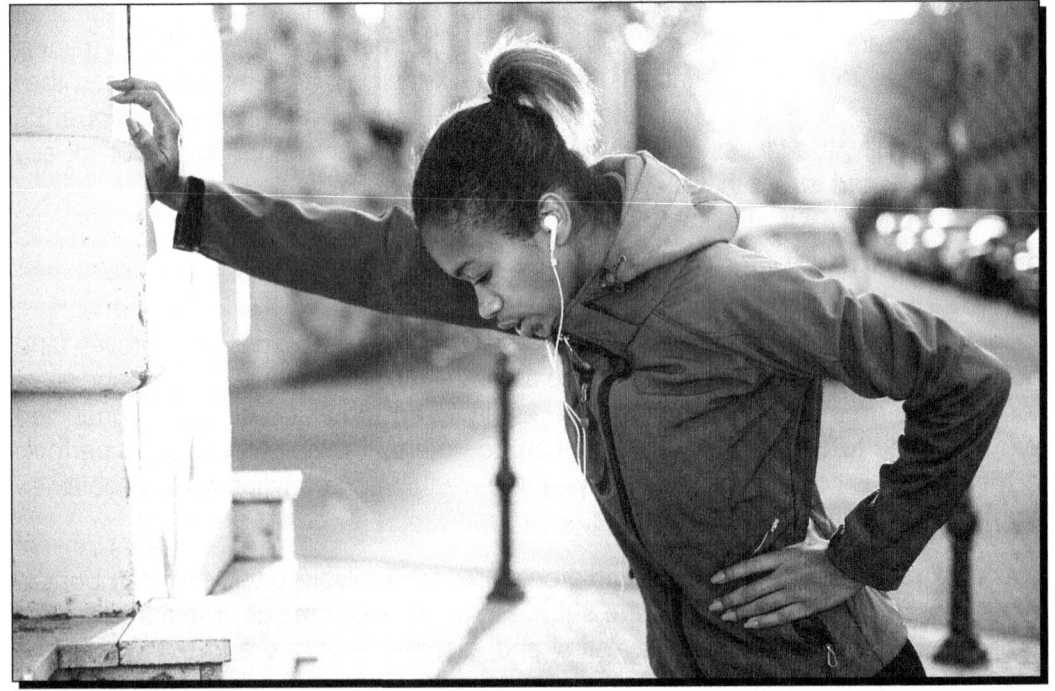

The most widely accepted measure of aerobic fitness is based on how much physical activity a person can do before they become fatigued.

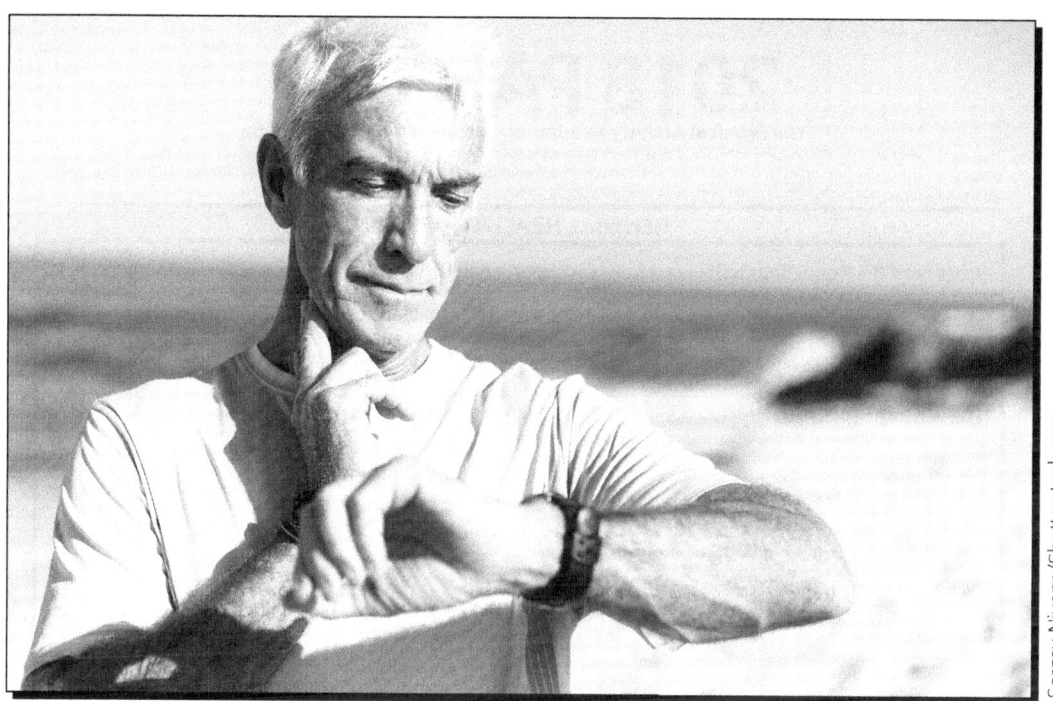

Simple, non-laboratory methods also exist for determining an individual's level of $\dot{V}O_2$max.

Simple, non-laboratory methods also exist for determining an individual's level of $\dot{V}O_2$max. One basic, simplified approach involves predicting a person's $\dot{V}O_2$max on the basis of how well they perform a specific task. For instance, how fast can the person walk or run a specific distance? How much does the person's heart rate change during submaximal exercise? Such fitness testing (and retesting) can also be useful to illustrate gains and improvements that have been made from an individual's particular exercise regimen.

Safety should always be paramount. Prior to taking a physically challenging exercise test, a person should take certain precautions, regardless of whether the testing is to take place in the office of their physician or in a health-related facility or neither. These precautions should involve completing a health/medical questionnaire, having their resting blood pressure and resting heart rate measured, and signing an informed consent form.

One of the most widely used health/medical questionnaires is the Physical Activity Readiness Questionnaire for Everyone (PAR-Q+), a relatively simple, yet quite valid, assessment that is used to screen individuals prior to their undergoing exercise testing or initiating an exercise program (a PAR-Q+ is shown in Figure 4-2). The PAR-Q+ has been widely used over the years to determine whether it is safe for an individual to engage in a physically demanding activity.

2018 PAR-Q+

The Physical Activity Readiness Questionnaire for Everyone

The health benefits of regular physical activity are clear; more people should engage in physical activity every day of the week. Participating in physical activity is very safe for MOST people. This questionnaire will tell you whether it is necessary for you to seek further advice from your doctor OR a qualified exercise professional before becoming more physically active.

GENERAL HEALTH QUESTIONS

Please read the 7 questions below carefully and answer each one honestly: check YES or NO.	YES	NO
1) Has your doctor ever said that you have a heart condition ☐ OR high blood pressure ☐?	☐	☐
2) Do you feel pain in your chest at rest, during your daily activities of living, **OR** when you do physical activity?	☐	☐
3) Do you lose balance because of dizziness **OR** have you lost consciousness in the last 12 months? Please answer **NO** if your dizziness was associated with over-breathing (including during vigorous exercise).	☐	☐
4) Have you ever been diagnosed with another chronic medical condition (other than heart disease or high blood pressure)? **PLEASE LIST CONDITION(S) HERE:** _____	☐	☐
5) Are you currently taking prescribed medications for a chronic medical condition? **PLEASE LIST CONDITION(S) AND MEDICATIONS HERE:** _____	☐	☐
6) Do you currently have (or have had within the past 12 months) a bone, joint, or soft tissue (muscle, ligament, or tendon) problem that could be made worse by becoming more physically active? Please answer **NO** if you had a problem in the past, but it *does not limit your current ability* to be physically active. **PLEASE LIST CONDITION(S) HERE:** _____	☐	☐
7) Has your doctor ever said that you should only do medically supervised physical activity?	☐	☐

If you answered NO to all of the questions above, you are cleared for physical activity.
Please sign the PARTICIPANT DECLARATION. You do not need to complete Pages 2 and 3.

- Start becoming much more physically active – start slowly and build up gradually.
- Follow International Physical Activity Guidelines for your age (www.who.int/dietphysicalactivity/en/).
- You may take part in a health and fitness appraisal.
- If you are over the age of 45 yr and NOT accustomed to regular vigorous to maximal effort exercise, consult a qualified exercise professional before engaging in this intensity of exercise.
- If you have any further questions, contact a qualified exercise professional.

PARTICIPANT DECLARATION
If you are less than the legal age required for consent or require the assent of a care provider, your parent, guardian or care provider must also sign this form.

I, the undersigned, have read, understood to my full satisfaction and completed this questionnaire. I acknowledge that this physical activity clearance is valid for a maximum of 12 months from the date it is completed and becomes invalid if my condition changes. I also acknowledge that the community/fitness centre may retain a copy of this form for records. In these instances, it will maintain the confidentiality of the same, complying with applicable law.

NAME _____ DATE _____
SIGNATURE _____ WITNESS _____
SIGNATURE OF PARENT/GUARDIAN/CARE PROVIDER _____

If you answered YES to one or more of the questions above, COMPLETE PAGES 2 AND 3.

⚠ **Delay becoming more active if:**
- You have a temporary illness such as a cold or fever; it is best to wait until you feel better.
- You are pregnant - talk to your health care practitioner, your physician, a qualified exercise professional, and/or complete the ePARmed-X+ at www.eparmedx.com before becoming more physically active.
- Your health changes - answer the questions on Pages 2 and 3 of this document and/or talk to your doctor or a qualified exercise professional before continuing with any physical activity program.

Copyright © 2018 PAR-Q+ Collaboration   1 / 4
01-11-2017

Reprinted with permission from the PAR-Q+ Collaboration (www.eparmedx.com) and the authors of the PAR-Q+ (Dr. Darren Warburton, Dr. Norman Gledhill, Dr. Veronica Jamnik, Dr. Roy Shephard, and Dr. Shannon Bredin).

Figure 4-2. Physical Activity Readiness Questionnaire for Everyone (PAR-Q+)

2018 PAR-Q+

FOLLOW-UP QUESTIONS ABOUT YOUR MEDICAL CONDITION(S)

1. Do you have Arthritis, Osteoporosis, or Back Problems?
If the above condition(s) is/are present, answer questions 1a-1c   If **NO** ☐ go to question 2

1a. Do you have difficulty controlling your condition with medications or other physician-prescribed therapies? (Answer **NO** if you are not currently taking medications or other treatments)   YES ☐ NO ☐

1b. Do you have joint problems causing pain, a recent fracture or fracture caused by osteoporosis or cancer, displaced vertebra (e.g., spondylolisthesis), and/or spondylolysis/pars defect (a crack in the bony ring on the back of the spinal column)?   YES ☐ NO ☐

1c. Have you had steroid injections or taken steroid tablets regularly for more than 3 months?   YES ☐ NO ☐

2. Do you currently have Cancer of any kind?
If the above condition(s) is/are present, answer questions 2a-2b   If **NO** ☐ go to question 3

2a. Does your cancer diagnosis include any of the following types: lung/bronchogenic, multiple myeloma (cancer of plasma cells), head, and/or neck?   YES ☐ NO ☐

2b. Are you currently receiving cancer therapy (such as chemotherapy or radiotherapy)?   YES ☐ NO ☐

3. Do you have a Heart or Cardiovascular Condition? *This includes Coronary Artery Disease, Heart Failure, Diagnosed Abnormality of Heart Rhythm*
If the above condition(s) is/are present, answer questions 3a-3d   If **NO** ☐ go to question 4

3a. Do you have difficulty controlling your condition with medications or other physician-prescribed therapies? (Answer **NO** if you are not currently taking medications or other treatments)   YES ☐ NO ☐

3b. Do you have an irregular heart beat that requires medical management? (e.g., atrial fibrillation, premature ventricular contraction)   YES ☐ NO ☐

3c. Do you have chronic heart failure?   YES ☐ NO ☐

3d. Do you have diagnosed coronary artery (cardiovascular) disease and have not participated in regular physical activity in the last 2 months?   YES ☐ NO ☐

4. Do you have High Blood Pressure?
If the above condition(s) is/are present, answer questions 4a-4b   If **NO** ☐ go to question 5

4a. Do you have difficulty controlling your condition with medications or other physician-prescribed therapies? (Answer **NO** if you are not currently taking medications or other treatments)   YES ☐ NO ☐

4b. Do you have a resting blood pressure equal to or greater than 160/90 mmHg with or without medication? (Answer **YES** if you do not know your resting blood pressure)   YES ☐ NO ☐

5. Do you have any Metabolic Conditions? *This includes Type 1 Diabetes, Type 2 Diabetes, Pre-Diabetes*
If the above condition(s) is/are present, answer questions 5a-5e   If **NO** ☐ go to question 6

5a. Do you often have difficulty controlling your blood sugar levels with foods, medications, or other physician-prescribed therapies?   YES ☐ NO ☐

5b. Do you often suffer from signs and symptoms of low blood sugar (hypoglycemia) following exercise and/or during activities of daily living? Signs of hypoglycemia may include shakiness, nervousness, unusual irritability, abnormal sweating, dizziness or light-headedness, mental confusion, difficulty speaking, weakness, or sleepiness.   YES ☐ NO ☐

5c. Do you have any signs or symptoms of diabetes complications such as heart or vascular disease and/or complications affecting your eyes, kidneys, **OR** the sensation in your toes and feet?   YES ☐ NO ☐

5d. Do you have other metabolic conditions (such as current pregnancy-related diabetes, chronic kidney disease, or liver problems)?   YES ☐ NO ☐

5e. Are you planning to engage in what for you is unusually high (or vigorous) intensity exercise in the near future?   YES ☐ NO ☐

Copyright © 2018 PAR-Q+ Collaboration   2 / 4
01-11-2017

Reprinted with permission from the PAR-Q+ Collaboration (www.eparmedx.com) and the authors of the PAR-Q+ (Dr. Darren Warburton, Dr. Norman Gledhill, Dr. Veronica Jamnik, Dr. Roy Shephard, and Dr. Shannon Bredin).

Figure 4-2. Physical Activity Readiness Questionnaire for Everyone (PAR-Q+) (cont.)

2018 PAR-Q+

6. **Do you have any Mental Health Problems or Learning Difficulties?** *This includes Alzheimer's, Dementia, Depression, Anxiety Disorder, Eating Disorder, Psychotic Disorder, Intellectual Disability, Down Syndrome*

If the above condition(s) is/are present, answer questions 6a-6b   If **NO** ☐ go to question 7

6a. Do you have difficulty controlling your condition with medications or other physician-prescribed therapies? (Answer **NO** if you are not currently taking medications or other treatments)   YES ☐ NO ☐

6b. Do you have Down Syndrome **AND** back problems affecting nerves or muscles?   YES ☐ NO ☐

7. **Do you have a Respiratory Disease?** *This includes Chronic Obstructive Pulmonary Disease, Asthma, Pulmonary High Blood Pressure*

If the above condition(s) is/are present, answer questions 7a-7d   If **NO** ☐ go to question 8

7a. Do you have difficulty controlling your condition with medications or other physician-prescribed therapies? (Answer **NO** if you are not currently taking medications or other treatments)   YES ☐ NO ☐

7b. Has your doctor ever said your blood oxygen level is low at rest or during exercise and/or that you require supplemental oxygen therapy?   YES ☐ NO ☐

7c. If asthmatic, do you currently have symptoms of chest tightness, wheezing, laboured breathing, consistent cough (more than 2 days/week), or have you used your rescue medication more than twice in the last week?   YES ☐ NO ☐

7d. Has your doctor ever said you have high blood pressure in the blood vessels of your lungs?   YES ☐ NO ☐

8. **Do you have a Spinal Cord Injury?** *This includes Tetraplegia and Paraplegia*

If the above condition(s) is/are present, answer questions 8a-8c   If **NO** ☐ go to question 9

8a. Do you have difficulty controlling your condition with medications or other physician-prescribed therapies? (Answer **NO** if you are not currently taking medications or other treatments)   YES ☐ NO ☐

8b. Do you commonly exhibit low resting blood pressure significant enough to cause dizziness, light-headedness, and/or fainting?   YES ☐ NO ☐

8c. Has your physician indicated that you exhibit sudden bouts of high blood pressure (known as Autonomic Dysreflexia)?   YES ☐ NO ☐

9. **Have you had a Stroke?** *This includes Transient Ischemic Attack (TIA) or Cerebrovascular Event*

If the above condition(s) is/are present, answer questions 9a-9c   If **NO** ☐ go to question 10

9a. Do you have difficulty controlling your condition with medications or other physician-prescribed therapies? (Answer **NO** if you are not currently taking medications or other treatments)   YES ☐ NO ☐

9b. Do you have any impairment in walking or mobility?   YES ☐ NO ☐

9c. Have you experienced a stroke or impairment in nerves or muscles in the past 6 months?   YES ☐ NO ☐

10. **Do you have any other medical condition not listed above or do you have two or more medical conditions?**

If you have other medical conditions, answer questions 10a-10c   If **NO** ☐ read the Page 4 recommendations

10a. Have you experienced a blackout, fainted, or lost consciousness as a result of a head injury within the last 12 months **OR** have you had a diagnosed concussion within the last 12 months?   YES ☐ NO ☐

10b. Do you have a medical condition that is not listed (such as epilepsy, neurological conditions, kidney problems)?   YES ☐ NO ☐

10c. Do you currently live with two or more medical conditions?   YES ☐ NO ☐

PLEASE LIST YOUR MEDICAL CONDITION(S) AND ANY RELATED MEDICATIONS HERE: _____

GO to Page 4 for recommendations about your current medical condition(s) and sign the PARTICIPANT DECLARATION.

Copyright © 2018 PAR-Q+ Collaboration
01-11-2017

Reprinted with permission from the PAR-Q+ Collaboration (www.eparmedx.com) and the authors of the PAR-Q+ (Dr. Darren Warburton, Dr. Norman Gledhill, Dr. Veronica Jamnik, Dr. Roy Shephard, and Dr. Shannon Bredin).

Figure 4-2. Physical Activity Readiness Questionnaire for Everyone (PAR-Q+) (cont.)

Lifestyle Medicine Handbook

2018 PAR-Q+

☑ **If you answered NO to all of the FOLLOW-UP questions (pgs. 2-3) about your medical condition, you are ready to become more physically active - sign the PARTICIPANT DECLARATION below:**
- It is advised that you consult a qualified exercise professional to help you develop a safe and effective physical activity plan to meet your health needs.
- You are encouraged to start slowly and build up gradually - 20 to 60 minutes of low to moderate intensity exercise, 3-5 days per week including aerobic and muscle strengthening exercises.
- As you progress, you should aim to accumulate 150 minutes or more of moderate intensity physical activity per week.
- If you are over the age of 45 yr and **NOT** accustomed to regular vigorous to maximal effort exercise, consult a qualified exercise professional before engaging in this intensity of exercise.

◯ **If you answered YES to one or more of the follow-up questions** about your medical condition:
You should seek further information before becoming more physically active or engaging in a fitness appraisal. You should complete the specially designed online screening and exercise recommendations program - the **ePARmed-X+ at www.eparmedx.com** and/or visit a qualified exercise professional to work through the ePARmed-X+ and for further information.

⚠ **Delay becoming more active if:**
- You have a temporary illness such as a cold or fever; it is best to wait until you feel better.
- You are pregnant - talk to your health care practitioner, your physician, a qualified exercise professional, and/or complete the ePARmed-X+ **at www.eparmedx.com** before becoming more physically active.
- Your health changes - talk to your doctor or qualified exercise professional before continuing with any physical activity program.

- You are encouraged to photocopy the PAR-Q+. You must use the entire questionnaire and NO changes are permitted.
- The authors, the PAR-Q+ Collaboration, partner organizations, and their agents assume no liability for persons who undertake physical activity and/or make use of the PAR-Q+ or ePARmed-X+. If in doubt after completing the questionnaire, consult your doctor prior to physical activity.

PARTICIPANT DECLARATION
- All persons who have completed the PAR-Q+ please read and sign the declaration below.
- If you are less than the legal age required for consent or require the assent of a care provider, your parent, guardian or care provider must also sign this form.

I, the undersigned, have read, understood to my full satisfaction and completed this questionnaire. I acknowledge that this physical activity clearance is valid for a maximum of 12 months from the date it is completed and becomes invalid if my condition changes. I also acknowledge that the community/fitness center may retain a copy of this form for records. In these instances, it will maintain the confidentiality of the same, complying with applicable law.

NAME _____ DATE _____

SIGNATURE _____ WITNESS _____

SIGNATURE OF PARENT/GUARDIAN/CARE PROVIDER _____

For more information, please contact
www.eparmedx.com
Email: eparmedx@gmail.com

Citation for PAR-Q+
Warburton DER, Jamnik VK, Bredin SSD, and Gledhill N on behalf of the PAR-Q+ Collaboration. The Physical Activity Readiness Questionnaire for Everyone (PAR-Q+) and Electronic Physical Activity Readiness Medical Examination (ePARmed-X+). Health & Fitness Journal of Canada 4(2):3-23, 2011.

Key References
1. Jamnik VK, Warburton DER, Makarski J, McKenzie DC, Shephard RJ, Stone J, and Gledhill N. Enhancing the effectiveness of clearance for physical activity participation; background and overall process. APNM 36(S1):S3-S13, 2011.
2. Warburton DER, Gledhill N, Jamnik VK, Bredin SSD, McKenzie DC, Stone J, Charlesworth S, and Shephard RJ. Evidence-based risk assessment and recommendations for physical activity clearance; Consensus Document. APNM 36(S1):S266-S298, 2011.
3. Chisholm DM, Collis ML, Kulak LL, Davenport W, and Gruber N. Physical activity readiness. British Columbia Medical Journal. 1975;17:375-378.
4. Thomas S, Reading J, and Shephard RJ. Revision of the Physical Activity Readiness Questionnaire (PAR-Q). Canadian Journal of Sport Science 1992;17:4 338-345.

The PAR-Q+ was created using the evidence-based AGREE process (1) by the PAR-Q+ Collaboration chaired by Dr. Darren E. R. Warburton with Dr. Norman Gledhill, Dr. Veronica Jamnik, and Dr. Donald C. McKenzie (2). Production of this document has been made possible through financial contributions from the Public Health Agency of Canada and the BC Ministry of Health Services. The views expressed herein do not necessarily represent the views of the Public Health Agency of Canada or the BC Ministry of Health Services.

Copyright © 2018 PAR-Q+ Collaboration 4 / 4
01-11-2017

Reprinted with permission from the PAR-Q+ Collaboration (www.eparmedx.com) and the authors of the PAR-Q+ (Dr. Darren Warburton, Dr. Norman Gledhill, Dr. Veronica Jamnik, Dr. Roy Shephard, and Dr. Shannon Bredin).

Figure 4-2. Physical Activity Readiness Questionnaire for Everyone (PAR-Q+) (cont.)

> **PAR-Q+ Citations:**
>
> Warburton DER, Jamnik VK, Bredin SSD, Shephard RJ, Gledhill N. The 2017 Physical Activity Readiness Questionnaire for Everyone (PAR-Q+) and electronic Physical Activity Readiness Medical Examination (ePARmed-X+). *Health & Fitness Journal of Canada* 2017;10(1):29-32.
>
> Warburton DER, Gledhill N, Jamnik VK, Bredin SSD, McKenzie DC, Stone J, Charlesworth S, Shephard RJ, on behalf of the PAR-Q+ Collaboration. The Physical Activity Readiness Questionnaire for Everyone (PAR-Q+) and electronic Physical Activity Readiness Medical Examination (ePARmed-X+): Summary of consensus panel recommendations. *Health & Fitness Journal of Canada* 2011;4:26-37.

Figure 4-2. Physical Activity Readiness Questionnaire for Everyone (PAR-Q+) (cont.)

A "no" answer to all of the seven questions on the PAR-Q+ questionnaire indicates that the individual has been cleared to engage in physical activity. In turn, a "yes" answer to one or more of those questions requires the individual to complete the series of follow-up questions that are detailed on pages 2 and 3 of the PAR-Q+. Based on the person's responses to those follow-up queries, guidelines about what to do next are listed on page 4.

Assessing aerobic fitness in a non-medical setting can vary somewhat from the testing that may be undertaken in a physician's office. Since laboratory testing of aerobic fitness is not cost-effective for the majority of individuals, several tests to predict $\dot{V}O_2$max have been developed that can be utilized in almost any setting. Among the more commonly employed tests are performance-based measures and tests that use a person's heart rate response to a submaximal walking or running exercise bout as the primary indicator.

HOW MUSCULARLY FIT IS THE PATIENT?

Daily living activities (at home, work, and play) require an individual to use their muscles. The muscles must be capable of doing particular movements on command for a particular duration of time. without sustaining an injury. This capability is typically referred to as muscular fitness.

A number of professionals in both the medical and the exercise science communities consider muscular fitness a combination of two distinct attributes: muscular strength and muscular endurance. Muscular strength is the ability of a muscle or a muscle group to exert a short-term maximum force, while muscular endurance, on the other hand, is the ability of a muscle or a muscle group to exert submaximal force for an extended period of time. Accordingly, the first step in assessing muscular fitness involves identifying which capability of muscular fitness is to be measured—strength or endurance.

Generally, muscular fitness is assessed using tests that either employ specific devices for measuring muscular strength and muscular endurance or involve performing calisthenic-type exercises. Calisthenic-type tests typically require little or no equipment, can be performed almost anywhere, and involve bodily movements that are somewhat more functional in nature.

Given the fact that individuals have their own unique genetic potential for achieving and demonstrating muscular fitness, comparing the muscular fitness assessment results of one person to another is of questionable value. A more logical approach would be to compare the results of muscular fitness testing to previous performances. Even accounting for the occasional glitch in testing results that might be attributed to emotional or physical factors, comparing the results of an individual's assessment efforts with their prior test scores should provide physicians and allied healthcare professionals with a reasonable basis for measuring the progress of their training efforts over time.

HOW FLEXIBLE IS THE PERSON?

Flexibility is the capacity of a skeletal joint to move through its full range of motion. This health-related fitness component is important for a number of reasons—not the least of which is that, all factors considered, a flexible muscle is less likely to be pulled or strained or to place undue pressure on a particular area of the body (e.g., the lower back, shoulders, etc.). The flexibility of a person is related to the relative "tightness" of the various soft tissues of their skeletal joints (joint capsule, muscles, tendons, ligaments). The musculature supporting a specific joint is the primary factor affecting how well that joint can move through its full range of motion.

The analogy of a muscle being like a rubber band can help explain a muscle's effect on the flexibility level of one of the body's skeletal joints. If someone pulls a little on the rubber band and then lets go, a certain amount of movement and energy is created. If, in contrast, someone pulls a lot, even greater movement and energy occur. On the other hand, if the person pulls too much or can't pull it at all, the rubber band (muscle) will either break or fail to generate any movement or energy at all.

Because flexibility is specific to a given joint, no general flexibility test exists for the total body. As a consequence, flexibility needs to be assessed separately for each of a patient's skeletal joints. Flexibility is sometimes assessed through a medical device specifically designed to measure the range of motion of a particular joint (using an instrument referred to as a goniometer). More typically, individuals tested in a health club setting, for example, often use a device called a sit-and-reach box, which allows the linear measurement of a joint's range of motion specific to the level of flexibility in the spine and posterior hip and leg muscles. This test is completed with an individual seated on the floor with their legs together, flat against the floor, and the toes of both feet pointing straight up in the air. The individual then tries to lean forward as far as possible, and a measurement is taken as to how far—either away from or past the toes—the person can reach.

HOW MUCH FAT IS TOO MUCH FAT?

Having an appropriate level of body composition (i.e., the ratio of fat to fat-free mass in the body) is important to a patient for a number of reasons—some physical, some mental. An excessive level of fat has been shown to be a major cause of several diseases, including diabetes, cardiovascular disease, and cancers. Too much body fat can also have a negative impact on self-perception and an individual's ability to interact with others in a social setting.

Perhaps, the most commonly employed and certainly one of the easiest methods for determining a person's relative level of body composition is for that individual to simply look at themselves in a full-length mirror, without any clothes on. This simple self-screen can help indicate whether the person may have too much fat on their body.

Quantitatively, body composition can be measured with a variety of methods. The most practical method of assessing body composition is to use one of the several non-laboratory options (e.g., skinfold testing, circumference measurements, bioelectrical impedance, waist-to-hip ratio, etc.):

❑ Skinfold Testing

Skinfold testing involves measuring the amount of skin and fat just beneath the skin at any given location on a person's body. This test is conducted by pinching the skin at a pre-selected site (everything but muscle) and then measuring the thickness of the pinch. Whoever is taking skinfold or circumference measurements should have practiced repeatedly to ensure accurate and reliable technique. Furthermore, any retesting should be conducted by the same individual.

The data from pre-selected skinfold site pinches (triceps, chest, abdomen, thigh) is then factored into specific equations that are designed to calculate a person's level of body composition. A number of different skinfold test equations exist. When working with someone to decide whether to use a particular equation, it should be noted that most equations are gender- and age-specific and are designed to be employed only with a population similar to that from which they were derived.

Each equation is based on data collected from specific body sites and requires precise techniques for measuring the skinfolds at each site. Even when performed by a trained health/wellness professional, with years of experience, for example, skinfold technique error rates can be as high as three to five percent. With an untrained professional or an individual with little experience, the skinfold technique is simply ineffective.

❑ Circumference Measurements

According to the circumference method for estimating percent body fat, large circumferences at certain sites on the body (e.g., waist, hips, etc.) indicate a higher level of percent body fat, while large circumferences at other sites (e.g., the neck) indicate a lower level of percent body fat. A number of equations employ circumference measurements, which are typically made with a cloth measuring tape that does not stretch when pulled. Each equation involves specific measurements and detailed techniques for taking those measurements. In general, calculated body fat percentage of 31 and 25, for women and men respectively, are considered acceptable.

❑ Bioelectrical Impedance Analysis

Bioelectrical impedance analysis (BIA), which is the preferred methodology to assess body fat level for some professionals, is based upon the principle that the conductivity of an electrical impulse is greater through lean muscle mass than fatty tissue. When a miniscule electrical charge is sent through the body, a computer measures the resistance between electrodes and computes body density, and therefore body composition. A device is required to measure body fat percentage using BIA. Although every one of these devices uses the same basic method, they range in price from less than $50 each to the tens of thousands of dollars. Purchase decisions are based on the features desired.

❑ Waist-to-Hip Ratio

A relatively easy-to-perform field test of a patient's fat distribution pattern is that person's waist-to-hip ratio (WHR). Simply stated, this ratio compares the narrowest portion of an individual's waist (the circumference of their body measured at the level of their navel) to the widest area of their hips (the circumference of their body measured at the largest protrusion of their buttocks). The larger the ratio, the higher the level of fat deposited on the waist. In turn, the larger the ratio, the higher the patient's risk of certain medical problems. A cut-off ratio of 0.80 for men and 0.95 for women has been established as the maximal WHR limit, above which the risk for heart disease becomes substantially higher. Waist circumference, alone, should be at or below 40 inches for men and 35 inches for women.

Many researchers have concluded that a person's level of percent body fat is probably not as important as where the fat is located on an individual's body. Collectively, where the fat is deposited on the body is often referred to as fat patterning. An individual's fat distribution patterns can predict the susceptibility to certain medical problems. Fat stored in the abdominal region, for example, as opposed to the legs, hips, and arms, indicates susceptibility to coronary disease, diabetes, and high blood pressure.

Fat patterning can also categorize individuals according to the "shape" of their bodies. For example, if a person tends to store excess fat on their chest and stomach areas (a characteristic of males), that individual is termed an "apple" (because an apple is wider at the top than at the bottom). If, on the other hand, the individual has excess fat below the waist (an attribute of women), that person is referred to as a "pear" (since a pear is wider at the bottom than at the top).

SETTING EXERCISE GOALS

Once it has been determined how fit a patient is, the logical next step is for the medical or allied healthcare professional to help that individual decide what goals they would like to achieve from the exercise efforts. Identifying a person's fitness goals provides a basis for determining what activities should be part of an individual's exercise regimen and also helps set up criteria for evaluating how well the program is working. It should be strongly emphasized to the patient that it didn't take two weeks for them to get into their current level of condition. Therefore, the hope to get "in shape" in two weeks is unrealistic.

Establishing an individual's personal fitness goals can be beneficial in other ways, as well. For example, determining the objectives a person plans to accomplish by exercising can help provide that individual with the motivation to make meaningful changes in physical activity level and to stick with those changes. On the other hand, knowing their fitness level is usually not enough. It is a good idea for people to explore where they want to be before creating a "road map." As such, the exercise program goals can help serve as the directional bridge between "what is" and "what can ultimately be," with regard to a person's level of fitness and health.

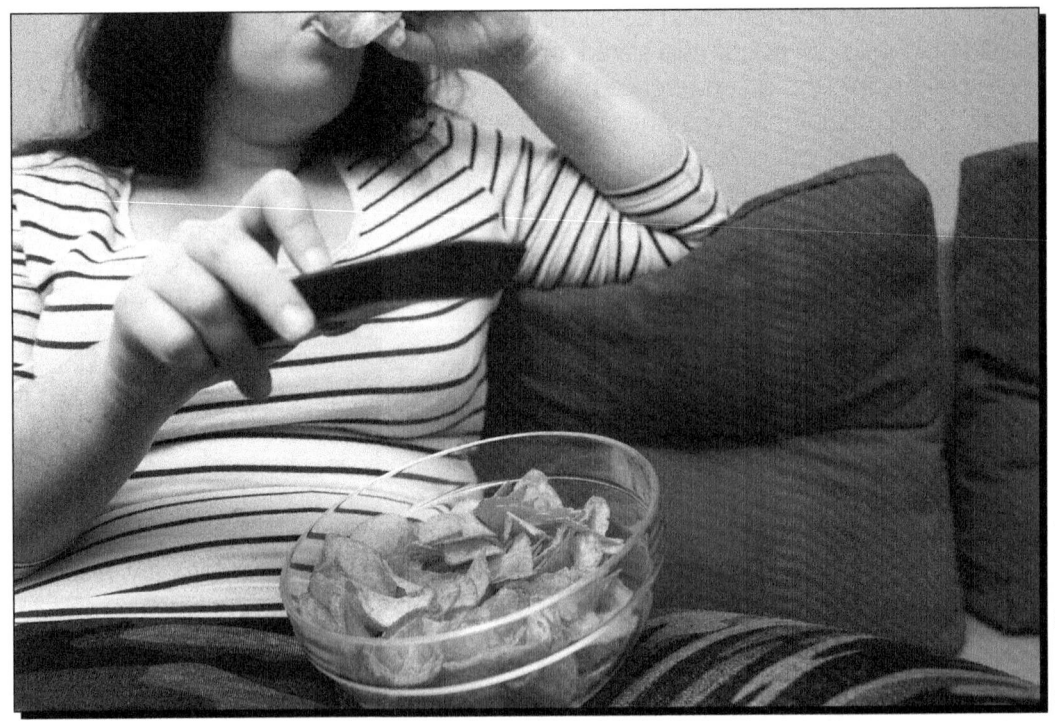

It should be strongly emphasized to the patient that it didn't take two weeks for them to get into their current level of condition. Therefore, the hope to get "in shape" in two weeks is unrealistic.

❏ What Is a Fitness Goal?

A fitness goal is simply a statement of results that a person wants to achieve from an exercise program. Establishing a fitness goal involves identifying some specific measurable accomplishment one hopes to achieve within specific time and resource constraints. Such an objective should address the following four major elements:
- An action or accomplishment verb
- A single, measurable, significant result
- A time period or date within which or by which the result is to be achieved
- The outlay of resources (time, money, etc.) that an individual expects or is willing to commit to making the desired result a reality

Using the aforementioned model as a guideline, the physician or allied healthcare professional can help a patient construct a fitness goal that will meet their unique objectives and situation, for example:
- To lose eight pounds within 30 days by monitoring dietary intake and working out on a treadmill three times per week, 20 minutes per session
- To lower blood pressure to within a normal range within six months by stopping smoking, making a conscious effort to eat a healthier diet, and exercising regularly at least four times a week for a minimum of 30 minutes per session
- To be able to do at least 10 properly performed push-ups non-stop by next year by engaging in a sound, total-body strength-training workout

It should be noted that none of the three aforementioned sample personal fitness goals includes a justification for its existence or a precise description of how it should be accomplished. As a rule, a fitness goal identifies only what, when, and how much exercise is involved. The "why" comes before, and the prescription for "how" comes afterward.

❏ How Should Fitness Goals Be Set?

Deciding what a person should achieve from their exercise efforts is a relatively personal matter. Obviously, a patient can and should consider feedback from someone who has both the training and the experience to give thoughtful advice. With regard to goal setting, the most commonly used technique is the SMART approach (which was discussed in Chapter 3). This practical acronym offers five basic criteria that each of a patient's fitness goals should meet:
- Specific: Each of a patient's fitness goals needs to identify exactly what objective they hope to achieve by exercising on a regular basis. Although an individual can have more than one goal, each particular goal should specify a single key result to be accomplished (e.g., lose weight, develop strength, lower resting heart rate, etc.). As such, each exerciser should be able to look at the one key objective and tell the extent to which the goal has been achieved.

- Measurable: Whenever possible, through the use of numbers or percentages, an individual's fitness goals should be quantitatively expressed (e.g., lose 10 pounds, bench press their body weight, lower their resting heart rate at least 5 bpm, etc.). Quantifying goals makes it easier to determine the relative extent to which a particular person's exercise efforts are successful.
- Action-oriented (and appropriate): Fitness goals are generally action-oriented. It is also critical to make sure that the goals are appropriate. Fitness goals should be appropriate to an individual's personal interests and needs. At the least, none of a patient's fitness goals should expose that individual to an undue likelihood of doing anything that might otherwise subject them to any injury or health problem (e.g., losing too much weight, losing a significant amount of weight too fast, placing too much stress on their joints, etc.). The point to keep in mind is that while a particular objective may be achievable, the objective itself may not be, in all instances, appropriate for an individual personally.
- Realistic: Since a fitness goal can and should serve as a source of motivation for a patient, it should be one that is within a person's reach, yet not too easy to accomplish. A goal that is well beyond an individual's reach can foster a negative attitude toward the exercise program and can diminish their desire to stick with the exercise regimen. On the other hand, all factors considered, a person can be better served if their fitness goals represent a meaningful challenge. Such intangibles as "meeting a challenge head on," "pride of accomplishment," "paying the price," etc. can have a positive impact on the effort expended to accomplish a fitness goal.
- Time-sensitive: A specific date or period of time for achieving a patient's fitness goal should be established. If individuals have multiple fitness goals, a timeline for accomplishing each particular goal should be created. From a practical standpoint, patients must be prepared to adjust the proposed schedules for achieving their fitness goals as circumstances change or as they develop a clearer, more realistic understanding of exactly what can be accomplished within a given time period.

The process of establishing fitness goals can be further enhanced if an individual takes three additional steps: write down the goals; if the goal is intangible, identify measurable indices that can provide a reliable indicator of progress toward achieving that goal; and confirm that the fitness goals are "big enough."

Because individuals tend to remember those things that turn out well and either forget or modify those things that are less than they had hoped, the patient should record their goals in writing. Written goals can serve as a constant reminder and provide patients with an effective tracking device to measure the progress of their exercise efforts.

If, for any reason, individuals want to achieve an intangible objective from the exercise program, they must establish measurable sub-objectives that might otherwise indicate whether their exercise efforts are effective in this regard. For example, if a person wants to reduce their stress levels by exercising, it would be important to identify what quantifiable "byproducts" of stress could be used as evaluative measures for that particular fitness goal (e.g., lessened number and diminished severity of headaches; number of restful hours of sleep attained per night; etc.).

Finally, fitness goals should be "big enough" to justify an individual's personal commitment of essential resources (time, energy, and money). Obviously, this step mandates that, to the degree possible, efforts should be focused on reality. The patient needs to determine what is best, and the lifestyle medicine practitioner needs to help the patient figure this out—"not too much," "not too little." In other words, every patient needs to keep the goals in perspective, as well as to root the goals in a positive, "can-do" attitude.

❑ How Can Fitness Goals Be Prioritized?

When it comes to a patient's exercise program, an individual has the option of choosing from a wide variety of fitness goals. Obviously, it could be counterproductive and a waste of time to enumerate too many goals. Furthermore, it is in the patient's best interest to establish some sort of priority order for their goals.

As with other aspects of the process for establishing fitness goals, a person has a great deal of subjective latitude when prioritizing personal fitness goals. In this regard, a number of factors may be taken into consideration. For example, does the patient have an underlying, burning desire to achieve a particular goal? Does a particular medical/health condition generate a sense of urgency to accomplish a specific goal? Are specific attitudes and values involved? Is their goal realistic given the patient's genetic makeup? Are the goals satisfying psychological needs? Does any underlying drive for achieving a particular goal exist in their subconscious?

❑ How Can the Target Be Hit?

The process of establishing appropriate fitness goals is not terribly complicated. The primary attribute that is needed in this regard is common sense. At a minimum, common sense concerning what the individual can realistically do either to improve their ability to perform their activities of daily living or to have a positive impact on their level of health. Bear in mind that an analogy can be drawn between a person setting goals and framing dreams. An individual's fitness goals, as well as their dreams, are like a road map to what they want to accomplish in life. To paraphrase Henry David Thoreau, "In the long run, individuals hit only what they aim at ..."

❑ A Health Account for Life

Each time patients exercise, they are making a deposit into their "health bank." With each fitness assessment, the patient is ensuring that the "health funds" will be there when needed in the future. The benefits of their actions, in this regard, are undeniable.

LIVE AND LEARN WITH DR. BETH FRATES

Let's go back to the first chapter in this book, when I related the story of my father. When he sprinted to make the train, his heart suddenly started beating quickly, demanding more oxygen. His coronary arteries, however, were blocked by plaque and could not supply the needed oxygen. Thus, a part of his heart muscle started to weaken and pump inefficiently. This situation led to severe damage and the death of portions of his heart muscle. This additional damage resulted in his heart beating asynchronously, which caused blood to pool in his atrium. A large blood clot formed in his atrium, a piece of which broke off and traveled to my father's brain, where it blocked blood flow to that area of his brain. This clot prevented blood from delivering oxygen to the part of my father's brain that controlled his left side—face, arm, and leg. Those brain cells died. As a result, he was left with paralysis on his left side.

Fortunately, the brain and heart can heal. The brain can form new connections, called synapses, and parts of the brain that are functioning properly can connect with the parts that are not. This type of rewiring is critical for the recovery of a stroke survivor, and exercise plays an important role in the rehabilitation process after a stroke.

Physical therapists work with the lower extremities to help increase strength and power in them, as well as to retrain the gait for steady walking. Occupational therapists work with the upper extremities and focus on activities of daily living (ADLs) to increase strength, power, and function in the arms and hands. Speech pathologists help people with their feeding, swallowing, and speech issues. Psychologists and social workers help patients to recover mentally and emotionally. Exercise is at the foundation of many of these treatments and helps recovery in a number of ways.

Another take-home point with this live and learn is that people who are sedentary—not exercising three days a week for 30-minute sessions for three months' duration—are at risk for a cardiac event if they go from sitting to a vigorous level of exercise, meaning going from sitting to sprinting. Vigorous level of exercise means the person cannot talk, while performing the activity. Moderate level means the person can talk but not sing when exercising. And low intensity exercise means the person can sing while doing the work. It is best to start out with a low intensity exercise and work up slowly. Start low and go slow when starting exercise.

CHOOSING THE "RIGHT" EXERCISE

How should a person exercise? Run? Swim? Zumba? Work out on a machine, such as a treadmill, exercise cycle, or a cross trainer? Does it really matter? It does. In fact, deciding which type of exercise an individual wants to engage in can be one of the more important decisions a patient can make concerning their exercise program.

Thoughtfully reached, such a decision can enhance the likelihood that a person can achieve their exercise-related goals and objectives. Carelessly reached, such an approach to the issue can have negative consequences. For example, if an individual selects a way to exercise that is incompatible with their needs and interests, this choice heightens the likelihood of having a diminished level of exercise compliance, which, in turn, reduces the levels of results that could be achieved from the exercise regimen. As a result, an unbridgeable conflict is created between expectations and the results achieved by working out. An inappropriately selected training modality can also increase their risk of sustaining an injury while exercising.

Unfortunately, some individuals don't purposefully consider their exercise options. Rather, they either address the matter in a relatively hasty manner or use a subjective "feeling" or "gut reaction" to make their choice of what modality to employ when exercising. As a result, they may compromise their exercise efforts.

❏ Making a Suitable Choice

Once a person decides that it is in their best interest to engage in the type of exercise that offers the best relative choice (all factors considered), they should then attempt to determine which exercise activity is, in fact, the "right" one for them. In essence, they should address the task as they would any other important personal decision in their life.

For example, the process of selecting which exercise tool to use should embody the fundamental steps normally inherent in a sound decision-making process—set a goal (e.g., ascertain the "right" exercise modality); identify possible solutions for achieving the specified goal (e.g., working out on a stair-climbing machine, roller blading, strength training, rowing, using a stationary exercise bike, jogging, swimming, etc.); establish criteria for evaluating each possible solution (e.g., safety, cost, etc.); apply the criteria to each alternative course of action; and make the appropriate decision (choice).

Of the various steps involved in the normal decision-making process, perhaps the most problematic is deciding which criteria the patient should use to assess the relative merits of various modality options. In this regard, the acronym "S.S.A.F.F.E.E." can provide them with meaningful guidelines for making such a decision. While assigning a priority ranking to each of the seven possible criteria is essentially a subjective (i.e., personal) matter, using "S.S.A.F.F.E.E." can help a person make an informed judgment concerning the "good" and "bad" aspects of each of their respective choices.

A brief overview of the seven criteria in the "S.S.A.F.F.E.E." acronym includes the following points:

- *Scientifically documented benefits:* All stated claims and counterclaims concerning a specific exercise modality should be scientifically corroborated. In this regard, such research should be independently (i.e., by an unbiased, outside research team) conducted on a double-blind basis, with an appropriate study design and control groups. Preferably, the results of this research would be published in a refereed professional journal. In other words, a patient's chosen mode of exercising should offer confirmed benefits (unlike many of the so-called exercise devices promoted on television—e.g., magnets, thigh machines, etc.).

- *Safe:* An exercise modality should not subject a patient to excessive force or stress on any part of the body. While no exercise activity can ever be considered 100 percent safe, some activities are obviously safer than others. For example, walking and machine-based stair climbing place lower orthopedic stress on a person's lower body than running.
- *Appropriate to a patient's unique needs and situation:* Every potential exercise tends to have qualities, characteristics, and idiosyncrasies that can affect the degree to which a particular exercise modality is appropriate for an individual. For example, the cost of engaging in a specific modality may preclude a patient from using a particular exercise mode if that person has limited financial resources. Convenience, lifestyle, and existing fitness level are examples of other factors that should be considered with regard to their potential impact on whether a specific exercise modality is appropriate for a particular patient.
- *Functionally sound:* All factors considered, the more functional the exercise experience, the more applicable and beneficial the consequences of that exercise bout to "real-life" activities. In recent years, the functionality of a given activity has been addressed by proponents of a movement theory that is popularly referred to as "closed chain exercise." It is much more beneficial, they claim, for a person to train in a "natural" manner that involves weight-bearing, multi-joint exercise. The less desirable (and less functional) way to exercise is to engage in non-weight-bearing activity—one that frequently stresses muscles or muscle groups in an isolated (i.e., "unnatural") manner.
- *Feel:* Depending on how they are engineered, exercise machines have a mechanical level of efficiency that affects the experiential "feel" of the machine. All factors considered, the larger the range of this level of efficiency, the greater the likelihood that an individual will be able to match their personal level of mechanical efficiency with the exercise modality they are using. In sports, this level of efficiency is sometimes referred to as an athlete's "wheelhouse" (e.g., a stroked tennis ball looks larger than normal when it is coming at an individual). In the exercise arena, this aspect is often perceived to affect the degree to which a person can get into their personal "comfort zone."
- *Effective:* Like everyone else, an individual's exercise efforts tend to be geared to achieve specific results. All factors being equal, the higher the level of particular results a person can gain from a specific type of exercise activity, the more desirable the modality. Furthermore, the results an individual achieves by exercising are typically the most important single factor in whether that person sticks with their exercise regimen.
- *Enjoyment:* Exercise can and should be fun. A beneficial exercise experience should not be perceived as a pointless grind and should not be painful. If it is, the likelihood of a patient sticking with their exercise regimen is greatly diminished.

Accordingly, activities should be selected that an individual enjoys or will quickly come to enjoy, thereby providing intrinsic motivation.

❑ Making the "Right" Choice

Once a patient decides to exercise, the patient usually has a number or options to choose from regarding which exercise modality to use. Nonetheless, such a choice should not be made in a haphazard manner. Rather, the actual modality selected should be the result of a thoughtful, well-considered process. While several modalities may meet most (if not all) of the suggested evaluative criteria, an individual has a personal responsibility to decide which modality is most "right" for them. They might need to try different exercises before they settle on the right fit. Anything less might compromise their exercise efforts. As an extrapolation of the traditional axiom might dictate, it is much better for a patient to be "S.S.A.F.F.E.E.," than sorry.

AVOIDING TURNING A POSITIVE INTO A NEGATIVE

In a sound exercise program, exercise tends to become a healthy obsession, a part of a person's daily routine. As a rule, other people, work, or life events do not generally take precedence over the need or desire to exercise. That being said, psychologically healthy exercisers are more than willing to take a day off from time to time. They are comfortable with taking a "vacation" from exercise, either when traveling or simply when the opportunity to work out is not available. They recognize the need to feed, fuel, and rest their bodies. They are also comfortable adjusting the intensity of their workout when they are injured or ill.

In contrast, compulsive exercisers feel tremendous guilt when they do not exercise as often or as intensely as usual. They struggle with irrational fears of weight gain, feelings of laziness, and low self-worth when they do not exercise. As such, they could be considered exercise "addicts" in the sense that they might prioritize exercise over meeting with a good friend visiting from far away for only one day or miss an important work outing on the weekend in order to complete their exercise. In addition, the amount of exercise necessary to feel good and worthwhile might increase over time. Since compulsive exercisers are often using their relationship with exercise, in part, to conquer other fears or problems they may be experiencing, this is not healthy. Seeing a psychologist or therapist might be the best way to overcome this pathological relationship with exercise. It is important for people to work on their issues rather than "run away" from them.

❑ Taking a Bite Out of Reality

Excessive physical activity is a common characteristic among patients with eating disorders. Estimates suggest that up to 80 percent of those individuals struggling with eating disorders exercise compulsively. Excessive exercise is associated with more serious psychopathology, poorer treatment outcome, and higher relapse risk among eating-disordered patients. Excessive activity is one of the last symptoms to improve with treatment and requires a longer period for recovery, which may be due to an intense drive for thinness, as well as a strong tendency toward perfectionism.

Exercise can also be used in an unhealthy manner as a compensatory behavior for overeating. "Exercise-bulimics" measure the amount of exercise they need to do by the amount of food they eat. Rather than exercising for their health and wellness, these individuals exercise primarily to compensate for binge eating. Their behaviors encourage increased binge eating and set in motion a vicious cycle of compulsive overeating and compulsive exercise.

Excessive exercise is used psychologically to contend with poor body image and dissatisfaction with weight, shape, or appearance. Recent research suggests that over-exercise also functions to regulate negative emotions, such as sadness, loneliness, anger, and anxiety. In more extreme cases, vigorous physical activity can be viewed as a punitive act in line with self-injurious behavior.

❏ More Is Not Better

Healthy exercisers recognize their physical limitations and respect the messages that their bodies give them. They listen to their sore muscles, fatigue, and emotions. They enjoy exercise, but do not feel depressed or dissatisfied on the days they cannot exercise. They are happy to move their bodies, raise their heart rates, and stretch their muscles. They do not abuse their bodies. They recognize that some workout sessions might be more difficult than others. They do not use exercise to feel superior to others or to fix other aspects of their lives.

❏ Too Much of a Good Thing

Exercise can be excessive with regard to amount, frequency, duration, or intensity. Compulsive exercise is ritualistic; it must be done at the same time, in the same way, for the same duration every day. The exercise feels obligatory in that an individual works out, despite circumstances that would preclude it for most people. Exercise is "abused" or used in a destructive manner. It becomes the primary means of coping with stress. It continues despite illness or injury. Withdrawal symptoms, such as moodiness, trouble concentrating, or a change in appetite will occur if exercise is reduced or abated. Excessive exercise can be dangerous. It may result in decreased sex hormone levels, poor bone density, stress fractures, musculoskeletal problems, decreased immune function, prolonged QT intervals, electrolyte imbalance, and cardiac arrhythmias, among others.

An individual can, in fact, be doing "too much of a good thing," with regard to exercise. Although exercise can be used in a healthy manner to combat fatigue, low mood, and stress, excessive reliance upon exercise to manage difficult emotions is unproductive. Individuals struggling with disordered eating or those who exercise compulsively should be referred to a mental health professional. A consult with a physician, psychiatrist, psychologist, or an allied healthcare professional with expertise in eating disorders is recommended as well.

PRESCRIBING EXERCISE

It is important to note that in numerous beneficial ways, exercise is, in fact, medicine. Similar to medication, the type and dosage of an exercise regimen may need to be modified, based on each patient's unique response. Some individuals may be able to tolerate more; others less. Some modalities may work well for one person, while a different approach may be required for another.

The American College of Sports Medicine has developed guidelines (10th Edition) that serve as the foundation for exercise prescription for both healthy persons and individuals with various chronic diseases and disabilities. A summary of those guidelines is detailed in Figure 4-3.

It is important to note that caution should always be used when introducing new exercise program elements to a patient. As such, the individual's response should be closely observed both during and after their exercise session. Furthermore, physicians and allied healthcare professionals should collaborate with other relevant members of the patient's healthcare team to ensure the best possible care for that individual.

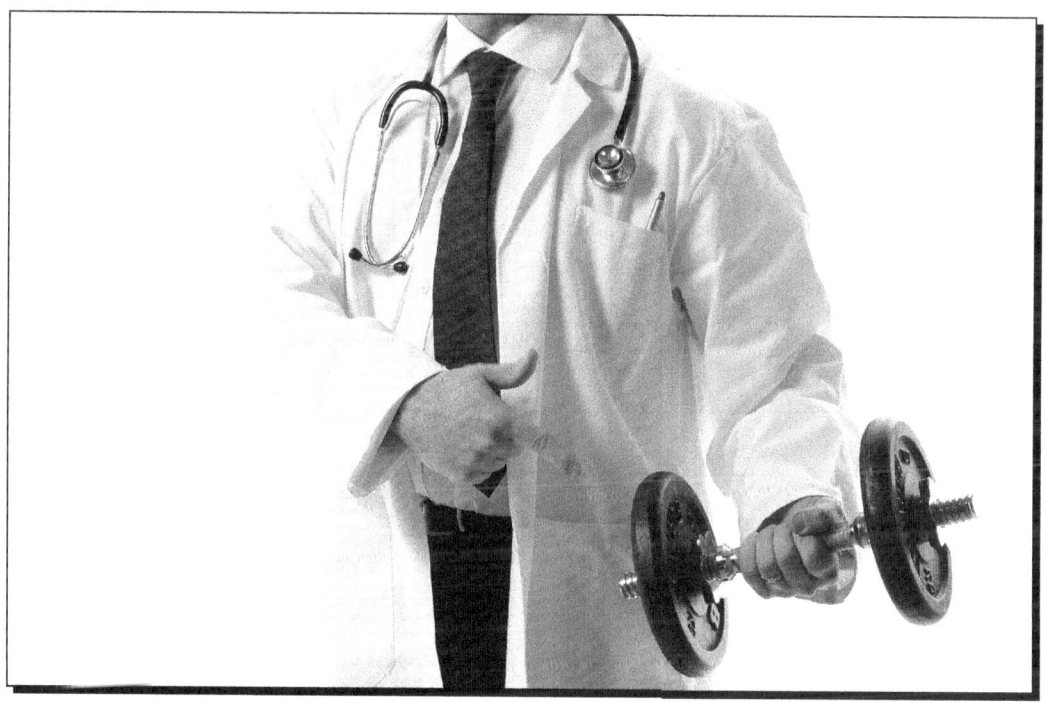

In numerous beneficial ways, exercise is, in fact, medicine.

	Aerobic Exercise	**Resistance Training**	**Flexibility**	**Neuromotor Skills Training**
Frequency	5 days/wk moderate intensity	2-3 days/wk	2-7 days/wk	2-3 days/wk
	3 days/wk vigorous intensity	48 hrs between same muscle group		
	or combination			
Intensity	40-59% HRR = moderate intensity	about 60-80% 1 RM	To point of tightness or slight discomfort	Unknown
	60-89% HRR = vigorous intensity	about 50% 1 RM when 15-25 reps and with deconditioned persons		
	30-39% HRR = light intensity for deconditioned persons			
	Interval training = varying intensities, fixed intervals			
Time	30-60 minutes daily, moderate intensity (>150 mins/wk)	N/A	10-30 sec/stretch	20-30 min
	20-60 minutes, vigorous intensity (>75 mins/wk)		30-60 sec/stretch for older adults	
	or a combination of above, >10 min bouts		PNF: 20-75% max voluntary contraction followed by 10-30 sec assisted stretch	
Type (Mode)	Rhythmic aerobic exercise involving large muscle groups	Multi-joint and single-joint exercises	Static, dynamic, or PNF stretching	Motor skills training to improve balance, agility, coordination, gait
		Major muscles groups, including core		Tai chi, yoga for fall prevention in older adults
		Opposing muscle groups		
Volume	>500 -1,000 MET-min.wk-1	8-12 repetitions, 2-4 sets	Total 60 sec/joint	Unknown
	7,000+ step count/day	2-3 min rest between sets		
		1 set, 10-15 reps for deconditioned persons		
Progression	Gradually increase duration, frequency, intensity	Gradually increase resistance, reps, frequency	Unknown	Unknown

Figure 4-3. A summary of ACSM's general exercise prescription (FITT-VP) guidelines (based on *ACSM's Guidelines for Exercise Testing and Prescription*, 10th edition)

RISK STRATIFICATION SYSTEM

Physicians are sometimes wary of telling people to exercise, because exercise acutely stresses the heart. Although the risks of having an acute cardiac event are very low, and there are significant benefits to be gained, there are some patients who require medical screening and clearance before beginning an exercise program.

The American College of Sports Medicine's Guidelines for Exercise Testing and Prescription, 10th edition, details a system of risk stratification that can help guide physicians and allied healthcare professionals in making an assessment of whether or not it is appropriate for a patient to exercise, and to what degree. ACSM cites three risk categories that should be considered—low, moderate, and high.

❑ A Low-Risk Patient for Initiating Exercise

Low-risk patients are men age ≤ 45 years old or women age ≤ 55 who have no symptoms of cardiovascular disease and have no more than one risk factor for cardiovascular disease. Positive risk factors include family history (such as a father who had a heart attack or stroke before 55 or a mother who had a heart attack before the age of 65), cigarette smoking, a sedentary lifestyle, obesity, an abnormal lipid profile, and pre-diabetes. A negative risk factor is a high HDL (good) cholesterol level.

Patients who fall into the low-risk category can be cleared for low-, moderate-, or vigorous-intensity exercise, without further intervention from a physician or cardiologist. It is always best, however, for the patient to see their own primary care physician before initiating an exercise program.

In general, people need to start out at low intensity level of exercise, especially if they are basically sedentary. It is also important to remember to progress slowly. Start low and go slow. Remember the example of Donald Pegg who was sedentary and sprinted for the train only to end up with a heart attack detailed in the Live and Learn in this chapter. One of the most dangerous times for exercise is a sedentary person moving right into vigorous intensity exercise.

❑ A Moderate-Risk Patient for Initiating Exercise

Moderate-risk patients are men > 45 years old and women > 55 years who are asymptomatic, but have two or more risk factors for cardiovascular disease. These patients can be cleared for low- and moderate-intensity exercise. Further evaluation by an exercise physiologist, cardiologist, or another physician is recommended, if the patient wishes to engage in vigorous-intensity physical activity. They might need an exercise stress test, depending on their specific disease processes and risk factors.

❑ A High-Risk Patient for Initiating Exercise

High-risk patients are individuals with one or more signs or symptoms of cardiovascular, metabolic, or pulmonary disease. This category includes patients who are diagnosed with diabetes, given that they are considered to have metabolic disease. Does this mean that someone with a history of heart attack or stroke should not exercise at all? No. However, they may need to go through cardiac rehabilitation and be cleared by a physician to exercise on their own. They may be required to perform a specific progression of exercises before switching to a home exercise routine that they can undertake safely.

Unlike patients who are at low- or moderate-risk, it is recommended that patients who are at high risk of having an adverse event while exercising receive further evaluation prior to initiating *any* noteworthy level of intensity of physical activity. Going directly from a sedentary lifestyle to vigorous exercise can be dangerous and could result in sudden cardiac arrest or myocardial infarction. With habitual vigorous exercise, however, it has been shown that the relative risk of a heart attack can be dramatically reduced.

AN EXERCISE MACHINE WITH HAIR

Dr. Egil Martinsen, a Norwegian psychiatrist, recommends that if someone is thinking of getting any piece of exercise equipment, they should get a dog. A Harvard Health Special Report titled *Get Healthy, Get a Dog* (http://www.health.harvard.edu/staying-healthy/get-healthy-get-a-dog), authored by Dr. Frates, further explores the benefits of man's best friend. In fact, burgeoning research suggests that people who have dogs not only exercise more often, they are also healthier. This observation makes intuitive sense, since most people get out two or three times a day to walk their dog.

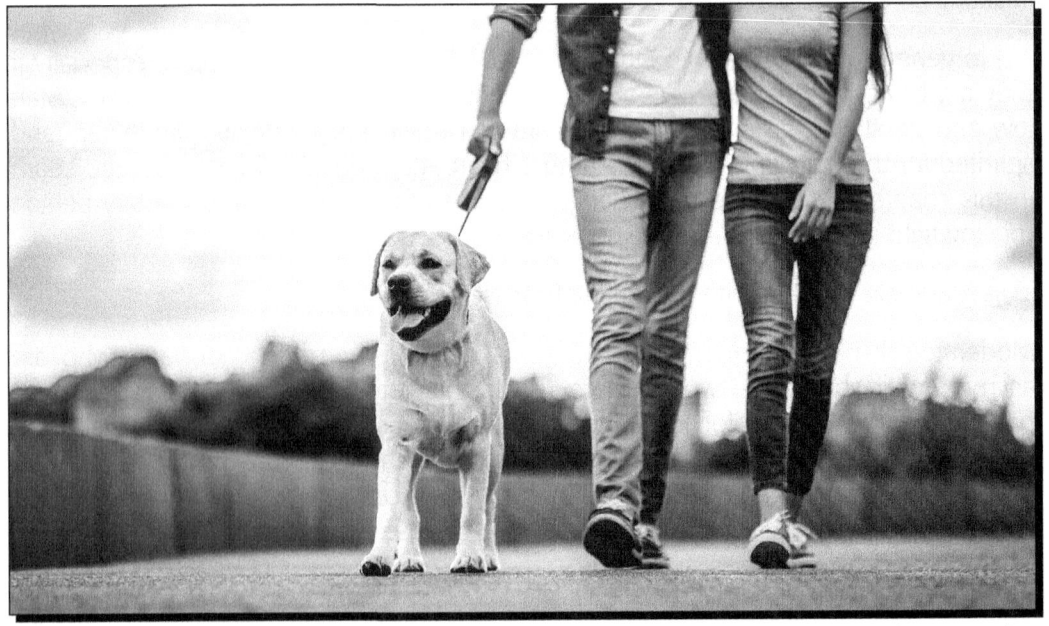

Research suggests that people who have dogs not only exercise more often, they are also healthier.

THE FRATES MOSS METHOD

The popular saying attributed to the Latin writer Publilius Syrus, "A rolling stone gathers no moss," inspired the creation of a lifestyle medicine framework, based on that quote called the Frates MOSS Method™ (M=Motivation, O=Obstacles, S=Strategies, and S=Strengths). This method can be used whenever a physician or allied health professional counsels a patient about exercise. Similar to a rolling stone that gathers no moss, if individuals are active, they gather no disease.

❑ Motivation

Motivators for exercise come in all shapes and sizes. One of Dr. Frates clients was a 74-year-old woman who wanted to exercise and lose weight. Her motivation for this was to feel comfortable wearing a bathing suit, when she visited a friend in Florida. It would not have occurred to most clinicians that this would be a goal for her, but it was. (Furthermore, she ended up losing weight and feeling so good about herself that she tried on bikinis at the store!)

In fact, one of the key issues attendant to ascertaining why someone might want to become physically active entails the question, how does a physician or an allied health professional discover what an individual patient's motivators are? The answer, in most instances, is relatively straightforward—by asking an open-ended question, such as "Is there something specific that happened recently to make you want to start exercising, if so what happened? or "What makes you want to start exercising now?"; "What is motivating you to start exercising? What benefits do you expect to achieve with exercise? or, "Is there any reason in particular that you want to start exercising?"

❑ Obstacles

Obstacles also come in all shapes and sizes, and tend to be specific to the individual. It is important to be aware that the obstacles facing a clinician may be different from those that a patient encounters. Furthermore, the obstacles that an individual faces today will likely be different than they were either two years ago or five years. Ironically, one person's motivation can be someone else's obstacles. For example, many mothers find that their children are motivators at times (wanting to be healthy and life a long time to enjoy them) and obstacles at other times (when they need rides to school and extracurricular activities). Many parents want to be good role models for their children, but they often feel that their responsibilities at home and at work are too great. So, they do not prioritize exercising.

One of the biggest obstacles for many people is not having a clearly defined motivation for exercising. If patients do not really know why they want to be more active, it will be difficult for them to start and maintain an exercise regimen. Not surprisingly, it is generally much easier to sit at home and watch television, while eating ice cream, than it is to go outside for a walk.

❑ Strategies

To overcome an individual's obstacles to exercising, a strategy needs to be developed that will work for that specific person. In reality, a wide variety of strategies are possible. The key is to understand that when it comes to exercising, one size does not fit all. For example, some people might be motivated if they have a partner to exercise with, while others may find a wearable tracker that counts their steps each day as motivating. A treadmill workstation, a standing desk, or a chair ball might be a great option for someone who works in an office. Other possible alternatives include scheduling walking meetings, having dance-party breaks at work (at 3 p.m., music is turned on for five minutes for people to dance), etc. Patients could also be directed to consider using a smartphone app, or website such as SparkPeople, or keeping a journal of their exercise efforts to help them be consistent.

❑ Strengths

It is important to work with a patient's strengths when creating an exercise plan. Patients often come to lifestyle practitioners feeling very defeated and hopeless about changing. They might say, "This isn't going to work. I don't even know why I'm here," to which the practitioner might respond, "Well, let's talk about you as a person." A lifestyle medicine practitioner might discover that the patient is a woman, who is divorced and has raised her children alone, is great at organizing and very capable of managing the house as well as her job. She clearly has strengths to work with that she may not be acknowledging or even appreciating herself. By using appreciative inquiry (discussed in Chapter 3) the lifestyle medicine practitioner can highlight the patient's strengths, what is going well, and hold a productive, positive conversation with the patient. Drawing out people's strengths with coaching strategies and the Frates COACH Approach using curiosity, openness, appreciation, compassion and honesty helps to build the patient's confidence and enables the physician or allied healthcare professional to help create meaningful SMART goals with patient.

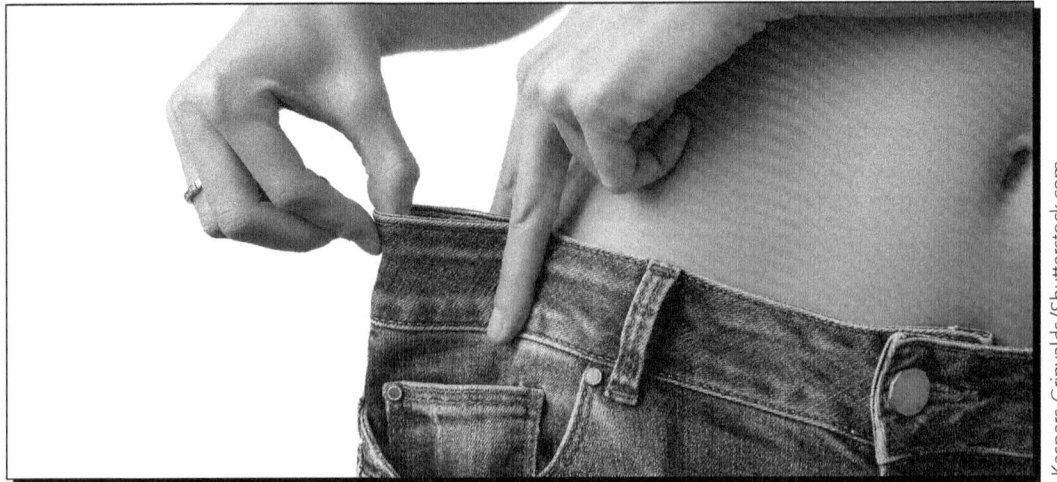

When it comes to exercising, one size does not fit all.

FITT PRESCRIPTIONS FOR EXERCISE/ PHYSICAL ACTIVITY

F—Frequency of exercise. The basic goal is to accumulate at least 150 minutes of moderate physical activity in the week. To achieve the benefits of exercising on a regular basis, the recommendation is to exercise five to six days of the week. This timetable can be adjusted to suit the schedule of the patient.

I—Intensity of the exercise. As reviewed in the chapter, it is recommended that people start their exercise regimen at a low level of intensity and work their way up to a moderate level. Prior to initiating a new exercise routine, it is best for the individual to get clearance from their primary physician. Depending on the medical history and the activity history of the patient, the patient may be ready for low-, moderate-, or vigorous-intensity exercise. Ultimately, the level of intensity needs to be individualized. How patients monitor their intensity levels is also a personal matter. Among the more popular options for monitoring exercise intensity are the talk test, Borg Rate of Perceived Exertion, and heart rate monitoring.

T—Time for exercise. As noted previously, the goal is to accumulate at least 150 minutes of moderate-intensity physical activity, depending on the patient's history and interests. Exercise sessions can range from 10 to 60 minutes or considerably more, depending on the schedule and fitness level of the individual. In fact, some evidence exists that even relatively brief bouts of 10 minutes can be helpful to the body.

T—Type of exercise. This aspect is a very important part of the exercise prescription. First and foremost, the individual needs to select an exercise that they enjoy, a factor that will vary for people. For most people, it is the key to sustaining exercise.

- An example of a FITT prescription for low intensity exercise:

    F—four days a week
    I—low
    T—10 minutes in both the a.m. and p.m
    T—stationary bicycle

- An example of a FITT prescription for low intensity exercise:

    F—four days a week
    I—low
    T—40 minutes each day (collectively)
    T—bicycling to and from work; walking the dog in the evening

❏ An example of a FITT prescription for moderate intensity exercise:

F—five days a week
I—moderate
T—accumulate 30 minutes each day
T—brisk walking—walk to and from work, as well as for 10 minutes at lunch

❏ An example of a FITT prescription for moderate intensity exercise:

F—five days a week
I—moderate
T—30 minutes each session
T—brisk walking or swimming laps

❏ An example of a FITT prescription for vigorous intensity exercise:

F—five days a week
I—vigorous
T—30 minutes a day
T—jogging

KEY POINTS/TAKEAWAYS FOR CHAPTER 4

❏ Chapter Review:

- Overall goal: Understand the impact that exercising regularly can have on a person's health.
- Application goal: Develop strategies that can help make physical activity a daily part of a patient's life.

❏ Discussion Questions:

- What are the primary obstacles that can otherwise preclude someone from exercising on a regular basis?
- Why is a sedentary lifestyle a controllable risk factor for health?
- What strategies can be employed to change a patient's mindset and behavior concerning exercise?
- What are the core elements of an exercise prescription?
- Why is exercise medicine?

	TITLE	AUTHORS	JOURNAL	YEAR	KEY FINDINGS
1	Personal exercise habits and counseling practices of primary care physicians: a national survey	Abramson S, et al.	Clinical Journal of Sport Medicine	2000	A cross-sectional survey of 298 random primary care physicians in the United States that sought to quantify physician exercise behaviors and its relationship to exercise counseling. It found that physicians who exercised were more likely to counsel their patients to exercise. It also identified inadequate time and knowledge/experience as the most common barriers to exercise counseling.
2	Exercise and acute cardiovascular events	AHA Scientific Statement	Circulation	2007	A scientific statement that endorses the beneficial effect of habitual physical activity on reducing coronary heart disease events but recognizes that vigorous activity can acutely and transiently increase the risk of sudden cardiac death and acute myocardial infarction in susceptible people. "The incidence of both acute myocardial infarction and sudden death is greatest in the habitually least physically active individuals .... Maintaining physical fitness through regular physical activity may help to reduce events because a disproportionate number of events occur in least physically active subjects performing unaccustomed physical activity."
3	Interventions to increase physical activity among healthy adults: meta-analysis of outcomes	Conn VS, Hafdahl AR, Mehr DR	American Journal of Public Health	2011	This meta-analysis comprised of 99,011 participants concluded that "interventions designed to increase physical activity were modestly effective. Interventions to increase activity should emphasize behavioral strategies over cognitive strategies."
4	Best practices statement, physical activity programs and behavior counseling in older adult populations	Cress ME, et al.	Medicine & Science in Sports & Exercise	2004	Key practices identified to promote physical activity in older adults included: having a multidimensional activity program, utilizing behavior change principles, managing risk by starting at low intensity and gradually increasing to moderate intensity physical activity, having an emergency plan in place for community-based programs, and monitoring aerobic intensity for progression and motivation.
5	Television viewing time and mortality: the Australian Diabetes, Obesity and Lifestyle Study (AusDiab)	Dunstan DW, et al.	Circulation	2010	A study of 8,800 Australians that found that each additional hour of television watched per day translated to an 11% increase in all-cause mortality.
6	The exercise pill—too good to be true?	Goodyear LJ	New England Journal of Medicine	2008	Discusses some of the complex changes that occur in skeletal muscle and the possibility of mimicking these molecular changes using pharmaceuticals. It ultimately concluded that: "It is unlikely that a single 'exercise pill' will ever supply most of the benefits of regular exercise."

Figure 4-4. Physical activity guidelines and prescription evidence

	TITLE	AUTHORS	JOURNAL	YEAR	KEY FINDINGS
7	Aerobic exercise improves hippocampal function and increases BDNF in the serum of young adult males	Griffin EW, et al.	*Physiology & Behavior*	2011	A study in Ireland that assessed baseline levels of brain-derived neurotrophic factor (BDNF) and memory performance of male college students. After showing participants photos of faces and names of strangers, they had half of the subjects ride a stationary bike until exhausted and half of the subjects rest quietly for 30 minutes. The exercise group exhibited improved performance on the memory test and had increased levels of BDNF as compared to the group that rested quietly.
8	Physical activity and public health: updated recommendation for adults from the American College of Sports Medicine and the American Heart Association	Haskell WL, et al.	*Circulation*	2007	"All healthy adults aged 18 to 65 yr need moderate-intensity aerobic (endurance) physical activity for a minimum of 30 min on five days each week or vigorous-intensity aerobic physical activity for a minimum of 20 min on three days each week …. In addition, every adult should perform activities that maintain or increase muscular strength and endurance a minimum of two days each week."
9	Dose response issues concerning physical activity and health: an evidence-based symposium	Kesaniemi YK, et al.	*Medicine & Science in Sports & Exercise*	2001	This symposium panel evaluated the dose-response relationship of physical activity to health outcomes and concluded that "there is an inverse and generally linear relationship for the rates of all-cause mortality, total cardiovascular, and coronary heart disease incidence and mortality and for the incidence of type 2 diabetes mellitus." Dose-responses were difficult to definitively evaluate for other health outcomes due to lack of high quality data. The panel also recognized that it is important to balance the health benefits with the potential risks associated with greater volume and intensity of exercise.
10	The evidence in support of physicians and health care providers as physical activity role models	Lobelo F, de Quevedo IG	*American Journal of Lifestyle Medicine*	2016	A review article that found a "significant positive association between healthcare providers' physical activity habits and counseling frequency, with odds ratios ranging between 1.4 and 5.7 (p<.05), in 6 studies allowing direct comparison."
11	Exercise and older patients: prescribing guidelines	Mayer J, Mernitz H	*American Family Physician*	2006	Discusses exercise prescription for older adults and recommends addressing frequency, intensity, type, time, and progression for aerobic activity, strength training, and flexibility exercises with patients. It also recognizes the importance of motivational strategies and social support.

Figure 4-4. Physical activity guidelines and prescription evidence (cont.)

	TITLE	AUTHORS	JOURNAL	YEAR	KEY FINDINGS
12	Recovery after an Ironman triathlon: sustained inflammatory responses and muscular stress	Neubauer O, König D, Wagner KH	European Journal of Applied Physiology	2008	A study of 19 well-trained male triathletes that evaluated muscle damage and inflammatory markers 19 days into recovery after an Ironman triathlon. It found that there are significant systemic inflammatory responses post-race, but these decline relatively quickly. "However, a low-grade systemic inflammation persisted until at least 5 days' post-race, possibly reflecting incomplete muscle recovery."
13	Exercise as a treatment for chronic low back pain	Rainville J, et al.	Spine Journal	2004	This literature search found that exercise was safe for individuals with back pain and that it did not increase their risk of further back injuries. "Most studies of exercise have noted overall reduction in back pain intensity that ranges from 10%-50% after exercise treatment." Furthermore, they found evidence that exercise "can lessen the behavioral, cognitive, affect and disability aspects of back pain syndromes."
14	Importance of assessing cardiorespiratory fitness in clinical practice: a case for fitness as a clinical vital sign: a scientific statement from the American Heart Association	Ross R, et al.	Circulation	2016	A review of 24 studies that "found consistent evidence supporting the notion that physically active physicians and other HCPs are more likely to provide PA counseling to their patients and can indeed become powerful PA role models. This evidence appears sufficient to justify randomized trials to determine if adding interventions to promote PA among HCPs, also results in improvements in the frequency and quality of PA preventive counseling and referrals, delivered by HCPs, to patients in primary care settings."
15	Role of counseling to promote adherence in healthy lifestyle medicine: strategies to improve exercise adherence and enhance physical activity	Stonerock GL, Blumenthal JA	Progress in Cardiovascular Diseases	2017	This article reviews psychological, behavioral, and environmental factors that contribute to adherence to healthy lifestyle behavior change. The authors provide examples and discuss how motivational interviewing and the transtheoretical model of behavior change can be used to increase patient physical activity levels.
16	Exercise, brain, and cognition across the life span	Voss MW, et al.	Journal of Applied Physiology	2011	A review article that found ample evidence to support exercise as "one of the most effective means available to improve mental and physical health, without the side effects of many pharmacological treatments." It also discusses current gaps in the literature and areas to consider for future research.

Figure 4-4. Physical activity guidelines and prescription evidence (cont.)

References

1. Abramson S, Stein J, Schaufele M, et al. Personal exercise habits and counseling practices of primary care physicians: a national survey. *Clinical Journal of Sport Medicine.* 2000;10:40-48.
2. AHA Scientific Statement. Exercise and acute cardiovascular events. *Circulation.* 2007;115:2358-2368.
3. Conn VS, Hafdahl AR, Mehr DR. Interventions to increase physical activity among healthy adults: meta-analysis of outcomes. *American Journal of Public Health.* 2011;101(4): 751-758.
4. Cress ME, et al. Best practices statement, physical activity programs and behavior counseling in older adult populations. *Medicine & Science in Sports & Exercise.* 2004;36:1997-2003.
5. Dunstan DW, Barr EL, Healy GN, et al. Television viewing time and mortality: the Australian Diabetes, Obesity and Lifestyle Study (AusDiab). *Circulation.* 2010;121:384-391.
6. Goodyear LJ. The exercise pill—too good to be true? *New England Journal of Medicine.* 2008;359:1842-1844.
7. Griffin EW, Mulally S, Foley C, et al. Aerobic exercise improves hippocampal function and increases BDNF in the serum of young adult males. *Physiology & Behavior.* 2011;104:934-941.
8. Haskell WL, Lee I-M, Pate RR, et al. Physical activity and public health: updated recommendation for adults from the American College of Sports Medicine and the American Heart Association. *Circulation.* 2007;116:1081-1093.
9. Kesaniemi YK, Danforth E Jr, Jensen MD, et al. Dose response issues concerning physical activity and health: an evidence-based symposium. *Medicine & Science in Sports & Exercise.* 2001;33:S351-S358.
10. Lobelo F, de Quevedo IG. The evidence in support of physicians and health care providers as physical activity role models. *American Journal of Lifestyle Medicine.* 2016;10(1):36-52. doi:10.1177/1559827613520120.
11. Mayer J, Mernitz H. Exercise and older patients: prescribing guidelines. *American Family Physician.* 2006;74(3):437-444.
12. Neubauer O, König D, Wagner KH. Recovery after an Ironman triathlon: sustained inflammatory responses and muscular stress. *European Journal of Applied Physiology.* October 2008;104(3):417-426. doi:10.1007/s00421-008-0787-6. Epub 2008 Jun 12.
13. Rainville J, Hartigan E, Martinez E, et al. Exercise as a treatment for chronic low back pain. *Spine Journal.* 2004;4:106-115.
14. Ross R, Blair SN, Arena R, et al. Importance of assessing cardiorespiratory fitness in clinical practice: a case for fitness as a clinical vital sign: a scientific statement from the American Heart Association. *Circulation.* 2016;134(24):e653-e699. Epub 2016 Nov 21.
15. Stonerock GL, Blumenthal JA. Role of counseling to promote adherence in healthy lifestyle medicine: strategies to improve exercise adherence and enhance physical activity. *Progress in Cardiovascular Diseases.* 2017;59(5):455-462.
16. Voss MW, Nagamatsu LS, Liu-Ambrose T, et al. Exercise, brain, and cognition across the life span. *Journal of Applied Physiology.* 2011;111:1505-1513.

Figure 4-4. Physical activity guidelines and prescription evidence (cont.)

REFERENCES

- Abramson S, Stein J, Schaufele M, Frates E, Rogan S. Personal exercise habits and counseling practices of primary care physicians: a national survey. *Clinical Journal of Sport Medicine.* 2000;10:40-48.
- AHA Scientific Statement. Exercise and acute cardiovascular events. *Circulation.* 2007;115:2358-2368.
- Almendrala A. This Specific Type of Exercise Improves Men's Fertility. HuffPost. December 7, 2016. Available at: https://www.huffingtonpost.com/entry/exercise-improve-sperm-quality_us_58476015e4b0d0df1836f796. Accessed August 2018.
- American College of Sports Medicine. *ACSM's Guidelines for Exercise Testing and Prescription.* 10th ed. Philadelphia: Lippincott Williams & Wilkins; 2017.
- American College of Sports Medicine. *ACSM's Health-Related Physical Fitness Assessment Manual.* 4th ed. Philadelphia: Lippincott Williams & Wilkins; 2014.
- American College of Sports Medicine. *ACSM's Resource Manual for Guidelines for Exercise Testing and Prescription.* 7th ed. Philadelphia: Lippincott Williams & Wilkins; 2014.
- Begot I, Peixoto TC, Gonzaga LR, et al. A home-based walking program improves erectile dysfunction in men with an acute myocardial infarction. *American Journal of Cardiology.* 2015;115(5):571-575. doi:10.1016/j.amjcard.2014.12.007.

- Cress ME, et al. Best practices statement, physical activity programs and behavior counseling in older adult populations. *Medicine & Science in Sports & Exercise.* 2004;36:1997-2003.
- Dunstan DW, Barr EL, Healy GN, Salmon J, Shaw JE, Balkau B, Magliano DJ, Cameron AJ, Zimmet PZ, Owen N. Television viewing time and mortality: the Australian Diabetes, Obesity and Lifestyle Study (AusDiab). *Circulation.* 2010;121:384-391.
- Egger G, Binns A, Rossner S. *Lifestyle Medicine: Managing Diseases of Lifestyle in the 21st Century.* North Ryde, N.S.W.: McGraw-Hill; 2010.
- Farrell PA, Joyner MJ, Caiozzo VJ. *ACSM's Advanced Exercise Physiology.* 2nd ed. Lippincott Williams & Wilkins; 2011.
- Frank E, Breyan J, Elon L. Physician disclosure of healthy personal behaviors improves credibility and ability to motivate. *Archives of Family Medicine.* 2000;9:287-290.
- Frates EP, Moore MA, Lopez CN, McMahon GT. Coaching for behavior change in physiatry. *American Journal of Physical Medicine & Rehabilitation.* December 2011;90(12):1074-1082. Available at: http://www.wellcoaches.com/images/pdf/Coaching-Am-Journal-Physical-Medicine-Dec-2011.pdf. Accessed September 2017.
- Gibbons L, et al. ACC/AHA guideline update for exercise testing. *Circulation* 2002; 106:1883-1892.
- Gomes D. 4 Exercises to Treat Erectile Dysfunction for Men Struggling With Impotence. Medical Daily. September 15, 2016. Available at: https://www.medicaldaily.com/4-exercises-treat-erectile-dysfunction-men-struggling-impotence-398026. Accessed August 2018.
- Gómez-Pinilla F, Ying Z, Roy RR, Molteni R, Edgerton VR. Voluntary exercise induces a BDNF-mediated mechanism that promotes neuroplasticity. *Journal of Neurophysiology.* 2002;88:2187-2195.
- Goodyear LJ. The exercise pill—too good to be true? *New England Journal of Medicine.* 2008;359:1842-1844.
- Griffin EW, Mulally S, Foley C, Warmington SA, O'Mara SM, Kelly AM. Aerobic exercise improves hippocampal function and increases BDNF in the serum of young adult males. *Physiology & Behavior.* 2011;104:934-941.
- Haskell WL, Lee I-M, Pate RR, Powell KE, Blair SN, Franklin BA, Macera CA, Heath GW, Thompson PD, Bauman A. Physical activity and public health. Updated recommendation for adults from the American College of Sports Medicine and the American Heart Association. *Circulation.* 2007;116:1081-1093.
- Hwang MY. Why you should exercise. *Journal of the American Medical Association.* 1999;281(4).
- Jonas S, Phillips E. *ACSM's Exercise Is Medicine: A Clinician's Guide to Exercise Prescription.* Philadelphia: Lippincott Williams & Wilkins; 2009.
- Kesaniemi YK, Danforth E Jr, Jensen MD, et al. Dose response issues concerning physical activity and health: an evidence-based symposium. *Medicine & Science in Sports & Exercise.* 2001;33:S351-358.

- Mayer J, Mernitz H. Exercise and older patients: prescribing guidelines. *American Family Physician.* 2006;74(3):437-444.
- Neubauer O, König D, Wagner KH. Recovery after an Ironman triathlon: sustained inflammatory responses and muscular stress. *European Journal of Applied Physiology.* October 2008;104(3):417-426. doi:10.1007/s00421-008-0787-6. Epub 2008 Jun 12.
- Rainville J, Hartigan E, Martinez E, Limke J, Jouve CA, Finno M. Exercise as a treatment for chronic low back pain. *Spine Journal.* 2004;4:106-115.
- Ratey J, Hagerman E. *Spark: The Revolutionary New Science of Exercise and the Brain.* New York: Little, Brown and Company; 2008.
- Sharma A, Madaan V, Petty FD. Exercise for mental health. *Primary Care Companion to the Journal of Clinical Psychiatry.* 2006;8(2):106.
- Shiraev T, Barclay G. A hydrothermally processed maize starch and its effect on blood glucose levels during high intensity interval exercise. *Australian Family Physician.* December 2012;41(12):960.
- Steiner JL, et al. Exercise training increases mitochondrial biogenesis in the brain. *Journal of Applied Physiology.* October 2011;111(4):1066-1071.
- U.S. Department of Health and Human Services. 2008 Physical Activity Guidelines for Americans. Available at: www.health.gov/paguidelines. Accessed November 2008.
- U.S. Department of Health and Human Services. *Physical Activity and Health: A Report of the Surgeon General.* Atlanta, GA: U.S. Department of Health and Human Services, Centers for Disease Control and Prevention, National Center for Chronic Disease Prevention and Health Promotion; 1996. Available at: http://www.cdc.gov/nccdphp/sgr/pdf/prerep.pdf. Accessed December 2008.
- Voss MW, Nagamatsu LS, Liu-Ambrose T, Kramer AF. Exercise, brain, and cognition across the life span. *Journal of Applied Physiology.* 2011;111:1505-1513.

CHAPTER 5

THE NUTRITION-HEALTH CONNECTION

Written in collaboration with Kayli Dice, MS, RDN

"Eat food, not too much, mostly plants."

—Michael Pollan
Author
Activist about the places where
nature and culture intersect

Disclosure:

Nutrition is arguably one of the most controversial and charged subjects in lifestyle medicine. Food plays such an integral role in our lives—not only physically, but socially, emotionally, and even spiritually for some. Regardless of an individual's particular situation, however, there is consistent and compelling evidence to support healthy eating patterns that are whole foods, plant-based (WFPB) for preventing, halting and reversing disease.

The following chapter is by no means intended to be a gospel of diet and nutrition dogma. Rather, it is intended to provide an overview of the common themes related to healthy eating patterns established by the best possible scientific evidence. It is our hope and intention to provide future editions that reflect updated information. This chapter takes into consideration the latest research and guidelines. It is designed to provide you with the information and evidence you need to effectively counsel patients about general healthy eating patterns.

❑ Chapter Goals:

- Develop an understanding of what constitutes a diet that promotes health.
- Explore the basics of a whole foods, plant-based diet.
- Consider the why, what, and how of a healthy diet
- Understand how to help patients stick to a healthy diet.
- Provide a basic overview of digestion, metabolism, and energy balance.
- Review basic strategies for effective weight management.

❑ Learning Objectives:

- To comprehend the role that nutrition plays in lifestyle medicine
- To grasp the key factors associated with a healthy eating pattern
- To be aware of the diet spectrum, ranging from the standard American diet (SAD) to the whole foods, plant-based (WFPB) diet
- To understand the power of plants
- To recognize the need to focus on behavior change, with regard to weight management

❑ Guiding Questions:

- Why is it important to consume a nutritious diet?
- What can people do to adopt and maintain healthy eating habits?
- What is the role of energy balance in body weight maintenance?

❑ Important Terms:

- *Nutrire* (Latin): To feed.
- *Nutrition* (a term initially used in the 15th century): The act or process of nourishing or being nourished. The sum of the processes by which an animal or plant takes in and utilizes food substances.
- *Diet* (derived from the Greek word "diatia," meaning a way of life): As a noun—food and drink regularly provided or consumed; habitual nourishment; the kind and amount of food prescribed for a person to eat for a special reason; a regimen of eating and drinking sparingly so as to reduce one's weight; as a verb—to eat less food or to eat only particular kinds of food in order to try and lose weight.
- *Nutritional science:* Nutritional science is the study of the effects of the components in food on the metabolism, health, and performance, as well as the resistance of humans and animals to disease. It also includes the study of human behaviors related to food choices.
- *Whole foods, plant-based (WFPB):* A dietary pattern centered on minimally processed vegetables, fruits, whole grains, and legumes with nuts and seeds in moderation. It minimizes or excludes meat (including poultry and fish), dairy, eggs, added sugar, and processed oils. It's an evidence-based dietary pattern centered

on whole, plant foods eaten as close to their natural state as possible for disease prevention, treatment, and reversal.
- *WFPB vs. vegan:* A vegan diet is defined only by what it excludes—all animal products. A person can eat a vegan diet and still be very unhealthy. For example, Oreos and potato chips are vegan! WFPB guidelines outline the foods to include for optimal health.
- *Standard American diet (SAD):* Also known as the Western diet, SAD represents the modern American diet that contributes to the chronic disease epidemic. It is high in refined flours, sugar, high-fat foods and oils, and highly-processed packaged foods; and low in fiber, fruits and vegetables, and other whole, plant foods.

Nutrition can play a substantial role in almost every aspect of a person's life. The word comes from the Latin term "nutrire," meaning to feed. Not only can inadequate nutrition have a negative impact on an individual's ability to engage in most of the tasks attendant to daily living, it can also affect that person's health in a number of ways. Accordingly, eating the right foods in the right amount, at the appropriate time—while generally avoiding the wrong ones—is absolutely essential.

In reality, there are many different definitions for the word diet. In this book, the term is used to reflect a healthy eating pattern. When you see the word diet, as in the WFPB diet, it really means healthy eating pattern. The word derives from the Greek word "diatia," which means way of life. In other words, this text is essentially going back to the origin of the word. Not only are these lifestyle medicine diets really healthy eating patterns, moreover, they are a way of life.

For physicians and allied healthcare professionals, as well as patients, the overriding issue is what constitutes the "right" approach to nutrition. Somewhat paradoxically, a mountain of information on the topic exists—some of it sound, much of it unfounded. The obvious key for anyone interested in the subject of nutrition is to make sure that whatever information is being considered is evidence-based and grounded in documented facts. The ACLM's dietary lifestyle position statement is as follows: For the treatment, reversal, and prevention of lifestyle-related chronic disease, the ACLM recommends an eating plan based predominantly on a variety of minimally processed vegetables, fruits, whole grains, legumes, nuts, and seeds. The ACLM is currently working on a Nutrition Position Paper due for release in 2019 which will spell out more detailed guidelines. The basics will be covered in this chapter.

Given the importance of nutrition in lifestyle medicine, it is inevitable that physicians and allied healthcare professionals will encounter situations in which they will need to discuss various nutritionally related issues with their patients. In order to be prepared when those scenarios occur, healthcare professionals will need to have a working understanding of various topics, including what constitutes a healthy diet; what are the foods known to nourish the body; how can people stick to a healthy diet; what are the basic factors involved in effective weight management; what can people do to stop overeating; how can people eat more plants which will help with reversal, treatment and prevention of disease as well as weight control and satiety; and why is behavior change the key to effective weight management.

WHAT CONSTITUTES A HEALTHY DIET?

In reality, a healthy diet is not overly complicated. It is the collective byproduct of a person's choices regarding what they eat and drink. In theory, the more often a person makes sound food choices, the healthier they will be. It's helpful to think of healthy eating as a spectrum. The more you move toward the ideal end of the spectrum, the greater results you reap. This factor is especially important for individuals eating for disease reversal, a topic which will be discussed later.

In 2014, a systematic review was published by Dr. David Katz, entitled "Can We Say What Diet is Best for Health?" that evaluated all of the eating patterns with sufficient research to evaluate: low carbohydrate, low-fat/vegetarian/vegan, low-glycemic, Mediterranean, mixed/balanced diet, and the paloelithic diet. It found that among the compatible elements that were included in all of these diets was an emphasis on whole plant foods, as well as a limitation on consuming refined starches, added sugars, and processed foods. It essentially concluded that the healthy eating pattern present in all of these diets was Michael Pollan's recommendation to eat real "food, not too much, mostly plants." This statement is sound advice, and most certainly promotes health and prevents disease.

With regard to healthy eating, there are certain underlying tenets of emphasis concerning the relationship between nutrition and lifestyle medicine to which ACLM is resolutely committed. For the treatment, reversal, and prevention of lifestyle-related chronic disease, the ACLM recommends an eating plan based predominantly on a variety of minimally processed vegetables, fruits, whole grains, legumes, nuts, and seeds. The true beauty of a whole foods, plant-based (WFPB) diet is its simplicity, as well as its impact on helping to prevent and even to reverse some onerous health-related conditions. A WFPB diet should be viewed as a dietary "north star." The closer individuals get to that "north star," the better. Individuals should be encouraged to consume foods that are best for their health as well as for the health of the environment. The focus should be on eating foods that are grown from the ground, in as close to nature's packaging as possible.

Individuals who adopt a predominantly plant-based dietary lifestyle can experience transformative results, in a relatively brief period of time. This metamorphosis can be extremely reinforcing, affirming, and motivating, given the impact of such immediate, positive results.

The ACLM dietary lifestyle message is straightforward and can be summed up in three simple words—EAT MORE PLANTS. As such, the more that an individual moves along the spectrum toward that "north star," the more transformative their results. In that regard, lifestyle medicine practitioners not only need to educate their patients on the power of plants and the WFPB diet, they should also work with them to empower them to move as close as possible to that north star.

NUTRITION BASICS

Before discussing the specifics of whole foods, plant-based nutrition, several basic concepts of nutrition science are worth reviewing, including the essential nutrients, energy balance, and the process of digestion.

THE SIX ESSENTIAL NUTRIENTS

The body requires six essential nutrients that it cannot synthesize on its own (or at least to the degree it needs them). These nutrients, which must be supplied by the diet, are grouped into two main categories—each with three separate entities. The nutrients without calories are water, vitamins, and minerals. Although the non-caloric nutrients do not directly provide energy, they have an essential role because they participate in energy-producing reactions. Without their presence, the body could not produce energy. The caloric nutrients are carbohydrates, protein, and fat. The nutrients with calories supply the energy an individual requires to perform their daily living activities. Carbohydrates and protein each provide four calories per gram, while fat provides nine calories per gram.

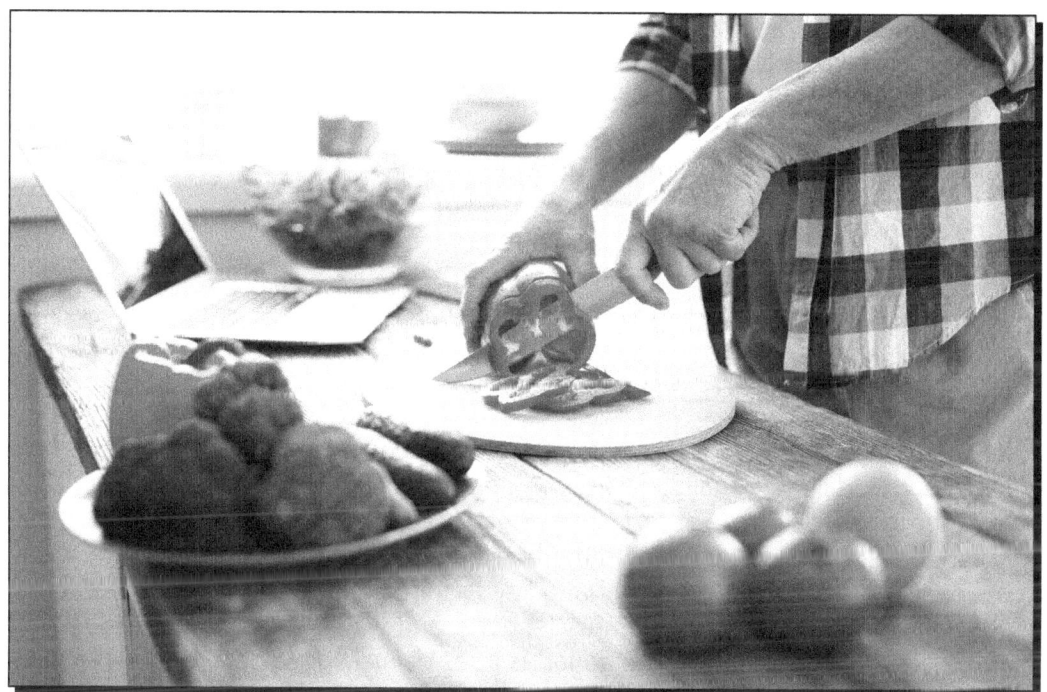

"Nutrition should be recognized as the wholistic effect of countless nutrients involving countless diseases working through countless mechanisms."

Although it is important to have a working understanding of these individual nutrients, the emphasis is often falsely placed on individual nutrient recommendations, instead of whole food recommendations. This erroneous practice is called "nutrition reductionism" and fails to acknowledge the incredible way that all of these nutrients work in concert inside the human body. T. Colin Campbell, PhD, author of *The China Study*, says that "Nutrition should be recognized as the wholistic effect of countless nutrients involving countless diseases working through countless mechanisms. Nutrition must be wholistic: looking at countless nutrients and mechanisms that control many diseases." Simply put, we eat food, not nutrients!

CALORIE AND ENERGY BALANCE BASICS

For a person to maintain body weight, there must be energy balance (a situation in which energy consumed equals energy expended). In that regard, if more energy is consumed than is used, weight will be gained; if more energy is expended than consumed, weight will be lost. However, numerous other factors contribute to and affect energy intake and expenditure, and it is not just about calories. Rather, it is more about quality of the diet than calories. (In a later section, a common sense approach to weight management that focuses on food quality, rather than counting calories, is discussed.)

Several factors affect energy intake, such as ethnic and religious practices, family traditions, childhood experiences (e.g., foods received as rewards), emotional comfort received from food, access, convenience, availability, variety, education, occupation, income, nutrition beliefs, media or peer influences, and the taste of food. Some factors may not be easily controllable—such as physical disability, injury or other form of activity restriction, and physical environment (e.g., living in an unsafe neighborhood)—while other factors, such as making time for exercise, may be.

❑ Components of Energy Expenditure

Total daily energy expenditure (TDEE) can be broken down into the following three components: resting metabolic rate (RMR), also known as resting energy expenditure (REE), thermic effect of food (TEF), also known as dietary induced thermogenesis (DIT), and energy expenditure due to physical activity (EEPA).

• Resting metabolic rate. RMR, the largest component of the TDEE, represents 60-75 percent of daily expenditure. It is the amount of energy the body expends on maintenance activities while at rest, such as growth and maintenance of tissues, organ function, breathing, circulation, and other bodily activities that keep people alive. Many years of scientific research indicate that a key factor correlated with RMR is lean body mass (LBM), which is made up of muscle, bone, and water. The common perception that "muscle burns more calories than fat" is true. Maintaining skeletal muscle requires approximately 13 kcal/kg per day, while adipose tissue requires only 4.5 kcal/kg per day. One effective way to increase RMR is to build skeletal muscle through resistance training. While organs also significantly contribute to RMR, their size or activity cannot be healthily influenced through training or lifestyle modifications.

- Thermic effect of food. TEF is the energy expended to digest and metabolize food. TEF is the smallest component of TDEE, representing only 5-10 percent of the total. Because many factors affect this component, TEF needs to be examined carefully. For example, the TEF is a little higher when digesting and metabolizing proteins and carbohydrates as compared to fats. However, this factor does not mean that unlimited quantities of protein or carbohydrate can be consumed without weight gain. Similarly, TEF is higher for a larger meal as compared with a small snack, but energy expenditure is not significant enough to warrant the frequent consumption of large meals.

Some fad-diet books claim that the timing and/or combinations of nutrient consumption will maximize TEF. While eating a diet that is higher in protein does increase TEF, the absolute number of additional calories burned is likely not clinically significant, particularly in the short term. The same factor goes for eating a few larger meals versus many smaller meals. It is likely easier for an individual to take the stairs at work or consume one less piece of hard candy, rather than preferentially try to increase the TEF. An emphasis needs to be placed on the larger picture: decreasing total energy intake and increasing energy expenditure via physical activity.

- Energy expenditure due to physical activity. EEPA represents all voluntary physical activity, including structured exercise, informal activities (e.g., gardening, running errands, housework), and even fidgeting. EEPA is the most variable of the three components of energy expenditure, typically representing 15-30 percent of the TDEE in most individuals. EEPA can also fall outside of this range. For example, EEPA in a very sedentary person may fall below 15 percent, while in an elite endurance athlete in training, it may be greater than 30 percent. Of the three components of TDEE, EEPA is the one that is most modifiable (unless there is a limiting physical disability present). EPPA is the component where physicians and allied healthcare professionals can be the most influential with helping their patients achieve their weight-management goals.

❑ Measuring Energy Intake and Expenditure

While food provides an important source of joy and pleasure, individuals are ultimately biological systems who must eat to live, rather than live to eat. The overarching goal of physicians and allied healthcare professionals in terms of weight management is helping their patients balance their energy intake with their energy expenditure. On the energy intake side of the balance equation, the role of physicians and allied healthcare professionals is to help their patients understand the energy content of the foods consumed and how to best determine this information. On the energy expenditure side, it is the role of physicians and allied healthcare professionals to determine the mode, frequency, intensity, and duration of physical activity to best meet a patient's weight-management goals. Given that they are knowledgeable in the area, not only can they help assess fitness levels, they can also develop an appropriate exercise regimen for the patient that is in accordance with their needs and interests. If the clinician does not feel comfortable discussing dietary habits and energy balance, the practitioner should recommend the patient work with a registered dietitian.

The energy content of food is measured by a laboratory technique called bomb calorimetry. A sample of dried food is burned and the amount of heat given off is measured in units called kilocalories (kcal). The kilocalories are in the form of gross energy, which does not take digestibility into consideration. However, because the energy values that appear on a food label or in a nutrient database do take digestibility factors into account, the information can be comfortably used by consumers. For example, foods high in fiber are not fully digested in a human body, but are completely combusted in a bomb calorimeter. Therefore, the amount of kilocalories shown on a food label or listed in the USDA nutrient database are invariably less than those measured in a bomb calorimeter. This represents an additional benefit to consuming fiber-rich foods.

Similar to how heat emission from food burned in a bomb calorimeter is used to determine its energy content, heat production during physical activity is used to estimate energy expenditure in a room calorimeter. This direct measure of energy expenditure is accurate. Due to its high cost and relative scarcity, however, it is rarely used in practice.

An alternative method to direct calorimetry involves the collection of inspired and expired air and subsequent analysis of oxygen consumption and carbon dioxide production during rest or physical activity. This method is used widely in both research and clinical practice.

A third method, called doubly-labeled water, is very accurate for measuring energy expenditure in a free-living environment for several days. Unlike the relative confinement of a room calorimeter, this method allows the estimation of energy expended as people live their normal lives, such as performing activities of daily living and formal, structured physical activity. It is, however, very expensive and few laboratories have the resources at this time to practice this method.

The physicians and allied healthcare professionals who want to help a patient achieve their weight-management goals must be able to program a suitable level of exercise to balance that person's energy-intake level. While performing a complete nutrition assessment may not be within the scope of practice for them, a patient's energy needs can be safely estimated, using the various equations that are available in many standard textbooks. It is important to emphasize that all of the equations give estimates, not exact energy requirements. The estimates are a good starting point to determine how much to eat in order to meet goals (i.e., weight loss or maintenance) or how many calories are burned during an exercise session. If weight gain or weight loss is occurring, then the person is not in energy balance, even if the equations indicate otherwise. The next step should be to adjust the exercise program or caloric intake accordingly.

The calorie conversation is less relevant when a person adopts a whole foods, plant-based diet, since they tend to lose weight, or maintain a healthy weight naturally when eating this way and plants tend to aid in this process. Most people following a whole foods, plant-based diet do not count calories, which is one of the benefits of this healthy eating pattern.

HOW FOOD IS DIGESTED: UNDERSTANDING THE BASICS

❏ The Digestive Tract

The digestive tract is a long hollow tube that begins in the mouth and ends at the anus. Nutrients from food must pass through the digestive tract to be absorbed into the bloodstream. Various stages of digestion occur at different parts of the digestive tract. A brief description of the primary digestive activities that occur along the length of the digestive tract can provide the basis for a better understanding of the digestive process.

❏ The Digestive Process

• *The mouth.* In the mouth, chewing serves to grind food into smaller pieces and increase the surface area upon which digestive enzymes can work. Many smaller pieces of food have a larger surface upon which enzymes can bind than does a single chunk of the same amount of that particular food. The larger surface area facilitates digestion, because virtually all digestive activities are driven by enzymatic reactions. In addition, saliva is released in the mouth. Saliva helps to moisten food, which allows for easier swallowing. Although food could be completely digested without first entering the mouth, gastrointestinal transit time is reduced when food is thoroughly masticated prior to swallowing.

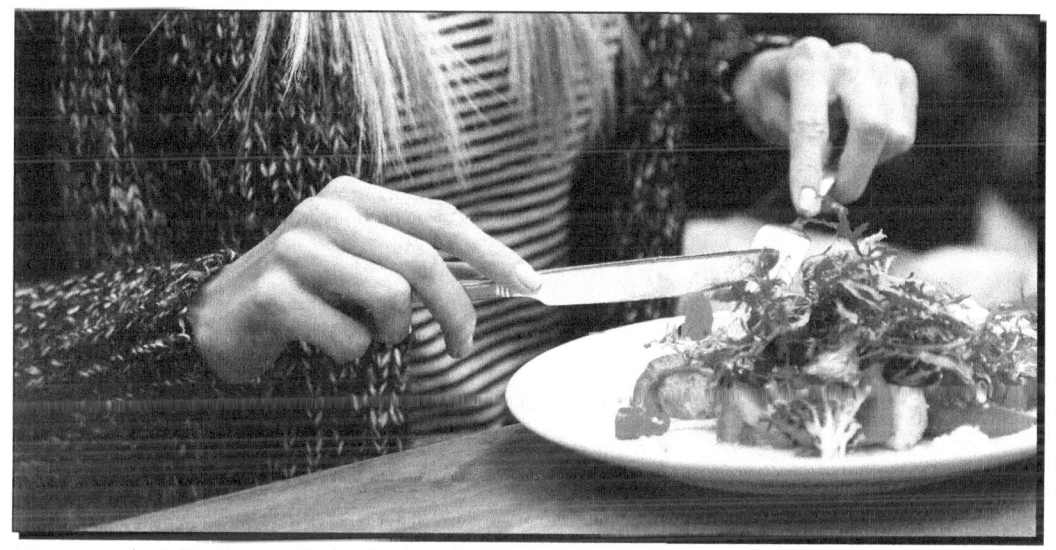

Most people following a whole foods, plant-based diet do not count calories, which is one of the benefits of this healthy eating pattern.

- *The esophagus.* Once food leaves the mouth, it travels to the stomach via a lengthy pipe in the digestive tract called the esophagus. While gravity helps the food travel to the stomach, it is not necessary due to involuntary, wavelike contractions along the entire digestive tract called peristalsis. Peristaltic contractions continually push food forward along the digestive tract. Reverse peristalsis, or vomiting, is the violent contractions of the stomach and esophagus in the opposite direction.

- *The stomach.* The stomach is a holding reservoir that churns food and secretes digestive juices containing acids and enzymes. Food generally stays in the stomach for approximately two to four hours, although a number of factors can affect this timeframe. For example, liquids leave the stomach faster than solids. Carbohydrates exit more rapidly than proteins, and proteins exit more rapidly than lipids. High-fiber carbohydrates stay in the digestive tract longer than simple carbohydrates.

- *The small intestine.* The small intestine is the primary site of digestion and absorption of nutrients into the body. In this part of the digestive tract, plentiful enzymes help break apart larger molecules into particles small enough to cross the intestinal cell wall into the bloodstream. After consumed food is churned and mixed with stomach acid and digestive enzymes in the stomach, it becomes a liquid substance known as chyme that enters the small intestine. Chyme typically remains in the small intestine for 3- 10 hours, depending on its nutrient composition. Of all the macronutrients, fat takes the longest to digest.

   The small intestine is more than just a smooth hollow tube. In fact, it contains villi and microvilli, or folds that significantly increase the surface area to approximately 600 times that of a simple cylinder. The cells that line the intestinal wall have a very short lifespan and completely recycle every three to five days. The small intestine is a "use it or lose it" organ. If a person goes for long periods of time without eating, those cells die. In fact, they are not replaced, because no demand exists for their use. The good news is that intestinal cells will regenerate over time with feeding. On the other hand, an individual cannot rapidly switch from fasting to overeating without some gastrointestinal distress. Until the cells grow back, nutrients will not be adequately absorbed, a situation that will often result in diarrhea.

- *The large intestine.* Any nutrient that is not broken down small enough to cross the small intestinal wall will continue into the large intestine (colon). In a healthy person, only approximately five percent of a meal reaches the colon, an amount that includes some vitamins and minerals. Contents can remain in the large intestine for 24-72 hours, depending on the fiber and fluid content of the meal. The large intestine contains water, sodium, potassium, small amounts of undigested starches, and microflora, which are bacteria that help keep the colon healthy. Colon bacteria are also responsible for producing gas as a by-product of their digestion of fiber or other waste. Diets adequate in fluid and fiber generally result in stools that are soft and easily passed through the rectum. Diets inadequate in fluid and fiber may result in hard, dry stools.

❑ Factors Affecting Digestion

Nervousness or stress can affect digestion time. In fact, no unequivocal rule exists as to whether stress speeds up or slows down digestion. For example, if an individual is nervous, consumed food may stay in the stomach longer than normal and produce an uncomfortable feeling. On the other hand, another person with the same level of stress might experience rapid digestion and the resultant case of diarrhea.

Nutrition science may seem complicated, but it's actually quite simple. As Susan Benigas, executive director of ACLM, co-author of the *Plant-based Nutrition Quick Start Guide*, founder of the Plantrician Project, and co-founder of the International Plant-based Nutrition Healthcare Conference, noted in a press release on August 29, 2018 (http://www.brooklyn-usa.org/nyc-health-hospitals-bellevue-and-bp-adams-announce-pilot-program-for-patients-to-adopt-plant-based-diet-reducing-risk-for-heart-disease-and-diabetes/): "Lifestyle medicine is about how one moves, thinks, sleeps, with what one eats being foundational, focused on a diet heavily comprised of that which grows from the ground in as close to nature's package as possible—nutrient dense, fiber-filled, health protecting and disease fighting." Another powerful quote from Susan Benigas is "Every bite we take is either a step toward health or a step toward disease." The crux of the underlying message that advocates consuming a healthy eating pattern from many sources is simply to eat more plants.

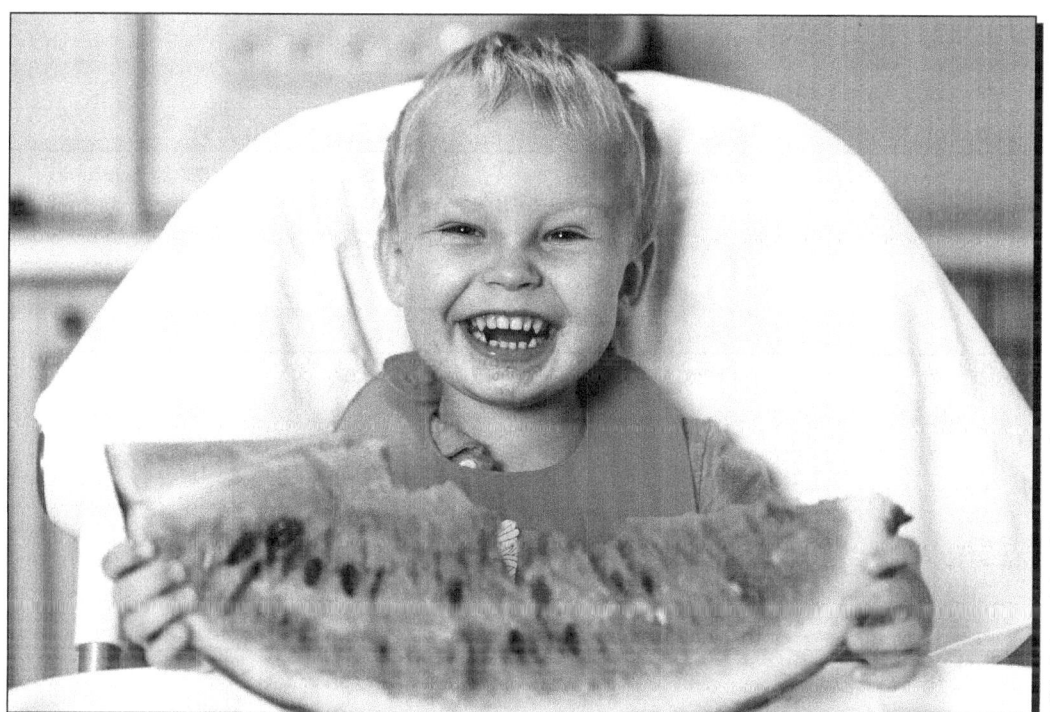

"Every bite we take is either a step toward health or a step toward disease."

Figure 5-1. Plant nutrients

THE POWER OF PLANTS

Plants are powerful. As a country, Americans do not consume fruit and vegetables in high enough quantities. According to the *CDC's Morbidity and Mortality Weekly Report,* only 1 in 10 adults meets the federal fruit or vegetable consumption recommendations. In reality, these recommendations are minimal, with guidelines of 1.5 cups of fruit per day and 2-3 cups of vegetables per day. More reasonable recommendations are to consume *at least* 7-9 servings of fruit and vegetables per day. Ideally, however, the majority of the diet (i.e., a major part of every meal) is made up of plants—fruits and vegetables.

The key is to focus on plant foods in their most complete form, with nothing bad added and nothing good taken away. For example, sugar and Oreo cookies are vegan, but that doesn't make them health foods. Furthermore, nuts, seeds, and avocados are higher fat foods, yet they are whole, unprocessed, and health-promoting. In other words, it's not the particular diet label or individual nutrient that matters. It is the overall quality of the food in the diet that matters, and whole, plant foods are the highest quality foods.

Most people are amazed to learn about all the nutrients packed into plants. Figure 5-1 reveals a summary of this information. Plants provide a powerful array of nutrients. All of the vitamins and minerals needed to be healthy (with the exception of vitamin B12) are found in vegetables, fruits, whole grains, nuts, seeds, and beans.

Nutrient	Deficiency Results In	Good Plant Sources	
Vitamin A	Blindness	Apricots Broccoli Cantaloupe Carrots Collards Mango	Romaine lettuce Spinach Squash Sweet potatoes Sweet red peppers
Calcium	Osteoporosis	Artichoke Broccoli Cheese Chinese cabbage Collards Clams Hummus Kale	Legumes Molasses Mustard greens Nuts Orange juice (fortified) Spinach Squash Turnip greens

Figure 5-1. Plant nutrients

Nutrient	Deficiency Results In	Good Plant Sources	
Vitamin C	Scurvy	Berries Broccoli Brussels sprouts Citrus fruits (oranges)	Dark green leafy vegetables Kiwi Peas Peppers (yellow) Tomatoes
Cobalamin (Vitamin B12)	Anemia	Fortified cereals Fortified nutritional yeast Tofu *Food sources should not be relied upon for adequate B12.	*Supplementation is recommended for those individuals who are eating a predominantly plant-based diet.*
Vitamin D	Rickets	Mushrooms Tofu	*Sunlight is perhaps the best source.*
Folate (Vitamin B9)	Anemia Birth defects	Asparagus Baked potatoes Beans Beets Broccoli Brussels sprouts Cabbage Collard greens Corn	Mustard greens Nuts Oranges Romaine lettuce Spinach Sweet potatoes Wheat grain breads and cereal
Iodine	Hypothyroidism	Baked potato Green beans White bread	Cranberries Dried seaweed Dried prunes
Iron	Anemia	Apricots Beans Broccoli Dried fruit, e.g., prunes, raisins Green pepper	Prune juice Pumpkin, sesame, or squash seeds Rice Spinach Soybeans Tofu
Magnesium	Convulsions Heart arrhythmias Weakness Tremor Tetany	Baked potato Black-eyed peas Beans Green leafy vegetables	Nuts Whole grains

Figure 5-1. Plant nutrients (cont.)

Nutrient	Deficiency Results In	Good Plant Sources	
Niacin (Vitamin B3)	Pellagra	Avocado Brown rice Green vegetables	Peanuts Sunflower seeds
Potassium	Heart arrhythmias Muscle weakness	Apricots Avocados Baked potato Bananas Cantaloupe Dates Honeydew melon Kiwi Nuts	Oranges and orange juice Peaches Prunes Raisins Spinach Tomatoes Winter squash
Thiamine (Vitamin B1)	Beriberi	Black beans Black-eyed peas	Sunflower seeds Wheat germ

Figure 5-1. Plant nutrients (cont.)

VITAMIN B12

Vitamin B12 aids in the development and production of nerve cells and red blood cells, as well as in DNA production. Deficiency is very serious, resulting in weakness, difficulty concentrating, anemia, and nervous system dysfunction.

B12 is the only nutrient that cannot be reliably obtained from a predominantly plant-based diet, not, however, because it is only sourced from animal products. Rather, B12 is actually made by bacteria. Animals obtain B12 by ingesting bacteria-containing dirt and water. Because of modern sanitation practices, humans rarely consume bacteria-containing B12. Accordingly, supplementation is recommended to ensure adequate intake. Patients can either take a B12 supplement daily of 10 micrograms, or consume a weekly B12 supplement of 2000 micrograms. Several foods are fortified with B12, such as plant milks (coconut, almond, cashew), soy products, and some breakfast cereals. If patients are consuming their B12 through these foods, it is recommended that they eat them two to three times a day in order to accumulate three micrograms a day.

CALCIUM: THE DAIRY MYTH

Whole, plant foods are superior packages for delivering calcium to the human body. The calcium in plant foods, like leafy greens and beans, are housed with other beneficial nutrients that improve calcium absorption and utilization.

It's a commonly believed myth that dairy products are superior and necessary sources of calcium. This belief is simply not true. In fact, cultures with the highest fracture risk also have the highest intakes of dairy products. In turn, countries that rarely or never consume dairy have the lowest rates of osteoporosis.

Dairy is high in saturated fat and cholesterol, and even fat-free dairy products still contain a protein called casein, which has been associated with prostate and breast cancers. Therefore, it is best to rely on plant foods to meet calcium needs.

While calcium is an important nutrient for skeletal health, a strong skeleton is more dependent on preserving calcium in the body than it is on consuming large amounts of calcium. The following are calcium-preserving tips that lifestyle medicine practitioners can share with their patients:
- Exercise regularly with weight-bearing activities, such as walking, jogging, and strength training.
- Avoid tobacco.
- Limit or avoid alcohol consumption.
- Limit highly processed, packaged, and restaurant foods, in order to manage sodium intake.
- Avoid excessive protein intake by eating a WFPB diet.
- Get an adequate intake of vitamin D via sun exposure, fortified plant milks, or supplementation, if needed.
- Eat calcium-rich plant foods, like dark leafy greens, lentils, and tofu.

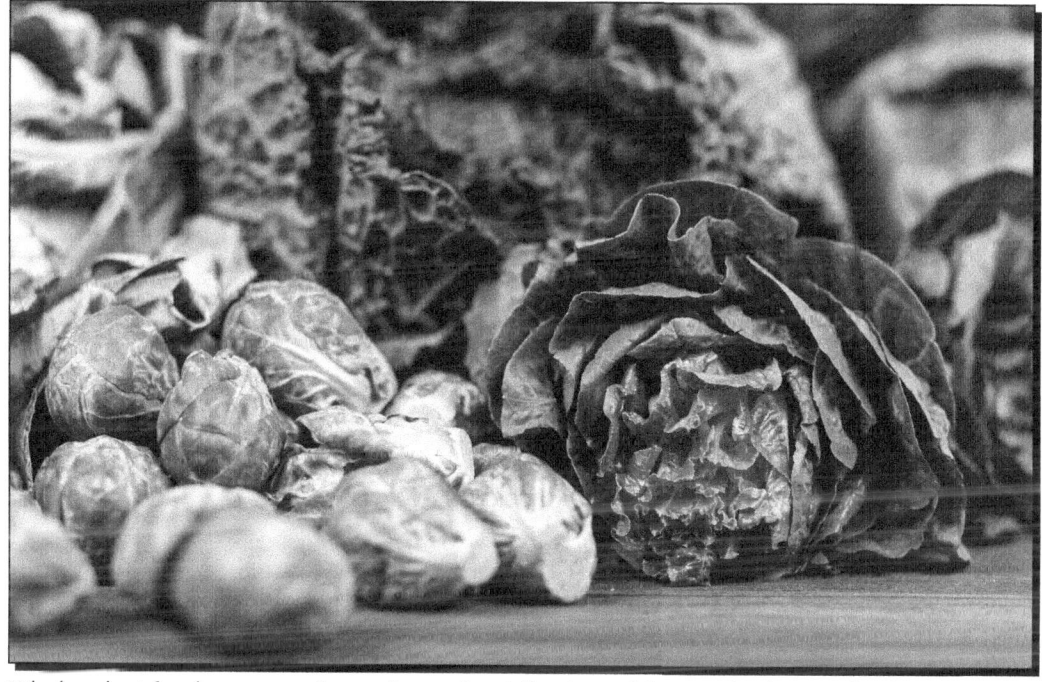

Whole, plant foods are superior packages for delivering calcium to the human body.

Vitamins and minerals are not the only important compounds in plants. Plants also have a plethora of phytonutrients that help to keep the body healthy and fight disease. The recommendation is to eat a rainbow of colors for variety, as well as to help ensure people are consuming as many different phytonutrients as possible. The different colors of the fruits and vegetables indicate that they have different phytonutrients in them. Figure 5-2 reviews this factor.

NATURAL HEALTHY
5 Colors of phytonutrients

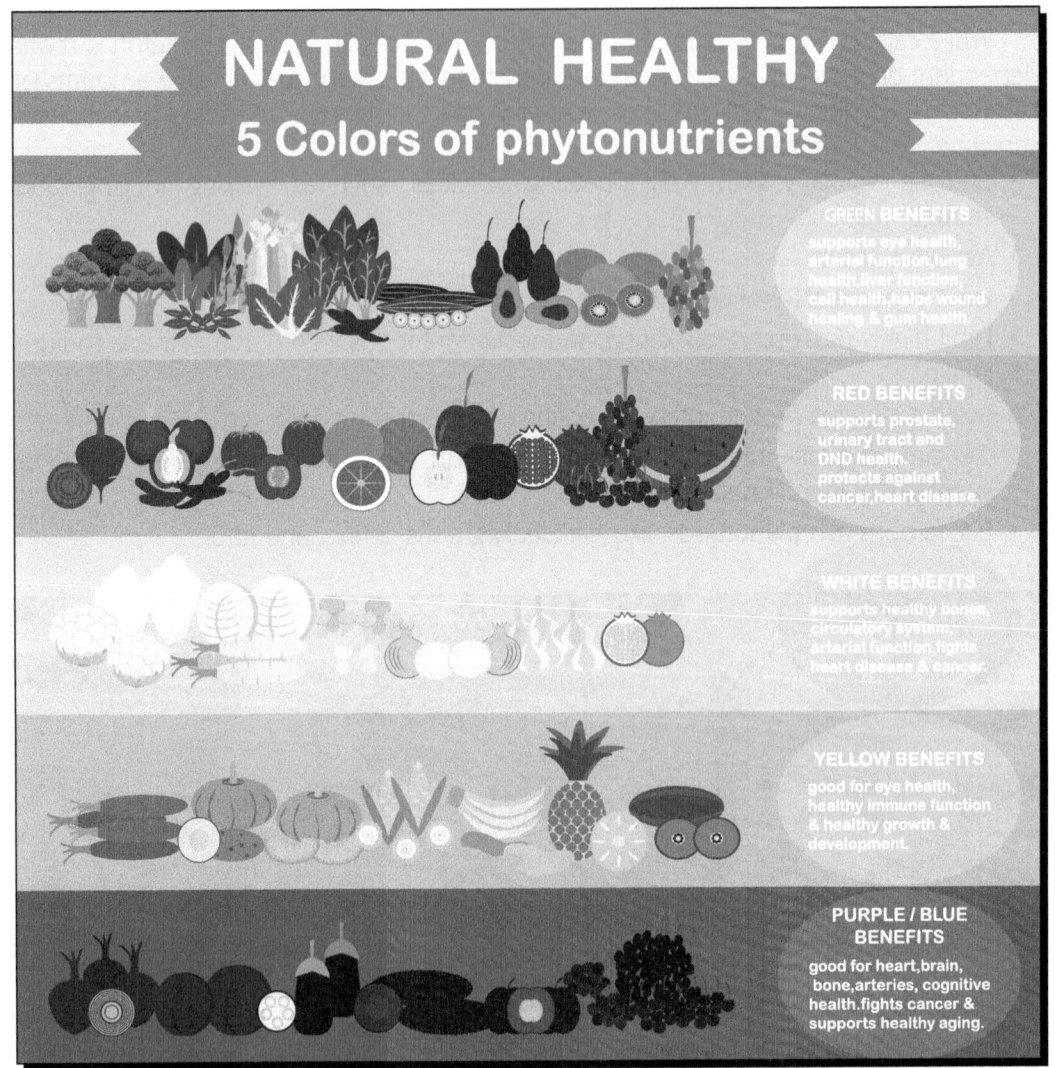

GREEN BENEFITS
supports eye health, arterial function, lung health, liver function, cell health, helps wound healing & gum health.

RED BENEFITS
supports prostate, urinary tract and DND health, protects against cancer, heart disease.

WHITE BENEFITS
supports healthy bones, circulatory system, arterial function, fights heart disease & cancer.

YELLOW BENEFITS
good for eye health, healthy immune function & healthy growth & development.

PURPLE / BLUE BENEFITS
good for heart, brain, bone, arteries, cognitive health, fights cancer & supports healthy aging.

Figure 5-2. Five colors of phytonutrients you should eat every day

PLANT PROTEIN

Plants are also great sources of protein. As such, individuals who eat only plants can easily achieve adequate amounts of protein each day. Just like calcium, plant protein comes packaged with countless other important vitamins, minerals, phytochemicals, fiber, and water. This is a stark contrast to the packaging of animal-based protein, which is delivered with unhealthy saturated fat and cholesterol. Western culture has become protein-obsessed, falsely believing that more is always better and that protein must come from animal-based foods. These are unfounded beliefs. The recommended protein intake is just 0.8 grams per kilogram of body weight (just 55 grams for a 150 lb. person). Excess protein is either stored as fat or excreted. Patients can meet their protein needs through plant-based foods, like beans, lentils, nuts, seeds, and whole grains. Figure 5-3 details a variety of plant sources with their protein content.

HEALTHY EATING BASICS

Physicians and allied health professionals can help their patients better understand the fundamental factors involved in a healthy, WFPB diet by offering them the following guidelines, while focusing on food groups vs. nutrients:
- Consume a variety of foods—no one food has every nutrient a person needs.
- Fill at least half your plate with vegetables and fruits in a rainbow of colors at every meal and even at snacks.
- Focus on whole grains—make whole grains the majority of the grains consumed daily. Avoid refined grains, like white breads, pastas, cookies, cakes, and pastries.
- Consume more beans, peas, and lentils.
- Include a portion controlled amount (a small handful) of nuts and seeds each day.
- Drink plenty of water to stay hydrated. Proper hydration is important for healthy immune, endocrine, cardiovascular, neural, gastrointestinal, muscle, and skeletal function.
- Reduce or work to eliminate red meat, poultry, and eggs.
- If consuming fish, limit it to twice a week, due to mercury contamination.
- Avoid trans fats—not only do they raise an individual's level of LDL (bad) cholesterol, they also lower their level of HDL (good) cholesterol.
- Limit highly processed and packaged foods, which tend to be high in sodium. Not only does excess sodium raise blood pressure, it may have other potentially harmful effects on certain chronic diseases. In contrast, potassium lowers blood pressure.
- Limit added processed oils. Unlike whole plant sources of fat, oils are extremely calorie dense and relatively nutrient poor.
- Do not rely on supplements as a substitute for real food. Supplements simply cannot provide the resultant "synergy" that occurs in the body that many nutrients require to be efficiently utilized in the body. In some instances of vitamin deficiency, a supplement might be recommended, depending on the level of deficiency.

Food	Amount	Protein (gm)	Protein (gm/100 cal)
Almond butter	2 Tbsp	7	3.4
Almonds	1/4 cup	8	3.7
Bagel	1 med. (3.5 oz)	11	4.1
Black beans, cooked	1 cup	15	6.7
Black-eyed peas, cooked	1 cup	13	6.7
Broccoli, cooked	1 cup	4	6.7
Bulgur, cooked	1 cup	6	3.7
Cashews	1/4 cup	5	2.9
Chickpeas, cooked	1 cup	15	5.4
Kidney beans, cooked	1 cup	15	6.8
Lentils, cooked	1 cup	18	7.8
Lima beans, cooked	1 cup	15	6.8
Peanut butter	2 Tbsp	8	4.1
Peas, cooked	1 cup	9	6.4
Pinto beans, cooked	1 cup	15	6.3
Quinoa, cooked	1 cup	8	3.7
Seitan	3 ounces	21	15.6
Soy milk, commercial, plain	1 cup	7	6.6
Soy yogurt, plain	8 ounces	6	4.0
Soybeans, cooked	1 cup	31	10.6
Spaghetti, cooked	1 cup	7	3.7
Spinach, cooked	1 cup	5	13.0
Sunflower seeds	1/4 cup	6	3.3
Tempeh	1 cup	34	10.6
Textured vegetable protein (TVP), cooked	1/2 cup	12	15.0
Tofu, extra firm	4 ounces	12	11.2
Tofu, regular	4 ounces	10	10.7
Veggie baked beans	1 cup	12	5.0
Veggie burger	1 patty	15	10.7
Veggie dog	1 link	10	20.0
Whole wheat bread	2 slices	8	5.4

Source: Reed Mangels, PhD, RD, *Simply Vegan*, The Vegetarian Resource Group, www.vrg.org. Used with permission.

Figure 5-3. Protein content of selected vegan foods

- Never overlook the calories in liquids—over one-fifth of the calories in the average American's diet comes from beverages (of all types).
- Never drink alcohol in excess—the basic rule of thumb is that women should be limited to one drink a day, and men to two drinks a day. There is some evidence that abstaining from alcohol is beneficial, especially with regard to cancer, specifically breast cancer. This decision is personal, one that needs to be made looking at the current research and the patient's personal risk factors. The American Heart Association recommends that if you don't drink, don't start.

BUILDING A BALANCED PLATE

After making nutrition recommendations to patients, it's vital also show them how to put those recommendations into action. The plate model, which is commonly used by many nutrition groups, is a great way to teach practical application. The plate graphic created by registered dietitians Brenda Davis and Vesanto Melina in their book *Becoming Vegan: Comprehensive Edition* aligns well with ACLM's nutrition recommendations (Figure 5-4). Although the graphic is titled "The Vegan Plate," utilizing the word "vegan," it employs the principles of a WFPB dietary pattern.

Becoming Vegan: Comprehensive Edition, Brenda Davis and Vesanto Melina, Book Publishing Co. 2014. Used with permission.

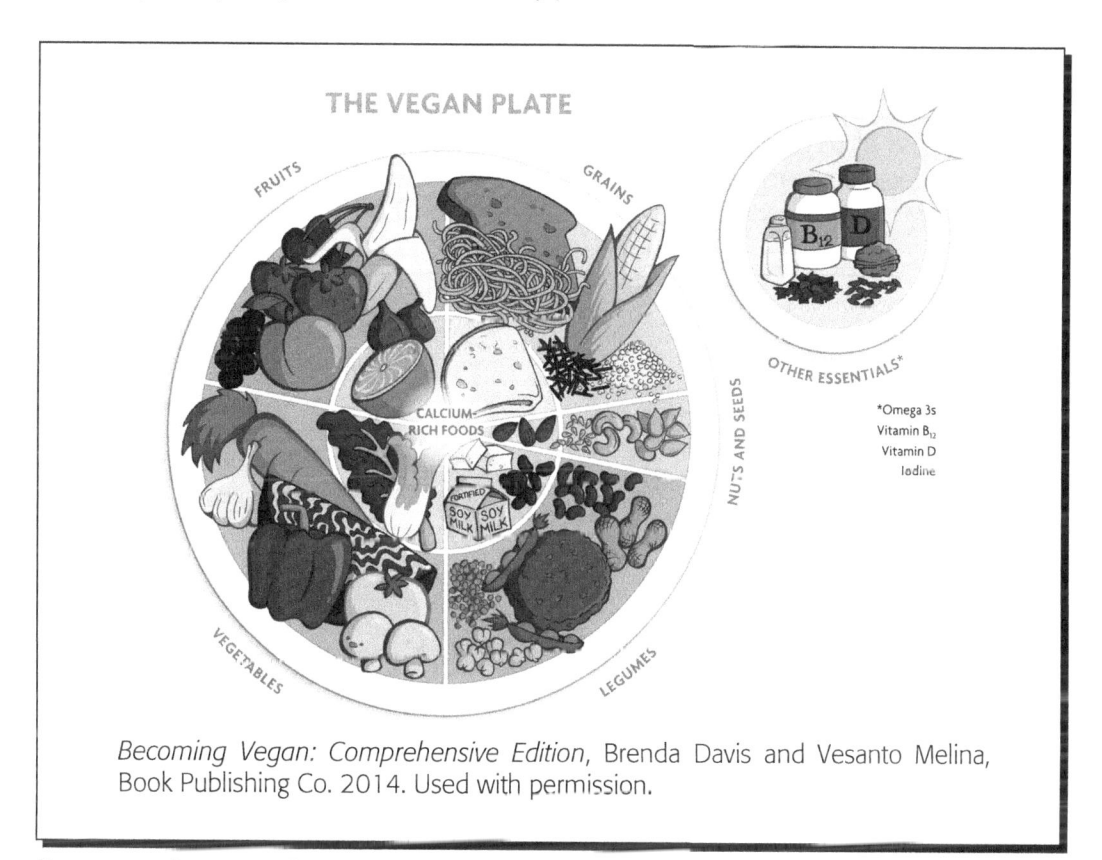

Figure 5-4. The Vegan Plate

ACLM advocates this eating pattern so that people will understand that healthy eating is not complicated. Every meal offers a choice to move further along the spectrum toward a predominantly WFPB diet. On occasion, individuals may make a conscious choice to deviate from their progression along the spectrum. In this instance, it is a choice, and they are aware of their digression. One meal or one snack that is not whole foods, plant-based does not mean all is lost. When the body receives the nourishing components of the plants again, the health promoting effects will start up again.

Every time someone eats plants, they take a step toward health. When people choose to consume highly processed, hyperpalatable foods they take a step away. It is a choice people make every day. Lifestyle medicine practitioners need to work to educate and empower people to choose whole foods, plant-based options.

PREVENTING, HALTING, AND REVERSING DISEASE

Evidence shows that a predominantly plant-based, whole foods dietary pattern has the power to prevent, arrest, and even reverse disease. In support of the whole foods, plant-based approach, Dr. Neal Barnard and colleagues published a paper in the journal *Nutrients*, in 2017, which reported on the cardiometabolic benefits of this type of plant-based diet. According to this article, plant-based diets may reduce the risk of coronary heart disease events by an approximately 40 percent and the risk of cerebral vascular disease events by approximately 29 percent. In addition, plant-based diets can reduce the risk of developing metabolic syndrome and type 2 diabetes by about 50 percent. Understanding the extensive evidence behind this well-documented approach to nutrition will help lifestyle medicine practitioners confidently educate patients.

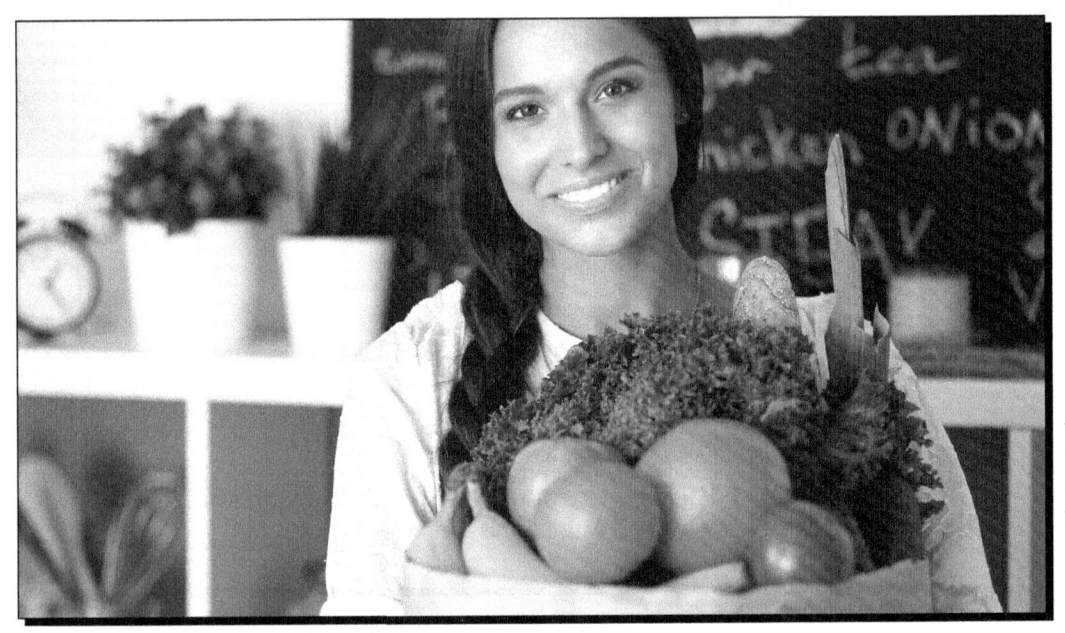

Healthy eating is not complicated.

THE FOUNDATION OF HEALTHY EATING

Walter Willett, MD, DrPH, MPH, former chair of the Harvard School of Public Health nutrition department, is one of the world's preeminent experts and researchers concerning the effects of a diet on the occurrence of major diseases. For almost four decades, he has investigated the long-term health consequences of food choices. Among his more noteworthy research findings are the following:

❑ The Importance of Fiber-Rich Whole Grains

Regarding fiber, Dr. Willett has found that a higher intake of fiber from green products is associated with a lower risk of coronary heart disease and diabetes. Furthermore, he suggests that substituting carbohydrate for saturated fat increases a person's level of the "good" cholesterol (HDL). HDL is a high-density lipoprotein, which, ideally, should be high. Furthermore, substituting monounsaturated fat for saturated fat diminishes LDL in an individual's bloodstream, without affecting HDL. In other words, it won't decrease HDL, but it will lower LDL, which is good, given that LDL (low-density lipoprotein) is the "bad" cholesterol.

❑ Reducing Red Meat to Reduce Disease Risk

Eating red meat, particularly processed meat, is associated with an increased risk of diabetes. Furthermore, lowering a person's intake of red meat will likely decrease the incidence of coronary heart disease, diabetes, colon cancer, and possibly premenopausal breast cancer.

❑ Reducing Salt Intake and Increasing Fruit and Vegetable Intake to Reduce Blood Pressure

Excess salt is irrefutably linked to high blood pressure. Researchers believe that individuals respond differently to salt, with some people being highly sensitive and others being able to tolerate higher intakes. For some people, lowering a person's intake of salt could potentially have significant beneficial effects. For example, it has been estimated at population level that a reduction of three grams per day of salt would reduce stroke by 22 percent and coronary heart disease by 16 percent. Furthermore, a higher intake of fruits and vegetables can have a positive impact on a person's risk of cardiovascular disease. The recommended daily intake of sodium is 1,500 milligrams per day, which is less than half of what the average American consumes each day.

HALTING AND REVERSING DISEASE WITH A WHOLE FOODS, PLANT-BASED DIET

Based on existing evidence and their own research, several luminary physicians, such as Caldwell B. Esselstyn, Jr., Dean Ornish, John McDougall, and Neal Barnard, have developed practical, specific dietary principles aimed at preventing and, most importantly, reversing a variety of diseases, including diabetes, heart disease, high cholesterol, hypertension, and obesity. Lifestyle medicine professionals should use these principles to shape their nutritional recommendations for patients.

The powerful disease-reversing approaches of each of these renowned physicians share many common threads. For example, they all recommend a predominantly whole foods, plant-based diet, including whole grains, vegetables, fruits, beans, and legumes. They also recommend keeping dietary fat intake low, around 10 percent of total calories, for disease reversal. This advice can be achieved by relying on the naturally-occuring fat found in the aforementioned plant foods, keeping portions of high-fat nuts, seeds, and avocados very small, as well as eliminating oil. Other common threads include limiting or eliminating added sugar and alcohol, animal products, and high-sodium foods, as well as staying adequately hydrated with plenty of unsweetened, non-caloric beverages like water and herbal teas.

The best-selling book *Prevent and Reverse Heart Disease* by Caldwell B. Esselstyn, Jr., MD, the renowned former Cleveland Clinic physician, outlines his dietary approach in detail. In addition to the aforementioned principles, Dr. Esselstyn heavily emphasizes eating dark leafy greens with every meal and eating rolled oats every day. With regard to avoiding all animal products, Dr. Esselstyn states that research suggests that digesting meat releases a byproduct, trimethylamine oxide (TMAO), that's an even stronger predictor of heart disease than cholesterol. Among the study participants who remained adherent to Esselstyn's diet, there was just a 0.6 percent recurrent cardiovascular event rate, compared to a 62 percent recurrent event rate in the nonadherent group.

Similar to the dietary approach advocated by Dr. Esselstyn, the dietary principles, developed by the renowned American physician and researcher Dean Ornish, are targeted at preventing the progression of coronary artery disease, as well as facilitating an actual improvement in coronary artery plaques. Dr. Ornish's diet and his lifestyle program have been tested and studied over the course of many years. In his Lifestyle Heart Trial, 82 percent of participants adhering to his diet saw an average change toward regression of their coronary artery disease. The evidence is so compelling that Dr. Ornish's program is one of the only endeavors that is covered by insurance for cardiac patients.

Along with Esselstyn and Ornish, Dr. John McDougall is a medical doctor and nutrition expert, who has been working and teaching in the area of nutrition for improved health and disease reversal for over 50 years. For 16 years, he operated an intensive in-hospital program at St. Helena Hospital and Health Center in Napa Valley. Currently, he conducts a 10-day residential clinic in Santa Rosa, California. More information about him and his program is available on his website (https://www.drmcdougall.com/health/education/free-mcdougall-program/introduction/).

Dr. Neal Barnard, founder of the Physicians Committee for Responsible Medicine, is well-known for his approach to reversing type 2 diabetes, which is outlined in his book

Dr. Neal Barnard's Program for Reversing Diabetes. Following the tenets of a low-fat, whole foods, plant-based diet, Dr. Barnard's research shows that adherents can lower their blood sugar levels and reduce medication use, compared to people following a standard diabetic diet protocol. They also see double the reduction in "bad" cholesterol levels, HbA1c levels, and body weight, compared to standard treatment protocol.

In addition to heart disease and diabetes, it is also worth mentioning that a whole foods, plant-based diet can prevent and slow cancer growth. Specifically, it reduces gastrointestinal cancers, as well as other cancers, such as ovarian and breast cancer. Plants are rich in cancer-fighting antioxidants and phytonutrients. According to the World Cancer Research Fund, lifestyle changes, including diet, could prevent as many as one-third of all cancer cases in the U.S.

The aforementioned luminary physicians are noteworthy instances of programs that have long, successful, evidence-based track records for helping patients reverse disease. The ACLM holds these diets up as standards of excellence for reversal, treatment, and prevention of disease. They are excellent examples of whole foods, plant-based diets, with a strong focus on consuming plants in their natural form, as close to the way they come out of the ground as possible.

TWO POPULAR DIETS ON THE SPECTRUM TOWARD WFPB

Patients face a million-dollar question: what diet can help them lose weight and keep it off, in addition to being good for their health? In that regard, a whole foods, plant-based diet is the appropriate choice. Two other popular diets consistently advocated by nutritional and health experts are the DASH diet and the Mediterranean diet. Because these diets are so commonly discussed, it is important to understand their underlying principles.

These diets both share some common threads with the north star WFPB diet. For, example, they emphasize plants and limit animal sources of food. The DASH diet allows six ounces of meat per day (three ounces is the size of a deck of cards). In reality, a number of Americans on the SAD diet are eating portions of meat that are practically three decks of cards for each meal, which would add up to 27 ounces per day. Accordingly, a limit of six ounces is a marked reduction. In addition, these diets emphasize vegetables, whole grains, nuts, seeds and legumes being front and center for all meals.

❏ DASH Diet

A dietary approach promoted by the U.S.-based National Heart, Lung, and Blood Institute (a part of the National Institutes of Health—an agency of the United States Department of Health and Human Services), the DASH diet is designed to help prevent and control hypertension. It can promote the loss of unwanted pounds, given that it can help guide a patient toward consuming healthier meals and snacks. It's guidelines may provide a helpful stepwise approach toward WFPB for patients who need it.

DASH, which is an acronym for *Dietary Approaches to Stop Hypertension*, is a diet rich in fruits, vegetables, whole grains, nuts, and beans, as well as consuming low-fat dairy foods. It includes the allowance of limited portions of meat, fish, and poultry, while limiting sugar-sweetened foods and beverages, sodium, red meat, and added fats. A sample breakdown for a 2,000 calories DASH diet is detailed in Figure 5-5.

Food Group	Servings per Day	What a Serving Size Equals
Grains	6-8	1 slice whole-wheat bread, 1 ounce (oz.) dry cereal, or ½ cup cooked cereal, rice, or pasta
Vegetables	4-5	1 cup raw leafy green vegetables or ½ cup cut-up raw or cooked vegetables
Fruit	4-5	1 medium fruit or ½ cup fresh, frozen, or canned fruit or 4 ounces of juice
Low-fat or fat-free dairy	2-3	1 cup skim or 1 percent milk, 1 cup yogurt, or 1 ½ oz. cheese
Lean meat, poultry, and fish	6 or less* *6 ounces or less a day	1 oz. cooked skinless poultry, seafood, or lean meat or 1 egg
Nuts, seeds, or legumes	4-5 per week	1/3 cup (1 ½ oz.) nuts, 2 tablespoons seeds, or ½ cup cooked beans or peas
Fats and oils	2-3	1 teaspoon vegetable oil, 1 tablespoon mayonnaise, or 2 tablespoons salad dressing
Sweets	Less than 5 servings per week	1 tablespoon sugar

Figure 5-5. Breakdown of the DASH diet for a 2,000 calorie daily ration

The following tips can be helpful to individuals who want to embrace the DASH diet:
- Include at least three whole grains each day.
- Consume a variety of fruits and vegetables.
- Consider eating raw veggies, such as mini peppers, mini cucumbers, and sugar snap peas.
- Add fruits and vegetables to smoothies, remembering that eating whole plant—fruit or vegetable—is the healthiest option.
- Eat fruit to curb sweet cravings.
- Eat legumes 4-5 times a week.
- Consider having a vegetarian meal at least once a week.

- Add beans to a side dish, soup, salad, or main dish.
- Add nuts or seeds to morning oatmeal, on a salad, or simply eat a serving for a snack.
- Try meatless recipes. If a person is just starting to focus on nutrition, they should try the meatless Monday approach.
- If a person chooses to consume dairy foods, choose low-fat or non-fat options.
- Consume foods that are relatively high in fiber (e.g., fruits, vegetables, whole grains, and legumes).
- Avoid eating processed foods that are high in sugar, salt, and fat.
- Reduce the amount of foods eaten that are high in saturated fat, cholesterol, and trans fat.

❏ Mediterranean Diet

People along the coast of the Mediterranean Sea, from the shores of Spain to the seaboard of Greece, have enjoyed the benefits of healthy eating for centuries. In recent years, their Mediterranean diet has garnered the intense interest of physicians and medical researchers. It has been found, in a number of well-conducted clinical studies, to successfully reduce weight, cholesterol levels, and cardiac risk. It has also been shown to lower the incidence of diabetes, cancer, Alzheimer's, and Parkinson's disease.

The founders of ACLM, back in 2004, established the American College of Lifestyle Medicine as the nation's preeminent medical professional society to fill the void of representing the field of medicine that uses lifestyle as a therapeutic intervention for the treatment and, often, reversal of disease—which is the underlying mission of ACLM. When lifestyle is prescribed in therapeutic doses adequate for treatment and reversal, then prevention is the natural byproduct. Accordingly, lifestyle medicine truly is what ACLM advocates become the foundation of all healthcare. When individuals speak to prevention and dietary lifestyle, whereas science is clear that treatment and reversal are facilitated by a low fat, plant-predominant way of eating, as well as when someone looks at the science that supports the efficacy of prevention, the Mediterranean diet is shown to be a healthful way of eating. The question then becomes, what is the clear definition of the Mediterranean diet?

The true Mediterranean diet is primarily focused on eating plant-based foods and foods that are fresh and unprocessed. Colorful vegetables and fresh fruits, whole grains, nuts, beans, and unsaturated fats, like olive oil, are consumed daily. Herbs and spices are used to flavor food, instead of salt. Fish and seafood are eaten a couple times per week. Portions of dairy products, poultry, and eggs are limited. Absent from the Mediterranean diet are packaged and processed foods. Simple sugars, sweets, and soda are also discouraged. In addition, greasy and fatty foods are avoided.

The Mediterranean diet is not something someone "goes on" or "does." Instead, it is a way of life that also includes physical activity and strong social relationships. It is important to note that no single, monolithic, traditional Mediterranean diet exists. Rather, there are several similarities among what the various countries in the Mediterranean typically eat. Accordingly, the traditional, healthy Mediterranean diet tends to encompass the following features:
- Emphasizes natural whole foods, while minimizing highly processed foods.
- Recommends eating an abundance of foods from plants daily (e.g., vegetables, fruit, beans, potatoes, nuts, seeds, and whole grain products).
- Encourages the use of "good" fats, including nuts, seeds, olives, avocados, and olive oil as the predominant fat (oil) for cooking and baking.
- Recommends consuming fish just twice per week.
- Limits milk products to mainly cheese and yogurt, in small amounts.
- Limits the number of eggs eaten weekly to four or less, and small portions of poultry.
- Allows wine to be consumed in low-to-moderate amounts, typically at mealtimes.
- Considers red meat and sweets "sometimes" foods that are only consumed on special occasions.

According to Oldways, a non-profit food and nutrition educational organization, committed to tradition-based eating patterns, the following tips can help enhance the efforts of someone who decides to adopt the Mediterranean diet:

- Fill at least half their plate with vegetables at lunch and dinner.
- If they choose to eat meat, think about red meat and poultry as condiments rather than the main course.
- Limit dairy to Greek or plain yogurt and cheese, in small portions.
- Eat seafood rich in omega-3 fatty acids twice per week.
- Start incorporating more vegetarian meals into their week, built from beans, whole grains, and vegetables.
- Flavor dishes with plenty of herbs and spices.
- Include "good" fats in their meals, like nuts, seeds, avocados, olives, and olive oil for cooking.
- Switch to whole grains, and try traditional Mediterranean grains, such as bulgur, barley, farro, and brown rice.

Although the aforementioned two diets are heavy on plants, they do allow for some meat, fish, and dairy consumption. The portions of these foods, however, are drastically smaller than what most Americans eat. Furthermore, unlike with whole plant foods, these diets communicate upper limits to all animal-based foods. In other words, recommendations are conveyed as eating "no more than"; in other words, consuming

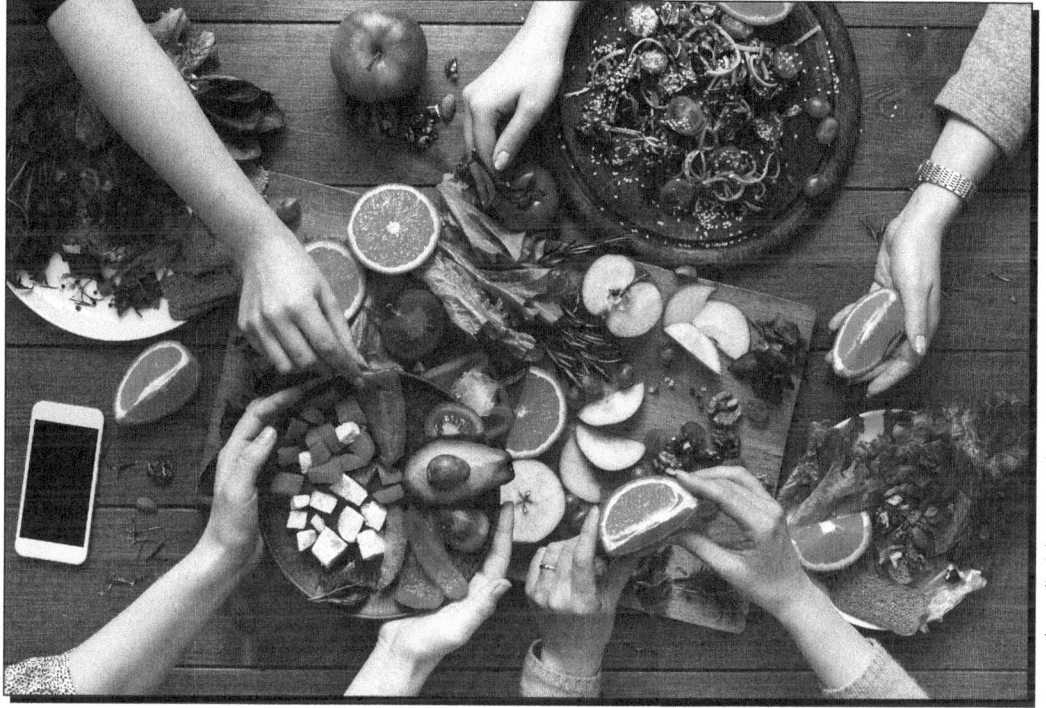

The only dietary pattern shown to reverse disease is a WFPB diet.

too much can have ill effects. In contrast, with whole plant foods, abundance and variety are key. These eating patterns are considered healthier than the SAD diet, and exist on the spectrum toward the north star WFPB diet. It is important to remember, however, that the only dietary pattern shown to *reverse* disease is a WFPB diet.

Because fish is a rich source of Omega 3 fatty acids, it's sometimes included as part of a predominantly whole foods, plant-based dietary lifestyle. Even research on individuals who reside in the blue zone regions of the world, those populations with the greatest longevity and lowest incidence of chronic disease, shows that these inhabitants consume small amounts of animal protein (just three to five times per month). These animal-based foods, however, are not required parts of their overall traditional diets. Dan Buettner, founder and president of Blue Zones, is often quoted saying, "Eat your beans!" because one factor that blue zone populations have in common is that they eat, on average, at least a cup of beans each and every day. The bottom line: making beans the center of an individual's meals instead of animal products is a wise and acceptable choice on any variation of a traditional, healthy diet. They are health-promoting and environmentally-friendly, as well as affordable.

NEED TO KNOW: 2015-2020 DIETARY GUIDELINES FOR AMERICANS

The most widely available nutrition recommendations are the *2015-2020 Dietary Guidelines for Americans*, developed by the U.S. Government. Because these recommendations are likely familiar to many patients, it is helpful to review the foundation of this document. This resource was designed as a tool for professionals to enable them to help enhance the ability of individuals to make healthy choices in their lives, as well as to enjoy a healthy diet.

In essence, the *Guidelines* serve as the evidence-based foundation for the nutrition education materials developed by the U.S. Government. Though no document is perfect, and there can be "contamination" or bias in any committee-created recommendations, these guidelines can be a useful resource for those patients who are currently consuming the SAD diet, full of processed foods, heavy in animal products, and light in plants. These guidelines set limits on the amount of meat and dairy. They also recommend limiting trans-fats, saturated fat, sugar, and salt.

Overall, the *Dietary Guidelines for Americans (DGA)* have remained fairly consistent, since they were initially released in 1980. However, new research on various dietary-related issues is being conducted and released all of the time. As such, the *Dietary Guidelines* are reviewed and updated every five years to reflect any new scientific evidence or clarification/understanding of previous information. The most recent *Guidelines* (2015-2020) have taken a big-picture approach, choosing to emphasize healthy eating patterns as a whole across the lifespan, as opposed to specific, individual nutrients.

The overarching theme of the *Dietary Guidelines* is that individuals need to build a healthy eating pattern. For example, people need to consume more fruits and vegetables, as well as more unrefined carbs and whole grains. Furthermore, the DGA Summary details safety recommendations concerning how to store and cook food.

Two of the core recommendations in the DGA were to (1) maintain caloric balance over time to achieve and sustain a healthy weight and to (2) focus on consuming nutrient-dense foods and beverages. The basic guidelines attendant to each aspect include the following:

- ❏ Maintain Calorie Balance Over Time to Achieve and Sustain a Healthy Weight:
  - Prevent/reduce excess weight through improved eating and physical activity (PA) behaviors.
  - Control total calorie intake to manage body weight.
  - Increase PA and reduce time spent engaging in sedentary behaviors.
- ❏ Focus on Consuming Nutrient-Dense Foods and Beverages:
  - Food and food components that should be reduced:
    - ✓ Less than 2300 mg daily of sodium, less than 1500 mg daily of sodium for high risk patients (2300 mg of sodium = one teaspoon and 1500 mg = ¾ of a teaspoon)
    - ✓ Less than 10 percent calories from saturated fats
    - ✓ Less than 10 percent calories from added sugars
    - ✓ Keep *trans* fat consumption as low as possible.
    - ✓ Reduce calories from solid fats and added sugars.
    - ✓ Limit consumption of refined grains.
    - ✓ If alcohol is consumed, do so in moderation (up to one drink/day for women and two drinks/day for men). According to the American Heart Association, a drink is one 12 oz. beer, 4 oz. of wine, 1.5 oz. of 80-proof spirits, or 1 oz. of 100-proof spirits.
  - Food and nutrients that should be increased:
    - ✓ Eat more fruits and vegetables, with an emphasis on variety and consuming whole fruits and vegetables.
    - ✓ Make sure that at least half of grains consumed are whole grains.
    - ✓ Consume fat-free and low-fat milk products
    - ✓ Vary the sources of protein—focus on plant proteins, including beans, peas, soy, unsalted nuts, and seeds. Animal proteins include seafood, poultry, lean meat, and eggs.
    - ✓ Replace proteins that are high in solid fat with more healthful choices.
    - ✓ Use oils to replace solid fats.
    - ✓ Choose foods with more potassium, fiber, calcium, and vitamin D.

USDA'S MYPLATE

In January 2011, the federal government launched MyPlate (Figure 5-6) to replace the previous daily caloric intake suggestion tool developed by the government, the Food Pyramid, which was introduced in 1991. The Food Pyramid was a colorful triangle that featured a variety of foods and specified how many servings of each food a person should eat each day.

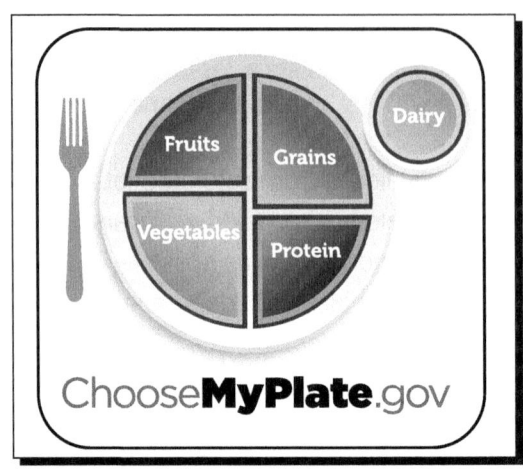

Figure 5-6. MyPlate

As the name MyPlate indicates, this resource is a plate—a plate full of the recommended combination of fruits, vegetables, protein, and grains that individuals should consume to keep them healthy. This revamped resource differed in several ways from its predecessor, including having less emphasis on grains, no mention of fats and oils, no mention of serving sizes, and the exclusion of nutrients. The focus was on the bigger picture of a healthy eating pattern. Moving away from filling the plate with just processed meats and French fries which is what many eat in the standard American diet (SAD). Ketchup, the only thing that adds color, is considered by some individuals as their serving of vegetable, which is perturbing. This plate, at least, is one step closer to a healthy eating pattern. Some patients might need to start here on their journey to the "north star" of the whole foods, plant-based diet (WFPB). This plate, however, is obviously not the same as the WFPB diet described previously.

Although the Dietary Guidelines align with ACLM's position on nutrition by emphasizing a variety of fruits, vegetables, and whole grains, ACLM does not endorse these guidelines, as a whole, due to the allowance of animal-based protein, dairy, and oils. The best way to counsel patients on adopting a healthy eating pattern is by focusing on the WFPB spectrum and helping them cultivate eating habits that move them along that spectrum toward the "north star."

HARVARD HEALTHY EATING PLATE

Approximately eight months later (September 2011), the Harvard School of Public Health released its own version of a plate, a new and improved version that featured considerably more detail (Figure 5-7). For example, it specifically suggests using oils from unsaturated fat sources, like olive and canola, for cooking, and consuming whole grains, rather than white bread.

HEALTHY EATING PLATE

Use healthy oils (like olive and canola oil) for cooking, on salad, and at the table. Limit butter. Avoid trans fat.

The more veggies – and the greater the variety – the better. Potatoes and French fries don't count.

Eat plenty of fruits of all colors.

STAY ACTIVE!

© Harvard University

Harvard School of Public Health
The Nutrition Source
www.hsph.harvard.edu/nutritionsource

WATER Drink water, tea, or coffee (with little or no sugar). Limit milk/dairy (1-2 servings/day) and juice (1 small glass/day). Avoid sugary drinks.

Eat a variety of whole grains (like whole-wheat bread, whole-grain pasta, and brown rice). Limit refined grains (like white rice and white bread).

Choose fish, poultry, beans, and nuts; limit red meat and cheese; avoid bacon, cold cuts, and other processed meats.

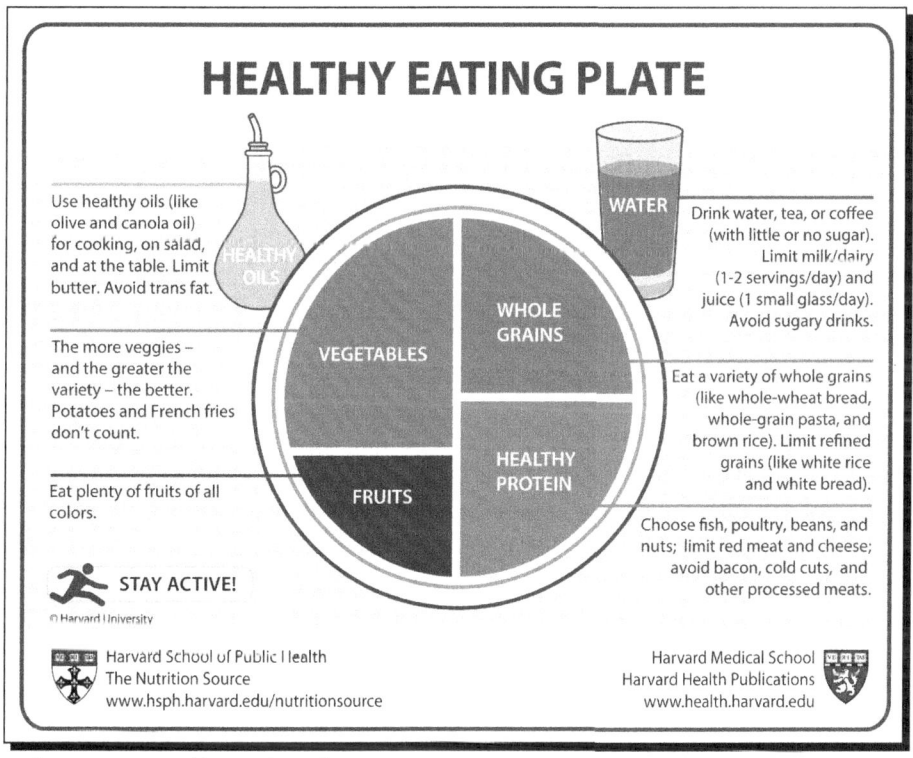

Harvard Medical School
Harvard Health Publications
www.health.harvard.edu

Figure 5-7. Healthy Eating Plate.

Developed by Dr. Walter Willett and his team at the Harvard School of Public Health, one of the more interesting features of the Healthy Eating Plate is that it is half full of veggies and fruits. This guideline is often eye-opening for patients. Some individuals think they eat really well, but they are shocked when they see the plate, given that the recommended amount of produce is considerably higher than what they actually consume.

One half of the Healthy Eating Plate is vegetables and fruits, while the other half of the plate is about equally divided between whole grains and healthy protein. Examples of appropriate whole grains are brown rice, quinoa, whole grain wheat bread, and whole grain pasta. Dr. Willett recommends that refined grains, such as white rice, white bread, and white pasta, be limited. The Healthy Eating Plate encourages getting protein from fish, poultry, beans, and nuts. Red meat, especially processed meat, should be restricted, in order to reduce an individual's risk of cancer.

Ultimately, striving for a diet of whole, plant-based foods should be the goal for everyone. In that regard, lifestyle medicine practitioners must meet the patient where these individuals are in their stage of change. As such, offering dietary options may help some patients find a diet that provides more plants, as well as one that works for them at their particular stage in their transition along the spectrum to a whole foods, plant-based lifestyle.

WEIGHT MANAGEMENT

The challenge of maintaining a healthy weight is something many people face. In America, 160 million people are either obese or overweight (approximately 75 percent of the men and 60 percent of the women). This situation has led to more than 45 million adults dieting to try and lose weight. Americans are spending more than $60 billion dollars a year on gym memberships, diet books, products, and services!

Concurrently, a number of people are also suffering from eating disorders, such as anorexia nervosa and bulimia. Unfortunately, too many individuals who are looking to lose weight are also seeking a "quick fix." They want a way to lose weight fast, with as little effort as possible. This quick-fix mentality has spawned a number of fad diets and practices, such as the starvation diet, fasting, the grapefruit diet, the high-protein/low-carbohydrate diet, the high-fat/low-carbohydrate diet, dietary pills, and expensive supplements, etc.

While millions of Americans have attempted to follow these types of diets and practices, few are able to maintain long-term weight loss success. Furthermore, repeated extreme dieting may have negative effects on metabolism. This consequence has been shown in a study done on the "Biggest Loser" contestants, which demonstrated that participants' metabolism was significantly slower, after having lost the weight, than otherwise would have been expected it to be for a person of that size and percent body fat. This situation, which has been termed adaptive metabolism or "set point," is one of the reasons that people struggle to keep weight off after they have lost it. If the vast array of popular diets and weight-loss practices don't work, what can people do to lose weight and to keep the weight off?

❑ Calorie Density: A Practical Approach to a Healthy Weight

As previously mentioned, one of the many side effects of adopting a WFPB lifestyle is weight loss and healthy weight maintenance, which is due to the low caloric density of most whole, plant foods. The calorie density approach to achieving and maintaining a healthy weight allows patients to eat a larger volume of food for fewer calories. It is also much more sensible and straightforward than fad diets and calorie counting, giving patients an opportunity to focus on real foods and food groups instead of nonsensical rules and numbers. Furthermore, following this approach maximizes the nutrient density of a patient's diet so they can obtain a healthy weight and improve their overall health, something that most weight loss diets cannot guarantee.

Calorie density is the measure of how many calories are in a certain weight of food. It is often expressed as number of calories per pound. Foods with a high calorie density contain a high number of calories in a relatively small amount of food, while foods with a low calorie density contain much fewer calories in the same weight of food. For example, a mini candy bar contains 150 calories, while a medium-size apple only has about 100 calories. In other words, a person can eat one and a half apples for the same "calorie cost" as one mini candy bar. Figure 5-8, created by Dr. Craig McDougall, MD, based on the calorie density work of Jeff Novick, MS, RD, provides a helpful chart to educate patients on this concept.

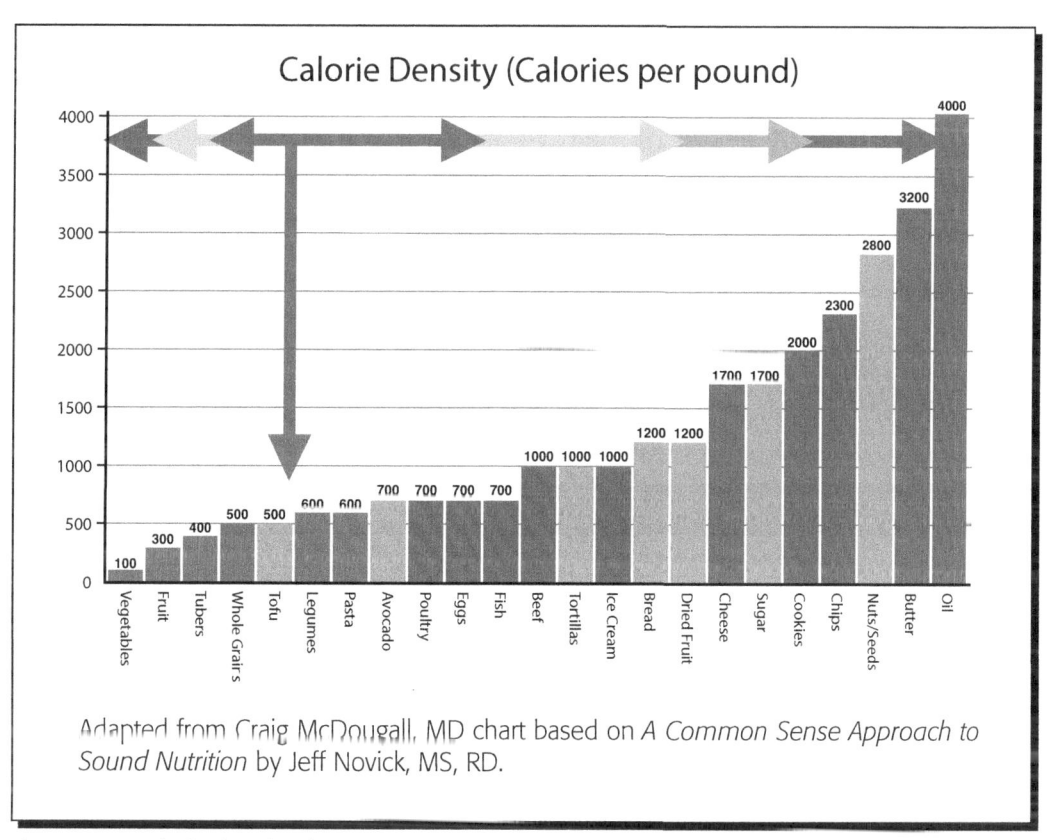

Figure 5-8. Calorie density chart

Low calorie-dense foods tend to be filling because of their fiber and water content. As a result, eating one and a half apples can be much more filling and satisfying than a mini candy bar. Because people tend to eat the same volume of food every day, reducing that volume, which is required by most weight loss plans, is a very challenging behavior to achieve. The volume of food a person eats contributes to feeling satisfied—visually by filling their plate (individuals eat with their eyes first) and physically by filling their stomach.

By adhering to the calorie density approach, people can continue to eat the same volume of food, but it will cost them fewer calories. Figure 5-9, from Jeff Novick, MS, RD, shows what 500 calories looks like in the stomach, when an individual consumes fruits and vegetables, compared to cheese and other options. This figure illustrates how low calorie-dense foods fill the stomach, trigger stretch receptors, and signal satiety to the brain. It costs a lot of calories to trigger this pathway with high calorie-dense foods, like animal products and oils.

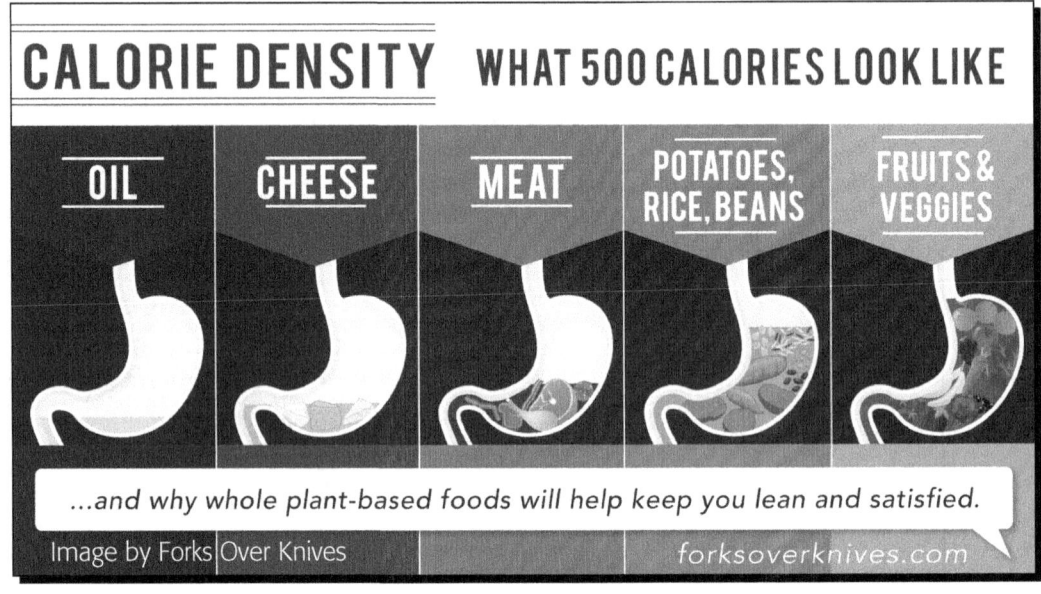

Figure 5-9. What 500 calories looks like

Another challenge in feeling satiated is that too many individuals rush when they eat, leading them to overconsume. This situation is particularly true if they are eating refined sugars. By the time their body tells their brain that it's full 20 minutes later, they will often have eaten everything in sight. If they took their time, however, sat down, ate mindfully, chewed every bite thoroughly, paused after each bite, and tried to enjoy their meal, they would be less likely to overeat. Gastric distention (i.e., bloating of the stomach) can also help with satiety. For example, when people fill up with water and fiber, not only is the fiber they consume nutritious, it also helps them feel full.

Knowing what to eat is critical. That's the quality part of the equation, which is more important than the quantity part of the equation. Energy balance, however, should also be considered, especially for those individuals having difficulty achieving their weight goals. How much food a person should eat depends on a variety of factors, including the person's age, height, weight, gender, and level of physical activity. In general, the basic guideline is to consume a sufficient amount of food to feel satisfied but not so much that they feel overly full. This factor is predicated on the idea that the person eating is paying attention to their level of satiety, a factor that is often dubbed "mindful eating."

Calorically, the number of calories that a person should consume a day also depends on the same aforementioned factors (i.e., age, height, weight, gender, and physical activity level). Caloric intake is also contingent on whether the individual wants to lose or gain weight. While the literature seems to be full of daily calorie estimators and suggested formulas to calculate caloric needs, no precise formula for calculating such a number in a non-laboratory setting currently exists. Every person is unique, to a degree, with regard to their caloric needs. As previously mentioned, when a person is on a whole foods, plant-based diet, they tend to lose excess weight naturally because of the low calorie density of these foods.

❏ How Much Should a Person Weigh?

The perceptions of many individuals about what constitutes an appropriate or ideal body weight tend to be somewhat distorted or misguided. This situation often leads to frustration regarding their inability (due to a perceived lack of willpower) to lose those final few pounds. These individuals can become obsessed with reaching some "mythical" ideal body weight. Their obsession is frequently manifested in a very counterproductive manner. Initially, at least, these individuals view "food" as their archenemy—something to be ingested only when their willpower cannot sustain them any longer. Many of them also exercise incessantly. Regrettably, most of these people suffer a relapse in their commitment to eat less and exercise more, which, in turn, causes them to feel like an incorrigible failure. Are these individuals really failures, or are they the victims of unrealistic goals and expectations?

To determine their ideal body weight, individuals shouldn't rely solely on numbers and perceived ideals. What represents a safe, realistic, and perhaps more importantly attainable body weight for them will depend (to a large extent) on the following factors:
- Medical history. A person's medical history, including a review of their personal health risk factors, is important when attempting to define their ideal body weight. For example, if their blood pressure is elevated, a modest weight reduction could be quite beneficial. Extra body mass means that their heart must work harder to pump blood through miles of extra capillaries that feed that extra tissue. Type II diabetes and blood lipid-lipoprotein profiles are other examples of medical conditions that can be positively affected by weight loss.

- Family history. Body weight, like most other physical characteristics, can be influenced by some genetic factors. There is active research in the area of genetics and obesity. Reports indicate that between 50-400 genes have an impact on obesity. It is estimated that if both of your parents are obese, you have an 80 percent chance of becoming obese. However, family habits, dietary customs, exercise routines, and time spent in front of the television also play a role. Working on all the ways to decrease your chances of obesity becomes paramount when there is a family history.
- Body fat distribution. As previously stated, body fat located in the abdominal region—specifically around the organs—is particularly damaging to a person's health. Accordingly, any person who possesses a high amount of belly fat as determined by waist-to-hip ratio (WHR), should strongly consider losing weight through a combined program of sensible eating and exercise. If the WHR is high and the BMI is a normal weight, it is still recommended that the patient work on losing the abdominal adipose tissue.
- Functional ability. If a patient's existing body weight inhibits their ability to either effectively and efficiently perform their activities of daily living or comfortably engage in the leisure-time pursuits of their choice, it is probably not at an ideal level.

❏ Winning the Losing Game

The answer to achieving a sensible weight is actually relatively simple: a patient must commit to a lifelong habit of healthy eating, a program of regular exercise, and a pattern of sensible behavior. In other words, losing weight should be an integral part of the plan of a patient who is overweight to become and remain healthy. As such, the essential elements of a person's strategy to lose weight and keep it off should be moving toward a predominantly plant-based diet, exercise, and behavioral modification (to facilitate their efforts to eat healthfully and sustain a routine exercise program), as well as adequate sleep (see Chapter 6). As many people can attest, this situation ends up being far more difficult than might otherwise be expected. With highly processed food available 24/7, little need for much daily physical activity, and numerous highly entertaining sedentary activities, it is no wonder weight loss and weight maintenance is so difficult!

A patient should keep in mind, however, that weight loss isn't something that can or should happen fast. It is essentially a relatively slow process that requires discipline, education, planning, and setting realistic goals. How much people eat, what they eat, and how much they exercise are factors over which they generally have significant control. There are some factors, however, over which people have little or no control. Patients need to learn to deal with these factors in an appropriate manner.

As noted previously, one of these factors is a person's genetics. The genes an individual is born with can affect whether they have a "weight problem." If both parents of a patient were overweight, there is a very good chance of that individual being overweight also. Accordingly, if a patient is genetically predisposed to weight gain, eating right and exercising regularly should definitely be a top priority for them. Furthermore, although genetics cannot be changed, there is evidence that genes can be modified via epigenetics. It's also worth noting that what might be seen as a genetic could actually be environmental, and therefor modifiable. In other words, a patient might have grown up in a household that promoted unhealthy habits that led to family health and weight issues. This is good news because a patient's environment is something they have control over.

How much a patient eats and their ability to lose weight may also be affected by certain psychological factors. These factors include all of the non-biological reasons that people eat. It should be noted that the feeling of being hungry is not always the reason for eating. For example, an individual's emotions often have a big effect on what and when that person eats. Any emotion, such as stress, boredom, loneliness, anxiety, depression, or fatigue may increase the likelihood of overeating.

Furthermore, a patient may simply eat out of habit, i.e., time to eat, being in the presence of people who are eating, and being exposed to the sight and smell of food. This factor is compounded by the fact that sugar, salt, and fat—the major ingredients in calorie-dense foods—trigger the reward circuits in an individual's brain, meaning these foods have definite addictive properties (see Chapter 11). During breaks at work or when watching television at night, some people routinely head for the breakroom, cupboard, or refrigerator. These behavioral patterns can be very hard to break. It requires careful planning ahead. For example, individuals should keep healthy foods readily available, limit the quantity and availability of high fat and high sugar foods, self-monitor the food they eat, and exercise.

Another factor to keep in mind with regard to weight loss is that calorie restriction negatively impacts metabolism. When insufficient calories are consistently being consumed, the body interprets this situation as starvation. In response, it will automatically reduce the rate at which it burns calories for energy (i.e., its metabolic rate), thus making losing weight more difficult.

This factor is further illustrated by understanding that a patient's resting metabolic rate represents the energy the body expends to maintain life and normal bodily operations, such as breathing, brain function, and digestion. About 60-75 percent of the calories that a person expends on a daily basis support these operations. When an individual limits their intake of calories, their resting metabolic rate eventually decreases because their body is trying to be as efficient as possible and conserve energy. Because the body must have fuel to maintain life and to perform certain essential bodily functions, it will do all that it can to conserve the calories that are consumed to ensure that these processes can continue. Alternatively, if the body receives a steady and adequate number of calories, it will recognize the fact that it doesn't have to worry about conserving fuel. In the process, it will continue to function as it normally does.

One of the primary modifiable factors that impacts metabolism is the amount of lean muscle mass a person has. The more lean muscle mass a patient has, the higher that individual's metabolic rate will be. Muscle tissue is much more metabolically active than fat tissue. One pound of muscle tissue burns about 13 calories a day, just to maintain itself; one pound of fat, on the other hand, burns only about 4.5 calories a day. By consistently working out and performing resistance/strength training, a person can usually (but not always) increase their amount of lean muscle mass, which will subsequently raise their metabolic rate.

❏ Sensible Eating

Often, one of the most difficult steps for a patient to master in their efforts to lose weight and keep it off is to adopt a sensible eating plan. An individual needs to keep in mind that there is a balance between reducing calories enough to lose weight versus diminishing their caloric intake too much, which will result in a marked decrease in metabolism and impairing normal bodily functions. With whole foods, plant-based eating, calorie intake tends to regulate itself. Patients can eat until comfortably full, and still maintain a calorie intake that's right for their goals.

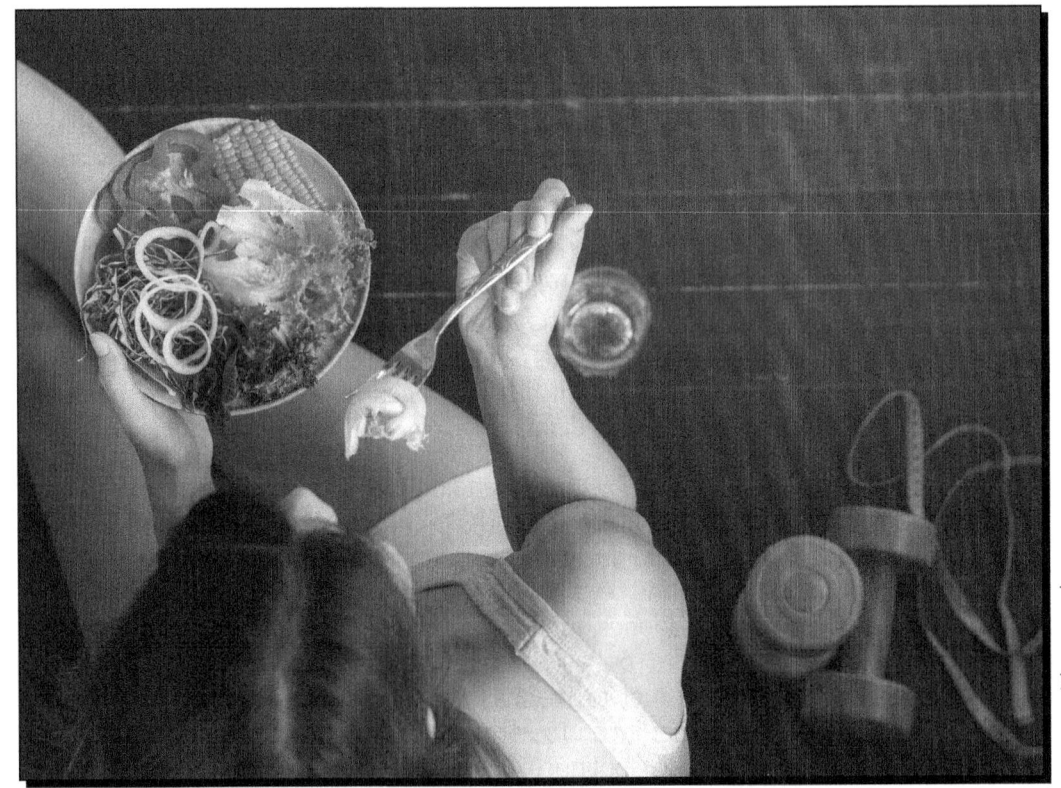

With whole foods, plant-based eating, calorie intake tends to regulate itself.

LIVE AND LEARN WITH DR. BETH FRATES

Most people have probably experienced the effects of not eating sensibly. Eating just because the food was there was part of an environmental or cultural pattern, and then became a habit. For me, this situation happened when I spent a year in England between my senior year in high school and college. In the US, I was an active athlete, playing three varsity sports in high school, including field hockey, basketball, and lacrosse. I had two-hour practices, every day after school. In addition, I often enjoyed running on the weekends.

Like most teenagers, I primarily ate my mom's homemade meals, except for lunches at school on weekdays. Well, all of this scenario changed when I went to England for the year and spent time there at a boarding school. First of all, the culture was different. There was tea time every day at 10:00 a.m., and desserts were available after lunch and dinner, every day. Furthermore, sports were not emphasized or glorified the way they were at my American high school. There were 1-hour practices, 2-3 times a week only.

Since I missed my regular routine of physical activity, I tried jogging on the streets in England. This practice, however, was not the norm in the mid 1980s in this country. In fact, during one of my jogging sessions, someone stopped and asked me if I needed help. Apparently, they thought that I was running away from something, running out of fear, as opposed to jogging for pleasure. Eventually, the combination of ginger cookies (probably 5-6 a day) at tea time, desserts almost every night (something that I rarely had at home in the US), and the lack of exercise took a toll on my body.

The result was a larger me. The change was so gradual that I didn't really notice it. When I returned home from England for Christmas, however, my grandmother was the first to inform me that I had changed. I vividly recall going to visit her at her house, ringing the doorbell looking forward to seeing her. When she opened the door, the first words out of her mouth were, "You got fat!" I was so surprised.

After my visit with her, I went home and weighed myself. Sure enough, I had gained about 10 pounds from September to December. This situation was alarming to me. On the other hand, if you think about it, it makes sense. I was not eating sensibly, and I had markedly reduced my level of exercise. This scenario proved to me, early on in my life, that my behaviors, as well as my food choices, would have a huge effect on my body.

I was home for three weeks and subsequently went back to my US routine of jogging and eating three home-cooked meals a day, with no desserts and no tea times. When I returned to England, I refrained from tea time, and I did aerobics/ calisthenics in my room (it was the 1980s). I managed to maintain my weight by altering my behaviors and eating patterns. There's nothing like a personal experience to reveal the power of lifestyle medicine.

❑ Sensible Program of Exercise on a Regular Basis

Because the two most important factors in keeping a person's weight at a desired level are sensible eating and regular exercise, an individual can take great strides to win the losing game by exercising on a regular basis. Exercise is reviewed extensively in Chapter 4. The U.S. Surgeon General reports that to be healthy, individuals should get about 30 minutes of moderate exercise on most, if not all, days of the week. This guideline is similar to the recommendations of the United States Health and Human Services Recommendations to accumulate 150 minutes of moderate intensity physical activity or 75 minutes of vigorous intensity exercise. In reality, most Americans do not even come close to this amount.

Statistics demonstrating that a sedentary lifestyle is the leading cause of weight-related issues in the United States help confirm the need to be physically active. In fact, too many people who have relatively sedentary desk jobs usually sit in front of a television set or at a computer when they come home from work at night. As a result, they burn fewer calories and store more fat than do more physically active people.

Exercise can have a positive impact on a patient's weight control efforts in a number of ways. For example, if they exercise on a regular basis, their body will burn calories faster. Furthermore, strength training can help build muscle mass, which will help keep a person's resting metabolic rate at a higher level. Recently released evidence indicates that routine aerobic exercise (like walking and/or jogging) can enhance an individual's level of self-control with regard to what they eat, for example, reducing cravings and impulsivity with sweets like cupcakes.

Exercise can also have an emotional impact on an individual. For example, exercise can help someone look better, even if they don't lose a lot of weight. Because muscle is more dense and heavy than fat, replacing fat with muscle will cause an individual to look more fit and trim. In some instances, a patient's waistline may be smaller, despite the fact that their total body weight remains unchanged. This situation is often noticed in the "belt test." This test is not an official or formal evaluation, obviously. However, many patients report that although the scale numbers didn't change, their belt loop went down one or two notches. Some even complain that their pants are falling down. The point that should be noted is that body composition can change, without a change in the scale—a scenario that is a healthy one.

Exercise needs to be something that patients find enjoyable or they are not going to want to do it. While any physical activity will improve health, the most effective exercise program for losing weight should include both aerobic conditioning and strength training, in conjunction with dietary changes. Aerobic conditioning not only burns calories and fat, it is also the best type of exercise for strengthening the heart muscle. Strength training may not burn as many calories during a workout as compared to aerobic exercise, but it does slightly increase metabolism after the workout and can help build and maintain lean muscle mass.

As discussed previously, increased muscle mass is highly metabolically active tissue. Maintaining muscle mass is critical when a person is in a caloric deficit, as losing lean muscle tissue further reduces an individual's metabolism. Resistance training has an optimal effect on body composition and metabolism—it helps maintain lean muscle tissue during weight loss and burns additional calories to help with fat loss.

When selecting aerobic exercises that will maximize a patient's efforts to lose weight, activities should be chosen that involve the largest muscle groups in the body, such as the legs and buttocks. Aerobic exercise should be rhythmic, should raise the individual's heart rate, and should slightly increase their rate of breathing. Among the examples of aerobic activities that are particularly appropriate for losing weight are walking, hiking, running, cycling, rowing, stair climbing, swimming, jumping rope, and dancing.

Considerable disagreement exists concerning which approach to aerobic exercise is better for weight loss: high-intensity activity for a short duration or low-intensity activity for a long duration. A common misconception is that low-intensity exercise is the best way to train if a person wants to lose weight, since a higher percentage of fat calories is being burned for fuel than is the case with high-intensity exercise. While it is true that a higher *percentage* of calories being burned comes from fat, working out at lower exercise intensities will burn fewer overall calories.

To illustrate this point, consider a hypothetical situation in which someone is working out for 30 minutes at a low level of intensity. They burn 150 calories, 70 percent of which is fat—equal to 105 "fat calories." The same individual then does a high intensity workout and burns 400 calories in the same amount of time (30 minutes). Since they are working out at a higher level of intensity, only 25 percent of the calories are fat, and 75 percent are carbohydrate. This situation equates to 100 "fat calories"—not only a similar amount of calories from fat being burned, but more than 2.5 times as many calories overall!

Exercising at a relatively low level of intensity offers two noteworthy benefits with regard to weight loss. First, because such activity is easier to do, a patient is more likely to stick with their exercise program. Second, because it tends to place a lower level of orthopedic stress on the joints of the body, it is safer and involves less physical discomfort. Both factors are especially important for individuals who are sedentary, who are unfit, who are overweight, or who are just starting an exercise program.

When a patient is attempting to lose weight, one of the main points that was briefly touched on previously is that it is the total number of calories they expend while exercising, not what percentage of those calories comes from either fat or carbohydrates. Although an individual may expend a higher percentage of fat calories at a lower level of exercise intensity, they will burn a higher number of fat calories, if they exercise at a higher level of intensity. The bottom line is that, all factors considered, the harder a person exercises, the more calories they burn

Strength training is another type of exercise that can greatly enhance a patient's weight-loss efforts. As noted previously, strength training can help an individual build and maintain his level of lean muscle, the tissue in the body that burns the most calories, because it is so metabolically active. All factors considered, the more lean muscle mass a person has, the easier it is for an individual to win the losing game.

❏ Sensible Behavior

Despite the fact that the number of individuals with weight-related health issues has evolved into a full-blown crisis over the past four decades, the efforts to address it share at least one thing in common—they have not worked. In reality, any attempt to provide a viable solution to the situation will require a new perspective. Recognizing the physiologic and behavioral basis of weight management offers a promising way forward.

In that regard, it is essential to note that weight is not a behavior. Rather, it is almost always a by-product of a series of behavioral choices made by someone. When physicians and allied healthcare professionals are working with patients who have weight management concerns, one of the major focuses should be on the behavior of the patients. Arguably, change their behavior—specifically their perception of themselves—change their weight.

Like almost everything else in life, people with weight management concerns tend to be motivated by different things. Accordingly, what may be an effective motivational

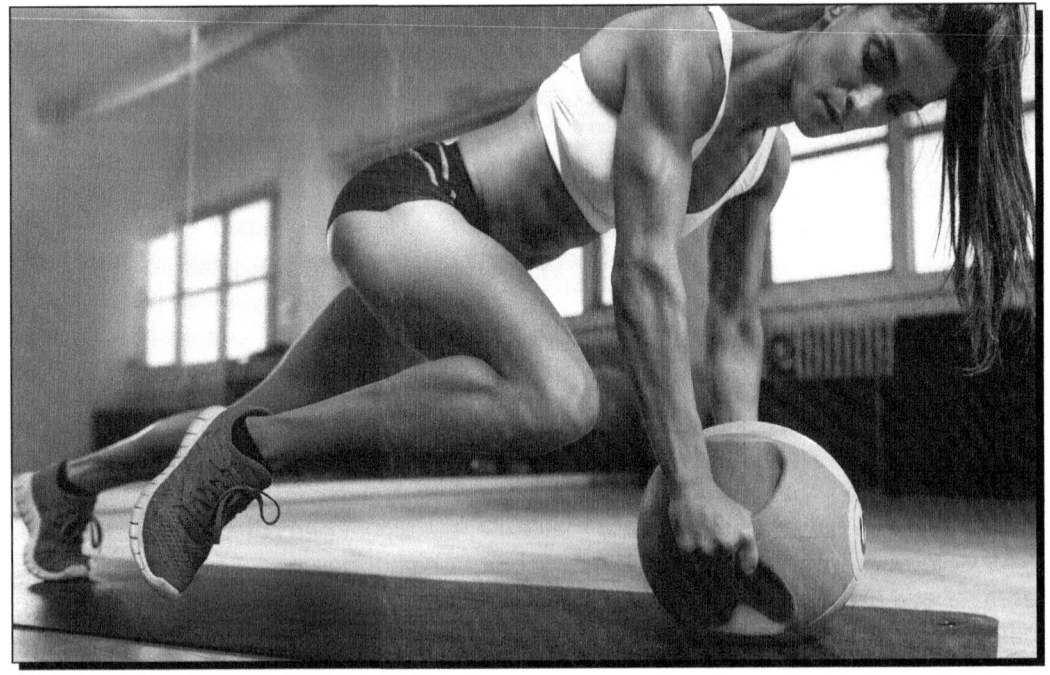

All factors considered, the more lean muscle mass a person has, the easier it is for an individual to win the losing game.

strategy for one person may not work as well for another. For example, asking a patient to lose an arbitrary number of pounds for a predetermined number of weeks may cause one individual to make positive, lifestyle-related changes in their behavior and could conversely lead to a counterproductive level of pressure in another.

Just as two individuals with weight-related issues are never exactly the same, the most effective way to treat such a person successfully is also not precisely the same from individual to individual. Any intervention with a patient should be tailored to meet the unique needs, interests, and goals of that particular person. It is the inherent responsibility of every physician and allied healthcare professional to ascertain what factors "distinguish" each of their weight-challenged patients, as an individual, and to respond accordingly.

Physicians and allied healthcare professionals should view their role as one that is grounded in active collaboration—interfacing with registered dietitians, certified exercise specialists, and other trained professionals, as needed and appropriate. The center of attention of everyone's efforts should be on what the patient can do to improve their health, as opposed to complying with some arbitrary numerical aspects of a weight management plan. Details of the Frates COACH Approach are discussed in Chapters 2 and 3.

When dealing with individuals who have weight concerns, one of the first tasks for physicians and allied healthcare professionals is to redefine success for each patient. Far too often, individuals (weight-challenged or not) view success, with regard to body weight, as a consequence of reaching an "external" goal, for example, losing a predetermined number of pounds or sculpting the body to attain a particular shape. In reality, being successful could be more appropriately perceived by these patients as achieving an enhanced level of health or sense of well-being.

Many physicians and allied healthcare professionals are often unduly concerned with the *failure* of these individuals to attain one or more of the numerical expectations that have been set for them. They're focusing on the wrong "F" word; instead of *failure*, they should be centering their attention on *fun*. In too many instances, the approach that they are taking with their patients is virtually devoid of any emphasis on *fun*. They overlook or ignore how challenging, dissatisfying, or outright distasteful patients may perceive this experience to be. This situation can drastically affect that individual's commitment to the endeavor.

One of the most effective resources in the toolbox of physicians and allied healthcare professionals can be to have an inventive open mind. They need to be creative with respect to changing the behavior patterns of their patients who need to lose weight. They need to ask themselves what they can do to help their patients actually achieve their weight management goals. This state of affairs often entails thinking outside of the box. Hence, the first C in the Frates COACH Approach is *curiosity*. (Remember that the other letters in the mnemonic stand for openness, appreciation, compassion and honesty.)

An important consideration for physicians and allied healthcare professionals to recognize with patients who are overweight is if any weight-related biases exist within the medical practice or in the practicing clinicians. This type of bias can have dire consequences. At a minimum, weight-related bias can impact the prism through which physicians and allied healthcare professionals view the issue of weight management. The resulting mindset can convey messages (both directly and indirectly) that are counterproductive, such as, "thin is beautiful;" "fat is ugly;" "the only reason people can't lose weight is that they don't try hard enough;" etc. Such narrow-mindedness can compromise their efforts to be part of the solution.

Lastly, individuals who want to manage their weight are to make informed choices about their behavior that affects their underlying weight-related goals, they need to receive advice and counsel that are based in science. Whatever guidance they are given should never be rooted in some "flavor-of-the-month" trend or diet craze.

❏ A Recipe for Success

It is quite evident that everyone cannot, and should not, be as thin as the proverbial "Hollywood" or "Madison Avenue" body type. Common sense and sound nutrition principles mandate that a person who wants to lose weight should avoid setting "hard and fast" body weight goals for themselves. Rather, an individual should strive for achieving a body weight that is compatible with a healthy lifestyle. In general, the body weight that results from adopting such a lifestyle should ultimately be considered as the ideal union between a person's wellness level, their genetic potential, and reality. In this regard, eating sensibly, exercising regularly, sleeping sufficiently, and keeping it fun is a sound recipe for losing weight and keeping it off.

❏ Choosing an Eating Plan

Over the years, there have literally been hundreds (if not thousands) of diets developed concerning how individuals can control what they weigh. One self-proclaimed dieting expert recommends one specific strategy, while another all-too-willing-to-offer-an-opinion food authority advocates the exact opposite approach (e.g., fat is good and carbohydrates are bad vs. carbohydrates are good and fat is bad). It should not be surprising to physicians and allied healthcare professionals that their patients are often in a quandary concerning what dietary plan they should follow to best address their own personal challenges with their weight.

While losing weight is typically a long-term process, selecting a particular diet regimen and sticking with it is an essential step to help ensure that whatever weight that is achieved is permanent. There are several factors that must be considered when choosing a diet. Above all else, the diet must be both safe and healthy. In other words, it needs to adhere to the keys for a healthy diet that were detailed previously in this chapter. The diet should also be one that is suitable to the needs, interests, and personality of the person trying to lose weight.

Lifestyle Medicine Handbook 211

The better the match, the greater the odds of achieving long-term success in the diet. To a degree, an individual can "customize" their diet plan—an effort that can enhance the likelihood that they will actually stick to their diet. For example, with regard to food, what are a person's triggers, what does the individual really care about, what are their behavioral patterns that tend to cause them to eat, what other factors do they find motivating, etc. The goal is to move away from the SAD diet and toward the whole foods, plant-based diet. Ultimately, the whole foods, plant-based diet will enable an individual to sustain their weight loss and maintain a healthy weight, as well as prevent, halt, and reverse disease.

❑ Food for Thought

In order to be able to handle situations with their patients involving their weight-loss efforts, physicians and allied healthcare professionals should develop a working understanding of several key nutrition-related issues (which have not been covered to this point in this chapter). Among the topics in that regard are portion distortion, the emotional and psychological elements of eating behavior, sugar cycle, and weight-loss plateaus.

• *Portion distortion.* It is virtually impossible for anyone not to notice that food portions have gotten larger, particularly in restaurants over the past two decades. Figure 5-10 illustrates how portion distortion has affected six common foods. The average intake of these foods 20 years ago and today is markedly different.

Portion *Distortion*

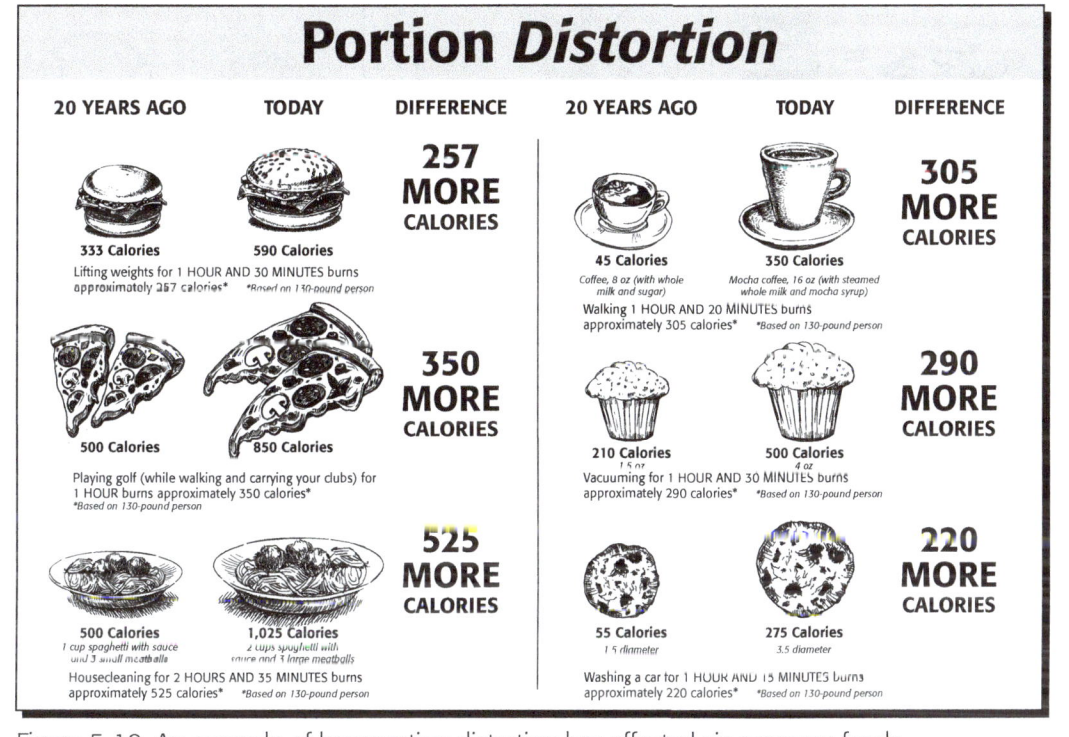

20 YEARS AGO	TODAY	DIFFERENCE	20 YEARS AGO	TODAY	DIFFERENCE
333 Calories	590 Calories	257 MORE CALORIES	Coffee, 8 oz (with whole milk and sugar) 45 Calories	Mocha coffee, 16 oz (with steamed whole milk and mocha syrup) 350 Calories	305 MORE CALORIES
Lifting weights for 1 HOUR AND 30 MINUTES burns approximately 267 calories* *Based on 130-pound person			Walking 1 HOUR AND 20 MINUTES burns approximately 305 calories* *Based on 130-pound person		
500 Calories	850 Calories	350 MORE CALORIES	210 Calories 1.5 oz	500 Calories 4 oz	290 MORE CALORIES
Playing golf (while walking and carrying your clubs) for 1 HOUR burns approximately 350 calories* *Based on 130-pound person			Vacuuming for 1 HOUR AND 30 MINUTES burns approximately 290 calories* *Based on 130-pound person		
500 Calories 1 cup spaghetti with sauce and 3 small meatballs	1,025 Calories 2 cups spaghetti with sauce and 3 large meatballs	525 MORE CALORIES	55 Calories 1.5 diameter	275 Calories 3.5 diameter	220 MORE CALORIES
Housecleaning for 2 HOURS AND 35 MINUTES burns approximately 525 calories* *Based on 130-pound person			Washing a car for 1 HOUR AND 15 MINUTES burns approximately 220 calories* *Based on 130-pound person		

Figure 5-10. An example of how portion distortion has affected six common foods

In reality, a portion, which is the amount of food that an individual chooses to eat for a meal can be big or small—it's their decision. One of the keys for a patient to effectively control how much they weigh is to consume appropriate portions of the food they eat. Figure 5-11 depicts several samples of what one serving should look like.

SIZE IT RIGHT
A guide (based on standards that most nutritionists follow) to what one serving should look like.

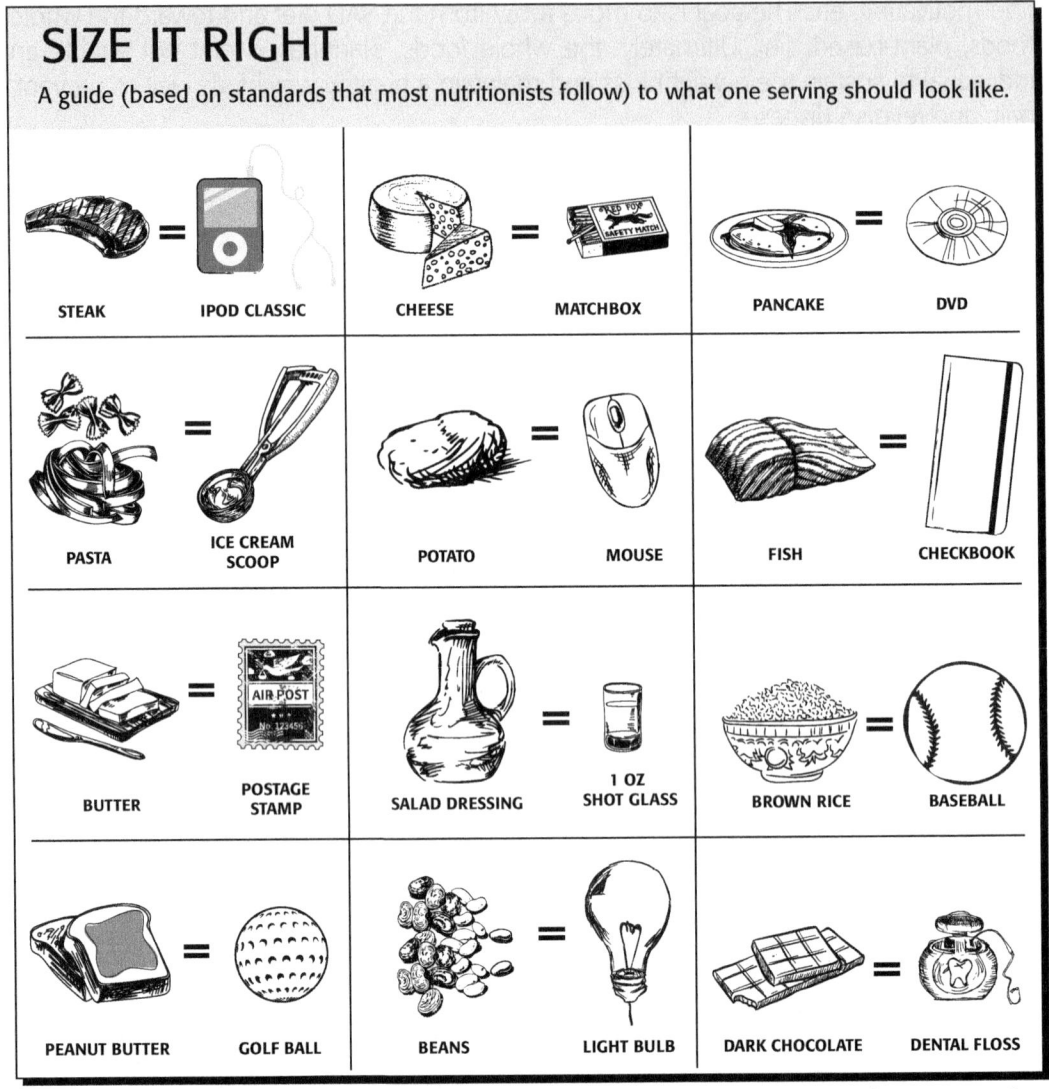

STEAK	IPOD CLASSIC	CHEESE	MATCHBOX	PANCAKE	DVD
PASTA	ICE CREAM SCOOP	POTATO	MOUSE	FISH	CHECKBOOK
BUTTER	POSTAGE STAMP	SALAD DRESSING	1 OZ SHOT GLASS	BROWN RICE	BASEBALL
PEANUT BUTTER	GOLF BALL	BEANS	LIGHT BULB	DARK CHOCOLATE	DENTAL FLOSS

Figure 5-11. A guide (based on standards that most nutritionists follow) to what one serving should look like

Another tool that can help a person to have a more realistic perception of what constitutes a suitable portion is a portion-size chart that details what a recommended portion might be, when it's compared to an object with which people are normally familiar (Figure 5-12). The portion size chart can be extremely useful for patients, as it is easy to remember. A fist represents about one cup, which would be suitable for

Lifestyle Medicine Handbook 213

a serving of rice, pasta, fruit, and veggies. A palm is about a three-ounce serving, if the individual is consuming meat, fish, and poultry. A handful is about a one-ounce serving for nuts and raisins. Two handfuls constitute an appropriate serving, if the patient is snacking on popcorn, for example. It should be noted that this chart is designed to provide patients with rough estimates.

HAND SYMBOL	EQUIVALENT	FOODS	CALORIES
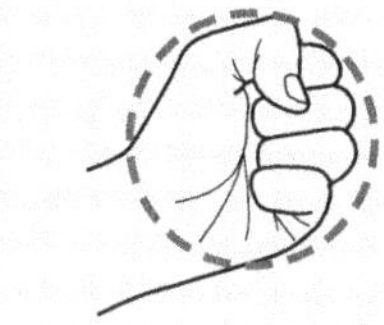	**Fist** 1 cup	Rice, pasta Fruit Veggies	200 75 40
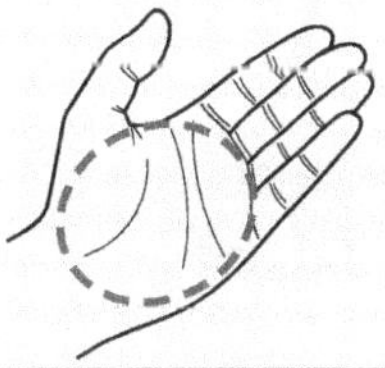	**Palm** 3 ounces	Meat Fish Poultry	160 160 160
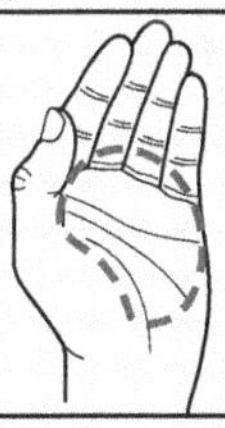	**Handful** 1 ounce	Nuts Raisins	170 85
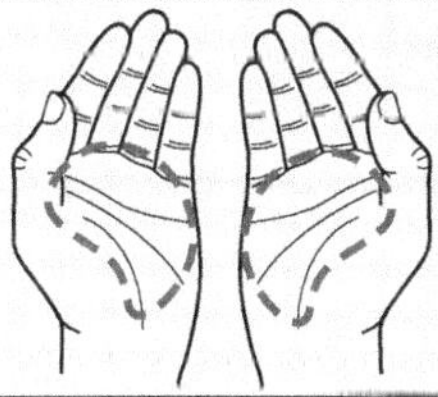	**2 Handfuls** 1 ounce	Chips Popcorn Pretzels	150 120 100
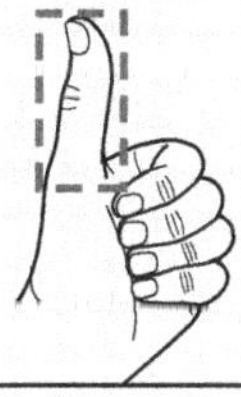	**Thumb** 1 ounce	Peanut butter Hard cheese	170 100
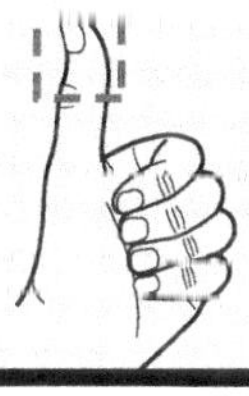	**Thumb tip** 1 teaspoon	Cooking oil Mayonnaise, butter Sugar	40 35 15

Figure 5-12. An example of a hand-based portion size chart

- *Sugar cycle.* Various hormones, including ghrelin and leptin, play a role in the sugar cycle, a cyclic form of sugar-related addictive-type behavior (Figure 5-13). Leptin is an appetite suppressor, while ghrelin increases hunger levels. One way to remember this is that leptin keeps a person lean, and ghrelin is the gremlin that invites an individual to keep on eating. The sugar cycle is really a balance between these and numerous other hormones in the hypothalamus.

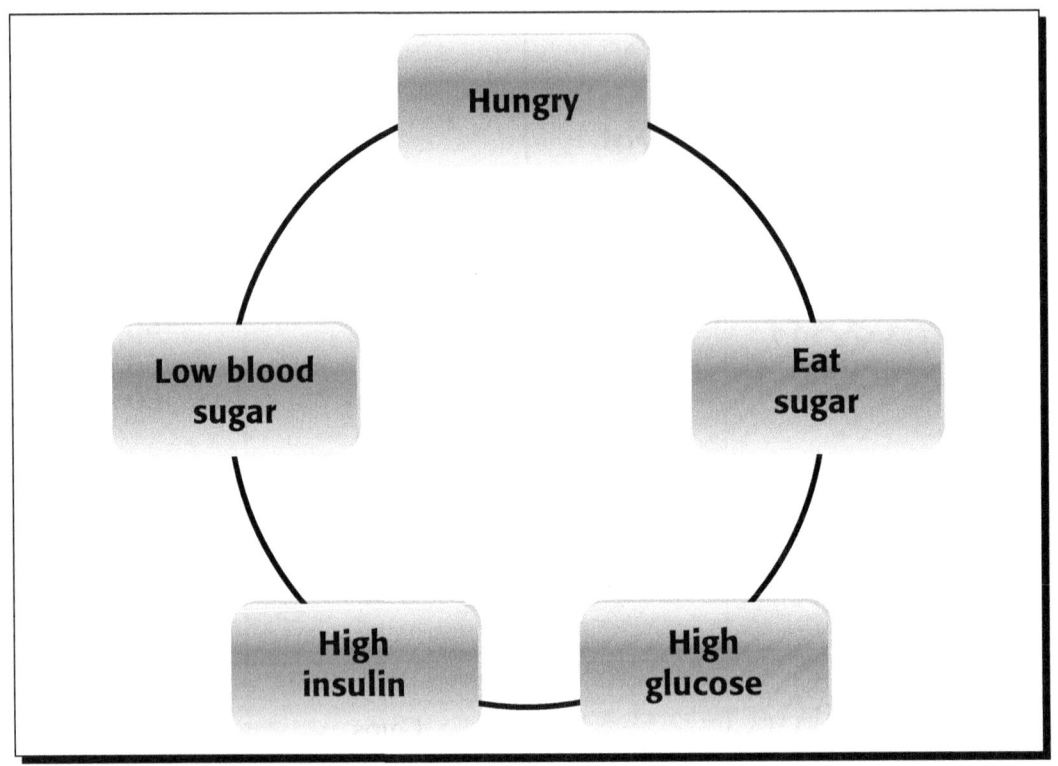

Figure 5-13. Sugar cycle

Patients may feel hungry, either because they have low blood sugar, or because of their normal routine of eating at a particular time (e.g. 12 o'clock is lunch time). They may reflexively reach for a refined carbohydrate, such as a cookie. Subsequently, they eat several of them, and enjoy each one; then at some point, they get a sugar high, a result of having a really high level of blood sugar. The body doesn't like this situation at all. In fact, it reacts as if it's an emergency, recruiting the pancreas to release insulin, because there is too much sugar in the blood stream.

The insulin (which is also a fat-storing hormone) helps to get the sugar out of the blood stream. This effort is the body's attempt to reach homeostasis. This process can actually cause too much insulin to be released with a resultant low blood sugar. This can lead the individual to feel hungry and want to eat again. The insulin will encourage the body to store fat, which is not helpful, especially when people are trying to lose weight.

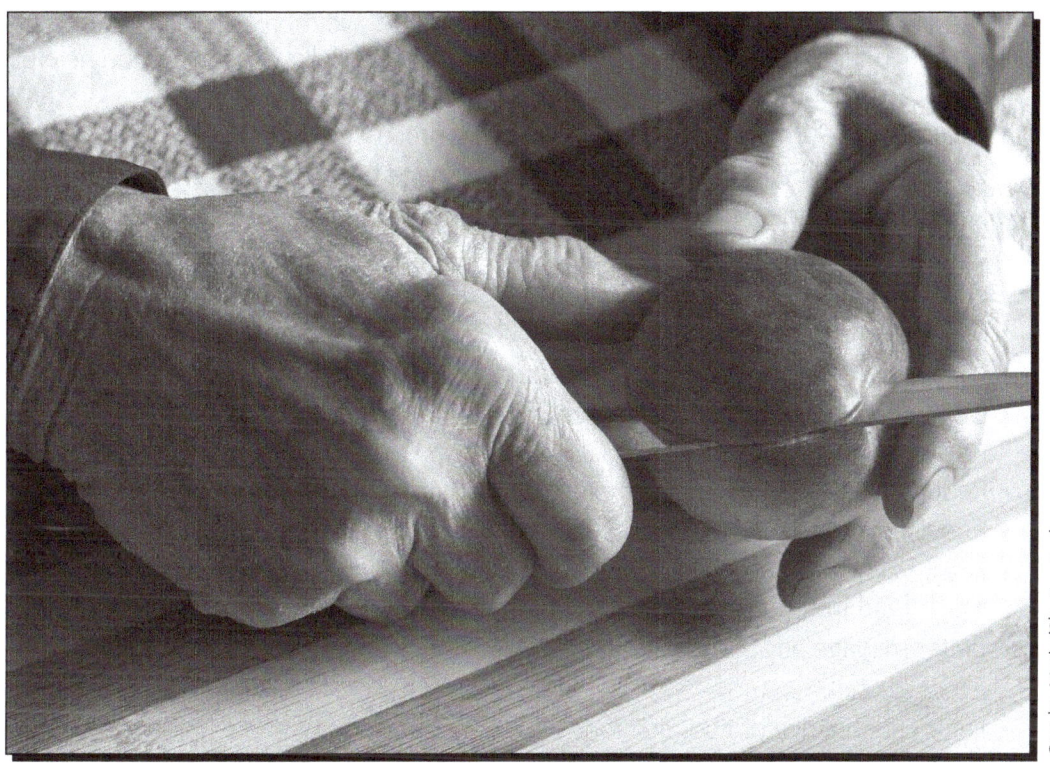

If a patient eats a diet that is rich in fiber (fruits, vegetables, as well as whole grains) their body will have a steady level of blood sugar, given that it takes much longer for the body to digest complex carbs and protein.

    The cycle keeps repeating, unless foods are eaten that help the body feel full. If a patient eats a diet that is rich in fiber (fruits, vegetables, as well as whole grains) their body will have a steady level of blood sugar, given that it takes much longer for the body to digest complex carbs and protein. This factor is the genesis of the suggestion to eat an apple with almond butter. Not only does the almond butter add some protein to the snack, it also requires added time for digestion. Eating complex carbs and proteins or a combination of the two also avoids the excessive insulin release and subsequent hypoglycemia. Unfortunately, it's simple for a person to just eat sugar, such as bread and pastries, which are not far from literally being sugar. The body doesn't have to work very hard to break down those foods and release the sugar into the bloodstream. It takes much longer for the body to digest protein and whole grains, like beans and brown rice. Of note, fat helps food to taste good and also adds to satiety.

• *Weight-loss plateaus.* One of the biggest motivation-killers someone on a diet may face is reaching a plateau concerning their weight-loss efforts. On occasion, despite an individual's best efforts to the contrary (exercising regularly and watching what they eat), their weight-loss program stalls. For no apparent reason, they've hit a weight-loss plateau. They shouldn't get discouraged, however. It's normal for a weight-loss regimen to slow and even stall.

The key, when this frustrating situation occurs, is to avoid backsliding and to try to break through the plateau by responding appropriately. The following tips can be helpful:
- Adjust caloric intake to match the body's current needs for weight loss.
- Focus on consuming quality foods (i.e., avoid processed foods).
- Get outside of their exercise comfort zone—change the routine to "shock" the body.
- Resist the urge to snack or to nibble, a little here and there.
- Check with a physician or allied healthcare professional to rule out having any underlying medical conditions that may be affecting their efforts to lose weight.
- Make sure they are getting a full night of restorative sleep.
- Make sure their body is properly hydrated (i.e., drink plenty of fluids).
- Do strength training to increase lean muscle mass (the body tissue that burns the most calories).
- Reduce their intake of refined grains.
- Exercise harder or more often.
- Keep track of what they eat to help ensure that they do not underestimate how much food they consume.
- Better manage any stress in their life.
- Avoid alcohol.
- Eat an abundance of fiber-rich foods like vegetables, fruits, and whole grains.
- Drink lots of water; avoid sugary beverages.
- Make vegetables a staple of every meal.
- Don't focus on the number on the scale; it may or may not be an accurate indicator of progress in their weight-loss efforts.

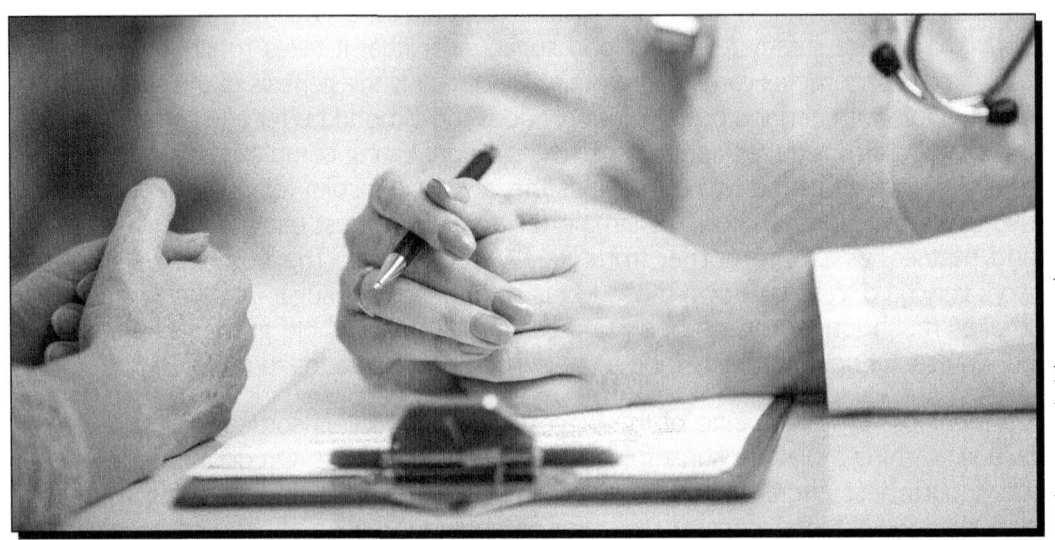

An individual who reaches a plateau concerning their weight-loss efforts should check with a physician or allied healthcare professional to rule out having any underlying medical conditions that may be affecting their efforts to lose weight.

LIVE AND LEARN WITH DR. BETH FRATES

One of my patients was trying to lose weight by increasing the amount that she exercised and modifying her diet. She had a sweet tooth and was working hard to find substitutes for her favorite 3 p.m. snack of pastries. I worked on using coaching skills and focused on using the Frates COACH Approach, demonstrating curiosity, openness, appreciation, compassion, and honesty during our visits.

This patient started using a stationary bicycle. While she enjoyed it, she was not losing weight. Ostensibly, this situation could have been due to her building muscle and losing fat, but she was disappointed. The disappointment compelled her to face her sweet tooth.

Since this patient really wanted to see her scale show a drop in her weight, she determined to make a goal that involved her pastries. She did not want to eat them anymore. I asked her what she would want to eat instead, and she wasn't sure. So, we engaged in a brainstorming session. We both shared ideas as to what she could eat at 3 p.m., if she got hungry. Options, like carrots with hummus, mixed nuts, and an orange, were considered.

Eventually, however, this patient gravitated to eating an apple and almond butter snack. She had not tried almond butter and was anxious to do so. Her goal was that she would buy apples and almond butter at the store on the way home and eat an apple a day at 4 p.m., on five of the days during the upcoming week. She was excited, and it seemed like a SMART goal.

The following week, the patient came to see me, and she looked upset. "It did not work," she proclaimed. I asked her to explain to me what she meant. She said, "I ate an apple with almond butter every day at 4 p.m., and I exercised every day for one hour on that stationary bike. But, I did not lose weight. It was a good week though, and I LOVED that almond butter. It is delicious. I like it so much, I can eat it plain right out of the jar. That is fine, right? You said almond butter was a "healthy choice."

It was then and there that I realized that I had not discussed portion size with her. So, I sheepishly asked, "It is great that you like almond butter, and it is a healthy choice. However, it is important to be careful with how much you eat. How much almond butter were you eating with each apple?" She looked at me with surprise and replied, "I loved it, as I told you. I don't know. Maybe I would eat about ¼ of the jar with each apple. I had to go back to the store to buy another jar after about four days."

This situation was a great learning moment for me. It is critical to go over portion information with patients when recommending a certain food. I had no idea that she would eat that much almond butter. So, we went over the fist serving size information, and she was pretty disappointed to find out that a serving size was the size of her thumb. This situation was an eye-opening experience for both of us.

ASSESSING A PATIENT'S NUTRITIONAL STATUS, WITH COACHING STRATEGIES

Before making prescriptive nutritional recommendations, lifestyle medicine professionals should perform a comprehensive nutrition assessment. This step is best undertaken in collaboration with a registered dietitian, well-versed in lifestyle medicine practices, given that dietitians are the experts in food and nutrition.

As discussed previously, physicians and allied healthcare professionals can employ coaching strategies when working with patients. This approach will help clarify what the patient's needs and interests are, as well as allow the clinician to encourage the individual to make appropriate lifestyle choices. For example, asking a person relevant questions about their nutrition-related practices and opinions can provide a wealth of information concerning what advice and guidance might best address their particular situation. At a minimum, the knowledge that is gained can serve as a logical starting point for whatever counseling that is deemed appropriate going forward.

A nutrition assessment involves four specific elements, including: an anthropometric assessment; a biochemical assessment; a clinical assessment; and a dietary assessment. These four factors are collectively reflected in the acronym "ABCD." As such, a typical nutrition assessment may include the following:

❏ Anthropometric Assessment

The first component of assessment is estimating an individual's body composition, including weight, height, and body mass index (BMI) classification, body measurements, and body composition. The formula for BMI is (body weight in kg) ÷ (height in meters)^2, which is used to classify a person as underweight, normal weight, overweight, or obese, and to help estimate a person's ideal weight range, using a height-weight table.

In reality, a number of problems exist with using height-weight tables to determine an individual's ideal body weight. For example, the body weights in these tables are considered to be desirable only on the basis that they had a positive correlation with longevity for the population studied. They do not take into account the health problems that are frequently associated with obesity.

The members of the first group studied for this purpose were subscribers to Metropolitan Life Insurance. This specific group of people is not representative of the general population (in fact, few minorities or individuals of lower socioeconomic status were included in the study). Furthermore, the body weights of these individuals were only measured once (if at all—since many individuals verbally reported their body weights and were never actually weighed). The information regarding the applicant's' body weights was only obtained at the time that the individuals initially applied for the life insurance. No information was obtained regarding changes in body weight or the subsequent development of health problems after the insurance policies were purchased. These issues aside, the fundamental weakness of height-weight tables is that they do not take into account body composition (i.e., the relative amount of body fat that comprises a person's total body weight).

A person's body fat percentage, rather than total weight, is what has important health implications. Some individuals believe that a specific ideal body weight can be established once an individual's percent body fat is known. Such a conclusion is a somewhat shortsighted view for a number of reasons. Because all of the available techniques for measuring body composition only provide an estimate of percent body fat, the resulting calculations are subject to error. In turn, any effort to utilize percent body fat calculations to ascertain a person's ideal body weight is impacted by those same limitations.

The issue is pervasive. For example, hydrostatic (underwater) weighing, the accepted "gold standard" for analyzing body composition, has a statistically acceptable margin of error of approximately plus or minus two to three percent. Even DEXA (dual energy X-ray absorptiometry), a very popular technique for assessing body fat, has a margin of error of plus or minus two to six percent. The more commonly employed techniques, such as skinfold measurements and bioelectrical impedance, have margins of error that are even higher (i.e., approximately plus or minus five to eight percent).

Unfortunately, even if a person's percent body fat could be accurately and precisely assessed, additional information would be needed to determine their ideal body weight. How much body fat an individual has may not matter as much as where it is located on their body.

As discussed previously in Chapter 4, considerable evidence indicates that the location of fat deposits on a person's body determines how easy it may be for them to lose weight, as well as increases their relative risk of developing a number of health related problems. The location of the fat that is deposited on the body is classified into two basic categories: male-pattern (android, graphically depicted as apple-shaped) and female-pattern (gynoid, graphically depicted as pear-shaped). Despite their illustrative names, each type of fat pattern can occur in both genders, although men usually tend to be "apples," and women are typically classified as "pears." "Apples" characteristically deposit high amounts of fat in the abdominal and trunk regions, while "pears" deposit high amounts of fat in the hip, buttocks, and thigh regions.

As noted in the previous chapter, the waist-to-hip ratio (WHR) is a simple, yet accurate, method for determining an individual's personal distribution pattern for body fat. The waist to hip ratio is determined by dividing an individual's waist circumference by their hip circumference. Waist circumference is defined as the smallest circumference between a person's rib cage and their belly button. Hip circumference is defined as the largest circumference of an individual's hip-buttocks region. Men with WHR values exceeding 1.00 are considered "apples," while women with WHR values above 0.80 are considered "pears." Available evidence suggests that individuals with fat distributed on their upper body (apples) are highly prone to "the deadly quartet" of risk factors for coronary heart disease—high blood pressure, type II (non-insulin dependent) diabetes, elevated levels of triglycerides (hypertriglyceridemia), and low levels of high density lipoproteins ("good cholesterol") in their blood. In general, the more of these risk factors that an individual has, the higher the person's risk of heart disease. All news is not bad for "apples," however. Weight loss (particularly fat loss) tends to be easier for "apples." Unfortunately, for individuals classified as "pears," it can be more difficult to lose the subcutaneous fat stored in the hips and thighs.

❏ Biochemical Assessment

Almost every lab test is impacted by nutritional status, some more dramatically than others. When reviewing lab results, it is important to do so in the context of the patient's overall status, including existing health conditions and hydration status. Biochemical assessment may include a lipid panel, urinalysis, and other specialty tests like B12 status based on the individual needs of each patient.

❏ Clinical Assessment

Clinical assessment helps identify signs and symptoms that indicate nutrition-related disease. Strategies include collecting a comprehensive medical history with a complete list of medications, vital signs, and conducting a physical assessment to observe signs of under- or over-nutrition and hydration status.

❏ Dietary Assessment

Although all components of nutrition assessment hold key pieces of data, dietary assessment is arguably the cornerstone. In order for recommendations and coaching to be successful, lifestyle medicine providers must first gain a clear understanding of what a patient's lifestyle is like at baseline. A solid understanding of a patient's eating habits, food preferences, schedule, family dynamics, economic situation, dieting history, and goals will result in a more effective plan to achieve those goals.

The first step of a complete dietary assessment is to establish an understanding of a patient's typical eating patterns. This step can be done by having patients complete a 3-day food record, typically two weekdays and one weekend day, of everything they eat and drink, or by completing a food frequency questionnaire which includes a list of questions aimed to capture broad eating patterns over the course of several months. A less intensive, yet still effective, way to understand dietary patterns is by conducting a 24-hour recall during the appointment.

In a recall, the lifestyle medicine professional simply asks the patient to describe in a step-by-step manner what they ate during the previous 24 hour period. It's helpful to take several passes through the 24-hour period, filling in more details with each pass. It's common for people to forget details, like beverages consumed, portion sizes, sauces, and other seemingly small but important specifics. Multiple passes, open-ended questioning, and props like measuring cups can help obtain the most accurate assessment.

Another important part of dietary assessment is a diet history, which includes assessing food allergies or intolerances, gastrointestinal health, and understanding any family, psychological, cultural, economic, or functional issues that impact food choices. Although much of the dietary assessment includes subjective and self-reported data, it is no less important.

Using the Frates COACH Approach to dietary assessment, among the questions that someone coaching a patient might ask are the following:
- What are your usual food choices for breakfast, lunch, and dinner?
- What did you eat yesterday?
- Do you often eat between meals? What, how much, and how often?
- How often do you eat out?
- How often do you eat fast foods?
- Do you really like to eat? In other words, how important is food to you?
- Are your food choices generally based on habit, cost, convenience, or taste? (pick one)
- Where do you shop for groceries? A supermarket, a farmers' market, your own garden? If you shop, do you consider making a healthy choice when purchasing a particular item?
- How many vegetables do you eat in a day? What and how many?
- How many fruits do you eat in a day? What and how many?
- What color foods are on your plate?
- What foods are typically in your refrigerator? Are they organized in any particular manner?
- What types of foods are in your cabinets?
- Do you reward yourself with certain foods? What, how much, and how often?
- How do you think your diet impacts your overall health?
- What is your most likely source of information on nutrition?

With the crucial information collected in this ABCD approach, a lifestyle medicine professional can begin to determine appropriate nutrition recommendations for a patient. Every patient is unique and will therefore need an individualized treatment plan. As mentioned previously, working with a registered dietitian at this stage can be tremendously helpful in setting up patients for long-term success.

When counseling patients on healthy eating patterns, it is best to use the Frates COACH Approach. As such, lifestyle medicine professionals should enter the room used for counseling with curiosity, openness, appreciation, compassion, and honesty. Every effort needs to be made to collaborate with the patient and work as a team. This approach will help clarify what the patient's needs and interests are as well as allow the clinician to encourage and empower the individual to make appropriate lifestyle choices. For example, asking a person relevant questions about their nutrition-related practices and opinions can provide a wealth of information concerning what advice and guidance might best address their particular situation. At a minimum, the knowledge that is gained can serve as a logical starting point for whatever counseling that is deemed appropriate going forward.

❑ Practical Strategies

A sensible eating plan should be focused on health-promoting foods that an individual enjoys, while not being overly restrictive when it comes to special occasions. When deciding what to eat in their diet, a patient should also consider what's right for their unique lifestyle, including expense, availability, and ease of preparation of the various foods. Furthermore, it is essential that a person adopts an eating plan that they likely will be able to stick with for an extended period of time. As lifestyle medicine practitioners guide patients on their journey to better health, the following is a summary of practical strategies for patients to incorporate into their WFPB eating plan.

• *Eat the rainbow.* Encourage individuals to consume a diet that has plenty of whole foods, in particular vegetables and fruits, in a variety of colors. Challenge them to build plates that feature foods of multiple colors.

• *Avoid or limit animal products.* Educate patients on the negative impact that animal products have on their health, and assist them in finding more appropriate sources of protein and calcium they enjoy, including beans, lentils, plant milks, and leafy greens.

• *Limit oils, sugar, and alcohol intake.* Emphasize the fact that, in general, a person should aim to keep their diet low in fat and cholesterol. Furthermore, added sugar, salt, and alcoholic beverages should be avoided or consumed in moderation.

• *Fill up on fiber-rich plant foods.* Point out that a patient should consume plenty of fiber-rich vegetables, fruits, seeds, and legumes. Fiber is important in the diet, because it fills the individual up and allows them to feel satisfied, while adding relatively few calories to their diet. Furthermore, fiber aids in moving food, nutrients, and toxins quickly through the digestive tract of the body, which lowers a person's risk of developing colon cancer, because those toxins are no longer present in that individual's digestive tract. The general goal should be to consume 25-40 grams of fiber a day. Fiber is only found in plant-based foods, which is one of the many reasons why plants are so important.

• *Stay hydrated.* Remind patients that sufficient water intake is another critical component to having a healthy diet. The body begins experiencing dehydration before an individual even knows that they're thirsty. When the systems of the body do not have enough water, the body's cells (which use water for every function they perform) will start extracting water from the bloodstream. When the blood is cycled back through the heart, the heart realizes that there is not enough water and triggers the thirst response that a person typically experiences. Once an individual starts replacing water in their system, it can be a bit late. The body has been dehydrated and has a lot of work to do to compensate for that condition. To prevent this situation from occurring, a person should drink water often, even when they don't feel thirsty.

Water intake can vary significantly among individuals. A simple way to monitor if a person is getting enough fluids is to look at the color of that individual's urine. It should be clear or a pale yellow color. Anything darker than that should prompt additional water intake. On days when an individual exercises or on very hot days, that person may need even more water to replace what they've lost through perspiration. It should be noted that fruits and vegetables have water in them naturally. As a result, when people are consuming a whole foods, plant-based diet with seven or more servings of fruits and vegetables a day, they are also taking in water while they eat.

Some people confuse hunger for thirst. They think they are hungry, but they are actually dehydrated and need water. Accordingly, a good tip is for patients to consider drinking a glass of water, if they feel hungry and they recently ate a meal.

- *Examine emotional factors.* Always remember that how much a patient eats and their ability to lose weight may also be affected by certain psychological factors. These factors include all of the non-biological reasons that people eat. It should be noted that the feeling of being hungry is not always the reason for eating. For example, an individual's emotions often have a big effect on what and when that person eats. Any emotion, such as stress, boredom, loneliness, anxiety, depression, or fatigue may increase the likelihood of overeating.

Furthermore, a patient may simply eat out of habit, i.e., time to eat, being in the presence of people who are eating, and being exposed to the sight and smell of food. This factor is compounded by the fact that sugar, salt, and fat—the major ingredients in calorie-dense foods—trigger the reward circuits in an individual's brain, meaning these foods have definite addictive properties (see Chapter 11). During breaks at work or when watching television at night, some people routinely head for the breakroom, cupboard, or refrigerator.

These behavioral patterns can be very hard to break. It requires careful planning ahead. For example, individuals should keep healthy foods readily available, limit the quantity and availability of high fat and high sugar foods, self-monitor the food they eat, and exercise. Help patients identify these pitfalls in their lives and establish effective strategies for bypassing them.

- *Keep portions in check.* Make sure that patients know that when eating high calorie dense foods, which inevitably happens in the course of life, keeping portions in check is key. For example, when eating a meal at home or in a restaurant, a person could limit themselves to consuming just one portion. They could also wrap up any leftovers right away to discourage nibbling. Because restaurant portions tend to be very large, eating just half of the entree and wrapping the other half up to take home can be a viable way to limit how much is eaten. Other tricks, when eating at home, include eating meals on smaller plates. Not only does this visual "deception" make it appear that the plate is overly full, rather than mostly empty, it has also been shown to reduce the number of calories consumed.

Mindful eating, including eating more slowly, taking smaller bites, and savoring each one can also help. It is important to understand that it takes the brain about 20 minutes to realize that the stomach is full. In this amount of time, most people tend to eat everything on their plates and have potentially already had seconds.

• *Eat until satisfied vs. full.* Suggest to patients that another way to aid in sensibly eating less is for them to forget about cleaning their plate. Rather than eating everything, a person should stop when they're full—even better at 80 percent of being full. When enjoying a meal, an individual should try to make that the only activity on which they're focusing. For example, watching television or reading, while eating, can lead to distractions. By sitting down and concentrating on their food, people are more likely to enjoy the meal, and won't be as likely to eat past the point of feeling full.

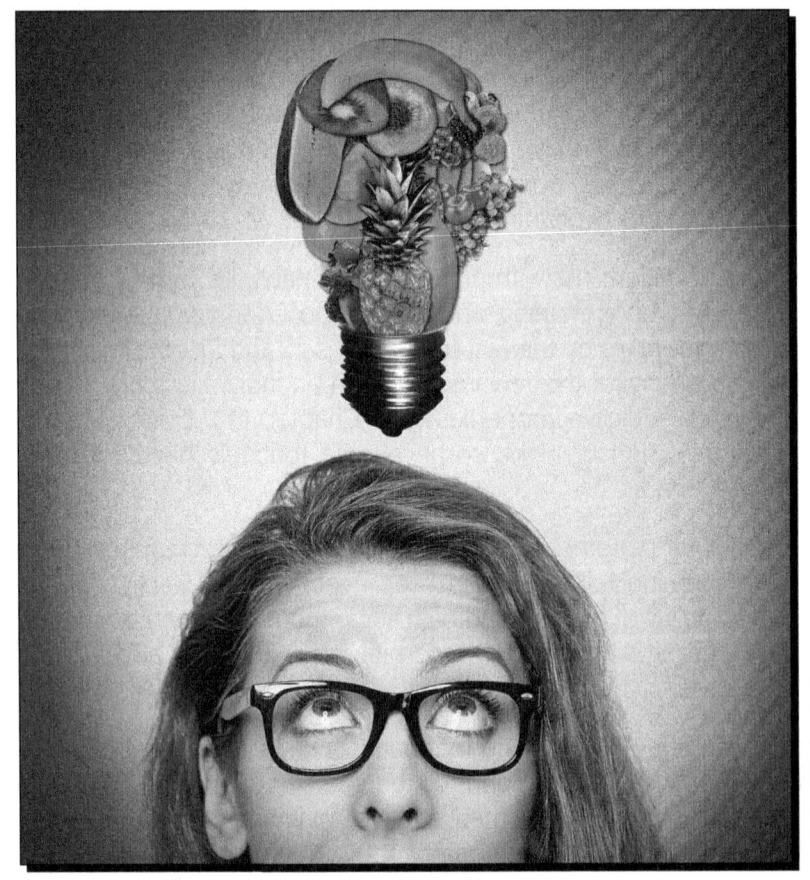

It is important to understand that it takes the brain about 20 minutes to realize that the stomach is full.

- *Curate a healthy food environment.* Draw attention to the fact that controlling what foods are in the house and available is also an effective means to facilitate sensible eating. If a person has a craving for high-fat foods or certain "junk foods," they should try to keep such foods out of the home entirely. If the rest of their family wants to eat cake and ice cream, they should try to keep those items and similar snacks in an out-of-the-way cupboard or deep in the freezer, where it is difficult to see or get to (i.e., out of sight, out of mind).

- *Balance meals throughout the day.* Stress the point that eating smaller amounts of food, but more frequently, may help with weight-loss efforts, *if* it helps an individual make healthier choices. Frequent eating requires planning and may discourage a person from stopping at a fast-food restaurant on the way home or going out to eat at lunch. In reality, there is no definitive data to suggest that eating less or more frequently will cause weight gain or weight loss. Some evidence, however, suggests that adequate calcium in the diet and adequate protein, both of which can be achieved on a plant predominant diet, can also help keep blood sugar levels stable and support continual weight loss.

Meal skipping is another relevant issue to consider with regard to healthy eating. Although associations exist between breakfast skipping and obesity, no causative relationship has been demonstrated. On the other hand, in obese individuals who have maintained a significant amount of weight loss, breakfast eating is one of the cornerstone behaviors identified. For weight maintenance, there is some evidence to suggest that a meal frequency routine that includes eating three regular meals a day, with two snacks, may be helpful.

- *Cook at home.* Have patients eat out less and learn how to stock their kitchens with healthy options. Making sure there are fresh fruits and vegetables, preferably in season available is key. Stocking cabinets with nuts and seeds, rather than potato chips and pretzels, is an example of an important swap for them to make. Encouraging patients to take cooking lessons, watch cooking shows, take cookbooks out of the library and perhaps consider buying ones that work best is highly recommended. Adding herbs and spices will help make these whole foods taste delicious. People do not need added sugar, salt, or fat to cook delicious foods. There are so many advantages to eating at home, such as saving money, reducing portion sizes, controlling the ingredients, and avoiding processed foods, as well as connecting with family at home around the dinner table. The following are cookbooks to try that can facilitate a person's journey to adhering to healthy eating habits. In reality, there are so many to explore:
    - ✓ *The Prevent and Reverse Heart Disease Cookbook,* by Ann Crile Esselstyn and Jane Esselstyn
    - ✓ *The How Not to Die Cookbook,* by Michael Greger, MD, FACLM
    - ✓ *Straight Up Food: Delicious and Easy Plant-Based Cooking Without Salt, Oil or Sugar,* by Cathy Fisher
    - ✓ *Forks Over Knives—The Cookbook,* by Del Sroufe

FITT PRESCRIPTIONS FOR NUTRITION

Just as there is a FITT prescription for exercise, there is a FITT prescription for nutrition. This is a simple framework that provides guidance for patients and providers, alike. First, select a focus for the prescription. In many instances, it will entail increasing the consumption of vegetables, with the goal of consuming six servings of vegetables a day. Next, use the Frates COACH Approach to collaborate with the patient and find a reasonable SMART goal to start with, such as consuming one serving of vegetables at lunch and dinner, five days over the course of the week. As the patient develops confidence and success with smaller goals, they can progress toward more challenging prescriptions.

F—Frequency: number of days per week
I—Intensity: number of servings
T—Time: which meal/snack times
T—Type: description of the food(s) to consume

❑ An example FITT prescription to work toward for consuming more vegetables:

F—every day
I—two servings
T—during meals
T—vegetables (including carrots, sweet potatoes, eggplant, cucumber, kale, lettuce, and tomatoes, with a concerted effort to eat the rainbow)

❑ An example of a FITT prescription to change from consuming sugar-laden desserts to fruit for dessert:

F—five days a week
I—one serving a day
T—dessert
T—enjoy a fruit for dessert (strawberries, watermelon, apple, orange, or another fruit of the individual's choice).

❑ An example of a FITT prescription for consuming healthy snacks:

F—7 days a week
I—one serving
T—3 p.m. snack
T—carrot and celery sticks with hummus

KEY POINTS/TAKEAWAYS FOR CHAPTER 5

❑ Chapter Review:

- Overall goal: Define sound nutritional practices.
- Application goal: Understand the nutrition-health connection.

❑ Discussion Questions:

- What role do you think nutrition plays in lifestyle medicine?
- What constitutes a healthy diet?
- What are the keys to a healthy diet?
- Are your nutritional habits consistent with current dietary guidelines?
- Which dietary plan do you prefer?
- What makes plants so powerful for maintaining and regaining health?
- What are the most essential factors involved in weight management?
- What strategy would you employ to get a weight-challenged patient to change their behavior?

	TITLE	AUTHORS	JOURNAL	YEAR	KEY FINDINGS
1	A low-fat vegan diet and a conventional diabetes diet in the treatment of type 2 diabetes: a randomized, controlled, 74-wk clinical trial	Barnard ND, et al.	American Journal of Clinical Nutrition	2009	A study of 99 subjects with type 2 diabetes that compared a low-fat vegan diet to a conventional diabetes diet. Both groups lost a significant amount of weight (-4 kg and -3 kg in the vegan and convention diet groups, respectively) and had significant improvements in total cholesterol and LDL cholesterol, as well as non-significant improvements in hemoglobin A1c. After adjusting for medication changes, a low-fat vegan diet appeared to improve glycemia and plasma lipids more than a conventional diabetes diet.
2	Effects of intensive diet and exercise intervention in patients taking cholesterol-lowering drugs	Barnard RJ, DiLauro SC, Inkeles SB	American Journal of Cardiology	1997	"Patients taking cholesterol-lowering drugs were placed on a very low fat, high-complex-carbohydrate diet with daily aerobic exercise and achieved 19%, 20%, and 29% reductions in total cholesterol, LDL-cholesterol and triglycerides, respectively."
3	Effects of a low-fat, high-fiber diet and exercise program on breast cancer risk factors in vivo and tumor cell growth and apoptosis in vitro	Barnard RJ, et al.	Nutrition and Cancer	2006	Researchers put overweight/obese postmenopausal women on a low fat (10-15% kcal), high-fiber (30-40 g per 1,000 kcal/day) diet and had them attend daily exercise classes for two weeks. They found significant reductions in serum estradiol, serum insulin, and insulin-like growth factor-I, with a significant increase in IGF binding protein-1. There were also in vivo serum changes that slowed the growth and induced apoptosis in serum-stimulate breast cancer cell lines in vitro.

Figure 5-14. Nutrition guidelines and prescription evidence

	TITLE	AUTHORS	JOURNAL	YEAR	KEY FINDINGS
4	Effect of lifestyle changes on erectile dysfunction in obese men: a randomized controlled trial	Esposito K, et al.	JAMA	2004	A randomized, single-blind trial of 110 obese men aged 35 to 55 years who had erectile dysfunction were assigned to either an intervention group receiving detailed information about how to achieve a weight loss of 10% or more, or a control group given general information about healthy food choices and exercise. BMI, interleukin 6, and CRP had decreased significantly more in the intervention group than in the control group. Physical activity increased more in the intervention group and erectile dysfunction index scores also improved in the intervention group as compared to the control group. Ultimately, researchers found that lifestyle changes were associated with improvement in sexual function in ~1/3 of obese men with erectile dysfunction at baseline.
5	Resolving the coronary artery disease epidemic through plant-based nutrition	Esselstyn CB	Preventive Cardiology	2001	"…Compelling data from nutritional studies, population surveys, and interventional studies support the effectiveness of a plant-based diet and aggressive lipid lowering to arrest, prevent, and selectively reverse heart disease …. The single biggest step toward adopting this strategy would be to have United States *dietary guidelines* support a plant-based diet."
6	Persistent metabolic adaptation 6 years after "The Biggest Loser" competition	Fothergill E, et al.	Obesity	2016	Fourteen "Biggest Loser" competitors had resting metabolic rate (RMR) and body composition measured at 30 weeks post-competition and six years later. At the end of the competition, average weight loss was 58 kg with a 610 kcal/day decrease in RMR. After six years, an average of 41 kg of weight was regained, while RMR was 704 kcal/day below baseline—a metabolic adaptation of -499 kcal/day ($p<0.0001$). They concluded that metabolic adaptation persists over time and is likely a proportional, but incomplete, response to contemporaneous efforts to reduce body weight.
7	Vegetarian diets: what do we know of their effects on common chronic diseases?	Fraser GE	American Journal of Clinical Nutrition	2009	A review of the evidence on the health effects of vegetarian diets on chronic disease. "There is convincing evidence that vegetarians have lower rates of coronary heart disease, largely explained by low LDL cholesterol, probable lower rates of hypertension and diabetes mellitus, and lower prevalence of *obesity*. Overall, their cancer rates appear to be moderately lower than others living in the same communities, and life expectancy appears to be greater. However, results for specific cancers are much less convincing and require more study." It also discusses how "vegetarian" as a dietary category is too broad and that further delineation of dietary components may be needed for a more complete understanding.

Figure 5-14. Nutrition guidelines and prescription evidence (cont.)

	TITLE	AUTHORS	JOURNAL	YEAR	KEY FINDINGS
8	Clinical events in prostate cancer lifestyle trial: results from two years of follow-up	Frattaroli J, et al.	*Urology*	2008	A one-year randomized controlled trial of 93 patients with early-stage prostate cancer who were undergoing active surveillance. Subjects were either encouraged to adopt a low-fat, plant-based diet, to exercise and practice stress management, and to attend group sessions, or placed in a control group of usual care. At the two-year follow-up 27% of control patients and 5% of experimental patients have undergone conventional prostate cancer treatment ($p<0.05$) without any other significant differences between groups in other clinical events.
9	An expanded model for mindful eating for health promotion and sustainability: issues and challenges for dietetics practice	Fung TT, et al.	*Journal of the Academy of Nutrition and Dietetics*	2016	A discussion of current studies of mindful eating health promotion and sustainability. "Promising results have been observed in the management of depression, stress, physical function, quality of life, and chronic pain." Describes the role mindful eating has in dietetics practice.
10	Bariatric surgery resistance: using preoperative lifestyle medicine and/or pharmacology for metabolic responsiveness	Gilbertson NM, et al.	*Obesity Surgery*	2017	This article raises a novel hypothesis that pre-bariatric surgery lifestyle interventions such as diet and exercise and pharmacology may reduce inflammation, improve insulin action, and increase physical function, subsequently reducing the number of people who are deemed resistant to bariatric surgery.
11	Environmental impact of dietary change: a systematic review	Hallstrom E, Carlsson-Kanyama A, Borjesson P	*Journal of Cleaner Production*	2015	A systematic review of 14 articles assessing the environmental impact of different dietary scenarios. It finds that dietary change in areas with affluent diet can reduce diet greenhouse gas emissions and land use demand by up to 50%.
12	Effects of a dietary portfolio of cholesterol-lowering foods vs lovastatin on serum lipids and C-reactive protein	Jenkins DJ, et al.	*JAMA*	2003	A randomized controlled trial done in 46 adults with hyperlipidemia that randomized subjects into one of three interventions for one month: a diet low in saturated fat (control), the same diet plus lovastatin (statin), or a diet high in plant sterols, soy protein, viscous fibers, and almonds (diet portfolio). Low-density lipoprotein was decreased by 8%, 30.9%, and 28.6%, respectively. C-reactive protein were 10%, 33.3%, and 28.2%. The significant reductions in the stat and dietary portfolio groups were all significantly different from changes in the control group, with no difference between the statin and dietary portfolio groups.

Figure 5.14. Nutrition guidelines and prescription evidence (cont.)

	TITLE	AUTHORS	JOURNAL	YEAR	KEY FINDINGS
13	Vegetarian diet improves insulin resistance and oxidative stress markers more than conventional diet in subjects with type 2 diabetes	Kahleova H, et al.	*Diabetic Medicine*	2011	A 24-week, randomized trial of 74 patients with type 2 diabetes that were assigned to receive either a vegetarian diet, or a conventional diabetic diet. All meals were provided to ensure that they were both isocaloric and calorie restricted (-500 kcal/day). Aerobic exercise was added to the second half of the study. Researchers found that "43% of participants in the vegetarian diet group and 5% of participants in the conventional diet reduced diabetes medication." Body weight decreased more in the vegetarian diet than in the conventional diet (-6.2 kg vs. -3.2 kg). The vegetarian diet had greater capacity to improve insulin sensitivity than the conventional diet, which may have been secondary to a greater loss of visceral fat, decrease in adipokines, and oxidative stress markers. Exercise further augmented the improved outcomes in the vegetarian diet.
14	Can we say what diet is best for health?	Katz DL, Meller S	*Annual Review of Public Health*	2014	This systematic review examined all mainstream dietary approaches and the published evidence pertaining to their impact on health. It found that "the fundamentals of virtually all eating patterns associated with meaningful evidence of health benefit overlap substantially." Furthermore, "A diet of minimally processed foods close to nature, predominantly plants, is decisively associated with health promotion and disease prevention and is consistent with the salient components of seemingly distinct dietary approaches."
15	Providing nutritional care in the office practice: teams, tools, and techniques	Kushner RF	*Medical Clinics of North America*	2016	An overview of the nutrition counseling process used in outpatient clinics. Emphasizes the importance of motivational interviewing, shared decision making, and collaboration between patients and providers. It also discusses multiple other models and theories of behavior change and their role in the counseling process.
16	Rapid reduction of serum cholesterol and blood pressure by a twelve-day, very low fat, strictly vegetarian diet	McDougall J, et al.	*Journal of the American College of Nutrition*	1995	Five hundred adults participated in a 12-day live-in program comprising of moderate exercise, stress management, and a strictly vegetarian, very low-fat diet. "During this short time period, cardiac risk factors improved: there was an average reduction of total serum cholesterol of 11% ($p<0.001$), of blood pressure of 6% ($p<0.001$) and a weight loss of 2.5 kg for men and 1 kg for women." Triglycerides were largely unchanged, except in two subgroups, and high-density lipoprotein cholesterol decreasing by 19%. "A strict, very low-fat vegetarian diet free from all animal products combined with lifestyle changes that include exercise and weight loss is an effective way to lower serum cholesterol and blood pressure."

Figure 5-14. Nutrition guidelines and prescription evidence (cont.)

	TITLE	AUTHORS	JOURNAL	YEAR	KEY FINDINGS
17	Increased telomerase activity and comprehensive lifestyle changes: a pilot study	Ornish D, et al.	Lancet Oncology	2008	A three-month study of 24 men with low-risk prostate cancer participated in a comprehensive lifestyle change program to see what effect it had on telomerase enzymatic activity. Researchers found that "comprehensive lifestyle changes significantly increase telomerase activity and consequently telomere maintenance capacity in human immune-system cells."
18	Healthful and unhealthful plant-based diets and the risk of coronary heart disease in U.S. adults	Satija A, et al.	Journal of the American College of Cardiology	2017	This study shows that eating more plant foods (versus animal foods) is associated with lower CHD risk, but eating more *healthy* plant foods is "associated with substantially lower CHD risk, whereas a plant-based diet index that emphasizes less-healthy plant foods is associated with higher CHD risk."
19	Plant-based dietary patterns and incidence of type 2 diabetes in US men and women: results from three prospective cohort studies	Satija A, et al.	PLoS Medicine	2016	"Our study suggests that plant-based diets, especially when rich in high-quality plant foods, are associated with substantially lower risk of developing T2D. This supports current recommendations to shift to diets rich in healthy plant foods, with lower intake of less healthy plant and animal foods."
20	Adherence to Mediterranean diet and health status: meta-analysis	Sofi F, et al.	British Medical Journal	2008	Found that adherence to a Mediterranean type of diet was associated with improvement in health status, reduction in overall mortality (9%), reduction in cardiovascular mortality (9%), decreased incidence of mortality from cancer (6%), and decreased incidence of Parkinson's disease and Alzheimer's disease (13%).
21	Analysis and valuation of the health and climate change cobenefits of dietary change	Springmann M, et al.	Proceedings of the National Academy of Sciences of the United States of America	2016	A comparative analysis of the health and climate change benefits of global dietary change that estimated that transitioning toward a more plant-based diet could reduce global mortality by 6% to 10% and food-related greenhouse gas emissions by 29% to 70% by 2050.
22	Climate benefits of changing diet	Stehfest E, et al.	Climatic Change	2009	An integrated assessment model that found that a global food transition to less meat or a complete switch to plant-based protein food would have a dramatic effect on reducing land use and methane and nitrous oxide emissions. "Dietary changes could therefore not only create substantial benefits for human health and global land use, but can also play an important role in future climate change mitigation policies."

Figure 5-14. Nutrition guidelines and prescription evidence (cont.)

	TITLE	AUTHORS	JOURNAL	YEAR	KEY FINDINGS
23	Global diets link environmental sustainability and human health	Tilman D, Clark M	*Nature*	2014	An analysis and discussion of the impact dietary choices have on the environment and human health. Researchers concluded that "alternative diets that offer substantial health benefits could, if widely adopted, reduce global agricultural greenhouse gas emissions, reduce land clearing and resultant species extinctions, and help prevent such diet-related chronic non-communicable disease. The implementation of dietary solutions to the tightly linked diet-environment-health trilemma is a global challenge, and opportunity, of great environmental and public health importance."
24	Usefulness of vegetarian and vegan diets for treating type 2 diabetes	Trapp CB, Barnard ND	*Current Diabetes Reports*	2010	Reviews the role that vegan and vegetarian diets play in diabetes prevention. Found that "research to date has demonstrated that a low-fat, plant-based nutritional approach improves control of weight, glycemia, and cardiovascular risk. These studies have also shown that carefully planned vegan diets can be more nutritious than diets based on more conventional diet guidelines…"
25	Nutritional update for physicians: plant-based diets	Tuso PJ, et al.	*Permanente Journal*	2013	A nutritional update on the utility of plant-based diets from the Kaiser Permanente Health system, which finds that "research shows that plant-based diets are cost-effective, low-risk interventions that may lower body mass index, blood pressure, hemoglobin A1c, and cholesterol levels. They may also reduce the number of medications needed to treat chronic diseases and lower ischemic heart disease mortality rates. Physicians should consider recommending a plant-based diet to all their patients, especially those with high blood pressure, diabetes, cardiovascular disease, or *obesity*."
26	Advanced glycation end products in foods and a practical guide to their reduction in the diet	Uribarri J, et al.	*Journal of the American Dietetic Association*	2010	Found that dry heat promotes the development of dietary advanced glycation end products (AGE) >10- to 100-fold above the uncooked state across food categories. Animal-derived foods that are higher in fat and protein are generally rich in AGE, whereas vegetables, fruits, whole grains, and milk contain relatively few AGE, even after cooking. "Frying, boiling, grilling, and roasting food yielded more AGE compared to boiling, poaching, stewing, and steaming."
27	Current evidence of healthy eating	Willett WC, Stampfer MJ	*Annual Review of Public Health*	2013	This article summarizes major findings in nutrition research from recent years and draws the following conclusions: "Good data now support the benefits of diets that are rich in plant sources of fats and protein, fish, nuts, whole grains, and fruits and vegetables; that avoid partially hydrogenated fats; and that limit red meat and refined carbohydrates. The simplistic advice to reduce all fat, or all carbohydrates, has not stood the test of science; strong evidence supports the need to consider fat and carbohydrate quality and different protein sources."

Figure 5-14. Nutrition guidelines and prescription evidence (cont.)

References

1. Barnard ND, Cohen J, Jenkins DJ, et al. A low-fat vegan diet and a conventional diabetes diet in the treatment of type 2 diabetes: a randomized, controlled, 74-wk clinical trial. *American Journal of Clinical Nutrition.* May 2009;89(5):1588S-1596S. doi:10.3945/ajcn.2009.26736H. Epub 2009 Apr 1.
2. Barnard RJ, DiLauro SC, Inkeles SB. Effects of intensive diet and exercise intervention in patients taking cholesterol-lowering drugs. *American Journal of Cardiology.* 1997;79:1112-1114.
3. Barnard RJ, Hong Gonzalez J, Liva ME, et al. Effects of a low-fat, high-fiber diet and exercise program on breast cancer risk factors in vivo and tumor cell growth and apoptosis in vitro. *Nutrition and Cancer.* 2006;55:28-34.
4. Esposito K, Giugliano F, Di Palo C, et al. Effect of lifestyle changes on erectile dysfunction in obese men: a randomized controlled trial. *JAMA.* 2004;291:2978-2984.
5. Esselstyn CB. Resolving the coronary artery disease epidemic through plant-based nutrition. *Preventive Cardiology.* 2001;4:171-177.
6. Fothergill E, Guo J, Howard L, et al. Persistent metabolic adaptation 6 years after "The Biggest Loser" competition. *Obesity (Silver Spring).* 2016;24:1612-1619.
7. Fraser GE. Vegetarian diets: what do we know of their effects on common chronic diseases? *American Journal of Clinical Nutrition.* 2009;89(5):1607S-1612S. doi:http://dx.doi.org/10.3945/ajcn.2009.26736K.
8. Frattaroli J, Weidner G, Dnistrian AM, et al. Clinical events in prostate cancer lifestyle trial: results from two years of follow-up. *Urology.* 2008;72:1319-1323.
9. Fung TT, Long MW, Hung P, et al. An expanded model for mindful eating for health promotion and sustainability: issues and challenges for dietetics practice. *Journal of the Academy of Nutrition and Dietetics.* July 2016;116(7):1081-1086.
10. Gilbertson NM, Paisley A, Kranz S, et al. Bariatric surgery resistance: using preoperative lifestyle medicine and/or pharmacology for metabolic responsiveness. *Obesity Surgery.* 2017;27(12):3281-3291. doi:10.1007/s11695-017-2966-1.
11. Hallstrom E, Carlsson-Kanyama A, Borjesson P. Environmental impact of dietary change: a systematic review. *Journal of Cleaner Production.* 2015;91:1-11.
12. Jenkins DJ, Kendall CW, Marchie A, et al. Effects of a dietary portfolio of cholesterol-lowering foods vs lovastatin on serum lipids and C-reactive protein. *JAMA.* 2003;290:502-510.
13. Kahleova H, Matoulek M, Malinska H, et al. Vegetarian diet improves insulin resistance and oxidative stress markers more than conventional diet in subjects with type 2 diabetes. *Diabetic Medicine.* 2011;28:549-559.
14. Katz DL, Meller S. Can we say what diet is best for health? *Annual Review of Public Health.* 2014;35(1):83-103. doi:10.1146/annurev-publhealth-032013-182351.
15. Kushner RF. Providing nutritional care in the office practice: teams, tools, and techniques. Medical Clinics of North America. 2016;100(6):1157-1168. doi:10.1016/j.mcna.2016.06.002.
16. McDougall J, Litzau K, Haver E, et al. Rapid reduction of serum cholesterol and blood pressure by a twelve-day, very low fat, strictly vegetarian diet. *Journal of the American College of Nutrition.* 1995;14:491-496.
17. Ornish D, Lin J, Daubenmier J, et al. Increased telomerase activity and comprehensive lifestyle changes: a pilot study. *Lancet Oncology.* 2008;9:1048-1057.
18. Satija A, Bhupathiraju SN, Spiegelman D, et al. Healthful and unhealthful plant-based diets and the risk of coronary heart disease in U.S. adults. *Journal of the American College of Cardiology.* July 25 2017;70(4):411-422.
19. Satija A, Bhupathiraju SN, Rimm EB, et al. Plant-based dietary patterns and incidence of type 2 diabetes in US men and women: results from three prospective cohort studies. *PLoS Medicine.* June 2016;13(6):e1002039.
20. Sofi F, Cesari F, Abbate R, et al. Adherence to Mediterranean diet and health status: meta-analysis. *British Medical Journal.* 2008;337:a1344. doi:10.1136/bmj.a1344.
21. Springmann M, Godfray HC, Rayner M, et al. Analysis and valuation of the health and climate change cobenefits of dietary change. *Proceedings of the National Academy of Sciences of the United States of America.* 2016;113:4146-4151.
22. Stehfest E, Bouwman L, van Vuuren DP, et al. Climate benefits of changing diet. *Climatic Change.* 2009;95:83-102.
23. Tilman D, Clark M. Global diets link environmental sustainability and human health. *Nature.* 2014;515:518-522.
24. Trapp CB, Barnard ND. Usefulness of vegetarian and vegan diets for treating type 2 diabetes. *Current Diabetes Reports.* 2010;10:152-158.
25. Tuso PJ, Ismail MH, Ha BP, et al. Nutritional update for physicians: plant-based diets. Permanente Journal. 2013;17(2):61-66. doi:10.7812/TPP/12-085.
26. Uribarri J, Woodruff S, Goodman S, et al. Advanced glycation end products in foods and a practical guide to their reduction in the diet. *Journal of the American Dietetic Association.* 2010;110(6):911-916.e12. doi:10.1016/j.jada.2010.03.018.
27. Willett WC, Stampfer MJ. Current evidence of healthy eating. *Annual Review of Public Health.* 2013;34(1):77-95. doi:10.1146/annurev-publhealth-031811-124646.

Figure 5-14. Nutrition guidelines and prescription evidence (cont.)

REFERENCES

- American College of Lifestyle Medicine, Turn the Tide Foundation. True Health Initiative. A Global Consensus on Lifestyle as Medicine. Available at: http://TrueHealthInitiative.org. Accessed January 2017.
- American Heart Association. Alcohol and Heart Health. Available at: http://www.heart.org/en/healthy-living/healthy-eating/eat-smart/nutrition-basics/alcohol-and-heart-health. Accessed September 2018.
- Appel LJ, Champagne CM, Harsha DW, et al. Effects of comprehensive lifestyle modification on blood pressure control: main results of the PREMIER clinical trial. *JAMA.* 2003;289.2083-2093.

- Appel LJ, Moore TJ, Obarzanek E, et al. The effect of dietary patterns on blood pressure: results from the Dietary Approaches to Stop Hypertension (DASH) trial. *New England Journal of Medicine.* 1997;336:1117-1124.
- Astrup A, Raben A, Geiker N. The role of higher protein diets in weight control and obesity-related comorbidities. *International Journal of Obesity (2005).* 2015;39(5):721-726. doi:10.1038/ijo.2014.216.
- Aune D, Rosenblatt DAN, Chan DSM, et al. Dairy products, calcium, and prostate cancer risk: a systematic review and meta-analysis of cohort studies. *American Journal of Clinical Nutrition.* 2015;101(1):87-117. https://doi.org/10.3945/ajcn.113.067157.
- Austin J, Marks D. Hormonal regulators of appetite. *International Journal of Pediatric Endocrinology.* 2009;2009:141753. doi:10.1155/2009/141753.
- Bachman JL, Phelan S, Wing RR, et al. Eating frequency is higher in weight loss maintainers and normal weight individuals as compared to overweight individuals. *Journal of the American Dietetic Association.* 2011;111(11):1730-1734. doi:10.1016/j.jada.2011.08.006.
- Barnard ND, Cohen J, Jenkins DJ, et al. A low-fat vegan diet and a conventional diabetes diet in the treatment of type 2 diabetes: a randomized, controlled, 74-wk clinical trial. *American Journal of Clinical Nutrition.* May 2009;89(5):1588S-1596S. doi:10.3945/ajcn.2009.26736H. Epub 2009 Apr 1.
- Barnard ND, Grogan BC. *Dr. Neal Barnard's Program for Reversing Diabetes: The Scientifically Proven System for Reversing Diabetes Without Drugs.* New York: Rodale Books; 2008.
- Barnard RJ, DiLauro SC, Inkeles SB. Effects of intensive diet and exercise intervention in patients taking cholesterol-lowering drugs. *American Journal of Cardiology.* 1997;79:1112-1114.
- Barnard RJ, Hong Gonzalez J, Liva ME, Ngo TH. Effects of a low-fat, high-fiber diet and exercise program on breast cancer risk factors in vivo and tumor cell growth and apoptosis in vitro. *Nutrition and Cancer.* 2006;55:28-34.
- BBC Productions. The Truth About Sugar [Video]. October 16, 2015. Available at: https://youtu.be/K4LzSH9qU_QYouTube. Accessed September 2017.
- Berardi J, Andrews R. Fruits and Vegetables. Precision Nutrition. Available at: https://www.precisionnutrition.com/color-chart. Accessed September 2018.
- Berthon BS, Wood LG. Nutrition and respiratory health—feature review. *Nutrients.* 2015;7(3):1618-1643. doi:10.3390/nu7031618.
- Bishop KS, Ferguson LR. The interaction between epigenetics, nutrition and the development of cancer. *Nutrients.* February 2015;7(2):922-947.
- Bouvard V, Loomis D, Guyton KZ, et al. Carcinogenicity of consumption of red and processed meat. *The Lancet Oncology.* 2015;16:1599-1600.
- Buettner D. *The Blue Zones: 9 Lessons for Living Longer From the People Who've Lived the Longest.* Washington, D.C.: National Geographic; 2012.

- Calorie Density. Available at: https://www.facebook.com/JeffNovickRD/photos/a.10155448872115125/10156061429660125/?type=1&theater. Accessed September 2018.
- Campbell TC, Campbell TM. *The China Study: The Most Comprehensive Study of Nutrition Ever Conducted and the Startling Implications for Diet, Weight Loss, and Long-Term Health.* Revised edition. Dallas, TX: BenBella Books; December 2016.
- Casazza K, Brown A, Astrup A, et al. Weighing the evidence of common beliefs in obesity research. *Critical Reviews in Food Science and Nutrition.* 2015;55(14):2014-2053. doi:10.1080/10408398.2014.922044.
- Centers for Disease Control and Prevention. Genes and Obesity. Available at: https://www.cdc.gov/genomics/resources/diseases/obesity/obesedit.htm. Accessed June 2018.
- Centers for Disease Control and Prevention. Only 1 in 10 Adults Get Enough Fruits or Vegetables [Press Release]. November 16, 2017. Available at: https://www.cdc.gov/media/releases/2017/p1116-fruit-vegetable-consumption.html. Accessed September 2018.
- Centers for Disease Control and Prevention. What Are the Risk Factors for Colorectal Cancer? Available at: https://www.cdc.gov/cancer/colorectal/basic_info/risk_factors.htm. Accessed June 2018.
- Choquet H, Meyre D. Genetics of obesity: what have we learned? *Current Genomics.* May 2011;12(3):169-179.
- Conviser J, Conviser J. *Unweighted Nation: Addressing the Obesity Crisis Through Cultural Change.* Monterey, CA: Healthy Learning; 2017.
- Craig WJ. Nutrition concerns and health effects of vegetarian diets. *Nutrition in Clinical Practice.* 2010;25:613-620. doi:10.1177/0884533610385707.
- Deshmukh-Taskar P, Nicklas TA, Radcliffe JD, et al. The relationship of breakfast skipping and type of breakfast consumed with overweight/obesity, abdominal obesity, other cardiometabolic risk factors and the metabolic syndrome in young adults. The National Health and Nutrition Examination Survey (NHANES): 1999-2006. *Public Health Nutrition.* 2013;16(11):2073-2082. pmid:23031568.
- Despres JP, Lemieux I. Abdominal obesity and metabolic syndrome. *Nature.* 2006;444:881-887.
- Dhurandhar EJ, Dawson J, Alcorn A, et al. The effectiveness of breakfast recommendations on weight loss: a randomized controlled trial. *American Journal of Clinical Nutrition.* 2014;100(2):507-513. doi:10.3945/ajcn.114.089573.
- Dwyer J. Nutrition 101: the concept of nutritional status and guides for nutrient intakes, eating patterns, and nutrition. In: Rippe JM, ed. *Lifestyle Medicine.* 2nd ed. Boca Raton, FL: CRC Press; 2013:103-118.
- Egger G, Pearson S. Fluid, fitness, and fatness. In: Egger G, Binns A, Rossner S. *Lifestyle Medicine: Managing Diseases of Lifestyle in the 21st Century.* 2nd ed. North Ryde, N.S.W.: McGraw-Hill; 2010:140-150.

- Erin F, Juen G, Lilian H, et al. Persistent metabolic adaptation 6 years after "The Biggest Loser" competition. *Obesity.* 2016;24:1612-1619.
- Esposito K, Giugliano F, Di Palo C, et al. Effect of lifestyle changes on erectile dysfunction in obese men: a randomized controlled trial. *Journal of the American Medical Association.* 2004;291:2978-2984.
- Esselstyn CB, Jr. Resolving the coronary artery disease epidemic through plant-based nutrition. *Preventive Cardiology.* 2001;4:171-177.
- Feskanich D, Bischoff-Ferrari HA, Frazier AL, et al. Milk consumption during teenage years and risk of hip fractures in older adults. *JAMA Pediatrics.* January 2014;168(1):54-60.
- Feskanich D, Willett WC, Colditz GA. Calcium, vitamin D, milk consumption, and hip fractures: a prospective study among postmenopausal women. *American Journal of Clinical Nutrition.* 2003;77:504-511.
- Fothergill E, Guo J, Howard L, et al. Persistent metabolic adaptation 6 years after "The Biggest Loser" competition. *Obesity* (Silver Spring). 2016;24:1612-1619.
- Fox CS, Massaro JM, Hoffmann U, et al. Abdominal visceral and subcutaneous adipose tissue compartments: association with metabolic risk factors in the Framingham Heart Study. *Circulation.* 2007;116:39-48.
- Frates EP. Interview with award winners from ACLM 2015, Nashville, Tennessee—Dean Ornish. *American Journal of Lifestyle Medicine.* 2016;10(5):341-344. doi:10.1177/1559827616642399.
- Frattaroli J, Weidner G, Dnistrian AM, et al. Clinical events in prostate cancer lifestyle trial: results from two years of follow-up. *Urology.* 2008;72:1319-1323.
- Fruits & Veggies—More Matters. What Are Phytonutrients? Available at: https://www.fruitsandveggiesmorematters.org/what-are-phytochemicals. Accessed September 2018.
- Fulkerson L. Forks Over Knives [DVD]. New York: Virgil Films & Entertainment; 2011.
- Fung TT, Long MW, Hung P, Cheung LW. An expanded model for mindful eating for health promotion and sustainability: issues and challenges for dietetics practice. *Journal of the Academy of Nutrition and Dietetics.* July 2016;116(7):1081-1086.
- Halton TL, Hu FB. The effects of high protein diets on thermogenesis, satiety and weight loss: a critical review. *Journal of the American College of Nutrition.* 2004;23(5):373-385.
- Hardy TM, Tollefsbol TO. Epigenetic diet: impact on the epigenome and cancer. *Epigenomics.* August 1 2011;3(4):503-518.
- Harvard Health Publications. Learn About Hidden Sugar in Foods [Video]. May 23, 2016. Available at: https://youtu.be/fVAEgzXXLVs. Accessed September 2017.
- Harvard Health Publishing. Why People Become Overweight. Available at: https://www.health.harvard.edu/staying-healthy/why-people-become-overweight. Accessed June 2018.

- He FJ, MacGregor GA. How far should salt intake be reduced? *Hypertension.* 2003;42:1093-1099.
- Herrero M, Havlík P, Valin H, et al. Biomass use, production, feed efficiencies, and greenhouse gas emissions from global livestock systems. *Proceedings of the National Academy of Sciences of the United States of America.* 2013;110(52):20888-20893. doi:10.1073/pnas.1308149110.
- Horikawa C, Kodama S, Yachi Y, et al. Skipping breakfast and prevalence of overweight and obesity in Asian and Pacific regions: a meta-analysis. *Preventive Medicine.* 2011;53:260-267.
- Jenkins DJ, Kendall CW, Marchie A, et al. Effects of a dietary portfolio of cholesterol-lowering foods vs lovastatin on serum lipids and C-reactive protein. *Journal of the American Medical Association.* 2003;290:502-510.
- Josse AR, Atkinson SA, Tarnopolsky MA, et al. Increased consumption of dairy foods and protein during diet- and exercise-induced weight loss promotes fat mass loss and lean mass gain in overweight and obese premenopausal women. *Journal of Nutrition.* 2011;141(9):1626-1634. doi:10.3945/jn.111.141028.
- Juhl CR, Bergholdt HKM, Miller IM, et al. Dairy intake and acne vulgaris: a systematic review and meta-analysis of 78,529 children, adolescents, and young adults. *Nutrients.* August 9 2018;10(8). pii: E1049.
- Kahleova H, Levin S, Barnard N. Cardio-metabolic benefits of plant-based diets. *Nutrients.* August 2017;9(8):848.
- Kahleova H, Matoulek M, Malinska H, et al. Vegetarian diet improves insulin resistance and oxidative stress markers more than conventional diet in subjects with type 2 diabetes. *Diabetic Medicine.* 2011;28:549-559.
- Katta R, Desai SP. Diet and dermatology: the role of dietary intervention in skin disease. *Journal of Clinical and Aesthetic Dermatology.* 2014;7(7):46-51.
- Katta R, Kramer MJ. Skin and diet: an update on the role of dietary change as a treatment strategy for skin disease. *Skin Therapy Letter.* January 2018;23(1):1-5.
- Katz DL, Colino S. *Disease-Proof: Slash Your Risk of Heart Disease, Cancer, Diabetes, and More—By 80 Percent.* New York: Plume; 2014.
- Katz DL, Meller S. Can we say what diet is best for health? *Annual Review of Public Health.* 2014;35(1):83-103. doi:10.1146/annurev-publhealth-032013-182351.
- Killoran E. Healthy Grocery Shopping Scavenger Hunt. Pritikin Longevity Center + Spa. Available at: https://www.pritikin.com/learn-healthy-grocery-shopping-skills. Accessed January 2017.
- King N, Egger G. Behavioral aspects of nutrition. In: Egger G, Binns A, Rossner S, eds. *Lifestyle Medicine: Managing Diseases of Lifestyle in the 21st Century.* 2nd ed. North Ryde, N.S.W.: McGraw-Hill; 2010:151-164.
- Know-It-All. Where do Fruits and Vegetables Get their Colors? Available at: https://empoweryourknowledgeandhappytrivia.wordpress.com/2015/08/18/where-do-fruits-and-vegetables-get-their-colors. Accessed September 2018.

- Kruskall LJ. *Fitness Professionals' Guide to Sports Nutrition and Weight Management.* Monterey, CA: Healthy Learning; 2010.
- Kulovitz MG, Kravitz LR, Mermier C, et al. Potential role of meal frequency as a strategy for weight loss and health in overweight or obese adults. *Nutrition.* 2014;30(4):386-392. doi:10.1016/j.nut.2013.08.009.
- LaComb RP, Sebastian RS, Wilkinson Enns C, et al. Beverage choices of U.S. adults: what we eat in America, NHANES 2007-2008. Food Surveys Research Group Dietary Data Brief No. 6. August 2011. Available at: https://www.ars.usda.gov/ARSUserFiles/80400530/pdf/DBrief/6_beverage_choices_adults_0708.pdf. Accessed August 2018.
- Laska MN, Hearst MO, Lust K, et al. How we eat what we eat: identifying meal routines and practices most strongly associated with healthy and unhealthy dietary factors among young adults. *Public Health Nutrition.* 2015;18(12):2135-2145. doi:10.1017/S1368980014002717.
- Leidy HJ, Clifton PM, Astrup A, et al. The role of protein in weight loss and maintenance. *American Journal of Clinical Nutrition.* 2015.
- Li D. Chemistry behind vegetarianism. *Journal of Agricultural and Food Chemistry.* 2011;59:777-784. doi:10.1021/jf103846u.
- Li JTC. Asthma: Does What You Eat Make a Difference? Mayo Clinic. Available at: https://www.mayoclinic.org/diseases-conditions/asthma/expert-answers/asthma-diet/faq-20058105. Accessed July 2018.
- LifespanHealth. Healthy Recipes Cooking Demonstration [Video]. November 2009. Available at: https://youtu.be/8mF0U546O84. Accessed September 2017.
- Marketdata Enterprises, Inc. The U.S. Weight Loss Market: 2014 Status Report & Market Research. Available at: http://www.marketresearch.com/Marketdata-Enterprises-Inc-v416/Weight-Loss-Status-Forecast-8016030/. Accessed June 2018.
- Martindale W. Is a Vegetarian Diet Really More Environmentally Friendly Than Eating Meat? The Conversation. February 6, 2017. Available at: http://www.cnn.com/2017/02/06/health/vegetarian-diet-conversation/. Accessed September 2017.
- McArdle WD, Katch FI, Katch VL. Chapter 9. *Exercise Physiology.* 5th ed. Baltimore, MD: Lippincott Williams & Wilkins; 2001.
- McDougall J, Litzau K, Haver E, Saunders V, Spiller G. Rapid reduction of serum cholesterol and blood pressure by a twelve-day, very low fat, strictly vegetarian diet. *Journal of the American College of Nutrition.* 1995;14:491-496.
- McDougall J, Thomas LE, McDougall C, et al. Effects of 7 days on an ad libitum low-fat vegan diet: the McDougall Program cohort. *Nutrition Journal.* 2014;13:99.
- McDougall JA, McDougall MA. *The McDougall Plan.* La Vergne, TN: Ingram Book Company; 1983.
- Merriam-Webster. Diet. Available at: https://www.merriam-webster.com/dictionary/diet. Accessed August 2018.
- Merriam-Webster. Nutrition. Available at: https://www.merriam-webster.com/dictionary/nutrition. Accessed August 2018.

- Murphy N, Norat T, Ferrari P, et al. Consumption of dairy products and colorectal cancer in the European Prospective Investigation into Cancer and Nutrition (EPIC). *PLoS ONE.* 2013;8(9):e72715. doi:10.1371/journal.pone.0072715.
- Nestle M. Corporate funding of food and nutrition research. *JAMA Internal Medicine.* 2016;176(1):13-14. doi:10.1001/jamainternmed.2015.6667.
- Ng M, Fleming T, Robinson M, et al. Global, regional, and national prevalence of overweight and obesity in children and adults during 1980-2013: a systematic analysis for the Global Burden of Disease Study 2013. *Lancet.* 2014;384:766-781.
- Nordqvist C. Nutrition: What Is It and Why Is It Important? Medical News Today. Available at: https://www.medicalnewstoday.com/articles/160774.php. Accessed June 2018.
- Nutrition.gov. Phytonutrients. Available at: https://www.nutrition.gov/subject/whats-in-food/phytonutrients. Accessed September 2018.
- NutritionFacts.Org. How Not to Die: The Role of Diet in Preventing, Arresting and Reversing Our Top 15 Killers [Video]. Available at: https://nutritionfacts.org/video/how-not-to-die/. Accessed May 2017.
- NWO BBC Horizon. The Truth About Vitamin Supplements [Video]. May 13, 2013. Available at: https://youtu.be/7i7gPyDZZv4.
- Oldways. Welcome to the Mediterranean Diet [Brochure]. Available at: https://oldwayspt.org/system/files/atoms/files/MedDietBrochure_0.pdf. Accessed September 2018.
- Ornish D, Brown SE, Billings J, et al. Can lifestyle changes reverse coronary heart disease?: The Lifestyle Heart Trial. *Lancet.* 1990;336:129-133.
- Ornish D, Lin J, Daubenmier J, et al. Increased telomerase activity and comprehensive lifestyle changes: a pilot study. *Lancet Oncology.* 2008;9:1048-1057.
- Ornish D, Scherwitz LW, Billings JH, et al. Intensive lifestyle changes for reversal of coronary heart disease. *Journal of the American Medical Association.* 1998;280:2001-2007.
- Ornish D, Smith A. *The Spectrum: A Scientifically Proven Program to Feel Better, Live Longer, Lose Weight, and Gain Health.* New York: Random House Publishing Group; 2008.
- Phillips T. The role of methylation in gene expression. *Nature Education.* 2008;1(1):116.
- Price JM, Egger G. Nutrition for the non-dietitian. In: Egger G, Binns A, Rossner S, eds. *Lifestyle Medicine: Managing Diseases of Lifestyle in the 21st Century.* 2nd ed. North Ryde, N.S.W.: McGraw-Hill; 2010:127-139.
- Protein in the Vegan Diet. Available at: http://www.vrg.org/nutrition/protein.php. Accessed June 2015.
- Public Broadcasting Service. How the Sugar Industry Paid Experts to Downplay Health Risks [Video]. 2016. Available at: http://www.pbs.org/video/2365841210/. Accessed September 2017.

- Redman LM, Smith SR, Burton JH, et al. Metabolic slowing and reduced oxidative damage with sustained caloric restriction support the rate of living and oxidative damage theories of aging. *Cell Metabolism.* 2018;27:805-815.e4.
- Reynolds G. How exercise might increase your self-control. *New York Times.* September 27, 2017. Available at: https://www.nytimes.com/2017/09/27/well/move/how-exercise-might-increase-your-self-control.html?action=click&contentCollection=health&region=rank&module=package&version=highlights&contentPlacement=2&pgtype=sectionfront&_r=0. Accessed October 2017.
- Rizzo NS, Jaceldo-Siegl K, Sabate J, et al. Nutrient profiles of vegetarian and nonvegetarian dietary patterns. *Journal of the Academy of Nutrition and Dietetics.* 2013;113(12):1610-1619.
- Rosenbaum M, Leibel RL. Adaptive thermogenesis in humans. *International Journal of Obesity (2005).* 2010;34(Suppl 1):S47-S55. doi:10.1038/ijo.2010.184.
- Satija A, Bhupathiraju SN, Rimm EB, et al. Plant-based dietary patterns and incidence of type 2 diabetes in US men and women: results from three prospective cohort studies. *PLoS Medicine.* June 2016;13(6):e1002039.
- Satija A, Bhupathiraju SN, Spiegelman D, et al. Healthful and unhealthful plant-based diets and the risk of coronary heart disease in U.S. adults. *Journal of the American College of Cardiology.* July 25 2017;70(4):411-422.
- Schoenfeld BJ, Aragon AA, Krieger JW. Effects of meal frequency on weight loss and body composition: a meta-analysis. *Nutrition Reviews.* 2015;73:69-82. doi:10.1093/nutrit/nuu017.
- Seimon RV, Roekenes J, Zibellini J, et al. Do intermittent diets provide physiological benefits over continuous diets for weight loss? A systematic review of clinical trials. *Molecular and Cellular Endocrinology.* 2015;418 Pt 2:153-172. doi:10.1016/j.mce.2015.09.014.
- Slavin J, Green H. Dietary fibre and satiety. *Nutrition Bulletin.* 2007;32(Suppl 1):32-42.
- Slavin JL, Lloyd B. Health benefits of fruits and vegetables. *Advances in Nutrition.* 2012;3(4):506-516. https://doi.org/10.3945/an.112.002154.
- Sofi F, Cesari F, Abbate R, Gensini GF, Casini A. Adherence to Mediterranean diet and health status: meta-analysis. *British Medical Journal.* 2008;337:a1344. doi:10.1136/bmj.a1344.
- Sofis MJ, Carrillo A, Jarmolowicz DP. Maintained physical activity induced changes in delay discounting. *Behavior Modification.* July 2017;41(4):499-528. doi:10.1177/0145445516685047. Epub 2016 Dec 29.
- Sroufe D. *Forks Over Knives—The Cookbook: Over 300 Recipes for Plant-Based Eating All Through the Year.* New York: The Experiment; 2012.
- Starke-Reed P, McDade-Ngutter C, Hubbard VS. Healthy people 2020: highlights in the nutrition and weight status focus area. In: Rippe JM, ed. *Lifestyle Medicine.* 2nd ed. Boca Raton, FL: CRC Press; 2013:119-130.
- Tantamango-Bartley Y, Jaceldo-Siegl K, Fan J, et al. Vegetarian diets and the incidence of cancer in a low-risk population. *Cancer Epidemiology, Biomarkers & Prevention.* February 2013;22(2):286-294.

- The Aspen Institute. Foods for Protecting the Body & Mind: Dr. Neal Barnard [Video]. August 19, 2015. Available at: https://youtu.be/BnHYHjchn6w. Accessed September 2017.
- The Endocrine Society. Cooking for Pleasure, Healthy for Life: Type 2 Diabetes Cooking Demonstration [Video]. September 21, 2012. Available at: https://youtu.be/oSBX2HLzIH8. Accessed September 2017.
- Trapp CB, Barnard ND. Usefulness of vegetarian and vegan diets for treating type 2 diabetes. *Current Diabetes Reports.* 2010;10:152-158.
- U.S. Department of Health and Human Services, U.S. Department of Agriculture. *2015-2020 Dietary Guidelines for Americans*. 8th ed. December 2015. Available at: http://health.gov/dietaryguidelines/2015/guidelines/. Accessed January 2017.
- U.S. Department of Health and Human Services, U.S. Department of Agriculture. Executive Summary. *2015-2020 Dietary Guidelines for Americans*. 8th ed. December 2015. Available at: https://health.gov/dietaryguidelines/2015/guidelines/executive-summary/. Accessed January 2017.
- U.S. Department of Health and Human Services, U.S. Department of Agriculture. Executive Summary. *Dietary Guidelines for Americans, 2010*. Available at: https://www.cnpp.usda.gov/sites/default/files/dietary_guidelines_for_americans/ExecSumm.pdf. Accessed January 2017.
- Walley AJ, Asher JE, Froguel P. The genetic contribution to non-syndromic human obesity. *Nature Reviews Genetics.* July 2009;10(7):431-442.
- Wang Z, Ying Z, Bosy-Westphal A, et al. Evaluation of specific metabolic rates of major organs and tissues: comparison between men and women. *American Journal of Human Biology.* 2011;23(3):333-338. doi:10.1002/ajhb.21137.
- WebMD. Phytonutrients. Available at: https://www.webmd.com/diet/guide/phytonutrients-faq#1. Accessed September 2018.
- Whole Foods Market. Healthy Cooking Techniques Videos [Video]. December 2015. Available at: http://www.wholefoodsmarket.com/healthy-eating/healthy-cooking-videos. Accessed September 2017.
- Willett WC, Stampfer MJ. Current evidence of healthy eating. *Annual Review of Public Health.* 2013;34(1):77-95. doi:10.1146/annurev-publhealth-031811-124646.
- Wing RR, Phelan S. Long-term weight loss maintenance. *American Journal of Clinical Nutrition.* July 2005;82(1 Suppl):222S-225S. https://doi.org/10.1093/ajcn/82.1.222S.
- Wiseman M. The second World Cancer Research Fund/American Institute for Cancer Research expert report. Food, nutrition, physical activity, and the prevention of cancer: A global perspective. *Proceedings of the Nutrition Society.* 2008;67:253-256.
- Wyatt HR, Grunwald GK, Mosca CL, et al. Long-term weight loss and breakfast in subjects in the National Weight Control Registry. *Obesity Research.* 2002;10:78-82.
- Zelman KM. Expert Q&A: Can Your Diet Help You Avoid Flu? WebMD. Available at: https://www.webmd.com/diet/features/expert-qa-can-your-diet-help-you-avoid-flu#2. Accessed July 2018.

CHAPTER 6

SLEEP MATTERS

"You're not healthy unless your sleep is healthy."

—Dr. William C. Dement
Founder, Sleep Research Center
Stanford University

❑ Chapter Goals:

- Be aware of how much sleep people need.
- Recognize the stages of sleep.
- Identify healthy sleep habits.
- Comprehend the connection between sleep and health.
- Be cognizant of factors that affect sleep.
- Be familiar with various sleep disorders.
- Know tips for falling asleep.

❑ Learning Objectives:

- To understand the basics of sleep
- To grasp the key factors that inhibit sleep
- To be aware of evidence-based information concerning sleep
- To be cognizant of the connection between sleep and health
- To recognize how to improve sleep through behavior change

❑ Guiding Questions:

- How can people get more sleep?
- How much sleep do people need?
- What are healthy sleep habits?
- What are the stages of sleep?
- What are the barriers to good sleep?
- How does a lack of sleep affect the body?
- How can people get more sleep?

❑ Important Terms:

- *Electroencephalography (EEG):* A recording of the electrical activity of the brain
- *NREM sleep:* The type of non-dreaming sleep that predominates over the course of a night's sleep
- *REM sleep:* Rapid eye movement sleep during which dreaming occurs
- *Sleep:* A natural periodic state of rest for the mind and body, in which the eyes usually close and consciousness is completely or partially lost, so that a decrease occurs in bodily movement and responsiveness to external stimuli. During sleep, the human brain undergoes a characteristic cycle of brain-wave activity that includes intervals of dreaming.

WHAT IS SLEEP?

Sleep matters. A lot. Sleep is foundational for health. Getting a good night's sleep is one of the most important things people can do for their overall health and well-being. The problem is that although all people need to sleep, how they experience sleep can be quite varied.

Sleep is a complex physiological process of restoration and renewal for the body. While sleep is often ignored and taken for granted, considerable research has shown that it is definitively a pillar of good health. The importance of sleep is underscored by the fact that a lack of sleep is often associated with a number of physical and emotional problems.

WHAT IS THE SCIENCE OF SLEEP?

In their book, *Sleep: A Very Short Introduction*, Steven W. Lockley and Russel G. Foster detail the behavioral criteria that are used to help describe sleep in people. They define sleep as a behavior characterized by a "rapidly reversible state of immobility with greatly reduced sensory responsiveness." According to Lockley and Foster, sleep can be distinguished from a coma or hibernation by its rapid reversibility. Furthermore, sleep is defined by increased arousal thresholds and decreased responsiveness to external stimuli. In other words, a noise or shaking may be needed to rouse someone from sleep. Humans have a preferred posture and place for sleep, choosing, for example, to sleep on a bed on their back, side, or stomach.

Under constant conditions, circadian regulation and persistence of an approximate 24-hour rhythm occurs in humans. Most people are awake for about 16 hours a day and sleep for around eight hours. Finally, and perhaps most importantly to the discussion of sleep in relation to lifestyle medicine, Lockley and Foster state that sleep is a behavior that is homeostatically regulated such that lost sleep is associated with an increased drive for sleep, with subsequent "sleep rebound."

Understanding the relationship between wakefulness and the brain can be helpful. Arousal centers exist in the brainstem and the hypothalamus that regulate sleep behaviors (refer to Figure 6-1). When people are awake, specific areas within their brainstem and hypothalamus send signals that stimulate the cerebral cortex. By keeping neurons in the cortex active, signals from these arousal centers maintain a person's alertness. Two neurotransmitters, orexin and hypocretin, are produced by these neurons, which stimulate these arousal centers to keep individuals awake.

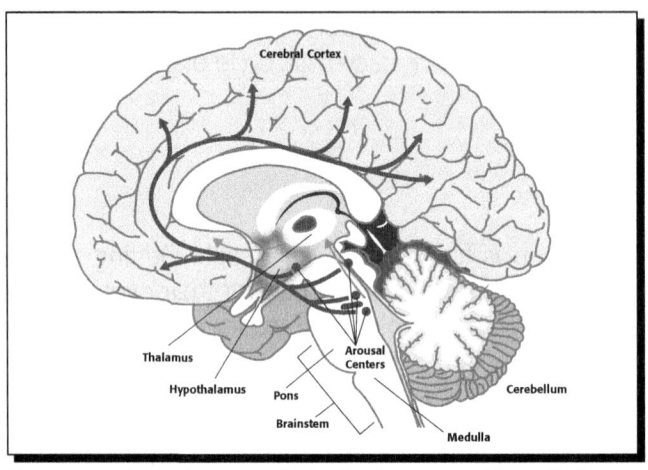

Figure 6-1. Arousal centers in the brainstem and hypothalamus

Conversely, neurons in an area of the brain known as the ventrolateral preoptic (VLPO) area help to promote sleep by inhibiting brain activity that maintains wakefulness (refer to Figure 6-2). Neurotransmitters released from the VLPO neurons reduce activity in the arousal regions of the brain, causing people to pass quickly into the unconscious state of non-REM sleep (the type of non-dreaming sleep that predominates over the course of a night).

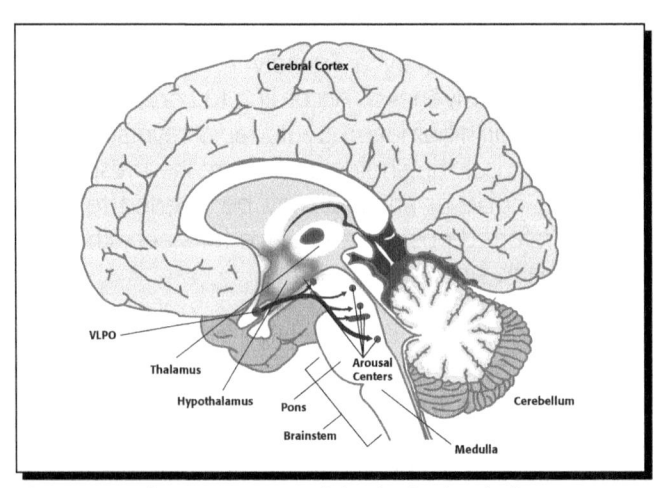

Figure 6-2. The VLPO area of the brain that helps to promote sleep

In the hypothalamus, a small group of brain cells known as the suprachiasmatic nucleus (SCN), often referred to as "the body's master clock," controls circadian cycles and influences many physiological and behavioral rhythms that occur over an approximately 24-hour period, including the sleep-wake cycle (refer to Figure 6-3). There are over 50,000 neurons in the SCN.

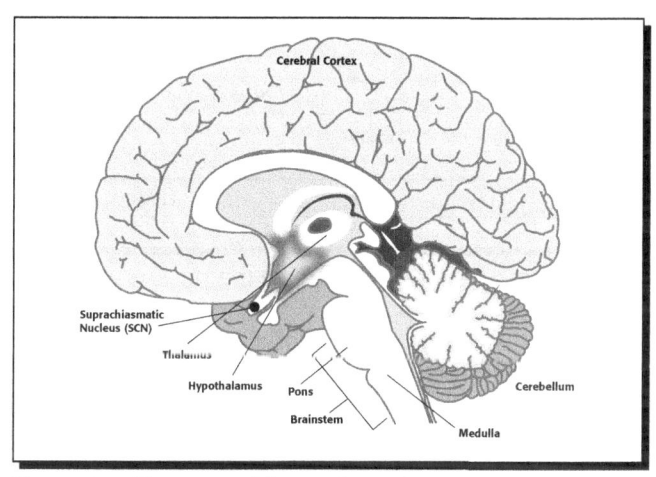

Figure 6-3. The suprachiasmatic nucleus

The SCN gets signals from the visual system—specifically, retinal ganglion cells (RGCs). In the presence of sunlight or light at 480 nm, the RGCs are stimulated to produce the photoreceptor melanopsin. Melanopsin signals daytime to the SCN, which, then signals the superior cervical ganglion, which induces the pineal gland to suppress the production of melatonin (the hormone that regulates the sleep-wake cycle). Melatonin levels rise coinciding with the onset of darkness, encouraging sleep to ensue. In contrast, when melatonin levels fall, concurrent with light exposure, wakefulness occurs. Collectively, this process is known as the circadian sleep drive.

There is also a homeostatic drive for sleep. This drive is related to the neurotransmitter adenosine, which is continuously released during the hours that people are awake and alert. Adenosine is produced when adenosine triphosphate (ATP), the driver of energy in the body, breaks down. As the body uses ATP, adenosine is released throughout the day. As adenosine accumulates it signals the need for sleep, which is why many people who wake up at 7 a.m. get sleepy around 11 p.m. (refer to Figure 6-4).

It is interesting to note that caffeine binds to the same receptor as adenosine, but it has the opposite effect. It increases cell activity, causing the pituitary gland to respond by producing adrenaline. Caffeine has a half-life of five-six hours (this means it takes five-six hours to metabolize half of the amount of caffeine that has been ingested). It generally takes five half-lives to be considered completely metabolized. In other words, it takes approximately 25-30 hours for one "dose" of caffeine to be completely metabolized!

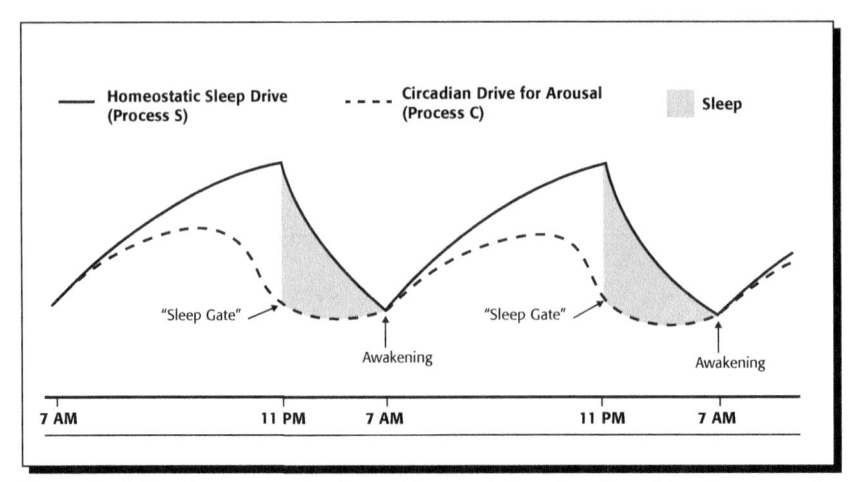

Figure 6-4. The homeostatic sleep drive and the circadian drive for arousal

While caffeine's effect is significantly dampened with each half-life iteration, it is often advised to minimize caffeine intake later on in the day due to the delayed effect that caffeine can continue to have that night. A general guideline of no caffeine after noon time is recommended.

STAGES OF SLEEP

It has historically been taught that sleepers experience five stages of sleep (stages 1, 2, 3, 4, and REM). However, the number of sleep stages has recently been consolidated into four stages of sleep (the previous stage 3 and stage 4 have been combined into a single stage N3, and they are all renamed as stage N1, N2, and N3 (referring to NREM), and stage REM). These stages generally progress cyclically from stage N1 through REM, although it does not have to proceed in a linear fashion. On average, a complete sleep cycle takes from 90 to 110 minutes. Furthermore, even as individuals cycle through the various stages of sleep, their sleep is naturally interrupted by brief awakenings. Known as "arousals," the awakenings only last a few seconds, such that people do not remember them the next morning.

Each of these stages can be assessed by electroencephalography (EEG), a measurement of the electrical activity of the brain. As Figure 6-5 indicates, the EEG recording is different for each stage of sleep.

❑ Stage N1

This stage occurs at the onset of sleep, when people are transitioning from wakefulness to sleep. Typically, it lasts between one and seven minutes. The depth of sleep is light, people are easy to arouse in this stage, and they may say they are still awake if awakened. A person's eyes fight to stay open. Muscle twitching might be observed. This stage is characterized by low-voltage, mixed-frequency EEG (electroencephalogram—

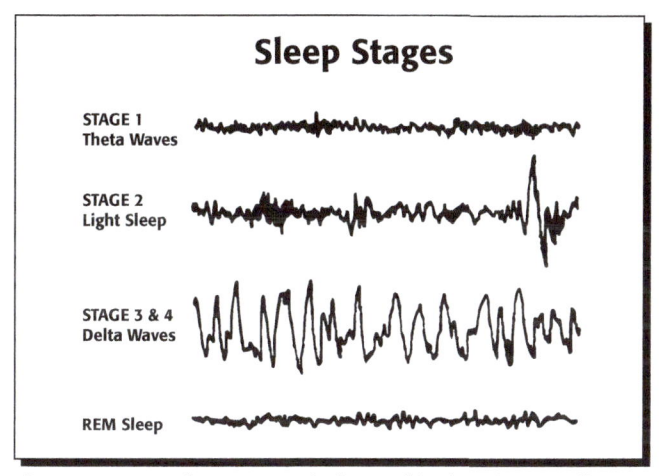

Figure 6-5. An electroencephalographic (EEG) recording of the four sleep stages

measures electrical activity of the brain) recordings, some slow, rolling eye movements, and some relatively higher EMG (electromyography—measures the activity of muscles) activity.

❑ Stage N2

Stage N2 usually lasts about 20 minutes. Over the course of the night, humans spend approximately 40 to 50 percent of their time sleeping in this stage. During this phase, the frequency of brain waves becomes slower, respiratory rate and heart rate slow down, and the body temperature tends to decline. The EEG is characterized by the presence of both sleep spindles (occasional bursts of rapid waves) and K-complexes (not unlike isolated delta waves). Collectively, stages N1 and N2 are often referred to as "light sleep."

❑ Stages N3

This stage is known as "slow-wave sleep" and "delta sleep." It is the beginning of deep sleep. During this period, the brain begins to produce high-amplitude, slow waves. The large delta waves are seen in all of the EEG and eye channels and muscle activity is reduced. Blood pressure falls, breathing slows, and body temperature declines further. It is more difficult to be awakened during this stage.

❑ Stage REM

Individuals enter this stage about 90 minutes after they initially fall asleep. During this phase of sleep, which occurs in increasing long episodes across the night for a total duration of 1.5 to 2 hours, the brain becomes more active. This stage is notable for rapid eye movements that are associated with dreaming. The eyes may move quickly in different directions. Heart rate and blood pressure increase. Breathing becomes faster, irregular, and shallow. This stage is when the brain consolidates and processes what it learned from the day before, so that it can be stored in a person's long-term memory.

❏ More Important Points Concerning Sleep Cycles

It should be noted that the four stages of sleep last for different durations at various ages in life. For example, sleep times and cycles for an infant will be quite different than that of an adult. The majority of sleep for people of all ages is non-REM sleep. Most non-REM sleep happens early in the evening. As the night progresses, the duration of the REM periods that an individual experiences increases, and the non-REM intervals get shorter.

LIVE AND LEARN WITH DR. BETH FRATES

When I was at Stanford Medical School, I was assigned to Santa Clara Valley Medical Center in San Jose for my surgery rotation in my third year. We were Q2 in those days, (i.e., we slept overnight in the hospital every second night). For example, over the course of a week we were on call Monday night, home Tuesday night to sleep, and back in the hospital again Wednesday night to sleep. Then, we were home for Thursday, but back in the hospital on Friday night to sleep. There was virtually no sleep when we were on call in the hospital at night. At the time, I thought I might go into surgery, and I was eager to help my residents and attending physicians with whom I was working. We were a team, and we wanted to be there to assist each other. Basically, we stayed up all night, monitored the patients, wrote our handwritten notes, checked labs, prepared for the next day's surgeries, or worked on research projects throughout the night.

I lived about a half-hour's drive from San Jose, close to the main Stanford campus. One day, after a long night on call, I felt exhausted. I could not wait to get home and go to bed. I considered taking a nap in the call room, because I was so sleepy, but I really wanted to get home. So, I got in the car and drove out of the hospital parking lot.

Once I got on the main road, I drove straight for a while, and then I reached a stop light. That's the last thing I really remember. I was at a light. All I know is I heard honking, and then I woke up startled. I didn't know where I was. Apparently, I went straight through the light and did not turn right, as I should have done in order to go home. I fell asleep. I could not believe it. It was so sudden. Thank goodness, I didn't hit anyone. In fact, I didn't hit anything. Frankly, that was one of the scariest things that has actually ever happened to me.

It was such a strange experience for so many reasons. I knew that I was too tired to drive, and that I was practically falling asleep standing up during our rounds, discussing patients that morning at 6 a.m. Furthermore, sleep deprivation affects your judgment, similar to the way alcohol affects a person's judgment about driving. In fact, studies show that moderate sleep deprivation produces impairments equivalent to those of alcohol intoxication. The average legal limit for commercial drivers is a blood alcohol content (BAC) of 0.04 percent. Yet, after 17 to 19 hours without sleep, performance was equivalent or worse than a BAC of 0.05 percent. Drunk people often proclaim "I'm fine. I'm okay to drive," even when it is clear to everyone around them that they are far from fine. Alcohol and sleep deprivation, however, change a person's perception of how they're actually functioning. They think they're doing better than they actually are. Just as you would not let a friend drive drunk, you should never allow a friend drive sleep deprived.

After that incident in San Jose, I vowed that if I were ever exhausted like that again, I would nap in the call room, before getting in my car to go home. It is worth a nap, which doesn't have to be greater than a half hour. In reality, a 20-to-30 minute nap can be very rejuvenating. I wish I had known that! When I became an intern at Mass General, I purposely moved to an apartment right across from the hospital, so that I would never have to drive post-call again.

The point to remember is that if you're feeling tired or fatigued, you need to either rest before you drive or pull off the road and take a nap in a safe location. I actually do this now when I feel my eyes getting heavy on a long drive. I was very lucky to have escaped that incident of falling asleep at the wheel unscathed. Now, I want to make sure that no one else gets behind the wheel too tired to drive.

HOW MUCH SLEEP DO PEOPLE NEED?

No official national guidelines for sleep exist. Several organizations, however, have developed sleep-related recommendations. For example, the National Institutes of Health (NIH) suggest that teenagers get 9 to 10 hours of sleep, and adults get seven to nine hours. The National Sleep Foundation (NSF) recommends that newborns get 12 to 18 hours of sleep, and that infants 3 to 11 months old get 14 to 15 hours a day. As kids age, the relative amount of sleep they need decreases (Figure 6-6). For example, young children (ages one to three) should get between 12 and 14 hours of sleep, while children three to five years of age should sleep for 11 to 13 hours. In turn, children between 5 and 17 years old should get from 8.5 to 11 hours of sleep a night. It is important to note that some degree of variance often exists between the different recommendations but all organizations recommend a minimum of seven hours, regardless of age.

AGE	SLEEP NEEDED (IN HOURS)
Birth to 2 months	12 to 18
3 to 11 months	14 to 15
1 to 3 years	12 to 14
3 to 5 years	11 to 13
5 to 10 years	10 to 11
10 to 17 years	8.5 to 9.5
17 or older	7 to 9

minimum recommendation

Source: National Sleep Foundation

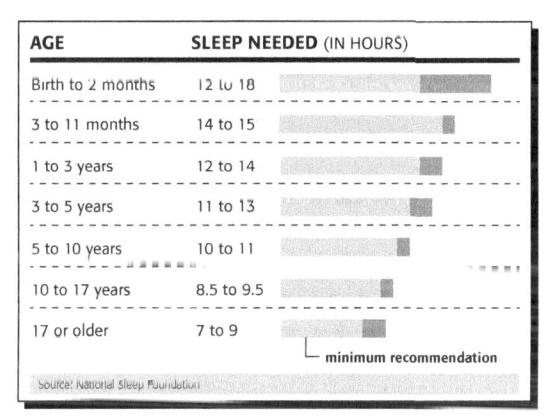

Figure 6-6. Sleep recommendations from the National Sleep Foundation, based on a person's age

In modern society, insufficient sleep (also called chronic partial sleep deprivation) based on sleeping for less than seven hours per night, may be the most common sleep disorder. Partial sleep deprivation over a series of nights has similar results to those seen after total sleep deprivation.

WHY IS SLEEP IMPORTANT?

Despite the aforementioned recommendations, considerable evidence indicates that many Americans don't get enough sleep on a regular basis. The impact of insufficient sleep entails more than feeling tired, irritable, and sluggish.

The long-term effects of sleep deprivation are significant. Not only does it drain a person's mental abilities, it also places their physical health at substantial risk, as well as dramatically lower their quality of life. For example, research indicates that sleeping less than six to eight hours a night increases the risk of early death by approximately 12 percent.

The most immediate and apparent impact of reduced sleep is increased sleepiness. Increasing sleepiness has numerous consequences for mood and performance. Increasing sleepiness is associated with increased reaction time, decreased short-term memory, and decreased performance on any task, with an included memory or response time component. For example, driving performance, after a night without sleep, is as poor as driving performance in individuals who are legally intoxicated. The implication is that driving after a night of lost sleep can have fatal consequences. Furthermore, because sleep deprivation decrements are also additive with the effects of alcohol, a person's risks are greatly increased in those individuals who have any degree of sleep deprivation and have consumed alcohol.

THE IMPACT OF SLEEP ON THE 11 SYSTEMS OF THE BODY

The body profoundly needs sleep, just as it needs oxygen and food to function at its best. When a person does not get enough sleep, it will have a negative impact on virtually all of the body's 11 systems.

❑ Circulatory System

Sleep impacts the processes that help keep the heart and blood vessels healthy, including a person's blood sugar, blood pressure, and inflammation levels. It also has a vital role in the body's ability to heal and repair itself, including the blood vessels and the heart. A lack of sufficient sleep decreases heart rate variability, makes an individual more prone to hypertension and cardiovascular disease, and increases a person's risk of heart attack and stroke.

❑ Digestive System

In addition to eating too much and not exercising enough (if at all), sleep deprivation is another risk factor for a person becoming overweight or obese. This factor is in part due to the impact of sleep on two hormones in the body—leptin and ghrelin. These hormones control an individual's feelings of hunger and fullness. Leptin tells the brain that it's had enough to eat, while ghrelin increases appetite. With insufficient sleep, the brain reduces leptin and increases ghrelin. This situation can lead to overeating and weight gain. In addition, given a person's impaired decision-making and impulse control in a sleep-deprived state, food choices often satisfy cravings for high calorie foods loaded with sugar, salt, and fat.

A lack of sleep can also lead to weight gain by decreasing energy levels, making it much harder to find the motivation to exercise. It can also prompt the body to release higher levels of insulin after meals. In turn, higher insulin levels can stimulate fat storage, as well as increase risk of type 2 diabetes.

❑ Endocrine System

The endocrine system of the body (the collection of glands that secrete hormones into the circulatory system, where they are transported to other systems) has a relatively complex relationship to sleep. For example, growth hormone is typically secreted during slow wave sleep (SWS). During sleep, the production of some hormones increases, while the secretion of others is inhibited. Insufficient sleep can result in a myriad of counterproductive changes to the body's delicate hormonal balances. For example, research has shown adults who report getting five or fewer hours of sleep a night are two and a half times more likely to have diabetes (due to unduly high levels of insulin production). Inexplicably, individuals who sleep too much (i.e., nine or more hours a night) are also at an enhanced risk for diabetes.

❑ Immune System

Sleep deprivation suppresses the ability of the body's immune system to function properly. During sleep, a person's immune system releases proteins called cytokines, some of which help promote sleep. Cytokines also play a role in fighting an infection or inflammation, or helping the body deal with stress. Sleep deprivation may lead to a decrease in the body's production of these protective proteins. Sleep deprivation decreases the effectiveness of vaccinations, such as flu vaccination. It can increase the risk of getting sick, and it can also lengthen the time it takes a person to recover from an illness.

❑ Dermatologic System

It appears that an inadequate level of sleep is correlated with reduced skin health, as well as an acceleration of skin aging. Not only do people who suffer from insomnia exhibit more signs of skin aging (e.g., fine lines, uneven skin pigmentation, reduced skin elasticity, etc.), they are less able to quickly recover from stressors to the skin, such as the sun and environmental toxins. Overall, a lack of adequate sleep weakens the ability of the skin to repair itself at night.

❑ Muscular System

Not only does sleep help the body recover from the demands imposed on it, it also helps stimulate muscle growth. For those individuals who work out or are trying to improve their body composition, they should remember that growth hormone is released predominantly during slow-wave sleep. Anything that reduces the amount of stage N3 sleep that a person is getting can impair this release and inhibit optimal recovery and impair performance. When an individual is able to properly recover, their body addresses the three Rs—replace, repair, and rebuild—all of which are essential for a healthy muscular system.

❑ Nervous System

The central nervous system is the information highway of the body. Sleep deprivation leaves the brain exhausted. As a result, it can't perform its duties as well as it usually does. For example, the individual will find it somewhat difficult to concentrate or learn new things. A person may find it challenging to remember any new information they may have learned. They may also feel more impatient or prone to mood swings. In addition, their ability to make decisions is impaired, and their level of creativity could be compromised. The bottom line is that sleep deprivation has major impact on basic function from reaction time to memory to mood, and the sleep-deprived individual may be only partially aware of their loss of function. Even momentary loss of attention during critical activities such as driving can be deadly. In addition, chronic sleep deprivation is strongly correlated with behavioral health issues, such as depression, anxiety, substance use, and attempted suicide.

❑ Reproductive System

Recent research has found a relatively clear connection between sleep deprivation and infertility. A lack of sleep diminishes a person's desire for sex, and can also decrease testosterone levels (affecting both quality and reproduction) in men, as well as interfere with a woman's capacity for reproduction. Furthermore, sleep deprivation appears to have a negative impact on the ability of a woman to have an orgasm.

❑ Respiratory System

A lack of sleep can make a person more vulnerable to a variety of respiratory infections, such as the common cold and the flu. It can also exacerbate symptoms in patients with chronic lung disease, while also increase snoring and the incidence of obstructive sleep apnea. These manifestations can interrupt an individual's sleep, diminish its quality, and magnify the impact of the sleep loss.

❏ Skeletal System

Sleep is crucial for bone health. Bones are constantly being broken down and repaired. This process of recovery happens primarily during sleep. A lack of adequate sleep disrupts the process. When sleep deprivation impacts remodeling, decreased bone density can result. Research on the sleep-bone health connection suggests that chronically inadequate levels of sleep affects bone metabolism and bone marrow composition. This factor has significant implications for skeletal development, bone healing and repair, blood cell differentiation, and aging.

❏ Renal/Urinary System

The urinary sequences of sleep-deprived individuals seem to exhibit an increased level of both urinary output and salt in the urine. The body's production of urine adheres to a circadian rhythm. During the day, people urinate more frequently. At night, their production of urine declines, enabling them to get uninterrupted sleep. A lack of sleep interrupts this pattern. Research suggests that irregular sleep patterns can increase the likelihood that a person will need to urinate at night. Sleep deprivation, particularly in children, can increase the probability of enuresis (involuntary urination). A degree of ambiguity exists regarding whether sleep-related factors lead to bladder control problems or vice versa.

WHAT ARE THE POSSIBLE BARRIERS TO SLEEP?

A number of factors can interfere with an individual's ability to get a sufficient amount of sleep. Current research has found that exercise does not have a negative impact on sleep quality in trained individuals. Among the possible barriers to sleep are the following:

- Excessively high level of blood sugar
- Thyroid problems
- Psychological factors (e.g., distress, anxiety)
- Failure to prioritize sleep
- Absence of a sleep routine
- Disturbances, either from the outside or from the inside of the body (e.g., noise, temperature, light, etc.)
- Watching the clock, while trying to fall asleep
- Medications and supplements that interfere with sleep (e.g. some beta blockers, antiarrhythmics, thyroid medications, steroids, diuretics, theophylline for asthma, stimulants for ADHD, nicotine replacement products, some SSRIs—selective serotonin reuptake inhibitors, and other medicines, including those with caffeine)
- Taking daytime naps that last longer than a half an hour
- Going to bed too hungry or too full
- Trying to catch up on lost sleep at odd hours of the day
- Consuming too much caffeine or alcohol

- Lack of self-awareness that a sleep-related problem exists
- Sleep disorders

DISORDERED SLEEP VS. SLEEP DISORDERS

While poor sleep certainly exacerbates conditions like obesity and diabetes, chronic sleep loss, in and of itself, is a public health problem. The percent of adults in the United States who on average sleep less than six hours per night has been rising steadily for the past few decades. The CDC has estimated that 50 to 70 million Americans suffer from sleep deprivation, and 4 percent of adults reported using a prescription sleep aid in the past month. In addition, there has been an increase in sleep loss, which is driven largely by broad societal changes, including greater reliance on longer work hours, shift work, and increased access to television and the Internet. In the workplace, sleep deprivation results in injuries and decreased productivity, an expense on the order of 18 billion dollars each year. Furthermore, as many as 1.2 million car crashes annually are caused by fatigued drivers. While specific sleep disorders have been classified and characterized (as discussed in the following section), it should be emphasized that the vast majority of sleep problems are issues of disordered sleep due to occupational and lifestyle changes, rather than clinical sleep disorders, per se.

WHAT ARE THE MOST COMMON TYPES OF SLEEP DISORDERS?

While many Americans do not get an adequate amount of sleep due to work, school, or an inability to get to bed on time, millions of other Americans (50 to 70 million at a recent count) are unable to obtain enough sleep due to an underlying chronic sleep disorder. Millions of other individuals are transiently or acutely affected by a sleep disorder, sometimes recurrently. A sleep disorder is a medical disorder that impacts sleep (cycle or quality). Currently, over 70 different types of sleep disorders have been defined, but the most common sleep disorders are insomnia, sleep apnea, and restless legs syndrome/periodic limb movements. Narcolepsy is a rare sleep disorder with significant consequences.

❑ Insomnia

Insomnia is a very common sleep disorder that affects millions of people. An estimated 30 to 40 percent of Americans report suffering from insomnia each year. People with this condition find it difficult to fall asleep or stay asleep Patients with clinical insomnia also report daytime symptoms, such as fatigue, poor concentration or memory, irritability, reduced motivation, increased errors, anxiety or depression, or worry about the negative impact of their poor sleep. Insomnia can be a life-long primary problem, but it is also frequently associated with many other stressors or medical disorders. Insomnia is currently defined as either short-term or chronic insomnia:

❑ Short-term insomnia: Symptoms that persist for less than three months. Short-term insomnia is often associated with an acute condition, such as a poor sleep environment (temperature, light, noise), acute pain or discomfort, grief or other acute emotional stress, or use of or withdrawal from stimulants, such as caffeine, alcohol, medications, or illegal drugs, such as cocaine.

Chronic insomnia: Symptoms that last for three months or longer. Long-term insomnia typically occurs at least three nights per week. It is often associated with mental health problems, such as depression or anxiety; medical illness that causes any kind of pain or discomfort; other sleep disorders; chronic use of some medications, caffeine or alcohol; or irregular sleep habits.

A number of treatments are available for insomnia. For example, in 2016, the American College of Physicians recommended that all adult patients receive cognitive behavioral therapy for insomnia (CBT-I) as the initial treatment for chronic insomnia. The diagnosis of insomnia is a clinical diagnosis that can be made by lifestyle medicine practitioners. CBT-I is a therapy that could be provided by lifestyle medicine practitioners trained in this therapy or by a closely allied health professional. CBT-I contains a number of therapy components, starting with achieving improved sleep hygiene (regular bedtime and wake time, providing an appropriate sleep environment, avoiding evening disturbance from caffeine, alcohol, blue light from computer screens, phones, or clocks, or stimulating activity). Specific components of CBT-I include training for patients in the following components:

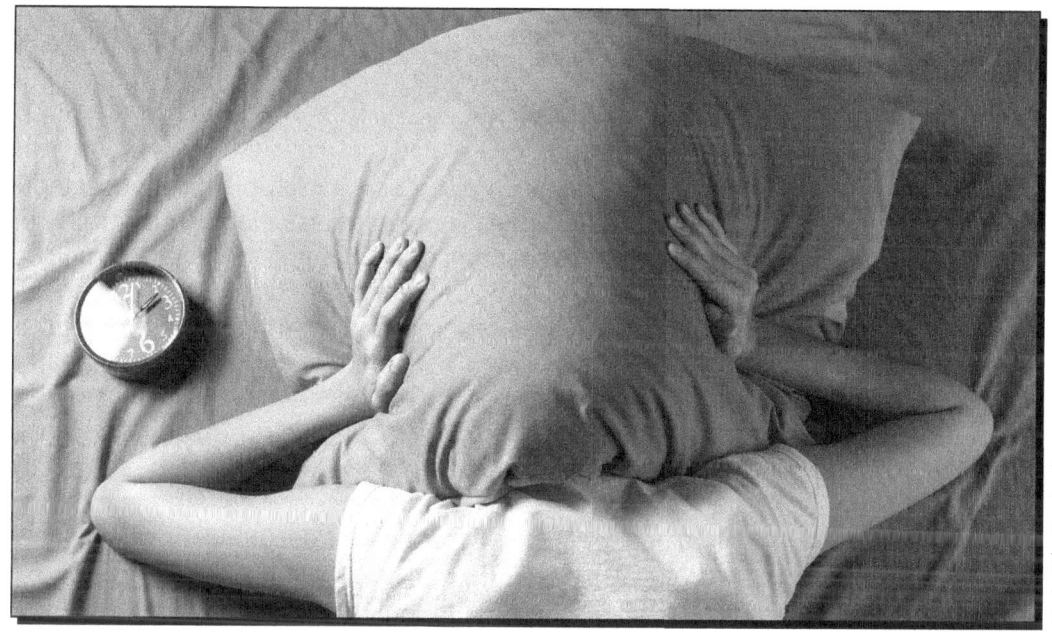

Long-term insomnia is often associated with mental health problems, such as depression or anxiety; medical illness that causes any kind of pain or discomfort; other sleep disorders; chronic use of some medications, caffeine or alcohol; or irregular sleep habits.

- Relaxation therapy—involves progressively relaxing muscle groups to prepare for sleep
- Stimulus control—provides rules for patients to limit time in bed awake (i.e., without being able to fall asleep) thereby improving the association of the bed as a place for sleep
- Sleep restriction—provides rules tracked with sleep logs to limit the amount of time patients are allowed to be in bed for sleep in an attempt to improve the probability of falling asleep and staying asleep during the desired sleep time
- Cognitive therapy—helps patients deal with cognitive arousal, such as the recurring thought that not being able to fall asleep will have negative consequences the next day, which subsequently worsens the ability of a person to fall asleep during the night

❑ Restless Legs Syndrome

Restless legs syndrome (RLS) is a condition characterized by a nearly irresistible urge to move the legs, particularly in the evenings. Also known as Willis-Ekbom disease, individuals with RLS experience abnormally uncomfortable sensations (e.g., crawling, creeping, drawing, pins and needles, prickly, pulling, tingling, etc.) in their lower legs. These symptoms typically occur in the afternoon or evening hours and are most severe when a person is at rest, sitting, or lying in bed. Approximately 10 percent of the adults in the United States are affected by this neurologic, sensorimotor disorder. Patients with restless legs typically continue to have limb movements after they have fallen asleep (then called periodic limb movements) that can disturb their sleep and/or bed partners. Patients may report waking up during the night and have difficulty returning to sleep, without realizing that their limb movements, which typically occur with a periodicity of about 30 seconds, continue to wake them as they try to return to sleep.

❑ Sleep Apnea

Sleep apnea is an increasingly common sleep disorder in which breathing repeatedly stops and starts. Individuals whose sleep apnea is untreated develop an obstruction in their upper airway while they are sleeping—sometimes hundreds of times each night. As a result of this potentially serious condition, their brain and body may not get enough oxygen, and they may become significantly sleep-deprived from the sleep disturbance associated with the effort to resume respiration. There are two types of sleep apnea:
- Obstructive sleep apnea (OSA): Occurs when the brain sends a signal to the muscles of the body, which make an effort to take a breath, but are unsuccessful because the airway becomes obstructed, preventing an adequate flow of air. Obesity greatly increases the risk of developing OSA. Apart from fatigue and complaints of falling asleep during the day, another symptom of obstructive sleep apnea is snoring.
- Central sleep apnea (CSA): Occurs when the brain does not send a signal to the body's muscles to take a breath, resulting in no muscular effort to take a breath.

LIVE AND LEARN WITH DR. BETH FRATES

One night, in 2010, not too far from where I worked, a car went right into a building. Given the situation, most people might conclude, "Oh, it must have been a drunk driver." The report in the local paper, "Driver reportedly sideswiped, illegally, idling car in front of a restaurant, CK Shanghai, before losing control, jumping the curb, lodging the Lexus in a wall between a pizza place and the neighboring Chinese restaurant. The driver and the two occupants in the automobile that sideswiped the car, as well as another person, were transported to Newton Wellesley Hospital." The article then went on to state, "The driver of the Lexus will be cited for marked lane violation and evaluated by the RMW to make sure he can safely operate a vehicle."

My first thought was that a little bit more was needed than to bring this gentleman to the RMV. It turned out that the driver of the Lexus was a very dear friend of mine. A fellow parent, our kids play hockey together. He is a very well-educated and very successful businessman.

Seeking to better understand what happened to him behind the wheel that day, he participated in a sleep study and discovered that he had an undiagnosed case of obstructive sleep apnea. He didn't know his diagnosis, but he knew he was exhausted. In fact, as I looked back at the situation, I remember that he usually had dark circles under his eyes. He was also overweight, as well as very hardworking.

It turned out that he hadn't been sleeping well, probably for years. Subsequently, he lost weight, which, in his case, helped him tremendously. He returned to full functioning and is back driving. The point to remember is that first appearances are not always what they appear to be. In reality, he didn't need an extended session at the RMV. What he really needed was to realize that he had a sleeping disorder and to then address it.

❏ Narcolepsy

Narcolepsy is a chronic sleep disorder that causes overwhelming drowsiness in the daytime. This condition is a neurological disorder that impacts the ability of a person to control sleep and alertness. Individuals with narcolepsy experience uncontrollable episodes of falling asleep during the daytime. Among other symptoms of this disorder are the loss of muscle tone in emotional situations (cataplexy), hallucinations when falling asleep (distorted perceptions), and an inability to move or talk (sleep paralysis) when awakening. All of the symptoms of narcolepsy may exist in various combinations and degrees of severity. An estimated 135,000 to 200,000 people in the United States have this disorder, although the number may be higher, since this condition often goes undiagnosed.

WHAT ADVICE CAN BE GIVEN TO ENHANCE A PERSON'S SLEEP?

Sleep may be a biologic necessity, but optimal sleep is a learned behavior, amenable to coaching and practice. Getting a good night's sleep is one of the most important things people can do for their overall health and well-being. Accordingly, physicians and allied healthcare professionals need to be able to ascertain why their patients may be having trouble sleeping and what can be done to alleviate or improve the situation.

With regard to the former, counseling the patient using coaching strategies and the Frates COACH Approach can be a very useful tool in unearthing the fundamental factors that are contributing to an individual's sleep-related problems. It is by asking open ended questions and listening attentively to the patient's sleep history that the lifestyle medicine practitioner will be able to help the patient solve their sleep problems. In order to identify a potential solution to the situation, physicians and allied healthcare professionals need to engage in an active, two-way (talk and listen) exchange of information with their patients.

Among the questions that can be asked of patients in this set of circumstances are the following:
- How rested do you feel when you get up in the morning?
- How is your energy level during the day?
- What is your bedtime routine, specifically noting what time you get into bed and what you are doing an hour prior to bed?
- What is your usual wake-up routine? Specifically, do you set an alarm, if so, for what time, and is it the same time weekdays and weekends? Do you snooze? Do you wake up on your own?
- Have you ever been told that you snore?
- Are you restless or uncomfortable during your sleep?
- What are your general eating habits before bedtime?
- Are your bed and bedroom a restful environment?
- Do you currently take any medicine that can affect your sleep?
- What are your current stress levels?
- How much caffeine do you consume in a day and when do you have your last caffeinated beverage?
- Do you drink alcohol in the evenings before going to bed?
- Do you only go to bed when you're tired?
- Do you watch the clock, once you go to bed?
- How long have you been experiencing problems with your sleep?
- What are your sleep troubles, specifically do you have difficulty falling asleep, staying asleep, or sleeping in the early morning?
- What do you do if you can't sleep? Do you get up and stay up until you become tired?

With regard to the aforementioned information that lifestyle medicine practitioners and allied healthcare professionals may collect, certain suggestions tend to apply to most patients. Counseling patients on how to achieve an optimal level of sleep can entail a variety of tips, which can be grouped into three convenient categories: preparation, environment, and timing.

❑ Preparation—Sleep is not passive; it requires a proactive routine:

- *Establish a regular sleep-wake routine, and adhere to it daily, even on weekends.* Go to bed at 11 p.m., if that is the routine, and wake up at 7 a.m. every day or go to bed at 10 p.m. and wake up at 6 a.m. Any reasonable schedule that has a bedtime prior to midnight and a wake time seven to eight hours after that is recommended.
- *Get regular physical activity in the morning or afternoon.* Exercising daily has been shown to promote good quality sleep. Morning exercise makes it easier to fall asleep at night and wake up in the morning. As long as an individual exercises regularly, it is okay to exercise in the evening. It is preferable to not do it immediately before bed, but current research has not shown that sleep is impaired.
- *Get daily exposure to outdoor light.* Remember that early morning light is the best way to keep a person's circadian rhythm synchronized.
- *Control caffeine and nicotine intake, and limit the consumption of alcohol.* Minimize caffeine intake later in the day (strive to drink coffee in the morning only). Limit alcohol consumption (no more than two drinks a day for men and one for women) and, if the individual drinks, try to consume alcohol during the dinner meal at least a couple of hours prior to bed. Both caffeine and alcohol can interfere with restful sleep. Caffeine can prevent a person from falling asleep, while alcohol may cause individuals to wake up during the night. Nicotine is a stimulant, which is best avoided entirely, if possible. It is also important to be cognizant of water or beverage intake just before bedtime, given that such an action may necessitate a visit to the bathroom in the middle of the night, which obviously disrupts sleep.
- *Power down before bedtime.* Read, meditate, do some deep breathing or gentle stretch yoga (not power yoga), or take a warm bath. Avoid watching television or being exposed to anything stimulating or that has bright lights, emitting blue wavelength light, which can block the production of melatonin. Keep the lights as dim as possible for the hour or two before bedtime. Blue light spectrum, emitted from smartphones, tablets, and televisions, increases cortisol and decreases the production of melatonin. At the present time, there are light bulbs that specifically avoid blue light. In addition, there are special apps and filters for phones that reduce the amount of blue light emitted and that can be switched on during the evening hours. There are also special sunglasses that block out the blue wavelength. Even with these special blue light blocking options, it is best to put the phone away after dinner time and avoid screen time (computer or TV) an hour or two prior to bed.

- ❑ *Environment*—Craft your surroundings to support optimal sleep:
  - *Keep the bedroom just for sleep and sex.* Don't watch television or use the computer/tablet/phone in the bedroom. Confine those activities to another room, so the only thing associated with the bedroom is sleep and sex. Furthermore, while it can be tempting to allow pets to sleep in the bed too, this practice is not recommended, as animals often take a great deal of space and move around at night, which can disrupt sleep. Designating a space specifically for a pet to sleep is recommended. This approach is safer and better for the animal and the owner.
  - *Get comfortable.* Turn the thermostat down to create a more optimal environment in which to sleep. A drop in core body temperature is another sleep signal for the body. A person can accelerate this natural process by setting the thermostat somewhere between 60-67 F. Wear socks to help with peripheral vasodilation (opening of the arteries in the feet and hands), which increases heat loss at the extremities and allows for the core temperature to drop. Make sure the room is completely dark, a step that may require the use of blackout curtains or an eye mask. It's best not to use a nightlight and to cover any lights being emitted by the clock or other devices. The room should also be quiet. People may have to wear ear plugs if there is external noise, or if their partner snores. Sometimes, white noise can help with sleep, given that it cancels out other distracting noises that can disturb sleep.
- ❑ *Timing*—Get the sleep you need, when you need it, as efficiently as possible:
  - *Eat wisely.* Eat dinner at least two hours before bedtime, so that the body has time to begin metabolizing and absorbing the food. If a person has insomnia, a small snack just before bedtime is acceptable. Calcium-containing foods, such as non-fat or low-fat milk, can be natural sleep aids. Foods that are high in tryptophan, which promotes sleep, are good options (e.g., dairy products [non-fat or low fat yogurt or milk], nuts, seeds, bananas, honey, eggs, oatmeal, or whole grain crackers). Carbohydrates work in conjunction with tryptophan to make it more accessible to the brain. This factor is likely why milk and cookies were a recommended sleep aid in the past. On the other hand, there are healthier options for the carbohydrate choice these days. Cherries (which are a natural source of melatonin), or unsweetened cherry juice are other good options. Research has found that cherries may be as effective as taking an over-the-counter melatonin supplement. High-protein, high-fat foods should be avoided, given that they are difficult to digest and may keep a person up. Chamomile tea doesn't contain caffeine and may help with relaxation. Inhaling the scent of lavender may also be relaxing and calming for patients which could help with sleep.
  - *If you nap, keep it to only 20 or 30 minutes.* Research studies have demonstrated that the naps of a short duration—even just nine minutes long—can be restorative. If naps are taken, they should be done in the early to mid-afternoon and last no more than 30 minutes. Napping for a short duration is important so that the person doesn't go into deep sleep, which can extend the duration of the nap (so-called sleep inertia), result in the person feeling sluggish, and interfere with night-time

sleep. If individuals are experiencing sleep problems, such as insomnia, naps can add to their problem, particularly if taken late in the day. For these people, napping should be limited and done only in rare circumstances. Remember that naps do not make up for chronic sleep loss or poor quality nighttime sleep.

EVEN MORE INFORMATION ABOUT SLEEP-RELATED MATTERS—COMMON QUESTIONS ANSWERED

- *What is a circadian rhythm?* A circadian rhythm is a 24-hour-interval clock that is operating in the background of a person's brain and varies alertness/sleepiness levels across the night and day. Sleep is easiest at low points in the circadian rhythm and more difficult at high points. People can have circadian problems when they try to fall asleep at a "bad" circadian time for sleep (during the evening for many people) or stay awake at a "good" circadian sleep time (often in the 4 to 6 a.m. time period).
- *What is the best time to go to bed?* The "best" time is often the habitual bedtime, since circadian rhythms adjust in a regular schedule in anticipation of sleep. In other words, there is significant variability of "best" times, as well as an opportunity for an individual to get on a "good" sleep schedule. Falling to sleep around 11 p.m. or before midnight, is often a good target time for those individuals who have a nine-to-five job and need to get out of the house by at least 8 a.m., because it allows for a wake-up time of 7 a.m., which allots an hour for breakfast, shower, and dressing.

    NREM sleep, which is deeper than REM sleep, dominates a person's slumber cycles in the early part of the evening, but tends to occur shortly after sleep onset, regardless of bedtime at night. REM sleep predominates later in the night, so that individuals who have chronically short sleep times become REM-deprived. This situation means that setting a sleep schedule is critical for optimal daytime functioning, productivity, and learning. On the other hand, these is no "right" or ideal bedtime for every person. Everyone has a unique chronotype, which is the behavior manifestation of underlying circadian rhythms determined by gene-environment interactions. Most people exist between the extremes of being "larks" and "owls."
- *How is sleep regulated?* The brain controls and regulates transitions that a person experiences between wakefulness and sleep. In reality, the transition is almost instantaneous. An individual is awake one moment and asleep the next. This alteration of consciousness entails a swift, but complex, interaction between various parts of the brain.
- *How important is a person's sleep environment?* The environment in which a person sleeps can have a significant impact on the quantity and quality of sleep that this individual gets. For example, too much light can shift a person's internal clock, making restful sleep difficult to achieve; too much noise can interrupt the sleep cycle. A temperature that is too hot or too cold can also be disruptive, particularly to REM sleep.

- *How does sleep change with age?* Adults experience several sleep-related changes as they age. The relative proportion of time spent in SWS is reduced, while time spent in the lighter NREM stages of sleep is increased. Older adults typically have increased awakenings during the night and are more likely to be affected by a variety of comorbid conditions (e.g., lung disease, heart disease, arthritis, etc.) that can have a disruptive effect on their sleep. In addition, they may undergo notable changes in their 24-hour circadian rhythm, which tends to weaken as they age. As a result, they may find themselves going to bed earlier and awakening earlier.
- *Why does jet lag disturb an individual's sleep pattern?* Jet lag results from the mismatch that occurs between an individual's external environment and her internal biological clock. In essence, the situation is due to circadian misalignment. A person's internal clock is out of sync with the actual time in the time zone in which the individual is located. In order to optimally manage jet lag, consider a few pointers. When travelling from east to west, try to stay awake until it is bedtime in the new location. On the other hand, when flying from west to east, try to get as much sleep as possible; and when you land, keep your sunglasses on for a few hours to help reset the body's clock.

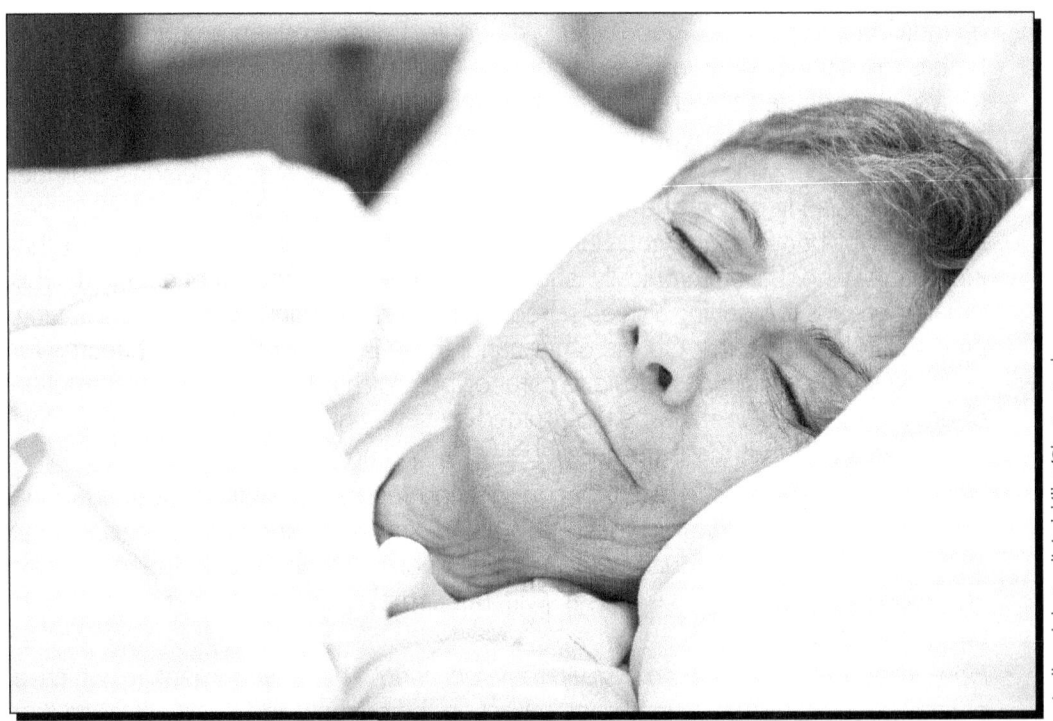

Adults experience several sleep-related changes as they age.

- *Why is having a sleep routine important?* The human body craves structure, e.g., going to bed at a regular time and waking up at the same time every day. Such a routine can make it easier to fall asleep, because the body tends to recognize the routine and then "powers down" on cue. This factor also reduces the amount of adrenaline and cortisol the body produces, as well as increases the level of sleep-inducing melatonin around the time that it expects the person to start winding down. It should be noted that while the body can handle spontaneous changes to its sleep routine, consistency is best on most days.
- *Why do people snore?* Snoring is the end result when a person can't move air freely through their nose and throat during sleep. It is caused by the tumultuous passage of air traveling over any structure in the snorer's mouth and throat (e.g., tongue, tonsils, and adenoids). This condition can be due to obstructive sleep apnea due to excessive weight or central sleep apnea from a malfunction in the brain circuitry.
- *What is a dream?* A dream is essentially stories and images that a person's mind creates during sleep. As such, it is a succession of images, ideas, emotions, and sensations that usually occur involuntarily in the mind during certain stages of sleep, primarily the REM stage.

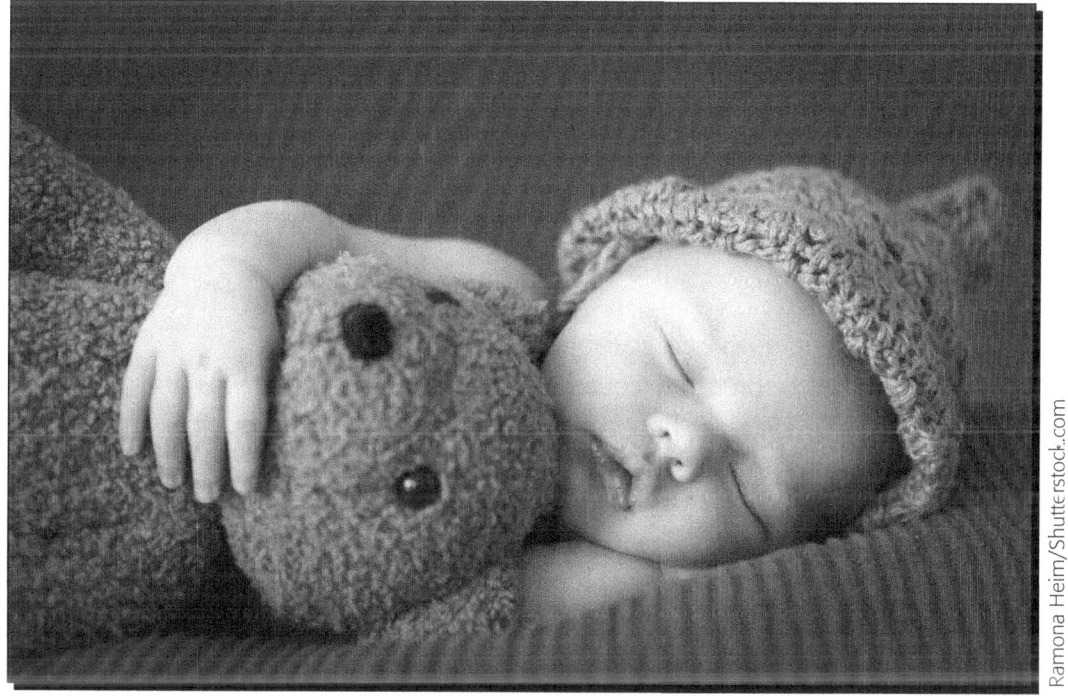

The human body craves structure, e.g., going to bed at a regular time and waking up at the same time every day.

FITT PRESCRIPTIONS FOR SLEEP

Just as there is a FITT prescription for exercise or nutrition, there is a FITT prescription for sleep. This prescription is a simple framework that provides guidance for patients and providers alike.

❑ An example FITT prescription to work toward for night time sleep:

    F—once in a 24 hour period
    I—deep restorative
    T—7 to 8 hours: 11 p.m. to 6 or 7 a.m.
    T—nighttime sleep

❑ An example FITT prescription for napping:

    F—once in the afternoon five days of the week
    I—light sleep
    T—30 minutes or less
    T—nap

KEY POINTS/TAKEAWAYS FOR CHAPTER 6

❑ Chapter Review:

- Overall goal: Explore the factors involved in getting sufficient sleep.
- Application goal: Understand the connection between sleep and health.

❑ Discussion Questions:

- How much sleep does a particular patient need?
- What is the best approach to counseling a patient about sleep?
- What is current evidence-based information concerning the external and internal factors that affect a patient's sleep?
- How does sleep affect each of the 11 systems of the body?
- What are healthy sleep habits?

	TITLE	AUTHORS	JOURNAL	YEAR	KEY FINDINGS
1	Effectiveness of lifestyle interventions on obstructive sleep apnea (OSA): systematic review and meta-analysis	Araghi MH, et al.	Sleep	2013	This systematic review and meta-analysis found that weight loss with lifestyle and diet resulted in improvements in obstructive sleep apnea measures but did not normalize them. It also concluded that more studies were needed to evaluate daytime sleepiness and other symptoms associated with obstructive sleep apnea.
2	The effects of bedtime and sleep duration on academic and emotional outcomes in a nationally representative sample of adolescents	Asarnow LD, McGlinchey E, Harvey AG	Journal of Adolescent Health	2014	Assessed the sleep patterns of 2,700 adolescents in grades seven through 12. It found that "late school year bedtime was associated with shorter total sleep time cross-sectionally, whereas late summertime bedtime was not." During the first wave of this study, late school year bedtime was associated with worse educational outcomes and emotional distress six to eight years later. In the first two waves of the study, >75% of adolescents surveyed who had late bedtimes reported sleeping fewer than the recommended nine hours.
3	Later school start time is associated with improved sleep and daytime functioning in adolescents	Boergers J, Gable CH, Owens JA	Journal of Developmental and Behavioral Pediatrics	2014	A study of 197 high school boarding students that surveyed the students' sleep habits before and after a 25-minute delay in school starting time that found that later school time was associated with improved sleep and daytime functioning in adolescents. "A modest (25 min) delay in school start time was associated with significant improvements in sleep duration, daytime sleepiness, mood, and caffeine use."
4	Sleep habits and patterns of college students: a preliminary study	Buboltz WC, Brown F, Soper B	Journal of American College Health	2001	A sample of 191 undergraduate students that found that only 11% of college students slept well consistently, with 73% experiencing occasional sleeping issues.
5	Sleep health: can we define it? does it matter?	Buysse DJ	Sleep	2014	Introduces the notion of sleep health and encourages a shift away from sleep disorders/problems and movement towards focusing on sleep and its role in promoting wellness, performance, and adaptation in individuals and populations.
6	Sleep duration predicts cardiovascular outcomes: a systematic review and meta-analysis of prospective studies	Cappuccio FP, et al.	European Heart Journal	2011	A systematic review that included 15 studies and found that both short (<5 hours) and long (>9 hours) duration sleep are predictors, or markers, of cardiovascular outcomes.
7	Recuperative power of a short daytime nap with or without stage 2 sleep	Hayashi M, Motoyoshi N, Hori T	Sleep	2005	A study of 10 healthy university students that found that naps of short duration, even nine minutes (six minutes of stage 1 and three minutes of stage 2) were restorative. It also found that three minutes of stage 2 sleep was more restorative than no stage 2 sleep in this study population.

Figure 6-7. Sleep and its effect on health and well-being evidence

	TITLE	AUTHORS	JOURNAL	YEAR	KEY FINDINGS
8	Age and sleep disturbances among American men and women: data from the U.S. Behavioral Risk Factor Surveillance System	Grandner MA, et al.	*Sleep*	2012	A cross-sectional analysis of 155,877 participants from the 2006 Behavioral Risk Factor Surveillance System that concluded that "advancing age was not associated with increased Self-Reports Sleep Disturbance OR Self-Reported Tiredness/Lack of Energy. These results suggest that the often-reported increase in sleep problems with age is a nonlinear phenomenon, mediated by factors other than physiologic aging."
9	Sleep symptoms associated with intake of specific dietary nutrients	Grandner MA, et al.	*Journal of Sleep Research*	2014	A cross-sectional study of 4,552 individuals that utilized the NHANES database to determine which nutrients were associated with sleep symptoms. As a hypothesis-generating study, there were a variety of novel associations found between sleep symptoms and diet/metabolism, potentially explaining association between sleep and cardiometabolic disease. Further studies are needed to see if these are correlations or causative relationships.
10	The effects of insomnia and sleep loss on cardiovascular disease	Kahn MS, Aouad R	*Sleep Medicine Clinics*	2017	Explores the relationship between insomnia and cardiovascular disease. It finds that "those who are sleep deprived or have insomnia have elevated cortisol levels, increased markers of sympathetic activity, increased metabolic rate, and endothelial dysfunction, all of which are correlated with increased risk of cardiovascular disease and risk factors. Both short sleep duration and insomnia are linked to the development of diabetes and hypertension. Insomnia is associated with increased risk of cardiovascular disease and mortality, although not all studies show consistent findings of a positive association."
11	Physiology: warm feet promote the rapid onset of sleep	Kräuchi K, et al.	*Nature*	1999	A novel study that showed that "the degree of dilation of blood vessels in the skin of the hands and feet, which increases heat loss at these extremities, is the best physiological predictor for the rapid onset of sleep."
12	Effects of vigorous late-night exercise on sleep quality and cardiac autonomic activity	Myllymaki T, et al.	*Journal of Sleep Research*	2011	Eleven physically fit young adults were monitored in a sleep lab twice, once after a vigorous late-night exercise session and once after a control day. Numerous physiologic parameters were measured: polysomnographic activity, actigraphic activity, cardiac autonomic activity, and subjective sleep quality. They found that "vigorous late-night exercise does not disturb sleep quality. However, it may have effects on cardiac autonomic control of heart during the first sleeping hours."

Figure 6-7. Sleep and its effect on health and well-being evidence (cont.)

	TITLE	AUTHORS	JOURNAL	YEAR	KEY FINDINGS
13	Memory for semantically related and unrelated declarative information: the benefit of sleep, the cost of wake	Payne JD, et al.	PLOS ONE	2012	A study of 2007 college students that examined the impact of sleep, wake, and the time of day on memory. It found that memory overall was superior following a night of sleep compared to a day of wakefulness. Memory was also superior when sleep occurred shortly after learning rather than following a full day of wakefulness.
14	Management of chronic insomnia disorder in adults: a clinical practice guideline from the American College of Physicians	Qaseem A, et al.	Annals of Internal Medicine	2016	Guidelines from the American College of Physicians based on a systematic review of randomized, controlled trials from 2004-2015. Recommendations on the management of chronic insomnia disorder in adults include the following:
15	Interactions between obesity and obstructive sleep apnea: implications for treatment	Romero-Corral A, et al.	Chest	2010	A review article that discusses the relationship between weight and obstructive sleep apnea (OSA). It notes that weight loss helps reduce the severity of OSA and attenuates the cardiometabolic abnormalities that exist in both diseases.
16	The role of sleep in the control of food intake	Shechter A, Grandner MA, St-Onge M-P	American Journal of Lifestyle Medicine	2014	Discusses the association between short sleep duration and its effect on energy intake. It appears that sleeping less than six hours tends to result in greater energy intakes, particularly of fat and possibly carbohydrates. This likely plays a role in the association between short sleep duration and obesity.
17	Association between light at night, melatonin secretion, sleep deprivation, and the internal clock: health impacts and mechanisms of circadian disruption	Touitou Y, Reinberg A, Touitou D	Life Sciences	2017	A review of evidence on the impact that exposure to artificial lights at night has on health. Discusses proposed countermeasures such as melatonin, bright light, and psychotropic drugs to improve adaptation to shift and night work
18	Moderate sleep deprivation produces impairments in cognitive and motor performance equivalent to legally prescribed levels of alcohol intoxication	Williamson A, Feyer A	Occupational and Environmental Medicine	2000	Thirty-nine subjects were subjected to 28 hours of sleep deprivation and alcohol intoxication up to about 0.1% blood alcohol concentration (BAC). Performance effects were measured and the researchers found that "after 17-19 hours without sleep, performance on some tests were equivalent or worse than that at a BAC of 0.05%. Response speeds were up to 50% slower for some tests and accuracy measures were significantly poorer than at this level of alcohol. After longer periods without sleep, performance reached levels equivalent to the maximum alcohol dose given to subjects (0.1% BAC)."

Figure 6-7. Sleep and its effect on health and well being evidence (cont.)

References

1. Araghi MH, Chen Y-F, Jagielski A, et al. Effectiveness of lifestyle interventions on obstructive sleep apnea (OSA): systematic review and meta-analysis. *Sleep.* 2013;36(10):1553-1562. doi:10.5665/sleep.3056.
2. Asarnow LD, McGlinchey E, Harvey AG. The effects of bedtime and sleep duration on academic and emotional outcomes in a nationally representative sample of adolescents. *Journal of Adolescent Health.* 2014;54(3):350-356. doi:10.1016/j.jadohealth.2013.09.004.
3. Boergers J, Gable CH, Owens JA. Later school start time is associated with improved sleep and daytime functioning in adolescents. *Journal of Developmental and Behavioral Pediatrics.* 2014;35:11-17.
4. Buboltz WC, Brown F, Soper B. Sleep habits and patterns of college students: a preliminary study. *Journal of American College Health.* 2001;50:131-135.
5. Buysse DJ. Sleep health: can we define it? does it matter? *Sleep.* 2014;37(1):9-17. doi:10.5665/sleep.3298.
6. Cappuccio FP, Cooper D, D'Elia L, et al. Sleep duration predicts cardiovascular outcomes: a systematic review and meta-analysis of prospective studies. *European Heart Journal.* 2011;32(12):1484-1492. doi:10.1093/eurheartj/ehr007.
7. Hayashi M, Motoyoshi N, Hori T. Recuperative power of a short daytime nap with or without stage 2 sleep. *Sleep.* 2005;28:829-836.
8. Grandner MA, Martin JL, Patel NP, et al. Age and sleep disturbances among American men and women: data from the U.S. Behavioral Risk Factor Surveillance System. *Sleep.* 2012;35(3):395-406. doi:10.5665/sleep.1704.
9. Grandner MA, Jackson N, Gerstner JR, et al. Sleep symptoms associated with intake of specific dietary nutrients. *Journal of Sleep Research.* 2014;23(1):22-34. doi:10.1111/jsr.12084.
10. Kahn MS, Aouad R. The effects of insomnia and sleep loss on cardiovascular disease. *Sleep Medicine Clinics.* 2017;12(2):167-177.
11. Kräuchi K, Cajochen C, Werth E, et al. Physiology: warm feet promote the rapid onset of sleep. *Nature.* September 2 1999;401:36-37. doi:10.1038/43366.
12. Myllymaki T, Kyrolainen H, Savolainen K, et al. Effects of vigorous late-night exercise on sleep quality and cardiac autonomic activity. *Journal of Sleep Research.* 2011;20:146-153.
13. Payne JD, Tucker MA, Ellenbogen JM, et al. Memory for semantically related and unrelated declarative information: the benefit of sleep, the cost of wake. *PLOS ONE.* 2012;7:e33079.
14. Qaseem A, Kansagara D, Forciea MA, et al. Management of chronic insomnia disorder in adults: a clinical practice guideline from the American College of Physicians. *Annals of Internal Medicine.* July 19 2016;165(2):125-133.
15. Romero-Corral A, Caples SM, Lopez-Jimenez F, et al. Interactions between obesity and obstructive sleep apnea: implications for treatment. *Chest.* 2010;137(3):711-719. doi:10.1378/chest.09-0360.
16. Shechter A, Grandner MA, St-Onge M-P. The role of sleep in the control of food intake. *American Journal of Lifestyle Medicine.* 2014;8(6):371-374. doi:10.1177/1559827614545315.
17. Touitou Y, Reinberg A, Touitou D. Association between light at night, melatonin secretion, sleep deprivation, and the internal clock: health impacts and mechanisms of circadian disruption. *Life Sciences.* 2017;173:94-106.
18. Williamson A, Feyer A. Moderate sleep deprivation produces impairments in cognitive and motor performance equivalent to legally prescribed levels of alcohol intoxication. *Occupational and Environmental Medicine.* 2000;57(10):649-655.

Figure 6-7. Sleep and its effect on health and well-being evidence (cont.)

REFERENCES

- Altman NG, Schopfer E, Jackson N, et al. Sleep duration versus sleep insufficiency as predictors of cardiometabolic health outcomes. *Sleep Medicine.* 2012;13(10):1261-1270. doi:10.1016/j.sleep.2012.08.005.
- Araghi MH, Chen Y-F, Jagielski A, et al. Effectiveness of lifestyle interventions on obstructive sleep apnea (OSA): systematic review and meta-analysis. *Sleep.* 2013;36(10):1553-1562. doi:10.5665/sleep.3056.
- Asarnow LD, McGlinchey E, Harvey AG. The effects of bedtime and sleep duration on academic and emotional outcomes in a nationally representative sample of adolescents. *Journal of Adolescent Health.* 2014;54(3):350-356. doi:10.1016/j.jadohealth.2013.09.004.
- Axelsson J, Sundelin T, Ingre M, et al. Beauty sleep: experimental study on the perceived health and attractiveness of sleep deprived people. *BMJ.* 2010;341:c6614. doi:10.1136/*bmj*.c6614.
- Bonnet MH, Arand DL. Patient Education: Insomnia (Beyond the Basics). UpToDate. Available at: http://www.uptodate.com/contents/insomnia-beyond-the-basics?source=search_result&search=insomnia&selectedTitle=1%7E18. Accessed September 2017.

- Buysse DJ. Sleep health: can we define it? does it matter? *Sleep.* 2014;37(1):9-17. doi:10.5665/sleep.3298.
- Cappuccio FP, Cooper D, D'Elia L, Strazzullo P, Miller MA. Sleep duration predicts cardiovascular outcomes: a systematic review and meta-analysis of prospective studies. *European Heart Journal.* 2011;32(12):1484-1492. doi:10.1093/eurheartj/ehr007.
- Cappuccio FP, D'Elia L, Strazzullo P, et al. Sleep duration and all-cause mortality: a systematic review and meta-analysis of prospective studies. *Sleep.* 2010;33(5):585-592.
- Centers for Disease Control and Prevention. Effect of Short Sleep Duration on Daily Activities—United States, 2005-2008. 2011;60(08):239-242. Available at: https://www.cdc.gov/mmwr/preview/mmwrhtml/mm6008a3.htm. Accessed June 2018.
- Chong Y, Fryar CD, Gu Q. Prescription sleep aid use among adults: United States, 2005-2010. NCHS data brief, no 127. Hyattsville, MD: National Center for Health Statistics; 2013. Available at: https://www.cdc.gov/nchs/data/databriefs/db127.pdf. Accessed June 2018.
- Cohen-Zrubavel V, Kushnir B, Kushnir J, et al. Sleep and sleepiness in children with nocturnal enuresis. *Sleep.* 2011;34(2):191-194.
- Dement WC, Vaughan C, Vaughn C. *The Promise of Sleep: A Pioneer in Sleep Medicine Explores the Vital Connection Between Health, Happiness, and a Good Night's Sleep.* New York: Random House Publishing Group; 2000.
- Division of Sleep Medicine at Harvard Medical School, WGBH Educational Foundation. Assess Your Sleep Needs. Get Sleep. Available at: http://healthysleep.med.harvard.edu/need-sleep/what-can-you-do/assess-needs. Accessed January 2017.
- Division of Sleep Medicine at Harvard Medical School, WGBH Educational Foundation. Finding Your Sleep/Wake Rhythm. Healthy Sleep. Available at: http://healthysleep.med.harvard.edu/interactive/circadian. Accessed January 2017.
- Division of Sleep Medicine at Harvard Medical School. Epworth Sleepiness Scale. Narcolepsy. Published 1997. Updated October 16, 2013. Available at: http://healthysleep.med.harvard.edu/narcolepsy/diagnosing-narcolepsy/epworth-sleepiness-scale. Accessed January 5, 2017.
- Foster RG, Lockley SW. *Sleep: A Very Short Introduction.* Oxford: Oxford University Press; 2012.
- Gozal D, Kheirandish-Gozal L. Childhood obesity and sleep: relatives, partners, or both?—a critical perspective on the evidence. *Annals of the New York Academy of Sciences.* 2012;1264(1):135-141. doi:10.1111/j.1749-6632.2012.06723.x.
- Grandner MA, Martin JL, Patel NP, et al. Age and sleep disturbances among American men and women: data from the U.S. Behavioral Risk Factor Surveillance System. *Sleep.* 2012;35(3):395-406. doi:10.5665/sleep.1704.
- Harvard Medical School Division of Sleep Medicine. Healthy Sleep. Available at: http://healthysleep.med.harvard.edu/healthy/science/how/neurophysiology. Accessed June 2018.

- Harvard Women's Health Watch. Medications That Can Affect Sleep. Harvard Health Publishing. Available at: https://www.health.harvard.edu/newsletter_article/medications-that-can-affect-sleep. Accessed October 2017.
- Havekes R, Park AJ, Tudor JC, et al. Sleep deprivation causes memory deficits by negatively impacting neuronal connectivity in hippocampal area CA1. eLife. 2016;5:e13424. doi:10.7554/eLife.13424.
- Hayashi M, Motoyoshi N, Hori T. Recuperative power of a short daytime nap with or without stage 2 sleep. *Sleep.* 2005;28(7):829-836. Available at: https://doi.org/10.1093/sleep/28.7.829. Accessed August 2018.
- HowSleepWorks.com. How Sleep Works—Sleep-Wake Homeostasis. Available at: https://www.howsleepworks.com/how_homeostasis.html. Accessed June 2018.
- IMS Institute for Healthcare Informatics. The Use of Medicines in the United States: Review of 2010. Available at: http://www.imshealth.com/deployedfiles/imshealth/Global/Content/IMS%20Institute/Static%20File/IHII_UseOfMed_report.pdf. Accessed June 2018.
- Jean-Louis G, Zizi F, Clark LT, et al. Obstructive sleep apnea and cardiovascular disease: role of the metabolic syndrome and its components. *Journal of Clinical Sleep Medicine.* 2008;4(3):261-272.
- Judd BG, Sateia MJ. Classification of Sleep Disorders. UpToDate. Available at: https://www.uptodate.com/contents/classification-of-sleep-disorders. Accessed June 2018.
- Jung CM, Khalsa SBS, Scheer FAJL, et al. Acute effects of bright light exposure on cortisol levels. *Journal of Biological Rhythms.* 2010;25(3):208-216. doi:10.1177/0748730410368413.
- Kahn MS, Aouad R. The effects of insomnia and sleep loss on cardiovascular disease. *Sleep Medicine Clinics.* 2017;12(2):167-177.
- Ko Y, Lee J-Y. Effects of feet warming using bed socks on sleep quality and thermoregulatory responses in a cool environment. *Journal of Physiological Anthropology.* 2018;37:13. doi:10.1186/s40101-018-0172-z.
- Kräuchi K, Cajochen C, Werth E, Wirz-Justice A. Physiology: warm feet promote the rapid onset of sleep. *Nature.* September 2 1999;401:36-37. doi:10.1038/43366.
- Lewis PA. *The Secret World of Sleep: The Surprising Science of the Mind at Rest.* New York: Palgrave MacMillan Trade; 2014.
- Moore RT, Kaprielian R, Auerbach J. Asleep at the Wheel: Report of the Special Commission on Drowsy Driving. 2009. Available at: https://sleep.med.harvard.edu/file_download/103. Accessed August 2018.
- Myllymaki T, Kyrolainen H, Savolainen K, et al. Effects of vigorous late-night exercise on sleep quality and cardiac autonomic activity. *Journal of Sleep Research.* 2011;20:146-153.

- National Institute of Neurological Disorders and Stroke. Narcolepsy Fact Sheet. Available at: https://www.ninds.nih.gov/Disorders/Patient-Caregiver-Education/Fact-Sheets/Narcolepsy-Fact-Sheet. Accessed June 2018.
- National Sleep Foundation. Food and Sleep. Available at: https://sleepfoundation.org/sleep-topics/food-and-sleep. Accessed October 2017.
- National Sleep Foundation. National Sleep Foundation Recommends New Sleep Times. Available at: https://sleepfoundation.org/press-release/national-sleep-foundation-recommends-new-sleep-times/page/0/1. Accessed June 2018.
- National Sleep Foundation. National Sleep Foundation Sleepiness Test. Available at: https://sleepfoundation.org/quiz/national-sleep-foundation-sleepiness-test. Accessed January 2017.
- Pigeon WR, Carr M, Gorman C, et al. Effects of a tart cherry juice beverage on the sleep of older adults with insomnia: a pilot study. *Journal of Medicinal Food.* 2010;13(3):579-583. doi:10.1089/jmf.2009.0096.
- Qaseem A, Kansagara D, Forciea MA, Cooke M, Denberg TD, Clinical Guidelines Committee of the American College of Physicians. Management of chronic insomnia disorder in adults: a clinical practice guideline from the American College of Physicians. *Annals of Internal Medicine.* July 19 2016;165(2):125-133.
- Rath T. *Eat Move Sleep: How Small Choices Lead to Big Changes.* New York: Missionday; 2014.
- Romero-Corral A, Caples SM, Lopez-Jimenez F, et al. Interactions between obesity and obstructive sleep apnea: implications for treatment. *Chest.* 2010;137(3):711-719. doi:10.1378/chest.09-0360.
- Rupavate S. 7 Scientific Reasons Why Lack of Sleep Can Be Bad for You. TheHealthSite. Available at: http://www.thehealthsite.com/diseases-conditions/7-scientific-reasons-why-lack-of-sleep-can-be-bad-for-you/. Accessed October 2017.
- Sleep Questionnaire. University of South Carolina School of Medicine, Department of Internal Medicine. Available at: http://internalmedicine.med.sc.edu/forms/Sleep%20questionnaire2.pdf. Accessed January 2017.
- Specker BL, Binkley T, Vukovich M, et al. Volumetric bone mineral density and bone size in sleep-deprived individuals. *Osteoporosis International.* 2007;18(1):93-99. Available at: https://doi.org/10.1007/s00198-006-0207-x. Accessed June 2018.
- Stevenson S. *Sleep Smarter: 21 Essential Strategies to Sleep Your Way to a Better Body, Better Health, and Bigger Success.* Emmaus, PA: Rodale Books; 2016.
- Taylor DJ, Kelly K, Kohut ML, et al. Is insomnia a risk factor for decreased influenza vaccine response? *Behavioral Sleep Medicine.* 2017;15(4):270-287. doi:10.1080/15402002.2015.1126596.
- Touitou Y, Reinberg A, Touitou D. Association between light at night, melatonin secretion, sleep deprivation, and the internal clock: health impacts and mechanisms of circadian disruption. *Life Sciences.* 2017;173:94-106.

- U.S. Department of Health and Human Services National Institutes of Health. Your Guide to Healthy Sleep. 2005 (updated 2011). Available at: https://www.nhlbi.nih.gov/files/docs/public/sleep/healthy_sleep.pdf. Accessed June 2018.
- U.S. Department of Health and Human Services National Institutes of Health and National Institute of Neurological Disorders and Stroke. Brain Basics: Understanding Sleep. 2008. Available at: https://education.ninds.nih.gov/brochures/Brain-Basics-Sleep-6-10-08-pdf-508.pdf. Accessed June 2018.
- Van Cauter E, Plat L. Physiology of growth hormone secretion during sleep. *Journal of Pediatrics.* 1996;128:S32-S37.
- WebMD. Foods That Help or Harm Your Sleep. Available at: https://www.webmd.com/sleep-disorders/ss/slideshow-sleep-foods. Accessed June 2018.
- WebMD. Sleep Disorders Guide. Available at: https://www.webmd.com/sleep-disorders/guide/sleep-disorders-symptoms-types. Accessed June 2018.
- West C, Egger G. To sleep perchance ... to get everything else right. In: Egger G, Binns A, Rossner S, eds. *Lifestyle Medicine: Managing Diseases of Lifestyle in the 21st Century.* 2nd ed. North Ryde, N.S.W.: McGraw-Hill; 2010:226-241.
- Williamson A, Feyer A. Moderate sleep deprivation produces impairments in cognitive and motor performance equivalent to legally prescribed levels of alcohol intoxication. *Occupational and Environmental Medicine.* 2000;57(10):649-655.
- Wojnar M, Ilgen MA, Wojnar J, et al. Sleep problems and suicidality in the National Comorbidity Survey Replication. *Journal of Psychiatric Research.* 2009;43(5):526-531. doi:10.1016/j.jpsychires.2008.07.006.
- Zick SM, Wright BD, Sen A, et al. Preliminary examination of the efficacy and safety of a standardized chamomile extract for chronic primary insomnia: a randomized placebo-controlled pilot study. *BMC Complementary and Alternative Medicine.* 2011;11:78. doi:10.1186/1472-6882-11-78.

CHAPTER 7

STRESS AND RESILIENCE

"It is not stress that kills us; it's our reaction to it."

—Hans Selye, MD, PhD
Endocrinologist
Pioneer researcher on the effects of
stress on the human body

❑ Chapter Goals:

- Understand the key aspects attendant to both stress and resilience.
- Gain an appreciation for the connection between stress and health.
- Acquire an understanding of the fight-or-flight response.
- Identify how stress impacts each of the systems of the body.
- Determine the factors (external and internal) that contribute to stress.
- Discuss the risk factors for stress.

❑ Learning Objectives:

- To understand the connection between stress and health
- To recognize inappropriate methods for coping with stress
- To become cognizant of the factors that contribute to stress
- To become familiar with the fight-or-flight response

❑ Guiding Questions:

- What is stress?
- What are the basic signs and symptoms of stress?
- How can stress, depending on the circumstances, be either bad or good for a person?
- How does the fight-or-flight response work in the modern era?
- How does chronic stress affect the mind and the body?
- What types of behaviors contribute to stress overload?
- How can chronic stress be relieved?

❏ Important Terms:

- *Eustress:* Beneficial stress that is either psychological, physical (exercise), or biochemical/radiological (hormesis)
- *Fight-or-flight response:* The body's combined physiological reactions to a stressor, leading to a cascade of hormonal changes and physiological responses that can assist an individual in fighting against the threat or fleeing it
- *Flow:* A concept attributed to psychologist Dr. Mihalyi Csikzentmihalyi that describes eustress in which the individual performing an activity is fully immersed in a feeling of energized focus, complete involvement, and joy in the task at hand
- *Relaxation response:* A concept attributed to Dr. Herbert Benson of Harvard that describes a situation in which the body is brought back to its pre-stress level—a state of calmness of the mind and body (e.g., a reduction in blood pressure and heart rate, as well as in cardiovascular disease)
- *Resilience:* The process of adapting well in the face of adversity, trauma, threats, or significant sources of stress (e.g., health problems, financial difficulties, workplace stressor, relationship issues, etc.)
- *Stress:* A state of mental or emotional strain or tension due to the perception of pressure (e.g., emotional or physical tension), as well as the body's response to it

Stress is a constant in peoples' daily lives. Furthermore, stress does not discriminate. It affects everyone from time to time. Men, women; rich, poor; at home, in the workplace, at play; overweight, skinny... it does not matter. No person is immune from stress.

Not surprisingly, over 43 percent of all adults suffer from the adverse effects of stress. Over three-fourths of all doctors' visits are for stress-related ailments and complaints. And stress costs the American economy more than $300 billion annually. Given the widespread prevalence of stress and the significant toll it can take on a person's health, it is essential that physicians and allied healthcare professionals fully understand this potentially harmful condition.

WHAT IS STRESS?

Dr. Hans Selye, a Hungarian-born researcher and clinician, was the first to coin the term "stress" in 1936. In an interview conducted with Dr. Selye at the National Institute of Stress on the topic of good and bad stress, he said: "The general public uses stress and distress as synonymous, but they are not. The stress of pain, of sorrow, of nervousness, of suffering—that is bad stress, distress. But the stress of creation, or the stress of being able to achieve by taking things in a resilient way, you don't want to eliminate that. Accordingly, there is good stress (technically 'eustress') and bad stress ('distress'). In fact, the response to any demand [on the body] is stress. There is always stress, so the only point is to make sure that it is useful to yourself and useful to others."

As evidenced by this definition, stress—a state of mental or emotional strain or tension, resulting from adverse or very demanding circumstances—can be a double-edged sword. Eustress is the term used to refer to "good stress," the physical and psychological kind that motivates you. Distress refers to "bad stress," the physical and psychological kind that is harmful and draining.

THE THEORETICAL ROOTS OF STRESS AND RESILIENCE

The theoretical framework of stress provides a pathway for physicians and allied healthcare professionals to analyze and ascertain how they can best provide counsel and advise on relevant health-related matters concerning stress. A variety of scientific theories involving stress and resilience have been developed and empirically tested over the years. Four of the most accepted theories are the general adaptation response theory, the Yerkes-Dodson law, the theory of flow, and the fight-or-flight response theory.

❑ Theory of General Adaptation Response

In 1936, Dr. Hans Selye developed the universally acclaimed theory of general adaptation response (GAS), which helps to explain the body's physiological response to stress. Selye hypothesized that the body experiences three predictable states (Figure 7-1) when it responds to stressors: alarm reaction (stage #1), resistance (stage #2), and exhaustion (stage #3). The first stage entails the body's immediate reaction to a stressor. During the second stage, the body adapts to the stressors to which it has been exposed. In the final (third) stage, the body's resistance to stress may either be gradually reduced, or it may collapse quickly. This situation may encompass the fact that the body's immune system, as well as its ability to resist disease, may be almost totally eliminated. It is at this stage when a person's health is in the most jeopardy.

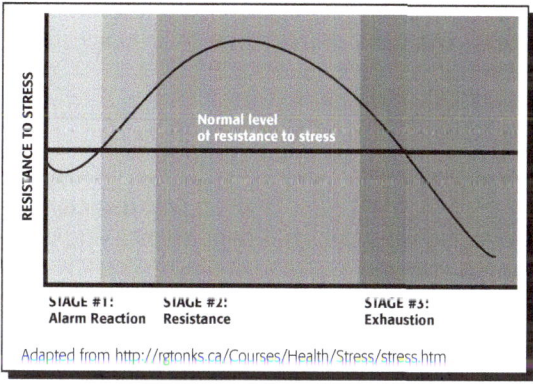

Figure 7-1. A graphic overview of Dr. Hans Selye's general adaptation syndrome

Selye also observed that individuals vary in their perceptions of the stressors they face. Furthermore, he believed that the stressors themselves present less of a risk to people's health than their maladaptive responses to them. Based on these observations, he categorized some diseases and mental disorders as "diseases of adaptation," resulting largely from errors in adaptive responses to the stressors, rather than the actual stressors themselves. Accordingly, physicians and allied healthcare professionals need to help their patients better understand, in each of their unique situations, what constitutes an appropriate response to their stressors. Also, identifying stress early and managing it will help prevent the progression from stage 1 to stage 3.

❑ Yerkes-Dodson Law

In 1908, two psychologists, Dr. Robert M. Yerkes and Dr. John D. Dodson, discovered that an empirical relationship exists between arousal (stress) and performance. They theorized that a person's performance level increases with physiological or mental arousal—but only up to a point. Accordingly, when the level of arousal or stress becomes too high, performance decreases. As Figure 7-2 indicates, human performance of any task varies with the level of arousal in a predictable parabolic curve. Essentially, a person could be too stressed to be productive or not stressed enough to perform a particular task.

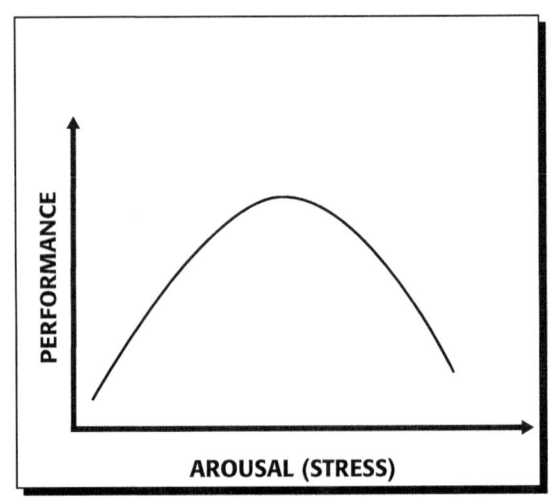

Figure 7-2. The Yerkes-Dodson law, depicting the relationship between performance and arousal (stress)

❑ Theory of Flow

In the 1960s, a noted psychologist, Dr. Mihaly Csikszentmihalyi, recognized and named the psychological concept of "flow," which refers to a highly focused mental state. When a person is in this mental condition, they are fully absorbed in what they are doing, often to a point where they lose a sense of time. Colloquially, a person who is experiencing flow is referred to as being "in the zone."

Flow is the state of concentration and engagement that can be realized by a person when performing a task that challenges his skills. This intense level of concentration leads to the production of both endorphins (the feel-good brain chemicals) and dopamine (the neurotransmitter that helps to regulate the pleasure and reward centers of the brain). This results in the individual experiencing feelings of joy.

Flow occurs when an individual's skill level is well-matched to the demands of the task that they are doing. However, if a mismatch exists between a person's skill level and the difficulty of the challenge, boredom or anxiety may predominate (Figure 7-3). For example, if an individual has a low level of skill and is facing a relatively large challenge, they will experience anxiety, rather than flow. If they have a high level of skill and are confronted with a relatively small challenge, they will experience boredom, rather than flow.

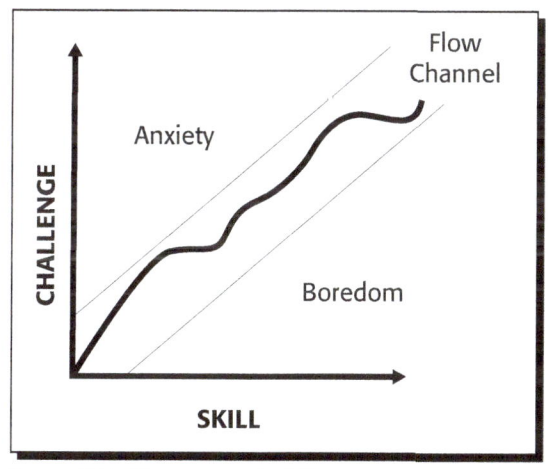

Figure 7-3. The concept of flow

Sharing this concept of flow with patients will help them to better understand how to handle situations when they are in the anxiety zone of the chart. In these situations, they can either work on increasing their skill level to meet the challenge, they can seek extra help from a person more skilled to fill the gap between their own skill level and the difficulty of the task, or they can alter the task. For example, if there is a deadline for a book chapter due in one day, and the author has only written two of twenty pages, they may feel paralyzed, because the challenge of writing eighteen pages in twelve hours is too great. To get out of the anxiety zone and attempt to get into the flow channel, the individual may try to renegotiate the deadline with the publisher so that the challenge is reduced. Alternatively, if the task at hand is to complete and collate papers for four hours, and a high level manager is relegated to perform this task, that manager might feel bored and even frustrated after the first 15 minutes. In that case, the manager can find someone else to do that task who is better suited for it, such as an administrative assistant or an intern.

Both the Yerkes-Dodson law and the theory of flow highlight the importance of eustress (good stress), as a motivating factor for good performance. They also point out that having either too much or not enough stress can detract from performance. There is a sweet spot for stress.

THE BENEFITS OF STRESS

The good side of stress is that it can help motivate individuals to prepare for or perform a particular task, e.g., take a test, interview for a job, go on a social date, etc. Furthermore, depending on the circumstances, it can also have life-saving implications. For example, in response to danger, a person's autonomic nervous system (Figure 7-4) mediates physiologic changes that are aimed to increase survival. For example, when confronted by an acute stressor, such as a lion in the hunter-gatherer era or a terror attack in the modern era, the sympathetic nervous system kicks into immediate action. The body ramps up its responses and devotes all of its energy to facing or avoiding the enemy. The heart rate increases so that more blood can be pumped to muscles, including the heart muscle. The respiratory rate increases to increase the supply of oxygen. Blood is diverted to the muscles, away from the organs. Glucose is released by the liver to provide energy for running or fighting. The stress hormones/brain chemicals adrenaline, epinephrine, norepinephrine, and cortisol are also released. The bladder relaxes, and the rectum contracts to prevent elimination. This sequence of physiologic changes is known as the flight-or-fight response and promotes a person's survival in the face of an existential threat.

THE DARK SIDE OF STRESS

Stress has a dark side when it simmers chronically in the background of the daily lives of people. This chronic stress can be harmful to an individual's health. In the modern era, the stresses that individuals face are not in the form of lions, tigers, and bears, but in the form of paperwork, colleagues, and information overload. In fact, people's minds often create existential threats where none actually exist by virtue of their thinking patterns. The mind can be so powerful that it can control the body's physiology. The body does not recognize the different sources of the stress response (i.e., project deadline vs. lion in the wild), it merely responds to the autonomic processes by releasing stress hormones, regardless of the physical situation.

The release of stress hormones is regulated by the hypothalamic pituitary adrenal (HPA) axis (Figure 7-5). In the presence of stress, the hypothalamus releases corticotropin-releasing hormone (CRH), prompting the pituitary to release adrenocorticotropic hormone (ACTH), which signals the adrenal gland to release the hormones cortisol along with epinephrine and norepinephrine into the blood. Cortisol is released for several hours after a stressful event before the body returns to a state of homeostasis (balance).

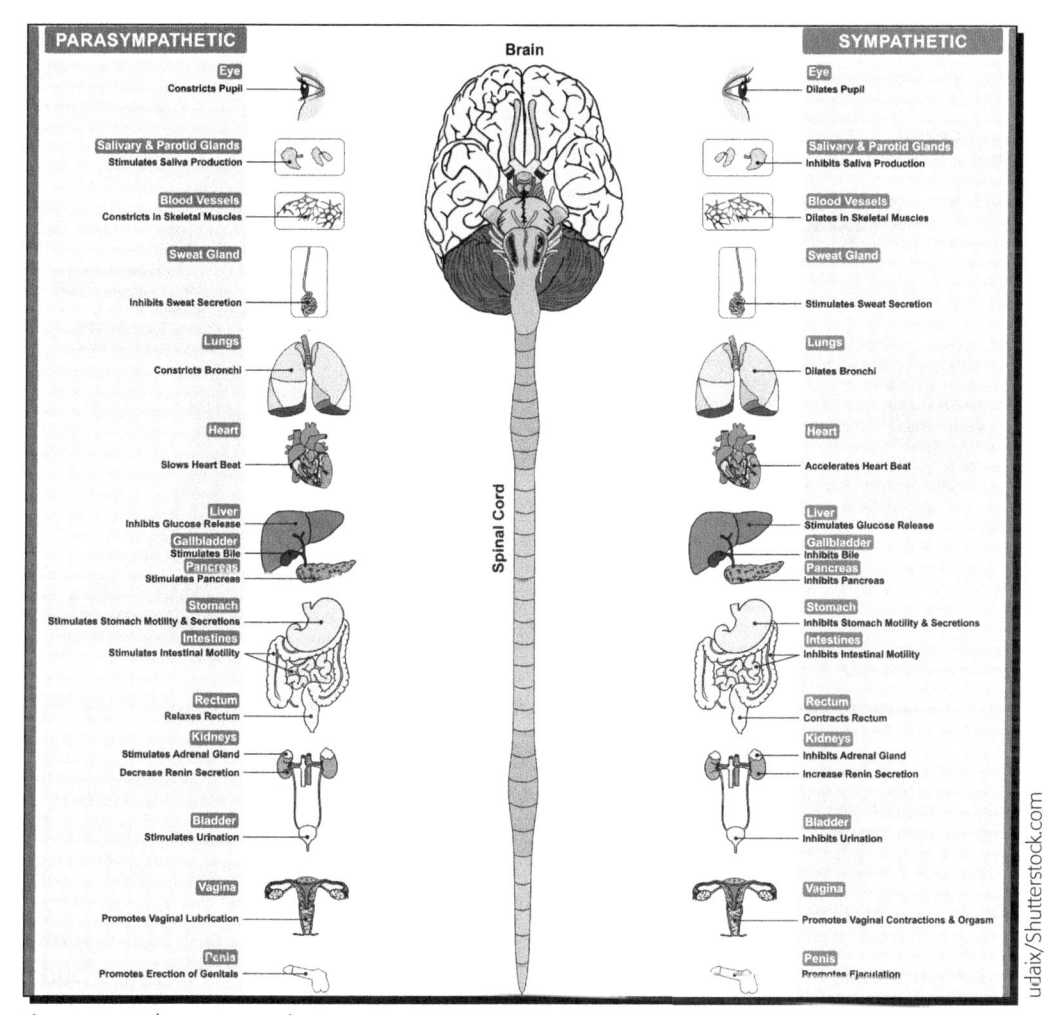

Figure 7-4. The autonomic nervous system

On the other hand, if stress is chronic, the body will habituate to the higher level of stress and the HPA axis will remain activated, which can have several negative consequences for the body. For example, chronic stress and an excess of cortisol can impair cognitive performance, dampen thyroid function, create a blood sugar imbalance such as hyperglycemia (too much sugar in the blood stream), decrease bone density, disrupt sleep, reduce muscle mass, elevate blood pressure, lower immune function, slow wound healing, and increase abdominal fat (which is more strongly correlated to heart problems than fat deposited in other areas of the body). It can also lead to heart attacks, strokes, higher LDL (the bad cholesterol) levels, and lower HDL (good) cholesterol levels, depression, and other health problems.

Excess cortisol can also damage the brain and block the formation of new connections in the hippocampus, which is the center of memory and learning. A study conducted by Lupien et al. in 1998 found that chronic stress can even reduce the

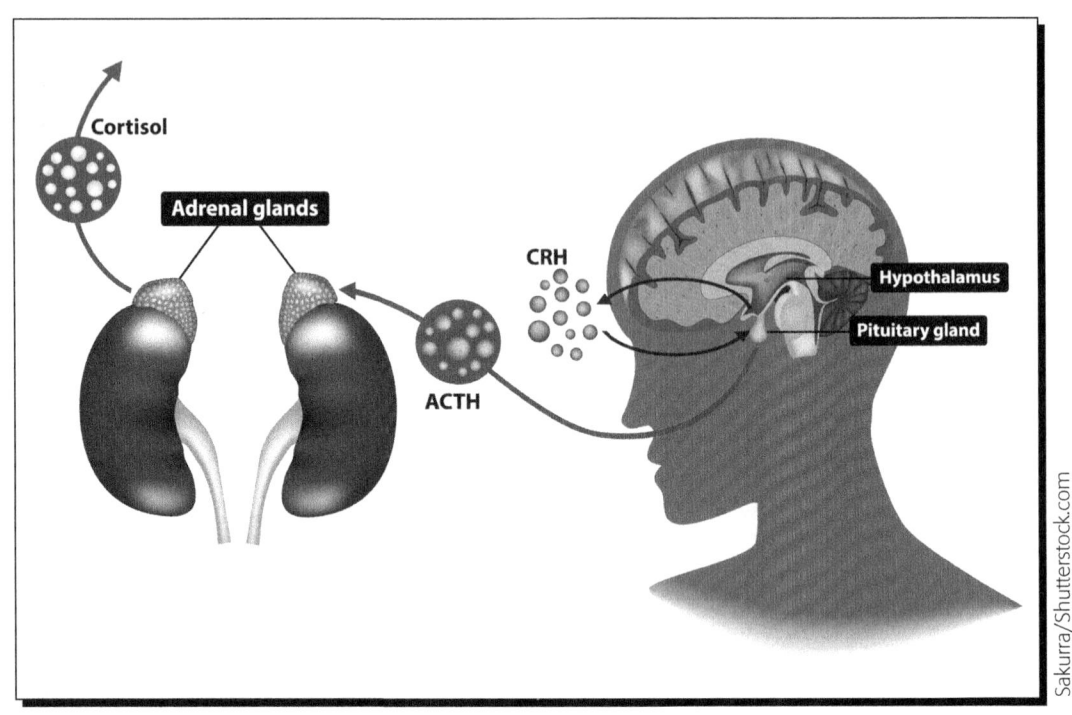

Figure 7-5. HPA axis

size of the hippocampus. These researchers looked at a group of elderly subjects and found on magnetic resonance imaging (MRI) that hippocampal size was reduced by 14 percent in those with significant and prolonged elevations in cortisol levels. They also had the subjects negotiate a maze, which showed that those individuals who had the highest levels of cortisol took the longest time to find their way out of the maze. In reality, if too little cortisol is produced, people may experience brain fog, cloudy-headedness, mild depression, low thyroid function, blood sugar imbalances such as hypoglycemia (too little sugar in the blood), fatigue, sleep disruption, low blood pressure, lowered immune function, and inflammation.

Like so many of the body's processes, the target is a fine line of delicate balance. Too much or too little of any one thing can be hazardous. The same life-saving responses in the body that were elicited by acute stress can become maladaptive responses when the stress becomes chronic. When this situation occurs, a person's health will suffer.

PSYCHOLOGICAL STRESS AND DISEASE

Until relatively recently, a number of people in the medical community were skeptical about the connection between psychological stress and disease. The tide turned as the evidence mounted in the medical literature. For example, a study published in *JAMA* in 2007 reviewed the literature and the way in which stress contributes to diseases such as clinical depression, cardiovascular disease, and human immunodeficiency virus

(HIV)/AIDS. Cohen et al. described psychological stress as occurring "when an individual perceives the environmental demands tax or exceed his or her adaptive capacity." They then went on to describe two pathways by which stress can induce disease:
- A behavioral pathway characterized by poor sleep, less exercise, less-than-optimal eating habits, a smoking habit, and non-adherence to medical treatments
- An endocrine pathway involving the HPA axis and the release of hormones that influence many organ systems and the immune system

With regard to depression, these authors cited social stressors, such as divorce, the death of a loved one, and the diagnosis of an illness or disease as connected to the development of depression. The mechanism by which this factor occurs appears to be that the increased stress level increases the cortisol level and decreases levels of neurotransmitters, such as serotonin, low levels of which are known to be associated with depression.

In reference to cardiovascular disease, they reported that chronic stress, such as workplace stress, is a contributor to cardiovascular disease because it raises norepinephrine levels, which increase the heart rate. Furthermore, with regard to HIV/AIDS, they reported that studies have shown a link between stress and the progression of AIDS. In fact, stress may even account for some of the variability seen in HIV progression from one patient to the next.

Other medical research articles have looked at stress, health, psychological, behavioral, and biological factors. For example, elevated levels of stress hormones, such as cortisol and norepinephrine, suppress immunity by altering the actions of cytokines—cell-signaling molecules that are produced by immune cells.

LIVE AND LEARN WITH DR. BETH FRATES

When I was a medical student, my professor, Dr. Michael Kay, instructed me to read through a study conducted by Alan Rozanski, et al., entitled "Mental Stress and the Induction of Silent Myocardial Ischemia in Patients with Coronary Artery Disease" that had been published in The New England Journal of Medicine *in 1988. He said we were going to replicate the experiment using me as the stressor.*

The researchers in the study enrolled several cardiac patients and put them through different mental stresses, asking them to do mental arithmetic or speak in public, for instance, and compared their responses on electrocardiogram (ECG) to those induced by exercise. The results showed that mental stress induced just as much myocardial ischemia—a reduction in blood flow to the heart that prevents the heart from receiving oxygen—as physical activity in these patients, and that ischemia was often "silent," meaning it didn't produce any symptoms. This type of ischemia is often a precursor to a heart attack.

To replicate this experiment Dr. Kay had me wear a white coat and go into a room with a person who had signed up for a study and was hooked up to an ECG machine. I was not to smile or make eye contact, which inevitably made the person uncomfortable and stressed, but that was part of the study. I was to say "Hello, I'm here to do the study with you. Are you ready?" When he or she replied, I was to ask the person to do an exercise called serial sevens, where you have to mentally subtract seven from 100 and so on. And I was to speed up the rate of the subtractions as the exercise went on, goading the person to do it faster. When the person gave a wrong answer, I had to say "No, do it again." This was actually very stressful for both the subject and for me—one person even cried.

Not surprisingly—at least from what we know today about psychological stress—the ECG results were similar to those seen in the study published in The New England Journal of Medicine: *The subjects had signs of silent ischemia. (I actually wish Dr. Kay had also hooked me up to an ECG machine; I wonder what my results would have been in this stressful situation!) I was very affected by this experiment and its results, and it solidified the value of mind/body medicine for me.*

THE IMPACT OF STRESS ON THE 11 SYSTEMS OF THE BODY

Although stress does not impact all 11 systems of the body equally, it does affect each of them to a degree, sometimes resulting in serious health-related consequences.

❑ Circulatory System

An acute stress, such as slamming on the brakes to avoid a traffic accident, causes an increase in the heart's rate and force of contraction, mediated by the release of cortisol, adrenaline, and noradrenaline. Blood is shunted away from the digestive system to the large muscles of the body (in preparation for running away). Heart rate increases as does blood pressure—all part of the flight-or-fight response. Chronic stress, however, may contribute to inflammation in the body's circulatory system, particularly in the coronary arteries, which increases the risk for hypertension, heart attack, and stroke.

❑ Digestive System

Stress can affect the body's digestive system in a number of ways. For example, it can cause the esophagus to go into spasms. It can also elevate the level of acid in the stomach, which can lead to indigestion. The stress of a serious illness can actually cause a medically defined "stress ulcer." Furthermore, while stress may not directly cause celiac disease or inflammatory bowel disease (e.g. Crohn's disease, ulcerative colitis), it can make all of these digestion-related diseases worse.

❑ Endocrine System

Stress leads to the release of the hormone cortisol, which is produced by the adrenal glands. Cortisol plays an important role in the regulation of blood pressure, as well as the normal functioning of several other systems of the body, including circulatory, respiratory, and reproduction. Excess cortisol can become taxing on the body and result in several negative endocrine changes, including, but not limited to, increased blood sugar, proteolysis (protein/muscle breakdown), and impairment of the immune system.

❏ Immune System

The increased cortisol discussed previously depresses the immune system. A number of the physical changes caused by depression (a condition correlated with stress), such as insomnia, are believed to weaken the body's immune system, as well. Furthermore, this factor can worsen any existing illnesses an individual may have.

❏ Dermatologic System

Stress can result in decreased blood flow to the skin, inelasticity of the skin, destabilization of glandular functions, and an interruption of tissue restoration. It can also slow wound-healing. In addition, stress increases the frequency of flares of eczema, psoriasis, and neurodermatitis, which causes severe itching of the skin.

❏ Muscular System

Stress can lead to the body's muscles being reflexively tense, which is characteristic of the body entering its fight-or-flight response. Essentially, chronic stress keeps the muscular system in a constant state of tightness and guardedness. When muscles are chronically tense, a person is more likely to experience tension-related conditions, such as headaches and migraines. Chronic muscle tension can also lead to stress-related pain in various areas of the body, including the shoulder, lower-back, upper-back, neck, hand/wrist, and elbow/forearm.

❏ Nervous System

The nervous system is comprised of the central nervous system (the spinal cord and brain) and the peripheral nervous system. The brain is the conductor of the stress response by first determining what is stressful and then sending the hormonal signals to trigger the flight-or-fight response in the other organs. There is enormous variation in the response to stress from person-to-person, based upon prior experiences, as well as some genetic variation. Brain regions, such as the hippocampus, prefrontal cortex, and amygdala, respond to acute and chronic stress and show changes in morphology and chemistry when activated.

The amygdala, part of a person's "primitive brain" or limbic system, activates emotions, such as anger or fear, in order to protect us from threats. In low or moderate stress situations, an individual's more "rational" or thinking brain—known as the prefrontal cortex—can override and calm the amygdala down, such that a person regains conscious control and decision-making ability. When the amygdala is triggered by extreme stress, however, it shuts off the prefrontal cortex and acts independently to stimulate an individual's behavioral response. This can be adaptive if a person's response is to dodge a reckless driver, but maladaptive, if an individual, for example, lashes out at colleagues, friends, and family.

The peripheral nervous system is further divided into the autonomic (ANS), somatic (controlling the muscles), and enteric (controlling the gastrointestinal tract) nervous systems. The ANS is comprised of the parasympathetic nervous system (PNS) and the sympathetic nervous system (SNS). The PNS is responsible for the state of rest and digestion, while the SNS is responsible for the state of fight or flight. Constant stress can lead to repeated cycles of the stress response, as well as deplete the body's resources over time.

❑ Reproductive System

Stress can be a drain on the reproductive system of both men and women. For men, evidence exists that mild-to-severe emotional stress not only depresses the production of testosterone, it can also interfere with spermatogenesis (the process of producing spermatozoa). Some indications also suggest that stress can have variable effects on testicular morphology.

For women, stress is believed to inhibit their reproductive functioning. It may also be responsible for "hypothalamic" amenorrhea. Furthermore, during the postpartum phase that pregnant women experience, stress is perceived as an indirect contributing agent for the occurrence of bouts of blues/depression and an increased level of autoimmune phenomena. In fact, stress, distraction, and fatigue may reduce sex drive and libido for both men and women.

❑ Respiratory System

Stress can affect the respiratory system of the body in a number of ways. For example, acute stress causes an individual to breathe faster, in an effort to quickly distribute oxygen-rich blood to the body. If an individual already has a respiratory-related problem (i.e., asthma, COPD, emphysema, chronic bronchitis, etc.), stress can make it more difficult to breathe. In addition, hyperventilation can trigger panic attacks.

❑ Skeletal System

Chronic stress can lead to a decreased level of bone density. Chronic stress alters the normal functioning of the hypothalamic-pituitary-adrenal signaling system, which controls levels of cortisol. High cortisol levels are considered a risk factor for bone loss, osteoporosis, and bone fracture.

❑ Renal/Urinary System

Stress can damage the kidneys. As the organs of the body that filter the blood, a person's kidneys are prone to problems with blood circulation and blood vessels. High blood pressure, which occurs when the body goes into fight or flight, can place an even greater burden on an individual's kidneys, especially if it lasts a long time and becomes a chronic condition.

The pathophysiology underlying the potential effect of stress on the urinary system remains unclear. An undue level of stress can lead to a variety of problems with urinary tract functioning, such as incontinence. In animal models, there is evidence that repeated psychological stress can affect urinary frequency and volume. Most people have probably experienced the sense of urgency to go to the bathroom before a big talk, a performance, or an examination of some kind. Some people have reported losing control of their bladder during a terrifying experience.

In fact, research demonstrates that there is a connection between overactive bladder (OAB) and psychological stress. The biology of the stress response, the fight-or-flight response, reveals that because the person who is fleeing from a frightening situation or getting ready to fight a lion will be too busy to urinate, the bladder will relax, and the urinary sphincter will constrict, keeping the urine in the bladder.

The urinary system is complicated. There are hormones released during a stressful event, which might be the reason that stress can have different effects on urination, depending on the person and depending on the level of danger and fear experienced by the individual.

In light of the biological effects of persistently elevated stress hormones, it makes sense that patients who suffer from chronic stress find themselves prone to more frequent and severe viral infections, as well as more serious health conditions, such as diabetes, heart disease, high blood pressure, and depression.

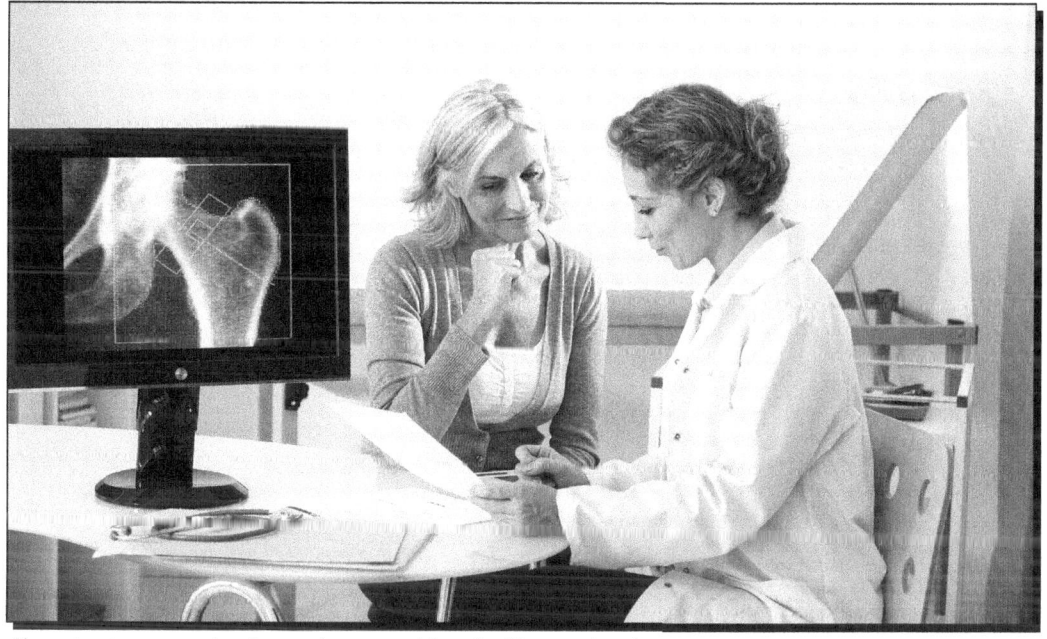

Chronic stress can lead to a decreased level of bone density.

RISK FACTORS AND SYMPTOMS OF CHRONIC STRESS

Stress can result from a variety of factors—external, internal, and physical, as well as psychological. The key is for the lifestyle medicine practitioner to ascertain what stressors are affecting a particular patient (yet another set of circumstances in which using the Frates COACH Approach with an emphasis on curiosity, open-mindedness, appreciation, compassion, and honesty could be very helpful), and then to develop an appropriate strategy for addressing the situation. Among the factors that can contribute to stress are the following:

- ❏ External Factors
  - Environmental issues
  - Everyday hassles
  - Family-related issues
  - Financial problems
  - Major life events
  - Other people
  - Work-related issues

- ❏ Internal Factors
  - Excessive caffeine
  - Insomnia
  - Highly processed food
  - Recreational drugs
  - Smoking

- ❏ Physical Factors
  - Excessive exercising
  - Illness
  - Injury
  - Lack of exercise
  - Obesity
  - Repetitive motion
  - Starvation

- ❏ Psychological Factors
  - An all-or-nothing attitude
  - Anxiety

- Being unduly pessimistic
- Fear
- Feelings of stress and pressure
- Reacting to life changes (e.g., the death of a loved one, divorce, etc.)
- Relationship issues
- Rigidity of thinking
- Taking things personally
- Unrealistic expectations

Furthermore, in the daily lives of patients, the effect of stress on an individual can manifest in a diverse array of symptoms. Being able to recognize the following symptoms can provide physicians and allied healthcare professionals with a relative jump on successfully managing them:

❑ Common Effects of Stress on the Body

- Change in sex drive
- Chest pain
- Fatigue
- Headache
- Muscle tension or pain
- Sleeplessness
- Upset stomach

❑ Common Effects of Stress on Mood (Thoughts and Feelings)

- Anxiety
- Feeling of being overwhelmed
- Irritability or anger
- Lack of focus or motivation
- Restlessness
- Sadness or depression

❑ Common Effects of Stress on Behavior

- Abusing drugs or alcohol
- Engaging in outbursts of anger
- Exercising less frequently
- Overeating or undereating
- Using tobacco
- Withdrawing socially

BUILDING RESISTANCE TO STRESS

Some individuals are better able to adapt well to the stress that they face (e.g., adversity, financial matters, health issues, relationship problems, trauma, tragedy, threats, workplace issues, etc.), than others. On the other hand, because people are relatively resilient to stress doesn't mean that they don't experience difficult times or stressful circumstances. Based on the data presented in this chapter, there is a need for lifestyle medicine practitioners to help their patients develop stress resiliency to fight the numerous symptoms and diseases associated with chronic stress.

For starters, Dr. Hans Selye offered several recommendations for living wisely:
- Adopt an attitude of gratitude.
- Be altruistic rather than self-centered.
- Retain a capacity for wonder and delight in life.
- Find a purpose in life.
- Keep a healthy sense of modesty about accomplishments and goals.

Other generalized recommendations to help cultivate resiliency include the following:
- Nurture a positive view of yourself.
- Treat problematic circumstances as a learning process.
- Develop a healthy sense of self-confidence.
- Embrace change.
- Form and maintain relationships.

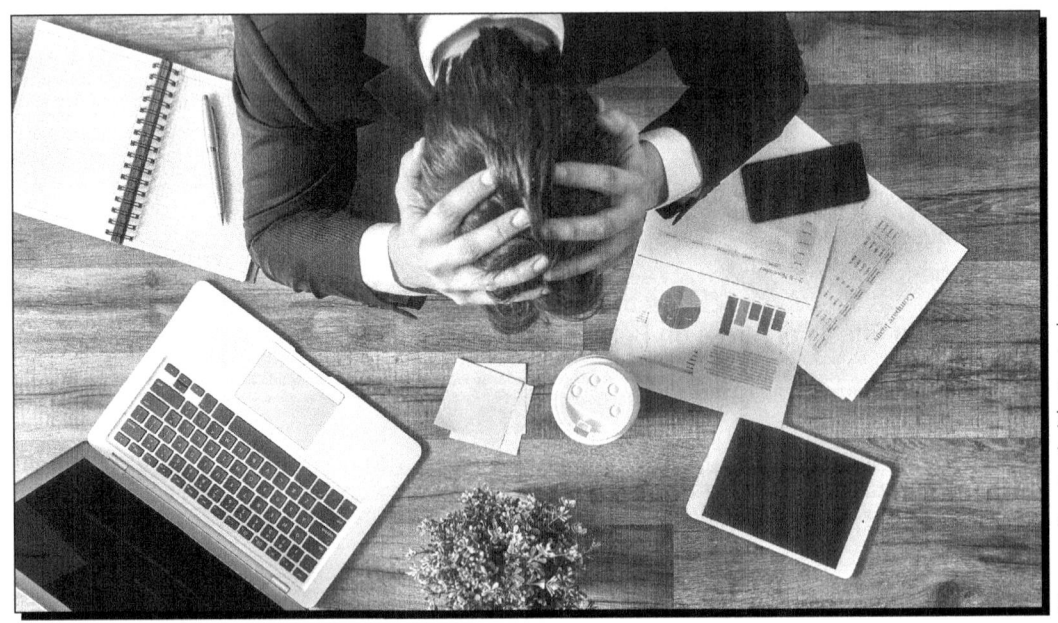

Because people are relatively resilient to stress doesn't mean that they don't experience difficult times or stressful circumstances.

- Learn to unwind (relax).
- Find time to move (exercise).
- Make an effort to find joy.
- Don't sweat the small stuff.
- Accept the fact that some things are beyond being controlled.
- Make sure to sleep seven to eight hours a night.
- Eat a healthy diet, focusing on consuming plants (vegetables, fruits, whole grains, nuts, seeds, beans, and legumes) and avoiding processed foods (sugar, white bread, white pasta, pastries, and processed/packaged foods).

LIVE AND LEARN WITH DR. BETH FRATES

When coaching a colleague who was struggling with a few excess pounds, he wanted to review his eating and exercise routines, right away. He felt confident that if he got on the right diet and found time to exercise, that he would get back to a normal BMI. He was a family physician with a hectic schedule and teenage boys at home. His wife was a great cook and got on board with the plant-based eating program right away. The patient started walking routinely after dinner and frequently took his wife and dog along on his daily excursion

Subsequently, all was going well, he had lost six pounds in three weeks, and was very pleased. Then, came his weekend of call. This situation is when the impact of stress on his eating habits became quite clear. We met the Monday morning after his call, and he was distraught. The first thing he said was, "Well, I blew it! All this hard work over three weeks, all to be undone with one weekend of call. I ate everything in the refrigerator, as well as all the cookies in the house."

He then went on to explain that similar episodes of "stress-eating" happened during his call weekends and during other events that were emotionally charged and stressful. I responded with, "This is good news!" He looked puzzled. I went on to explain that it was great that we uncovered this problem, while working together and that now we can brainstorm solutions around it for the future. Not only would this effort reduce stress, it would also help control these unhealthy eating binges, and thus, reduce his weight. He seemed surprised by my excitement.

Once we got into the "meat and potatoes" of the problem, he started to better understand the impact of this particular stressful weekend of call. Subsequently, we spent a great deal of time discussing deep breathing and empowering self-talk that he could use in the moment when he felt overwhelmed by a stressful situation. In addition, we created a specific plan for his call weekends. His house would be devoid of cookies, ice cream, and processed foods. Instead, it would be full of vegetables, fruits, nuts, seeds, and some dark chocolates (greater than 85 percent cocoa) that he could use in a homemade nut mix. The menus for the weekends (breakfast, lunch, and dinner) would be planned out. Furthermore, stress-relieving activities, like walks, listening to his favorite music, watching a good movie, and other relaxing activities, were planned. He picked up playing bridge with his wife, which became a favorite activity during stressful weekends. Accordingly, in this case, the difficulty with weight control was directly related to his difficulty with managing stress.

To reiterate, everyone is at risk for stress. The key is for a person is to avoid allowing stress to become chronic and to reach a level that is harmful to their health.

In the next chapter, the relaxation response, meditation, yoga, and mindfulness-based stress reduction will be reviewed in detail. These techniques help people to manage stress in the moment and to build stress resilience.

FITT PRESCRIPTIONS FOR STRESS RESILIENCY

Adopting an attitude of gratitude, finding the beauty and wonder in the world, and identifying a purpose in life can really help people build stress resiliency. The following are sample prescriptions for fostering stress resiliency. Chapter 8 features a focus on relaxation, meditation, and mindfulness, all of which are wonderful tools for stress management and stress resiliency.

❑ Find a purpose:

   F—one evening in the week
   I—spend focused quality time alone for contemplation
   T—one hour
   T—write down your strengths, gifts, and talents and how you can use them to make the world a better place. Work to craft a personal mission statement that reflects your unique purpose in this world.

❑ Express gratitude:

   F—five nights in the week
   I—focus on the things for which you feel gratitude
   T—spend 5 to 10 minutes
   T—write down two to three things for which you are grateful in a gratitude journal

❑ Finding the beauty in the world around you:

   F—once a week
   I—focus on the flowers, birds, or trees where you live
   T—10 to 20 minutes
   T—make careful observations of the nature that surrounds you. Use all of your senses whenever possible. Consider either writing down any observations that you make or drawing a picture of what you see. What are you curious about? What questions come to mind as you engross yourself in nature?

KEY POINTS/TAKEAWAYS FOR CHAPTER 7

❑ Chapter Review:

- Overall goal: Review the factors that lead to stress.
- Application goal: Understand the connection between stress and health.

❑ Discussion Questions:

- How does stress affect a person's health?
- What are some of the best pieces of advice that could be given to a patient who is suffering from chronic stress?
- What impact does stress have on each of the body's 11 systems?
- What does the fight-or-flight response entail?
- What are some of the risk factors and symptoms associated with chronic stress?

	TITLE	AUTHORS	JOURNAL	YEAR	KEY FINDINGS
1	Psychological stress and disease	Cohen S, Janicki-Deverts D, Miller GE	JAMA	2007	A commentary that defined psychological stress occurring "when an individual perceives that environmental demands tax or exceed his or her adaptive capacity." It further discusses how stress contributes to depression, cardiovascular disease, and progression of HIV/AIDS.
2	Counting blessings versus burdens: an experimental investigation of gratitude and subjective well-being in daily life	Emmons RA, McCullough ME	Journal of Personality and Social Psychology	2003	A series of three small studies of undergraduate students that suggest that "the gratitude-outlook groups exhibited heightened well-being across several, though not all, of the outcomes measured across the studies, relative to the comparison groups" (i.e., more gratitude, greater sense of feeling connected to others, increased optimism and positive feelings, less depression, higher sleep quality). The interventions seemed to have the largest effect on positive affect.
3	Optimism and the experience of pain: benefits of seeing the glass as half full	Goodin BR, Bulls HW	Current Pain and Headache Reports	2013	This review article explores the health-promoting effects of having an optimistic outlook. It finds that optimism is linked to "enhanced physiological recovery and psychosocial adjustment to coronary artery bypass surgery, bone marrow transplantation, postpartum depression, traumatic brain injury, Alzheimer's disease, lung cancer, breast cancer, and failed in vitro fertilization." Furthermore, "optimism seems to benefit the pain experience and its course of treatment."

Figure 7-6. Stress resilience evidence

	TITLE	AUTHORS	JOURNAL	YEAR	KEY FINDINGS
4	High evening cortisol level is associated with low TBS and increased prevalent vertebral fractures: OsteoLaus study	Gonzalez Rodriguez E, Lamy O, Stoll D	*Journal of Clinical Endocrinology and Metabolism*	2017	A cross-sectional study of 608 post-menopausal women that found that having a high evening salivary cortisol level was associated with a low trabecular bone score and an increased prevalence of radiologic vertebral fractures independently of other risk factors.
5	Correlation between psychological stress levels and the severity of overactive bladder symptoms	Lai H, et al.	*BMC Urology*	2015	A study of 51 subjects diagnosed with an overactive bladder that compared stress levels in these individuals to stress levels in patients diagnosed with interstitial cystitis/bladder pain syndrome (n=27) and healthy controls (n=30). They found that stress levels in subjects with an overactive bladder and interstitial cystitis/bladder pain syndrome were significantly higher than healthy controls. "There was a positive correlation between perceived stress levels and urinary incontinence symptoms, and its impacts on quality of life among overactive bladder patients."
6	The grateful disposition: a conceptual and empirical topography	McCullough ME, Emmons RA, Tsang JA	*Journal of Personal Sociology and Psychology*	2002	Researchers examined the correlates of the disposition toward gratitude in a series of four studies. Using a gratitude questionnaire, they found that higher scores (6-7) on the questionnaire were associated with increased positive emotions, life satisfaction, vitality, optimism, capacity to be empathetic, and levels of generosity, along with lower depression and stress. Higher scores of gratitude enhanced good feelings better than it decreased unpleasant emotions. Furthermore, the authors found that grateful people do not deny or ignore negative emotions, feelings, or events.
7	Mechanisms of stress in the brain	McEwen BS, et al.	*Nature Neuroscience*	2015	Discusses some of the underlying mechanisms of plasticity and vulnerability of the brain to help provide a "basis for understanding the efficacy of interventions for anxiety and depressive disorders as well as age-related cognitive decline."

Figure 7-6. Stress resilience evidence (cont.)

	TITLE	AUTHORS	JOURNAL	YEAR	KEY FINDINGS
8	Mental stress and the induction of silent myocardial ischemia in patients with coronary artery disease	Rozanski A, et al.	New England Journal of Medicine	1988	A study of 39 patients with coronary artery disease and 12 controls that assessed the causal relationship between acute mental stress and myocardial ischemia. They had patients perform a series of mental tasks and compared the responses to those induced by exercise using radionuclide ventriculography. It found that "the magnitude of cardiac dysfunction induced by the speaking task was similar to that induced by exercise," and that "personally relevant mental stress may be an important precipitant of myocardial ischemia—often silent—in patients with coronary artery disease."
9	Stress and health: psychological, behavioral, and biological determinants	Schneiderman N, Ironson G, Siegel SD	Annual Review of Clinical Psychology	2005	Explores the relationship between stress and health and found that chronic stress results in increased basal levels of stress hormones, suppressed immunity via cytokines, and increased pro-inflammatory cytokine production.
10	The effects of acute and chronic psychological stress on bladder function in a rodent model	Smith AL, Leung J, Kun S	Urology	2011	A study of 24 rats that sought to evaluate the effect that psychological stress has on bladder function. Researchers found that "repeated psychological stress results in lasting alterations in micturition interval, and volume."

References

1. Cohen S, Janicki-Deverts D, Miller GE. Psychological stress and disease. *JAMA.* 2007;298:1685-1687.
2. Emmons RA, McCullough ME. Counting blessings versus burdens: an experimental investigation of gratitude and subjective well-being in daily life. *Journal of Personality and Social Psychology.* 2003;84:377-389.
3. Goodin BR, Bulls HW. Optimism and the experience of pain: benefits of seeing the glass as half full. *Current Pain and Headache Reports.* 2013;17(5):329. doi:10.1007/s11916-013-0329-8.
4. Gonzalez Rodriguez E, Lamy O, Stoll D. High evening cortisol level is associated with low TBS and increased prevalent vertebral fractures: OsteoLaus study. *Journal of Clinical Endocrinology and Metabolism.* July 1 2017;102(7):2628-2636. doi:10.1210/jc.2016-3804
5. Lai H, Gardner V, Vetter J, et al. Correlation between psychological stress levels and the severity of overactive bladder symptoms. *BMC Urology.* 2015;15:14.
6. McCullough ME, Emmons RA, Tsang JA. The grateful disposition: a conceptual and empirical topography. *Journal of Personal Sociology and Psychology.* 2002;82:112-127.
7. McEwen BS, Bowles NP, Gray JD, et al. Mechanisms of stress in the brain. *Nature Neuroscience.* October 2015;18(10):1353-1363.
8. Rozanski A, Bairey CN, Krantz DS, et al. Mental stress and the induction of silent myocardial ischemia in patients with coronary artery disease. *New England Journal of Medicine.* 1988;318:1005-1012.
9. Schneiderman N, Ironson G, Siegel SD. Stress and health: psychological, behavioral, and biological determinants. *Annual Review of Clinical Psychology.* 2005;1:607-628. doi:10.1146/annurev.clinpsy.1.102803.144141.
10. Smith AL, Leung J, Kun S. The effects of acute and chronic psychological stress on bladder function in a rodent model. *Urology.* October 2011;78(4):967.e1-967.e7.

Figure 7-6. Stress resilience evidence (cont.)

REFERENCES

- AdrenalFatigue.org. Cortisol & Adrenal Function. Available at: http://adrenalfatigue.org/cortisol-adrenal-function/. Accessed June 2018.
- American Heart Association. Stress Management. Available at: http://www.heart.org/HEARTORG/HealthyLiving/StressManagement/Stress-Management_UCM_001082_SubHomePage.jsp. Accessed September 2017.
- American Psychological Association. How Stress Affects Your Health. Available at: http://www.apa.org/helpcenter/stress.aspx. Accessed September 2017.
- American Psychological Association. Stress. Available at: http://www.apa.org/topics/stress/index.aspx. Accessed September 2017.
- Benson H. *The Relaxation Response.* New York: William Morrow; 2000.
- Cohen S, Janicki-Deverts D, Miller GE. Psychological stress and disease. *JAMA.* 2007;298(14):1685-1687. doi:10.1001/jama.298.14.1685.
- Csikzentmihalyi M. *Flow: The Psychology of Optimal Experience.* New York: HarperCollins Publishers; 1991.
- Egger G, Binns A, Rossner S. Stress. In: Egger G, Binns A, Rossner S, eds. *Lifestyle Medicine: Managing Diseases of Lifestyle in the 21st Century.* North Ryde, N.S.W.: McGraw-Hill; 2010.
- Fernandez A, Goldberg E, Michelon P. *The SharpBrains Guide to Brain Fitness.* San Francisco: SharBrains; 2013.
- Genazzani AD. Neuroendocrine aspects of amenorrhea related to stress. *Pediatric Endocrinology Reviews.* 2005;2:661-668.
- Gonzalez Rodriguez E, Lamy O, Stoll D. High evening cortisol level is associated with low TBS and increased prevalent vertebral fractures: OsteoLaus study. *Journal of Clinical Endocrinology and Metabolism.* 2017;102(7):2628-2636. doi:10.1210/jc.2016-3804.
- Hardy R, Cooper MS. Adrenal gland and bone. *Archives of Biochemistry and Biophysics.* November 1 2010;503(1):137-145.
- Harvard Health Publications. Stress. Available at: https://www.health.harvard.edu/topics/stress. Accessed September 2017.
- *Health and Wellness for Life.* Champaign, IL: Human Kinetics; 2010.
- Healthline. The Effects of Stress on Your Body. Available at: http://www.healthline.com/health/stress/effects-on-body. Accessed September 2017.
- Helpguide.org. Stress Symptoms, Signs, and Causes. Available at: https://www.helpguide.org/articles/stress/stress-symptoms-signs-and-causes.htm. Accessed September 2017.
- Henneicke H, Li J, Kim S. Chronic mild stress causes bone loss via an osteoblast-specific glucocorticoid-dependent mechanism. *Endocrinology.* June 1 2017;158(6):1939-1950. doi:10.1210/en.2016-1658.

- Lai H, Gardner V, Vetter J, Andriole GL. Correlation between psychological stress levels and the severity of overactive bladder symptoms. *BMC Urology.* 2015;15:14.
- Lupien SJ, de Leon M, de Santi S, et al. Cortisol levels during human aging predict hippocampal atrophy and memory deficits. *Nature Neuroscience.* 1998;1:69-73.
- Mayo Clinic. Stress Basics. Available at: http://www.mayoclinic.org/healthy-lifestyle/stress-management/basics/stress-basics/hlv-20049495. Accessed September 2017.
- Mayo Clinic. Stress Symptoms: Effects on Your Body and Behavior. Available at: http://www.mayoclinic.org/healthy-lifestyle/stress-management/in-depth/stress-symptoms/art-20050987. Accessed September 2017.
- McEwen BS, et al. Mechanisms of stress in the brain. *Nature Neuroscience.* October 2015;18(10):1353-1363.
- McGrady AV. Effects of psychological stress on male reproduction: a review. *Archives of Andrology.* 1984;13:1-7.
- MedicineNet.com. Stress. Available at: http://www.medicinenet.com/stress/article.htm. Accessed September 2017.
- Merriam-Webster. Resilience. Available at: https://www.merriam-webster.com/dictionary/resilience. Accessed June 2018.
- Mönnikes H, Tebbe JJ, Hildebrandt M, et al. Role of stress in functional gastrointestinal disorders. *Digestive Diseases.* 2001;19(3):201-211.
- Nani BD, Lima PO, Marcondes FK. Changes in salivary microbiota increase volatile sulfur compound production in healthy male subjects with academic-related chronic stress. *Public Library of Science One.* Mar 20 2017;12(3):e0173686.
- National Institute of Mental Health. 5 Things You Should Know About Stress. Available at: https://www.nimh.nih.gov/health/publications/stress/index.shtml. Accessed September 2017.
- Rosch PJ. Reminiscences of Hans Selye, and the Birth of "Stress." The American Institute of Stress. Available at: https://www.stress.org/about/hans-selye-birth-of-stress/. Accessed June 2018.
- Rozanski A, Bairey CN, Krantz DS, et al. Mental stress and the induction of silent myocardial ischemia in patients with coronary artery disease. *New England Journal of Medicine.* 1988;318(16):1005-1012.
- Schneiderman N, Ironson G, Siegel SD. Stress and health: psychological, behavioral, and biological determinants. *Annual Review of Clinical Psychology.* 2005;1:607-628. doi:10.1146/annurev.clinpsy.1.102803.144141.
- Selye H. Stress and the general adaptation syndrome. *British Medical Journal.* 1950;1(4667):1383-1392.
- Selye H. *Stress Without Distress.* New York: Penguin Publishing Group; 1975.
- Selye H. *The Stress of Life.* Englewood, NJ: McGraw-Hill Education; 1978.
- Smith AL, Leung J, Kun S. The effects of acute and chronic psychological stress on bladder function in a rodent model. *Urology.* October 2011;78(4):967.e1-967.e7.

- Stress and Coping. Available at: http://rgtonks.ca/Courses/Health/Stress/stress.htm. Accessed July 2018.
- Teigen KH. Yerkes-Dodson: a law for all seasons. *Theory and Psychology.* 1994;4:525-547.
- The American Institute of Stress. Stress Effects. Available at: https://www.stress.org/stress-effects/. Accessed September 2017.
- Total Body Psychology. The Stress Response...and How It Relates to the HPA Axis! Available at: http://www.total-body-psychology.com.au/stress-response---hpa-axis.html. Accessed August 2018.
- Tsigos C, Kyrou I, Kassi E, et al. Stress, endocrine physiology and pathophysiology. [Updated 2016 Mar 10]. In: De Groot LJ, Chrousos G, Dungan K, et al., eds. Endotext [Internet]. South Dartmouth (MA): MDText.com, Inc.; 2000-. Available at: https://www.ncbi.nlm.nih.gov/books/NBK278995/. Accessed August 2018.
- WebMD. Stress Management Health Center. Available at: http://www.webmd.com/balance/stress-management/default.htm. Accessed September 2017.
- WebMD. The Effects of Stress on Your Body. Available at: https://www.webmd.com/balance/stress-management/effects-of-stress-on-your-body. Accessed June 2018.

CHAPTER 8

PEACE OF MIND WITH MEDITATION, MINDFULNESS, AND RELAXATION

*"Whoever values peace of mind and the health
of the soul will live the best of all possible lives."*

—Marcus Aurelius
Emperor of Rome
161 to 180

❑ Chapter Goals:

- Define meditation, mindfulness, and relaxation techniques.
- Discuss the similarities and differences between meditation, mindfulness, and relaxation techniques.
- Introduce the concept of meditation.
- Explore different types of mindfulness.
- Explore the Relaxation Response.
- Understand how meditation, mindfulness, and the Relaxation Response affect the brain.

❑ Learning Objectives:

- To understand the connection between peace of mind and health
- To grasp the commonalities and difference among mindfulness, meditation, and relaxation
- To become familiar with the Relaxation Response
- To recognize the barriers to having peace of mind

❑ Guiding Questions:

- What is meditation?
- What is mindfulness-based stress reduction?
- What is the Relaxation Response?

- How does meditation affect the mind and the body?
- What is the evidence that meditation, mindfulness, and relaxation techniques have positive effects on health and stress reduction?

❏ Important Terms:

- *Meditation:* The *Merriam-Webster Dictionary Online* states that meditation is an act or process of spending time in quiet thought. The authors of *SharpBrains*, on the other hand, describe meditation as "[a] capacity-building technique to manage stress and build resilience."
- *Mindfulness:* The quality or state of being mindful, and the practice of a person maintaining a nonjudgmental state of heightened or complete awareness of their thoughts, emotions, or experience on a moment-to-moment basis
- *Mindfulness-based stress reduction (MBSR):* A program developed by Dr. Jon Kabat-Zinn that has been proven to have powerful benefits for health and well-being
- *Relaxation:* The ability to become or cause something to become less tense, tight, or stiff; to stop feeling nervous or worried; to spend time resting or doing something enjoyable, especially after you have been doing work
- *Relaxation Response:* A relaxation technique developed by Dr. Herbert Benson, who describes it "as your personal ability to encourage your body to release chemicals and brain signals that make your muscles and organs slow down and increase blood flow to the brain." The Relaxation Response, which has been validated in many clinical studies, has been shown to be beneficial in reducing stress and preventing cardiac and other events.

Stress is a fact of life in 21st century America. Excessive stress occurs for a variety of reasons, and results in a variety of sequelae. For example, people may not sleep well, or they may stop exercising because they do not have the time. They may eat to relieve their level of stress or use alcohol or drugs to escape stress. Individuals may avoid social interactions and gatherings and may become reactive when they do interact with others. People may also perceive their world in a negative light, and find it difficult to appreciate humorous situations. On occasion, many of these responses occur within the same person.

As discussed in Chapter 7, it is known that the stress reaction can have a deleterious effect on our bodies. The question becomes how can an individual diminish these harmful effects and build stress resilience? Some stress-relieving practices include exercise, which helps to develop new neurons and connections, and relaxation practices such as meditation, tai chi, yoga, and walking. Connecting and maintaining close relationships with friends and loved ones is also a great way to relieve stress, as is touch—giving and/or receiving a hug, for instance. Feeling empowered and in charge of what is occurring in a person's life is also beneficial in reducing stress as it increases their perceived locus of control. Other practices that have been shown to reduce stress are positive thinking, laughter, and humor. In fact, even imagining laughter can reduce self-reported sadness. Stress can also be managed via nutrition and the foods we eat.

Another stress-relieving practice can be creating and writing in a gratitude journal. Gratitude journals are used as part of the treatment of depression and have been shown to improve mood and reduce stress if used regularly. For instance, when treating a person with depression, the clinician can invite the person try writing down three things for which they are grateful every day. This practice can also be used when working with a person who is feeling stressed.

STEPS TO HELP CREATE PEACE OF MIND

Peace of mind can be obtained in a variety of ways. Depending on the patient and the circumstances, some options for creating peace of mind can be more effective than others, as well as less challenging or more difficult than others. The key is to match the strategy for developing peace of mind with the unique needs and characteristics of each patient. Among the possible suggestions that could be shared with a patient, are the following:

- Learn to relax and trust yourself. More often than not, everything tends to work out over time.
- Focus on the end game. Don't allow yourself to be distracted by mistakes or setbacks.
- See and accept things as they are, rather than what you would like or expect them to be. Have an understanding of what you can and can't control.
- Empower yourself with hope. Strive and grow, even when their circumstances may not be what you would like them to be.
- Channel your energy on moving forward. Be positive. Reject negativity.
- Be introspective. Think about how to proceed. Don't let current difficulties cloud your judgment.
- Be patient. Take life one step at a time. As a rule, life tends to be an incremental process.
- Have a view to the future. Look forward, not backward.

In addition to the coaching techniques reviewed in Chapters 2 and 3, it is useful for the lifestyle medicine practitioner to be armed with validated stress reduction techniques that have been shown to reduce distress, improve relaxation, and cultivate peace of mind. This chapter details three strategies, or "paths," that are gaining both scientific evidence and mainstream acceptance to help manage the pervasive and often unavoidable stress of our daily lives.

THREE PATHS TO REDUCE STRESS AND ATTAIN A PEACEFUL MIND

Considerable research suggests that managing stress and achieving peace of mind is one of the most important things that patients can do to enrich their health, as well as their sense of well-being. Meditation, mindfulness, and relaxation techniques are three paths that can be used to reduce stress and create a peaceful mind. This chapter explores how these practices are similar and different from one another, as well as some of the research that substantiates their time-tested effectiveness. Arguably, of the various commonalities and dissimilarities, the most noteworthy is the fact that all three can be powerful tools for achieving a variety of health-related benefits—for both mind and body.

PATH #1: MEDITATION

There are a variety of ways to define meditation. Going back to Latin roots, the word "meditation" originates from *meditationem*, which means "a thinking over." The *Merriam-Webster Dictionary Online* states that meditation is a discourse intended to express its author's reflections or to guide others in contemplation. This definition follows along the lines of "a thinking over." Interestingly, when used in the realm of stress reduction, the act of meditation involves clearing your mind of routine day-to-day worries and focusing on your breath, a number, or a mantra. It has also been described by Alvaro Fernandez and Dr. Elkhonon Goldberg, the authors of *The SharpBrains Guide to Brain Fitness*, as "[a] capacity-building technique to manage stress and build resilience." They further define it as an activity or process during which people "[go] beyond [their] automatic thinking to get to a deeper or more grounded state."

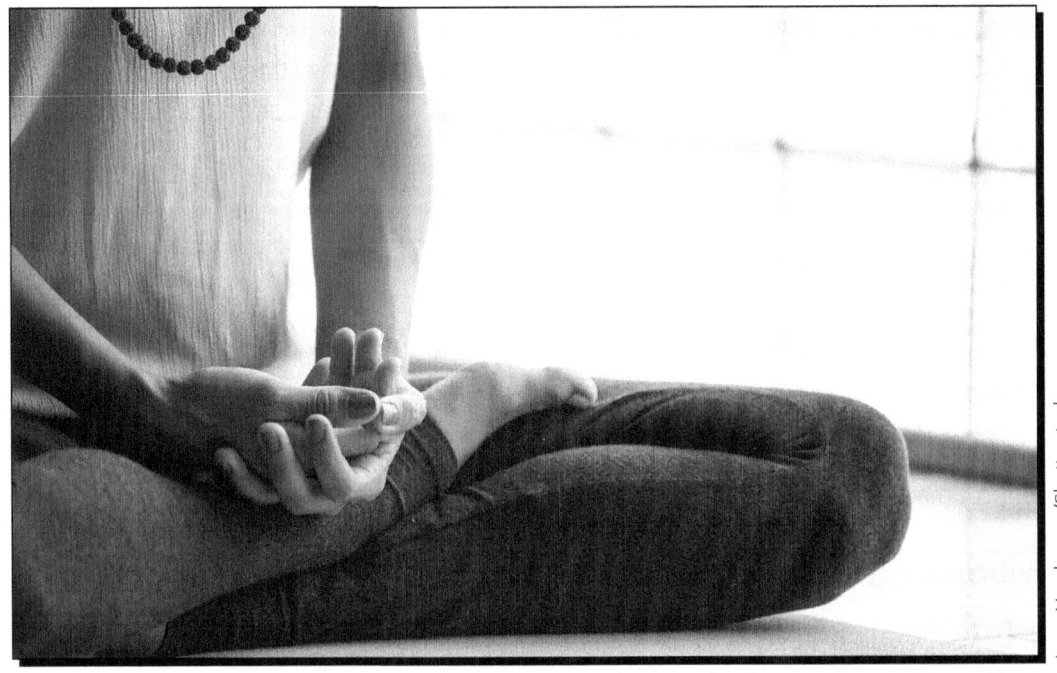

Meditation, mindfulness, and relaxation techniques are three paths that can be used to reduce stress and create a peaceful mind.

Meditation is an open practice, adaptable by the person studying it or practicing it, and hence, not amenable to confining definitions. How would you define meditation? For some individuals, meditation might be when they go for walks with their dogs, while for other people, it might entail praying. For still others, it might be sitting with a cup of warm tea and watching the sunrise.

Some individuals see meditation as a way to pay attention, cultivate awareness, and tend to what is going on within themselves. Others find engaging in sports, such as swimming, to be a form of meditation, because of the great amount of concentration and repetitive motion that is required of them to perform the sport. One lifestyle medicine student once stated that a phrase that worked best for her was to "be still," and then go deeper and be still there, and subsequently, to go deeper again and be still there—all the way to her center. This insight is profound.

For many people, meditation is not easy. It is a process without a final destination. It is a practice that you improve at each time you engage with it. Ultimately, the end goal of nearly all types and traditions of meditation is similar—to train and tame the mind, such that inner silence and higher modes of consciousness are accessible. This undertaking enables deeper and deeper self-discovery.

The practice of meditation has been ongoing for thousands of years, most notably among Buddhists. Only recently has meditation been scientifically researched and explored by the medical community as it relates to human health and disease. Two people have brought the concept of meditation to the forefront of lifestyle medicine: One of those individuals was cardiologist Dr. Herbert Benson, who developed the Relaxation Response technique, as well as founded the Mind/Body Medical Institute at Massachusetts General Hospital. The other pioneer in this field was Professor Emeritus Dr. Jon Kabat-Zinn, who has a PhD in molecular biology. A deep thinker, Dr. Kabat-Zinn, who has meditated on (thought over) states of consciousness, the mind, and how to be fully present in your life, ultimately created the technique of mindfulness-based stress reduction (MBSR).

MEDITATION IN MODERN CULTURE

Meditation is often considered a complementary health approach, fitting into the arena of CAM or complementary and alternative medicine. Many, but not all, of the approaches listed in this survey also fall into lifestyle medicine. For example, homeopathy is not part of mainstream lifestyle medicine. The bar graph in Figure 8-1 depicts the use of meditation and other complementary health practices by adults in 2012. It shows that 8 percent practice meditation, while another 10.9 percent practice deep breathing. There is also some evidence that children are practicing meditation, which can be helpful for developing their executive function. At the time of this research, more people were reporting meditating than were reporting getting a massage.

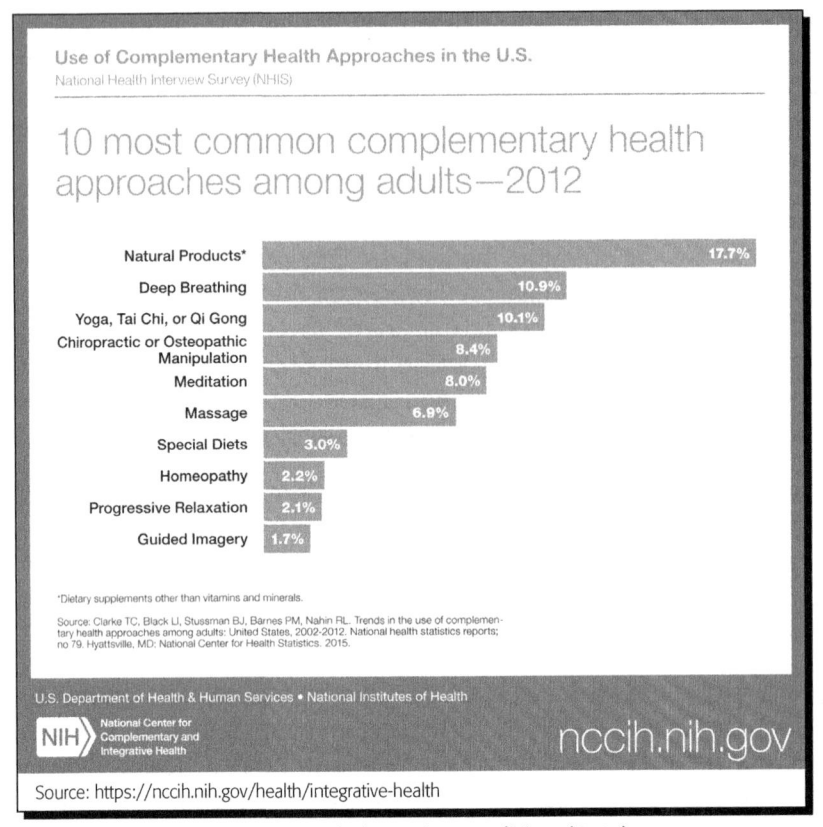

Figure 8-1. Complementary and alternative medicine (CAM) use among American adults in 2012

TYPES OF MEDITATION

There are a variety of types of meditation for patients. One common way to classify meditation is based on the practitioner's focus of attention. Either the attention is set on a specific focal point, or attention is distributed openly.

❏ Focused Attention Meditation

Focused meditation is the practice of a person focusing their attention on a single object throughout the session, such as a candle, a sound, a mantra, or an internal object, like a body part or the breath. As the practitioner advances, the ability to maintain focus and attention on the singular object increases and distractions become less frequent.

❏ Open Monitoring Meditation

Rather than focusing the attention on any one object, the practitioner remains open to any and all aspects of the present experience. This factor could come in the form of external sounds and sensations or internal thoughts, feelings, or cravings.

Other popular forms of meditation include:

❑ Activity-Oriented or Movement Meditation

This type is a form of meditation in which you engage in a repetitive activity, such as walking or practicing yoga. Even running is a form of meditation. When you are running methodically, you can direct your attention to the sound of your feet hitting the ground, the sound of your breath as you inhale and exhale, and the sensation of the air running across your limbs. Nothing else is going on, and you transition into a meditative state of mind. This form is considered movement meditation. Many people also practice walking meditation. Mazes can be used for this type of meditation as well.

❑ Mindfulness Meditation

Mindfulness meditation is the practice of becoming more fully aware and mindful of the present moment versus thinking about the past or future. It is currently one of the most popular forms of meditation, because it is one of the simplest to perform. You start by focusing on your breath, which, by definition, is the present moment. Inevitably, thoughts will come to mind, and emotions will arise. Rather than emptying your mind of all thought, you notice these thoughts and feelings. You are the watcher of your thoughts and feelings, which enhances self-awareness. Rather than getting caught up or hooked by these thoughts and emotions, you acknowledge them at a distance and then let them flow by you. You return your focus to the breath, each time building more concentration. The practice combines awareness with concentration.

❑ Transcendental Meditation (TM)

Perhaps the most widely practiced and scientifically studied form of medication, TM is a specific form of mantra meditation. It involves the use of a sound or mantra for 15 to 20 minutes twice per day.

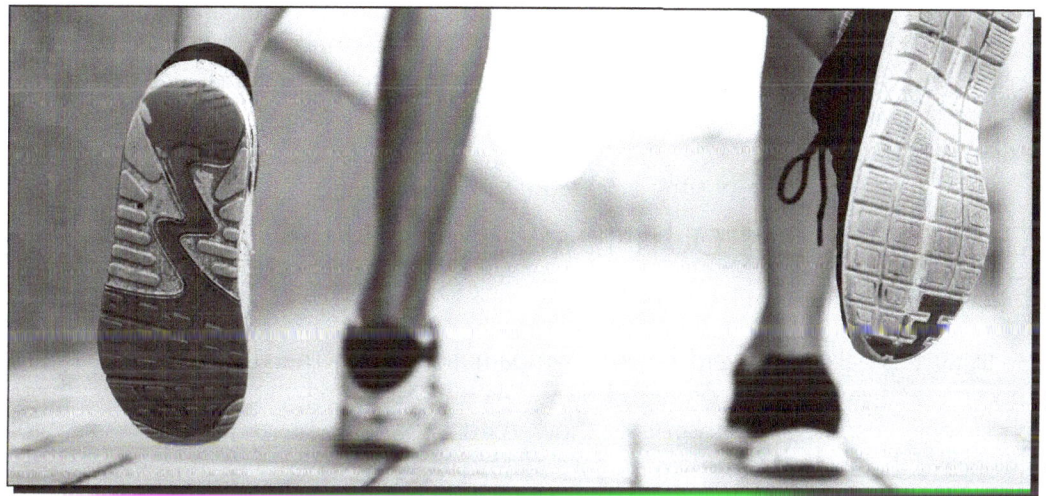

Running is a form of meditation.

THE FOUR ELEMENTS OF MEDITATION

The NCCIH website states that there are four main elements of meditation. These four elements are common to other types of relaxation practices that incorporate meditation, including MBSR and the Relaxation Response:
- A quiet location without distractions
- A specific, comfortable posture
- A focus of attention
- An open attitude

CURRENT UNDERSTANDING OF THE BIOLOGICAL BASIS OF MEDITATION

The exact mechanisms of how meditation works are not completely known, but they are an active focus of research. Chapter 7 included a discussion of stress, resiliency, the fight-or-flight response, and the actions of the sympathetic and parasympathetic nervous system (Figure 7-4), which is relevant in this situation. It has been hypothesized that meditation and relaxation work by increasing activity in the parasympathetic nervous system and decreasing activity in the sympathetic nervous system.

Breathing air into the lungs temporarily blocks the influence of the parasympathetic nervous system's influence on the heart rate, and breathing air out of the lungs reinstates this parasympathetic influence on the heart rate, causing your pulse to go down. Much of the time, people forget to breathe when they are stressed out, and they hold their bodies in tense and tight postures. When they begin to breathe and take long, slow, deep inhales and exhales, however, their bodies relax. Their muscles relax. Their heart rate decreases.

Some people emphasize their exhale to maximize the influence of the parasympathetic nervous system on the heart. A deep exhalation can be similar to a valsalva movement, which can trigger the vagus nerve and turn on the parasympathetic system. Vagal maneuvers are utilized when a cardiac patient is experiencing an extremely rapid heart rate.

THE IMPACT OF ROUTINE MEDITATION ON THE 11 SYSTEMS OF THE BODY

By tilting the balance toward the parasympathetic system, meditation impacts bodily function and systems in profound ways. As the following overviews show, these physiologic responses demonstrate how meditation can be a powerful single or adjunctive therapy for numerous disease states:

❏ Circulatory System

Helps to lower blood pressure. Slows the heart. Reduces pulse and heart rate. Lowers the risk of cardiovascular disease.

❏ Digestive System

Helps to stimulate digestion. Enhances the production of saliva and enzymes in the mouth. May enhance the ability to select healthier food choices through improved awareness.

❏ Endocrine System

Helps to normalize endocrine activity. Facilitates a restful sleep pattern. Promotes appropriate hormonal levels, which helps the body's immune system return to a balanced state.

❏ Immune System

Helps to manage stress. Improves immunity. Helps to reduce markers of inflammation. Diminishes the likelihood of experiencing anxiety and depression.

❏ Dermatologic System

Stress increases the production of skin sebum (the oily discharge that can lead to clogged pores and aggravate acne). Diminishes inflammation in the body, which can result in a worsening of skin conditions like eczema. Helps prevent the onset of cold sores (caused by the herpes simplex virus, on or around the lips).

❏ Muscular System

Helps to prevent muscle tension. Decreases the incidence of various stress-related disorders, such as a headache.

❏ Nervous System

Helps to ensure that the autonomic nervous system of the body continues to operate smoothly. As aforementioned, preferentially increases parasympathetic activity and promotes its far-reaching effects on the body. For more on this topic, refer to the section "Meditation and the Mind."

❏ Reproductive System

Helps to maintain the orderly balance of the hormones involved in the reproductive system. For women, stress can cause irregular menstrual cycles, sexual dysfunction, and other menstrual problems. In men, chronic stress can impair testosterone and sperm production.

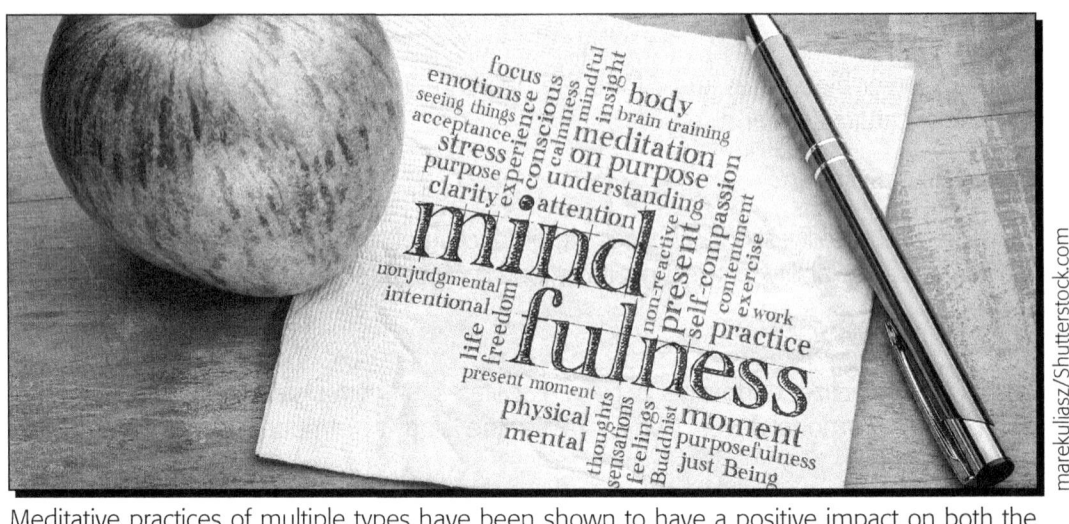

Meditative practices of multiple types have been shown to have a positive impact on both the mind and the body.

❑ Respiratory System

Helps to lower the rate of breathing. Because stress is a common asthma trigger, has been shown to reduce asthma symptoms and improve quality of life.

❑ Skeletal System

Helps to minimize the stress placed on bones and joints. Helps to prevent muscular tension, which can lead to a loss of flexibility, as well as aches and pains in commonly tensed muscles, such as those in the neck, upper back, and shoulders.

❑ Renal/Urinary System

Helps to treat overactive bladder symptoms in women.

THE HEALTH BENEFITS OF MEDITATION

In an increasing number of studies, meditative practices of multiple types have been shown to have a positive impact on both the mind and the body. For example, a recent review of 41 trials (most of them randomized, controlled studies), which collectively involved 3,515 participants of meditation programs that were designed to reduce psychological stress and improve well-being that was published in *JAMA Internal Medicine*, concluded that "Clinicians should be aware that meditation programs can result in small-to-moderate reductions of multiple negative dimensions of psychological stress." In particular, mindfulness meditation programs had moderate strength of evidence for improvements in anxiety, depression, and pain; low strength of evidence for improvements in stress/distress and mental health-related quality of life; and low strength of evidence or no effect or insufficient strength of evidence of an effect for positive mood, attention, substance use, eating, sleep, and weight.

With regard to the health of the body, meditation has been shown to reduce the risk of heart disease and stroke. This finding may be mediated by a reduction in blood pressure, which has also a validated effect of meditation. Smaller studies have also shown that meditation reduces cellular level inflammation and boosts immunity. Hence, meditation may have a complementary role in the management of inflammatory disorders. At this time, stronger study designs are needed to determine the effects of meditation programs on improving the positive dimensions of mental health, stress-related behavioural outcomes, bodily function, and health outcomes.

MEDITATION AND THE MIND

In addition to the observable and measurable effects of meditation and relaxation practices on the body, mind, and physical symptoms, there are also effects on the structure of the brain itself, as well as neurocognitive performance. In that regard, there are four areas of the brain that may be affected by meditation (Figure 8-2):

- *The prefrontal cortex:* Dictates complex behavior, executive functioning (the ability to plan, organize, focus, and think before responding), emotion, and behavioral functioning.
- *The insula:* Modulates self-awareness, perception, and cognitive functioning.
- *The amygdala:* Regulates emotional control.
- *The hippocampus:* Helps modulate cortical arousal and responsiveness as part of the limbic system, as well as being involved in memory and learning.

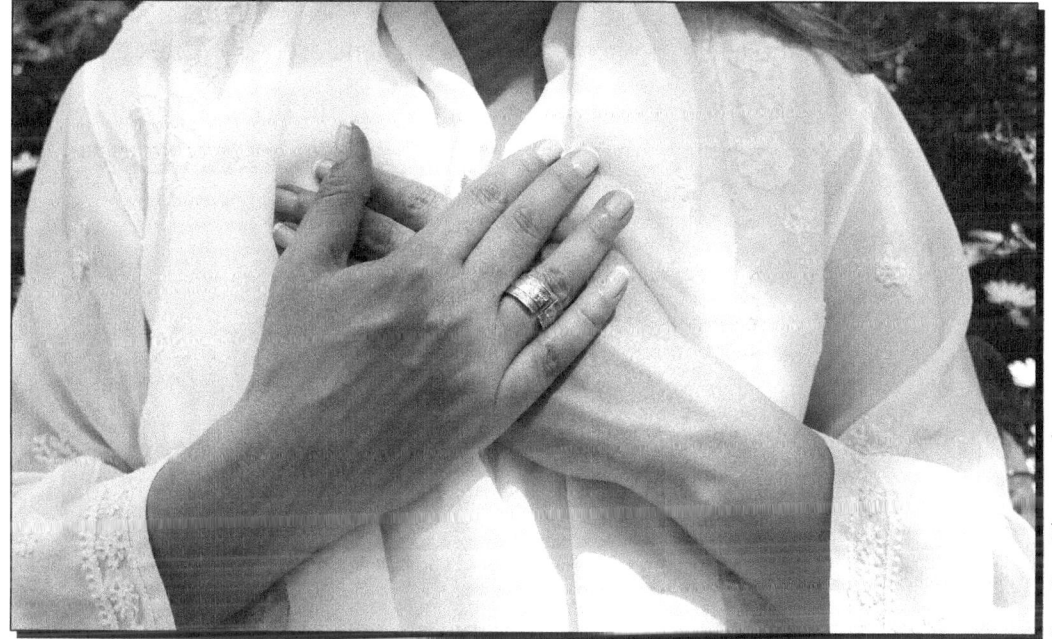

With regard to the health of the body, meditation has been shown to reduce the risk of heart disease and stroke.

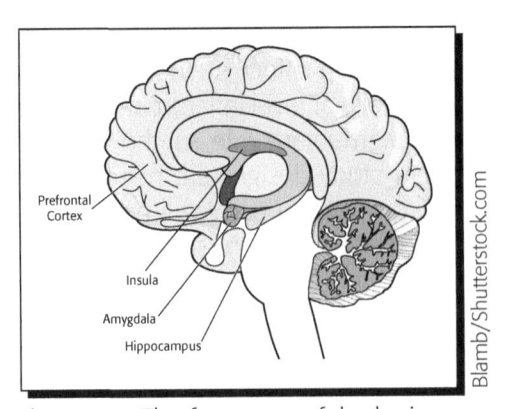

Figure 8-2. The four areas of the brain that may be affected by meditation

Dr. Sara Lazar, a psychologist at Harvard, studies the impact of yoga and meditation on the brain, in terms of cognition and behavior. She and her team have found evidence that the practice of meditation may actually slow the shrinkage of the brain that commonly occurs with aging.

In 2005, Dr. Lazar and her colleagues conducted a landmark correlational study, "Meditation experience is associated with increased cortical thickness." They enrolled 20 experienced meditators who practiced daily with 15 people who had no experience with either meditation or yoga. They then compared their brains on magnetic resonance imaging (MRI) scans and found that the cortical areas of people who meditated were thicker than those in control subjects, regardless of age (Figure 8-3). Meditators also had more activity in the insula, prefrontal cortex, and somatosensory cortex than nonmeditators (Figure 8-3).

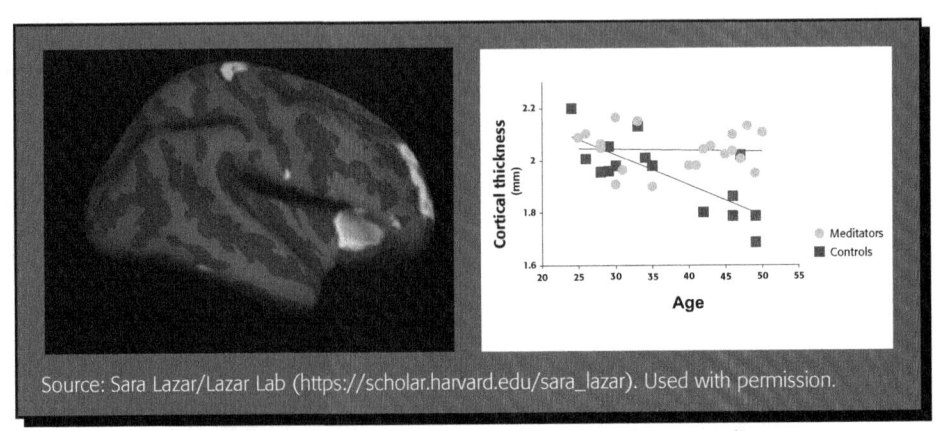

Figure 8-3. Comparison of cortical areas in meditators and nonmeditators

In 2010, Dr. Lazar led another study that reported on how the practice of mindfulness changes the brain. In this study, titled, "Stress reduction correlates with structural changes in the amygdala," she and her team asked 26 stressed, but healthy, subjects to partake in an eight-week long MBSR program. Prior to the study, participants took a survey that measured their level of perceived stress and underwent an MRI. The team found that subjects perceived less stress after the MBSR intervention, which correlated with decreases in the gray matter density in the amygdala—and it is thought that the smaller the amygdala, which is the center of emotions, the less stress and anxiety that is felt.

In a subsequent study, Dr. Lazar's team explored how the eight-week MBSR intervention changes various areas of the brain and affects memory, sense of self, empathy, and stress. They took MRI scans of 16 subjects who had never practiced meditation before and a control group at two weeks before and after the intervention. The researchers, who had the subjects do MBSR for 27 minutes, found that they had an increase in grey matter in their hippocampus, the site of memory and learning, as well as an area of the brain that is a contributor to emotional regulation.

Neurocognitive testing has shown that meditation improves focus, information processing, decision making, and allocation of attention and brain resources.

GETTING STARTED WITH MEDITATION

There are many examples of commonly employed meditation tactics that can help achieve the benefits that meditation has to offer. Some people need to start slowly and ramp up gradually with their meditation practice. Many people feel intimidated by the word meditation, and they think of Buddha or other Buddhist priests sitting perfectly still, quietly breathing for hours. This situation seems simply unattainable. In that regard, lifestyle medicine professionals should discuss the variety of ways that patients can meditate to help them to be more amenable to this powerful practice. Among the simple techniques to get started are the following:

- Perform a one-minute breath meditation. Ask the patient to take a deep breath in and out and focus only on the air coming in and out of their nose and mouth. One minute of conscious breathing can bring clarity to a person's world.
- Try a walking meditation. Instead of walking to get to a destination, engage the senses and enjoy the journey.
- Engage in a meditative yoga flow to release tension in the low back and reduce stress to the body. Flow from the yoga poses cat, to cow, to extended child's pose. Move at a slow pace and move with the breath.
- Cultivate strength and balance in the lower body with a standing yoga flow. Pay attention to the ground beneath the feet to improve proprioception.
- Perform lying down meditation. Continue this practice until the body and mind have reached a relaxed state.
- Use Zen meditation to be "at one" with the present moment. Employ conscious awareness of momentary experiences to lead to a more open mind.

- Focus on the self and others with unconditional love in the practice of loving kindness meditation. This practice extends feelings of compassion and caring to oneself and others.
- Release negative thoughts and feelings with a mantra. Choose a mantra to focus the mind on what it needs.
- Try concentration meditation. Focus the mind on a single point, such as their breath, a mantra, or phrase.
- Practice insight meditation (vipassana) to gain insight into reality, a process that can develop wisdom and compassion.
- Pay attention to a simple activity as a way to meditate. Choose a different activity to focus on every day for a week to train the mind to live in the moment.
- Use coloring as a way to bring the mind into focus and inspire creativity. For example, mandala-coloring (typically involving coloring in a series of geometric designs) can help bring one to the present moment.

LIVE AND LEARN WITH DR. BETH FRATES

Bringing meditation, mindfulness, and relaxation practices into my wellness workshops was an exciting opportunity for me. I remember the first time I planned to discuss "inner peace" and meditation. I prepared my slides and even brought some relaxation music on a CD that I could play on my CD player. I set everything up and put the music on before any of the patients entered the room. I loved the mellow music and hoped they would too.

The first gentleman arrived with his father. The group is for stroke survivors and caregivers. The father said, "Where's that elevator music coming from? I don't like it. We don't usually have this playing." So, I was off to a rough start.

The session, however, went really well. I discussed my personal experience with mindfulness-based stress reduction, which is described in detail in the next Live and Learn. Basically, I shared my journey with various other methods of finding inner peace, like mindfully eating a raisin, which we tried together, and relaxing with a body scan, which we also tried together.

As research shows, we, as practitioners, are more likely to counsel on exercise if we exercise. It makes sense that if we are comfortable with meditation, mindfulness, and relaxation techniques, then we would be more likely to counsel on them. If we are practicing them ourselves, then we can speak from the head and the heart about the benefits, the difficulty starting, and the possible ways to get started.

For me, it felt awkward at first to focus on these mind body techniques, because it was clear that some of the workshop participants were skeptical. On the other hand, it ended really well. In fact, one patient shared that she had tried "mediation" before, but felt that she felt "goofy," while doing it, and thought that it was "ineffective." Many of the participants were intimidated by it. This time, she stopped judging herself and just tried to focus on the activity, like chewing the raisin or relaxing her feet first, then her ankles, and subsequently her calves, as we did in the body scan.

In the end, all the participants reported that it was a useful session. Each of them said they had tried something new that they were willing to try at home. Sharing methods of meditation, mindfulness, and relaxation helps to increase your own inner peace, as a practitioner. That reminds me of the quote from Saint Francis of Assisi, "It is in giving that we receive." I went out of my comfort zone by trying to teach the patients about meditation, and it turned out to be a learning experience for me too. I gained confidence in my ability to run these sessions. I also obtained perspective about how patients feel about including these mind body techniques into their daily practice. It was a win-win for the patients and for me.

A WORD OF CAUTION

While there is very little downside to meditation, for some people, when they try to clear their mind, they may keep coming back to negative thoughts and feelings. While this is part of the meditation experience, those individuals, particularly people with psychiatric illness, may not be ready to open themselves up to meditation. In rare cases, it may make them feel worse at a certain stage of life or phase of their health journey. It is important to keep this factor in mind and to be respectful of patients who say the technique is not benefiting them.

PATH #2: MINDFULNESS-BASED STRESS REDUCTION (MBSR)

One of the most prominent and commonly practiced forms of meditation today, as well as one of the most scientifically validated, is MBSR. In 1979, Dr. Jon Kabat-Zinn founded the world-renowned MBSR Clinic at the University of Massachusetts-Amherst. Then, in 1995, he founded the Center for Mindfulness in Medicine, Health Care, and Society at the University of Massachusetts-Worcester. He has published two popular and important books on MBSR: *Full Catastrophe Living* and *Wherever You Go, There You Are*. His MBSR program can be taken in person as a five-day intensive course or online over eight weeks. Furthermore, a number of healthcare facilities offer this program to their clinicians, as well as to their patients.

Mindfulness is a term can have different meanings for different people. For Dr. Kabat-Zinn, mindfulness means paying attention in a particular way on purpose in the present moment and nonjudgmentally. There is no one correct way to practice MBSR and meditation. It is all about the individual person and their breath. Nothing else. No one else. Just the breath and the peaceful silence. The MBSR program empowers individuals to respond consciously, rather than automatically, to circumstances by pausing and breathing before they respond.

A review of 17 studies of MBSR as a stress management technique for healthy individuals was published in the *Journal of Evidence-Based Complementary Alternative Medicine*. Sixteen of the 17 articles examined demonstrated positive changes in psychological or physiological outcomes related to anxiety and/or stress when people practiced MBSR. Accordingly, the authors concluded that MBSR appears to be a promising modality for stress management, although randomized, controlled trials with larger sample sizes are needed to confirm these findings.

Likewise, mindfulness meditation has been found to be of benefit in reducing stress among caregivers. For example, in one medical journal article, the authors, Haines et al., discussed the stress caregivers of lung transplant patients' experience, given that since there is a high rate of rejection in lung transplants, caregivers do not know if the transplant was successful or not. In other words, there is a lack of control over the situation, because no one knows if the patient will survive.

In this study, 30 caregivers were asked to watch an MBSR DVD and to practice the technique for 5 to 15 minutes a day, for four weeks in their homes. The authors looked at the Perceived Stress Scale and the State Trait Anxiety Scale, finding that caregivers who watched the entire DVD and practiced MBSR, as instructed, reported reduced levels of perceived stress, state anxiety, and trait anxiety. (The "state of anxiety" refers to how the patient feels in that moment, that state. In contrast, "train anxiety" is more of an indicator of how anxious a person is on a day-to-day basis over time.) Scores for these same tests for those individuals who did not watch the DVD or only watched some of it did not change significantly. In fact, a number of other studies have been conducted on the positive impact of MBSR for various conditions, including chronic pain and sleep problems. As such, research continues to uncover its benefits.

LIVE AND LEARN WITH DR. BETH FRATES

I learned the value of MBSR on purpose in a time of crisis for myself. When my father died, I learned that my mother had cognitive difficulties. She had memory problems and was experiencing cognitive decline, also known as dementia. Because she was locking herself out of the house and forgetting about dinner dates with friends, she was distressed. I was deeply disturbed and worried about her future, as well as her day-to-day welfare. So, she moved in with me and my family. Living with two teenage boys can be stressful by itself, but adding a mother who really can no longer take care of herself into the mix can be overwhelming, which is exactly what it became after a year.

Feeling exhausted and very stressed, I looked up stress reduction techniques for caregivers of people with dementia, and found some interesting research studies. The first was on a form of chanting—I tried that and it was beneficial, but I thought I needed more. So, I performed another PubMed search on caregivers of dementia patients. I found a study discussing the benefit of MBSR for this population. I had wanted to participate in one of Jon Kabat-Zinn's programs for years, but could not find the time. Well, this was the time. I made the time. I took a five-day continuing medical education (CME) course on MBSR, and it was life-altering. I continue to practice MBSR to some extent each day.

I was always reluctant to attend these conferences, because I knew that there was one full day when no one could talk. Participants at the conference could not speak; the day was spent in silence. Silent mindfulness-based stress reduction, silent walking meditation, silent mindful eating, and silent sitting. As a person who enjoys talking, this scenario seemed like a nightmare. As it turned out, however, it was a very pleasant experience. In fact, I would relish the opportunity to spend another day in silence like that. I will admit it was difficult for me and a little uncomfortable at first. I kept trying to communicate with people with my body language, eyes, and facial expressions. Most people, however, were following the rules and simply being silent, totally silent. Once I accepted that, it was fine.

What I loved best was that the MBSR leaders kept repeating, "There is no way to do this wrong. You cannot fail. Furthermore, you are not getting graded. Just sit quietly, try to focus on your breathing and only on your breathing. Feel the air going into your lungs and coming out. Think only about your breath. If other thoughts enter your mind, it is ok. That is fine. Just gently bring your attention back to your breath. If you start running through your to-do list, that is fine. But, gently bring your focus back to your breathing." This practice was refreshing. It was really wonderful.

Most of the other participants in the training were physicians or other healthcare providers, getting their continuing education credits. There were patients, teachers, and lawyers there as well. One lawyer kept raising his hand exclaiming, "I can't do this. I don't get it. I am not doing it right." The leaders would repeat, "There is no right or wrong. Simply try to focus on your breath, if you are trying then that is all you can do." After five days, the lawyer raised his hand, "This was a waste. I still cannot do this. I cannot do mindfulness-based stress reduction." The leaders repeated their usual response, but the lawyer was not satisfied. I, however, was very satisfied, as were many other doctors whom I met. We were there to learn about MBSR to help our patients and our practice, but truly, most of us were there to help ourselves.

The first day of the conference, we were asked to share our names and what had brought us to the MBSR training. Most people said they had a healthcare practice and wanted to help their patients relax. I was toward the back of the room, and by the time they got to me, I had heard the same answers enough, so I spoke my truth. "I am here because my father died, and I am now caring for my mother who is living with me and my family—two teenage boys and a loving husband. I am also seeing patients, teaching, and writing. I am overwhelmed, and I need help. I am hopeful that what I learn can help me, and then I can help my patients."

After I shared my story, others who had already given their reasons for being at the conference raised their hands, and they then shared their own personal reasons for *being there—their truths. In this way, we all bonded. Most people left the conference feeling like they learned a great deal and had some level of mastery of MBSR. We were excited to share what we learned with our patients, family, and friends.*

PATH #3: RELAXATION AND THE RELAXATION RESPONSE

Meditation began to be scientifically explored in the United States in 1969, starting with work done by Dr. Herbert Benson, with studies on relaxation at Harvard University. The terms "relax" and "relaxation" can have different meanings for different people, and initially, they were understood to simply mean "resting." As noted previously, a common definition of the term "to relax" is the ability to become or cause something to become less tense, tight, or stiff; to stop feeling nervous or worried; to spend time resting or doing something enjoyable, especially after you have been doing work.

In 1975, Dr. Benson's book *The Relaxation Response* was published, in which he described the Relaxation Response as "your personal ability to encourage your body to release chemicals and brain signals that make your muscles and organs slow down and increase blood flow to the brain." In addition, Dr. Benson did a great deal of work on the mind/body connection. His findings were not readily accepted at first, but have since expanded globally and become a central tenet of lifestyle medicine. In reality, the mind/body connection has often been referred to by different names, such as stress management, learned relaxation, and hypnotic suggestion.

In 1992, Dr. Benson wrote another book *The Wellness Book—The Comprehensive Guide to Maintaining Health and Treating Stress-Related Illness*, which discussed general health and further elaborated on the concepts of *mind/body medicine*. In 2001, Harvard Health Publications released a *"Mind/Body Medicine"* special report, which provided an overview of Dr. Benson's work. Furthermore, one of his first continuing medical education (CME) courses on *mind/body medicine* was held in 2002.

Dr. Benson published his first research paper, "A wakeful, hypometabolic physiologic state," with two of his colleagues in the *American Journal of Physiology* in 1971. In this initial study, he enrolled 36 subjects between the ages of 17 and 41 years old. Twenty-eight of the participants were men, and eight were women. All of the participants had some experience with meditation, which ranged from less than one month to nine years, with an average of two to three years. The participants served as their own controls, and during each session spent 20 to 30 minutes in a quiet, premeditative state, 20 to 30 minutes in meditation, and 20 to 30 minutes in postmeditation. Dr. Benson and his team continuously monitored each participant's blood pressure, heart rate, respiratory rate, and electroencephalogram (EEG) readings, and took blood samples for oxygen concentration and carbon dioxide elimination throughout these sessions.

The practice was a form of TM, which was developed by Maharishi Mahesh Yogi as a standardized technique, in which meditators sit comfortably with their eyes closed. Dr. Benson described the process as "a systematic method that [the subject has been

Lifestyle Medicine Handbook 315

taught, which allows him to perceive] a 'suitable' sound or thought. Without attempting to concentrate specifically on this cue, he allows his mind to experience it freely, and his thinking, as the practitioners themselves report, rises to a 'finer and more creative level in an easy and natural manner.'"

Figures 8-4 to 8-7 show the oxygen and carbon dioxide measurements Dr. Benson and his team recorded, as they changed over the course of a meditation session. These figures demonstrate the balance of oxygen and carbon dioxide that exists during a meditative state. During this state, the body requires less oxygen and clears

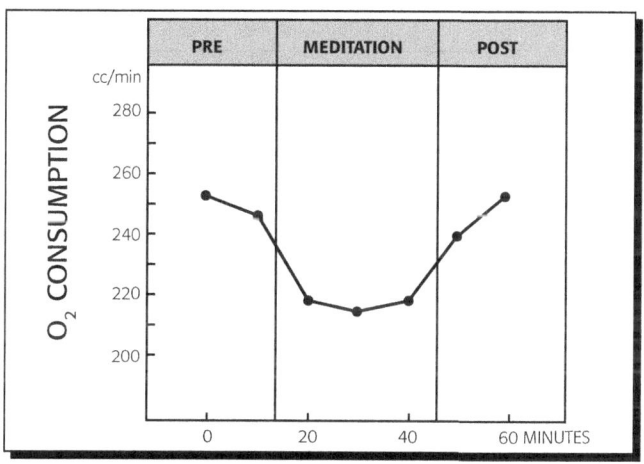

Figure 8-4. Oxygen consumption decreases during meditation

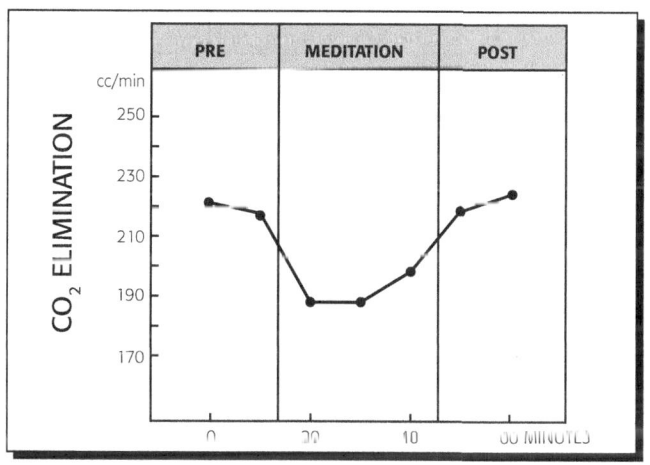

Figure 8-5. Carbon dioxide input decreases during meditation

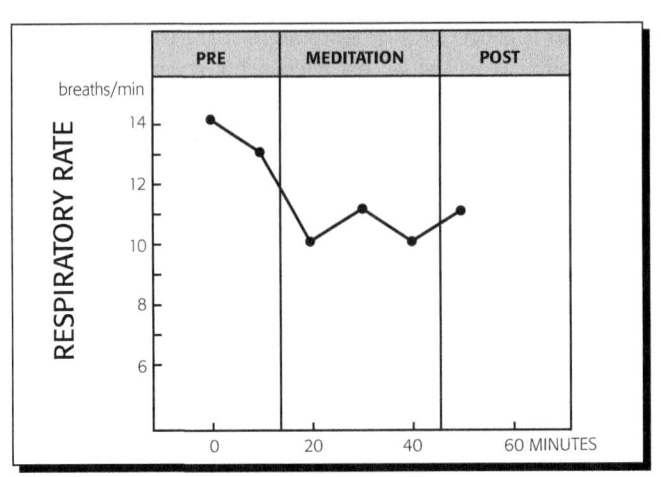

Figure 8-6. The rate of breathing decreases during meditation

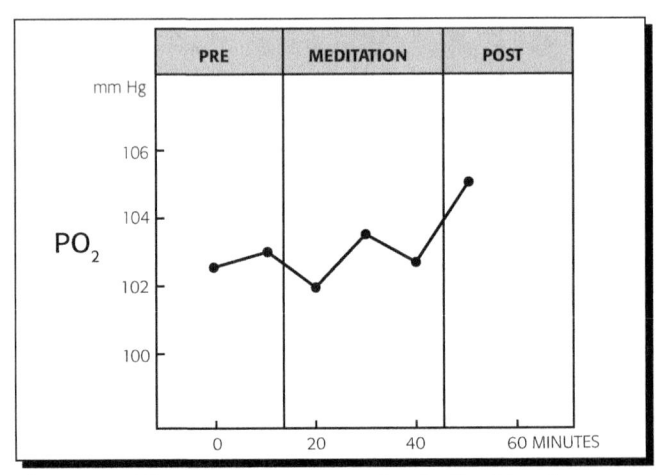

Figure 8-7. The oxygen concentration in the blood remains constant and even increases slightly during meditation

less carbon dioxide, but maintains a high level of oxygen in the blood. Dr. Benson defined this as the "hypometabolic state" and dubbed it the Relaxation Response. To achieve this state, a person must:
- Sit quietly in a comfortable position.
- Close the eyes.
- Progressively and deeply relax each muscle group in the body.
- Breath through the nose and silently repeat the word "one" with each breath. (Dr. Benson suggests the word "one," but any mantra can be used.)
- Continue with this practice for 10 to 20 minutes.

If thoughts bubble up as an individual is attempting to go into the hypometabolic state, Dr. Benson says not to worry about it, but rather just keep breathing and repeating the chosen word or mantra. It is important not to dwell on the thoughts. The person should acknowledge them and then go back to repeating the chosen word. He also says not to be concerned about whether or not a deep state of relaxation is being achieved. Instead, the individual should adopt a passive attitude and permit the relaxation to happen at its own pace.

DELETERIOUS EFFECTS OF STRESS

There is a definitive link between mental stress and deleterious health effects. For instance, Dr. Alan Rozanski and his team published the article "Mental stress and the induction of silent myocardial ischemia in patients with coronary artery disease" in *The New England Journal of Medicine* in 1988. This paper indicated that when subjects were placed under mental stress by being asked to perform "a personally relevant, emotionally arousing speaking task," they exhibited signs of cardiac dysfunction, as measured on radionuclide ventriculography. The Live and Learn from Chapter 7 reviewed the replication of this study that Dr. Frates performed for her senior thesis in college.

There is also a definitive link between the Relaxation Response and reduction in cardiac risk. In a review of 27 studies of patients recovering from ischemic heart disease who were taught relaxation therapy, reductions in resting heart rate and increases in heart rate variability, exercise tolerance, and HDL (good) cholesterol levels were found. The researchers also found a reduction in both anxiety and depression. The frequency of angina pectoris (chest pain) and arrhythmia (irregular heartbeats) was reduced, as well, along with exercise-induced ischemia (lack of oxygen to the heart muscle). Furthermore, the participants in these studies returned to work sooner, and cardiac events and cardiac deaths occurred less frequently in those that were taught the Relaxation Response. The more intensive the intervention, the greater the effect on cardiac health.

The authors concluded that relaxation therapy is effective as an adjunct to medical care, as well as standard cardiac rehabilitation, and that intensive programs have better results. They also concluded that relaxation is particularly beneficial for the emotional and physical state of the patient, and adds another dimension to rehabilitation and recovery. The results confirmed the findings of previous studies that had examined the important role of stress management and psycho-education for cardiac patients. Limitations of this research included small sample sizes and that there were only 10 randomized studies in the review.

While relaxation can be a secondary effect of some types of meditation, few forms of meditation are anything but relaxing. Determining the potential connection between relaxation and meditation entails considering the intention and purpose of various techniques involved. True relaxation is a mind/body state that is defined by the stimulation of the Relaxation Response.

In reality, any effort to relax can be enhanced by adhering to the following guidelines:
- Make a commitment to devote an uninterrupted period of time each day in which to practice relaxation techniques.
- Choose a quiet place in which to practice her relaxation techniques.
- Get into a comfortable body position.
- Concentrate on the repetition of a single focal point (e.g., a word, sound, mantra) or the breath, flowing in and out.
- Foster a positive state of mind.

A number of steps can be undertaken to help a person become attuned to their own body and achieve an appropriate degree of deep relaxation, including the following:
- Listening to music
- Art therapy
- Guided imagery (visualization)
- Cognitive therapy
- Biofeedback
- Progressive muscle relaxation
- Breathing exercises
- Herbal therapy
- Aromatherapy
- Mindfulness meditation
- Rhythmic movement

MINDFUL MOVEMENT

Dr. Sang Kim, a PhD in exercise physiology, has been doing research on movement and its effect on patients with post-traumatic stress disorder (PTSD). Dr. Kim, who himself has been practicing meditation and mindfulness-based movements for many years, wondered if he could help PTSD patients reduce stress and boost mental energy via physical movement. He designed and delivered the "Mindful Movement and Deep Breathing as a Self-Care Tool (MBX)," which consists of 12 movements to invigorate person's inner energy channels, or meridians.

In his article "PTSD symptom reduction with mindfulness-based stretching and deep breathing exercise," published in the *Journal of Clinical Endocrinology and Metabolism*, Kim and his colleagues describe a randomized, controlled trial performed with 28 female nurses and one male nurse. They instructed the study subjects to control their attention and awareness, and then to direct that awareness by utilizing their bodies and gradually creating a certain flow of physical movement that integrated with their mental awareness. Results show that the MBX program improved PTSD symptoms in four to eight weeks,

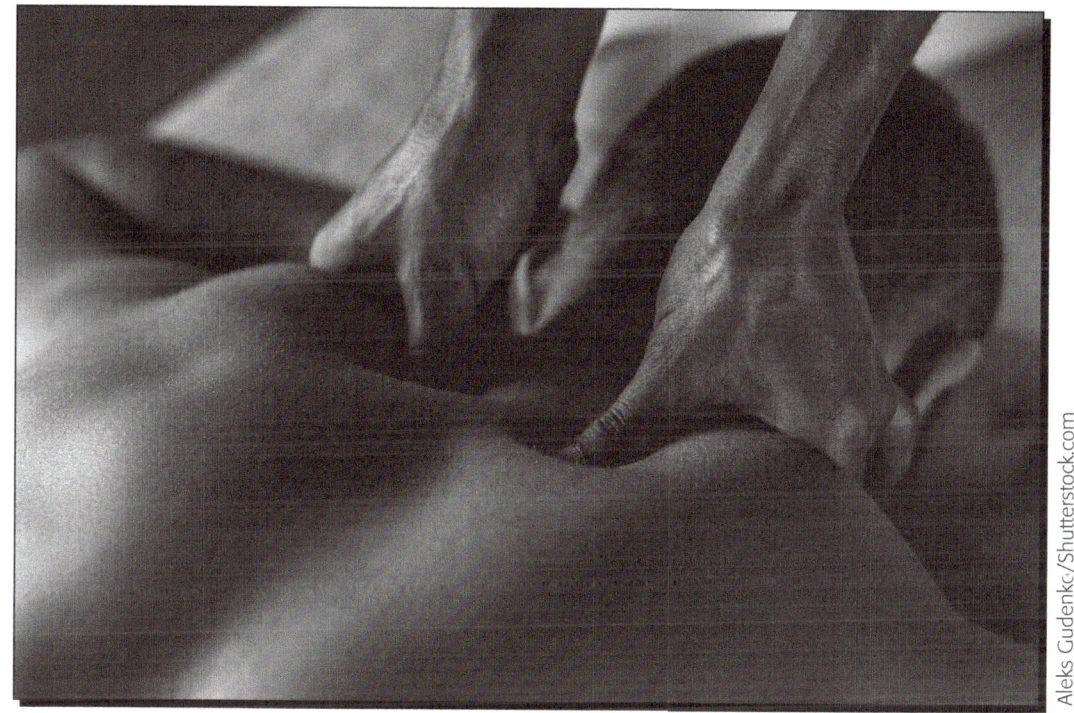

A number of steps can be undertaken to help a person become attuned to their own body and achieve an appropriate degree of deep relaxation.

and normalized levels of the stress hormone cortisol, as compared with control subjects. This study is just one example of ongoing research in the area of mind body medicine.

FITT PRESCRIPTIONS FOR MIND/BODY WORK (MEDITATION/MBSR/RELAXATION)

The following FITT prescriptions for the mind/body approaches need to be personalized with specific instructions for each patient. The FITT framework provides the lifestyle medicine practitioner with a general guideline to follow. For mind/body approaches, the frequency, time, and type elements are relatively clear, but intensity requires more detailed description. There can be a mild state of relaxation in which the patient feels less anxious and less stressed. Deep intensity is similar to a vigorous intensity for exercise. With deep mind/body work (meditation/MBSR/relaxation), the patient might experience a lasting quiet calm that allows for a greater sense of well-being immediately after the session and for hours later. Moderate intensity is somewhere in the middle. The patient is looking for more than a little stress relief but not expecting the long lasting effects experienced with deep intensity. The following are two examples of FITT prescriptions for mind/body.

❑ An example of a simple beginner's FITT prescription:

  F—once a day for two days of the week
  I—mild relaxation
  T—five minutes
  T—walking meditation. Walk outside, with specific attention paid to your feet touching the ground. Use all the senses you can—for example, listen to the noise your shoes make, feel your heels hit the ground, smell the flowers as you pass by them, and look at your feet as you are walking. On the other hand, also be careful to be aware of your surroundings.

❑ An example of a more advanced FITT prescription:

  F—five times a week
  I—deep relaxation, promoting long lasting stress resiliency
  T—20 to 30 minutes
  T—mindfulness-based stress reduction—focus on your breathing and let thoughts come in and out, without judging them. Continue to bring your thoughts to your breath.

KEY POINTS/TAKEAWAYS FOR CHAPTER 8

❑ Chapter Review:

- Overall goal: Review the factors that impact peace of mind.
- Application goal: Understand the connection between peace of mind and health.

❑ Discussion Questions:

- How does peace of mind affect a person's health?
- What is mindfulness?
- What are examples of mindfulness practices?
- What is meditation?
- What are examples of meditation practices?
- What is relaxation?
- What are examples of relaxation practices?
- How does the Relaxation Response impact a person's mental state?

	TITLE	AUTHORS	JOURNAL	YEAR	KEY FINDINGS
1	Meditation programs for psychological stress and well-being	Goyal M, Singh S, Sibinga EM	JAMA Internal Medicine	2014	An article evaluating the strength of evidence of mindfulness meditation programs that found moderate evidence that they improve anxiety, depression, and pain. There was low strength of evidence to support that mindfulness meditation programs had an effect on or improved stress/distress, mental health-related quality of life, positive mood, attention, substance use, eating, sleep, and weight.
2	Reducing stress and anxiety in caregivers of lung transplant patients: benefits of mindfulness meditation	Haines J, et al.	International Journal of Organ Transplantation Medicine	2014	A study of 26 subjects utilizing an eight-week mindfulness-based stress reduction intervention that found reductions in perceived stress scores, which correlated positively with decreases in amygdala grey matter density.
3	Mindfulness practice leads to increases in regional brain gray matter density	Hölzel B, et al.	Psychiatry Research	2011	Seventeen participants underwent an eight-week study utilizing an MBSR intervention to explore changes in brain regions. MRIs done prior to and after the MBSR intervention revealed increases in gray matter concentration in brain regions involved in learning and memory processes, emotion regulation, self-referential processing, and perspective taking.
4	Stress reduction correlates with structural changes in the amygdala	Holzel BK, et al.	Social Cognitive and Affective Neuroscience	2010	A longitudinal MRI study in 26 healthy individuals who participated in an eight-week mindfulness-based stress reduction intervention. They found that perceived stress scale (PSS) scores were significantly reduced after the intervention and that reductions in perceived stress correlated positively with decreases in amygdala gray matter density.
5	Mindfulness, self-compassion and empathy among health care professionals: a review of the literature	Raab K	Journal of Health Care Chaplaincy	2014	A literature review that found that reducing stress in healthcare workers can increase compassionate patient care. It suggested that MBSR could be used to develop self-compassion, which holds promise for reducing perceived stress and increasing effectiveness of clinical care.
6	Mental stress and the induction of silent myocardial ischemia in patients with coronary artery disease	Rozanski A, et al.	New England Journal of Medicine	1988	A study of 39 patients with coronary heart disease and 12 controls that assessed the causal relation between acute mental stress and myocardial ischemia using radionuclide ventriculography. In 59% of patients with coronary heart disease, 59% of them had wall motion abnormalities during periods of mental stress and 36% had a fall in ejection fraction of more than 5%. "The magnitude of cardiac dysfunction induced by the speaking task was similar to that induced by exercise." It concluded that "personally relevant mental stress may be an important precipitant of myocardial ischemia—often silent—in patients with coronary artery disease."

Figure 8-8. Relaxation, mindfulness, and meditation evidence.

	TITLE	AUTHORS	JOURNAL	YEAR	KEY FINDINGS
7	Stress reduction in the secondary prevention of cardiovascular disease: a randomized, controlled trial of transcendental meditation and health education in blacks	Schneider RH, et al.	*Circulation: Cardiovascular Quality and Outcomes*	2012	This randomized controlled trial of 201 black men and women with coronary heart disease found a 48% risk reduction in all-cause mortality, myocardial infarction, and stroke in the transcendental meditation group (HR 0.52; 95% CI 0.29-0.92; p-0.025) as compared to the health education group. The transcendental meditation group also showed a significant reduction of 4.9 mm Hg in systolic blood pressure and improved psychosocial stress factors.
8	Mindfulness-based stress reduction as a stress management intervention for healthy individuals: a systematic review	Sharma M, Rush S	*Journal of Evidence-Based Complementary and Alternative Medicine*	2014	Sixteen of the 17 articles included in this review demonstrated positive changes in psychological or physiological outcomes related to anxiety and/or stress. The authors noted that "despite the limitations of not all studies using randomized controlled design, having smaller sample sizes, and having different outcomes, mindfulness-based stress reduction appears to be a promising modality for stress management."
9	Relaxation therapy for rehabilitation and prevention in ischaemic heart disease: a systematic review and meta-analysis	van Dixhoorn J, White A	*European Journal of Cardiovascular Prevention and Rehabilitation*	2005	A review of 27 studies involving relaxation therapy that graded the intensity of interventions and looked at associations between physiologic, psychologic, and cardiac parameters. Overall, they found that full traditional relaxation training relaxation therapy reduced resting heart rate, increased heart rate variability, improved exercise tolerance, increased HDL cholesterol, and reduced anxiety and depression. Cardiac effects included a decreased frequency of angina pectoris occurrences, fewer arrhythmias, a reduction in exercise-induced ischemia, and fewer cardiac events and cardiac deaths. Abbreviated relaxation training only showed a decrease in resting heart rate.
10	Exercise, brain, and cognition across the life span	Voss MW, et al.	*Journal of Applied Physiology*	2011	A review article that found ample evidence to support exercise as "one of the most effective means available to improve mental and physical health, without the side effects of many pharmacological treatments." It also discusses current gaps in the literature and areas to consider for future research.
11	A wakeful hypometabolic physiologic state	Wallace RK, Benson H, Wilson A	*American Journal of Physiology*	1971	Physiologic parameters were studied in 36 adults (ages 17-41) during meditation. The physiologic changes included a decreased respiratory rate, blood pH, an increase in skin resistance and alpha waves, and unchanged blood pressure and rectal temperature. These changes differed from those seen during sleep, hypnosis, and other hypometabolic physiologic states.

Figure 8-8. Relaxation, mindfulness, and meditation evidence (cont.)

References

1. Goyal M, Singh S, Sibinga EM. Meditation programs for psychological stress and well-being. *JAMA Internal Medicine.* 2014;174(3):357-368.
2. Haines J, Spadaro K, Choi J, et al. Reducing stress and anxiety in caregivers of lung transplant patients: benefits of mindfulness meditation. *International Journal of Organ Transplantation Medicine.* 2014;5:50-56.
3. Hölzel B, Carmody J, Vangel M, et al. Mindfulness practice leads to increases in regional brain gray matter density. *Psychiatry Research.* 2011;191(1):36.
4. Holzel BK, Carmody J, Evans KC, et al. Stress reduction correlates with structural changes in the amygdala. *Social Cognitive and Affective Neuroscience.* 2010;5(1):11-17.
5. Raab K. Mindfulness, self-compassion and empathy among health care professionals: a review of the literature. *Journal of Health Care Chaplaincy.* 2014;20(3):95-108.
6. Rozanski A, Bairey CN, Krantz DS, et al. Mental stress and the induction of silent myocardial ischemia in patients with coronary artery disease. *New England Journal of Medicine.* 1988;318:1005-1012.
7. Schneider RH, Grim CE, Rainforth MV, et al. Stress reduction in the secondary prevention of cardiovascular disease: a randomized, controlled trial of transcendental meditation and health education in blacks. *Circulation: Cardiovascular Quality and Outcomes.* 2012;5:750-758.
8. Sharma M, Rush S. Mindfulness-based stress reduction as a stress management intervention for healthy individuals: a systematic review. *Journal of Evidence-Based Complementary and Alternative Medicine.* 2014;19(4):271-286.
9. van Dixhoorn J, White A. Relaxation therapy for rehabilitation and prevention in ischaemic heart disease: a systematic review and meta-analysis. *European Journal of Cardiovascular Prevention and Rehabilitation.* 2005;12:193-202.
10. Voss MW, Nagamatsu LS, Liu-Ambrose T, et al. Exercise, brain, and cognition across the life span. *Journal of Applied Physiology.* 2011;111:1505-1513.
11. Wallace RK, Benson H, Wilson A. A wakeful hypometabolic physiologic state. *American Journal of Physiology.* September 1 1971;221:795-799. Available at: http://ajplegacy.physiology.org/content/221/3/795. Accessed October 2017.

Figure 8-8. Relaxation, mindfulness, and meditation evidence (cont.)

REFERENCES

- Abbasy SA, Michelfelder A, Kenton K, et al. Home-based cognitive therapy for overactive bladder. *Journal of Urology.* April 1 2009;181(4):561.
- American Psychological Association. Stress in America: Stress and Gender. Available at: http://www.apa.org/news/press/releases/stress/2010/gender-stress.pdf. Accessed July 2018.
- Amihai I, Kozhevnikov M. The influence of Buddhist meditation traditions on the autonomic system and attention. *BioMed Research International.* 2015;2015:731579. doi:10.1155/2015/731579.
- Babauta L. Meditation for Beginners: 20 Practical Tips for Understanding the Mind. Zen Habits. Available at: https://zenhabits.net/meditation-guide/. Accessed October 2017.
- Ben-Shahar T. *Choose the Life You Want: The Mindful Way to Happiness.* New York: The Experiment; 2012.
- Benson H. *The Relaxation Response.* New York: Harper Collins Publishers; 1975.
- Benson H. *The Wellness Book: The Comprehensive Guide to Maintaining Health and Treating Stress-Related Illness.* New York: Simon & Schuster; 1992.
- Bhasin MK, Denninger JW, Huffman JC, et al. Specific transcriptome changes associated with blood pressure reduction in hypertensive patients after relaxation response training. *Journal of Alternative and Complementary Medicine.* May 2018;24(5):486-504.
- Bhongade MB, Prasad S, Jiloha RC, et al. Effect of psychological stress on fertility hormones and seminal quality in male partners of infertile couples. *Andrologia.* 2015;47:336-342. doi:10.1111/and.12268.

- Borreli L. A Life Hack for Sleep: The 4-7-8 Breathing Exercise Will Supposedly Put You to Sleep in Just 60 Seconds. Medical Daily. Available at: http://www.medicaldaily.com/life-hack-sleep-4-7-8-breathing-exercise-will-supposedly-put-you-sleep-just-60-332122. Accessed October 2017.
- Chen Y, Lyga J. Brain-skin connection: stress, inflammation and skin aging. *Inflammation & Allergy Drug Targets*. 2014;13(3):177-190. doi:10.2174/1871528113666140522104422.
- Cleveland Clinic. Stress & Asthma. Available at: https://my.clevelandclinic.org/health/articles/9573-stress--asthma. Accessed July 2018.
- Cleveland Clinic. Stress and Women. Available at: https://my.clevelandclinic.org/health/articles/4935-stress-and-women. Accessed July 2018.
- Cresswell DJ, et al. Alterations in resting-state functional connectivity link mindfulness meditation with reduced interleukin-6: a randomized controlled trial. *Biological Psychiatry*. July 1 2016;80(1):53-61.
- Edozien LC. Mind over matter: psychological factors and the menstrual cycle. *Current Opinion in Gynecology and Obstetrics*. 2006;18(4):452-456.
- Egger G, Binns A, Rossner S. *Lifestyle Medicine*. Australia: McGraw-Hill; 2008.
- Emmons RA, Mishra A. Why gratitude enhances well-being: what we know and what we need to know. In: Kennon M, Sheldon KM, Kashdan TB, eds. *Designing Positive Psychology: Taking Stock and Moving Forward*. New York: Oxford University Press; 2011.
- Fernandez A, Goldberg E, Michelon P. Chapter 7. In: Fernandez A, Goldberg E, eds. *The SharpBrains Guide to Brain Fitness*. San Francisco: SharpBrains Inc.; 2013: 121-146.
- Fredrickson B. The Positivity Self Test. Positivity Ratio. Available at: https://www.positivityratio.com/single.php. Accessed October 2017.
- Getting In. Anti-Social Personality Disorder (APD)—The Causes. Available at: http://www.getting-in.com/guide/gcse-psychology-development-of-personality-antisocial-personality-disorder-and-the-causes. Accessed October 2017.
- Gotink RA, Meijboom R, Vernooij MW, et al. 8-week Mindfulness Based Stress Reduction induces brain changes similar to traditional long-term meditation practice: a systematic review. *Brain and Cognition*. October 2016;108:32-41.
- Goyal M, Singh S, Sibinga EM. Meditation programs for psychological stress and well-being. *JAMA Internal Medicine*. 2014;174(3):357-368.
- Goyal M, Singh S, Sibinga EMS, et al. Meditation Programs for Psychological Stress and Well-Being. Comparative Effectiveness Review No. 124. (Prepared by Johns Hopkins University Evidence Based Practice Center under Contract No. 290-2007-10061-I.) AHRQ Publication No. 13(14)-EHC116-EF. Rockville, MD: Agency for Healthcare Research and Quality; January 2014. Available at: www.effectivehealthcare.ahrq.gov/reports/final.cfm. Accessed August 2018.

- Grossman P, Niemann L, Schmidt S, et al. Mindfulness-based stress reduction and health benefits: a meta-analysis. *Journal of Psychosomatic Research.* 2004;57:35-43.
- Haines J, Spadaro K, Choi J, Hoffman L, Blazeck A. Reducing stress and anxiety in caregivers of lung transplant patients: benefits of mindfulness meditation. *International Journal of Organ Transplantation Medicine.* 2014;5:50-56.
- Harvard Health Publishing. Mindful Eating. Available at: https://www.health.harvard.edu/staying-healthy/mindful-eating. Accessed July 2018.
- Harvard Medical School. The Herbert Benson, MD Course in Mind Body Medicine. Available at: https://mindbody.hmscme.com/. Accessed July 2018.
- Hayes S. *Get Out of Your Mind and Into Your Life: The New Acceptance and Commitment Therapy.* Oakland, CA: New Harbinger Publications; 2005.
- Hölzel B, Carmody J, Vangel M, et al. Mindfulness practice leads to increases in regional brain gray matter density. *Psychiatry Research.* 2011;191(1):36.
- Holzel BK, Carmody J, Evans KC, et al. Stress reduction correlates with structural changes in the amygdala. *Social Cognitive and Affective Neuroscience.* 2010;5(1):11-17.
- Kabat-Zinn J, Hanh TN. *Full Catastrophe Living: Using the Wisdom of Your Body and Mind to Face Stress, Pain, and Illness.* New York: Random House; 1990.
- Kabat-Zinn J. Guided Mindfulness Meditation Series 1 [Video]. Available at: https://www.youtube.com/watch?v=8HYLyuJZKno. Accessed October 2017.
- Kabat-Zinn J. Guided Mindfulness Meditation Series 3 [Video]. Available at: https://www.youtube.com/watch?v=4Thh-n5qD64. Accessed October 2017.
- Kabat-Zinn J. Mindfulness Guided Meditation: The Power of Now [Video]. Available at: https://www.youtube.com/watch?v=422n7tzAxEI.
- Kabat-Zinn J. *Wherever You Go, There You Are.* New York: Hyperion; 1994.
- Kachur T. Hate/Love. Science in Seconds. Available at: http://www.scienceinseconds.com/blog/Hate-Love. Accessed October 2017.
- Kim SH, Schneider SM, Bevans M, et al. PTSD symptom reduction with mindfulness-based stretching and deep breathing exercise: randomized controlled clinical trial of efficacy. *Journal of Clinical Endocrinology and Metabolism.* 2013;98:2984-2992.
- Kim SH. Mindful Movement and Deep Breathing a Self-Care Tool: MBX-12 at Harvard. One Mind One Breath. Available at: https://onemindonebreath.com/2014/12/02/mindful-movement-and-deep-breathing-a-self-care-tool-mbx-12-at-harvard-extension-course/. Accessed July 2018.
- Lazar S. Lazar Lab. Available at: http://scholar.harvard.edu/sara_lazar. Accessed October 2017.
- Lazar SW, Kerr CE, Wasserman RH, et al. Meditation experience is associated with increased cortical thickness. *Neuroreport.* 2005;16(17):1893-1897.

- Louie D, Brook K, Frates E. The laughter prescription: a tool for lifestyle medicine. *American Journal of Lifestyle Medicine.* July 2016;10(4):262-267.
- Lyons KE, Delange J. Mindfulness matters in the classroom: the effects of mindfulness training on brain development and behavior in children and adolescents. In: Schonert-Reichl K, Roeser R, eds. *Handbook of Mindfulness in Education.* New York: Springer; 2016.
- Mayo Clinic. Relaxation Techniques: Try These Steps to Reduce Stress. Available at: http://www.mayoclinic.org/healthy-lifestyle/stress-management/in-depth/relaxation-technique/art-20045368. Accessed October 2017.
- Meditation-MP3.org. Brain Waves and States of Consciousness. Available at: http://www.meditation-mp3.org/brainwave-entrainment/. Accessed February 2017.
- Merriam-Webster. Definition of Antidote. Available at: https://www.merriam-webster.com/dictionary/antidote. Accessed October 2017.
- Merriam-Webster. Definition of Meditation. Available at: https://www.merriam-webster.com/dictionary/meditation. Accessed July 2018.
- Merriam-Webster. Definition of Mindfulness. Available at: https://www.merriam-webster.com/dictionary/mindfulness. Accessed October 2017.
- Merriam-Webster. Definition of Relax. Available at: https://www.merriam-webster.com/dictionary/relaxing?show=0&t=1413887872. Accessed October 2017.
- Mindfulnet.org. What Is Mindfulness? Available at: http://www.mindfulnet.org/page2.htm. Accessed October 2017.
- Mitchell M. Dr. Herbert Benson's Relaxation Response. Psychology Today. Available at: http://www.psychologytoday.com/blog/heart-and-soul-healing/201303/dr-herbert-benson-s-relaxation-response. Accessed October 2017.
- National Institutes of Health. National Center for Complementary and Integrative Health. Complementary, Alternative, or Integrative Health: What's In a Name? Available at: https://nccih.nih.gov/health/integrative-health. Accessed July 2018.
- National Institutes of Health. Stress and Your Health. MedlinePlus. Available at: https://medlineplus.gov/ency/article/003211.htm. Accessed July 2018.
- Porcari J, Bryant C, Comana F. *Exercise Physiology.* Philadelphia: FA Davis; 2015.
- Raab K. Mindfulness, self-compassion and empathy among health care professionals: a review of the literature. *Journal of Health Care Chaplaincy.* 2014;20(3):95-108.
- Rippstein-Leuenberger K, Mauthner O, Bryan Sexton J, et al. A qualitative analysis of the Three Good Things intervention in healthcare workers. *BMJ Open.* 2017;7:e015826. doi: 10.1136/bmjopen-2017-015826.
- Rozanski A, Bairey CN, Krantz DS, et al. Mental stress and the induction of silent myocardial ischemia in patients with coronary artery disease. *New England Journal of Medicine.* 1988;318:1005-1012.
- Sainz B, Loutsch JM, Marquart ME, et al. Stress-associated immunomodulation and herpes simplex virus infections. *Medical Hypotheses.* March 1 2001;56(3):348-356.

- Schneider RH, Grim CE, Rainforth MV, et al. Stress reduction in the secondary prevention of cardiovascular disease: a randomized, controlled trial of transcendental meditation and health education in blacks. *Circulation: Cardiovascular Quality and Outcomes.* 2012;5:750-758.
- Seligman ME. *Flourish: A Visionary New Understanding of Happiness and Well-being.* New York: Free Press; 2011.
- Sharma M, Rush S. Mindfulness-based stress reduction as a stress management intervention for healthy individuals: a systematic review. *Journal of Evidence-Based Complementary and Alternative Medicine.* 2014;19(4):271-286.
- Spadaro JH, et al. Reducing stress and anxiety in caregivers of lung transplant patients: benefits of mindfulness meditation. *International Journal of Transplant Medicine.* 2014;5(2):50-58.
- Stahl B, Goldstein E, Santorelli S, Kabat-Zinn J. *A Mindfulness-Based Stress Reduction Workbook.* Oakland, CA: New Harbinger Publications; 2010.
- Teasdale JD, Williams MG, Segal ZV, Kabat-Zinn J. *The Mindful Way Workbook: An 8-Week Program to Free Yourself from Depression and Emotional Distress.* New York: The Guilford Press; 2014.
- The American Institute of Stress. Stress Effects. Available at: https://www.stress.org/stress-effects/. Accessed September 2017.
- Thomas M, et al. Breathing exercises for asthma: a randomised controlled trial. *Thorax.* 2009;64:55-61. doi: 10.1136/thx.2008.100867.
- Total Body Psychology. The Stress Response...and How It Relates to the HPA Axis! Available at: http://www.total-body-psychology.com.au/stress-response---hpa-axis.html. Accessed August 2018.
- van Dixhoorn J, White A. Relaxation therapy for rehabilitation and prevention in ischaemic heart disease: a systematic review and meta-analysis. *European Journal of Cardiovascular Prevention and Rehabilitation.* 2005;12:193-202.
- VIA Institute on Character. VIA Character Survey. Available at: https://www.viacharacter.org/www/. Accessed October 2017.
- Vinik AI. The conductor of the autonomic orchestra. *Frontiers in Endocrinology.* 2012;3:71. doi:10.3389/fendo.2012.00071.
- Voss MW, Nagamatsu LS, Liu Ambrose T, et al. Exercise, brain, and cognition across the life span. *Journal of Applied Physiology.* April 28 2011;111(5):1505-1513.
- Wallace RK, Benson H, Wilson A. A wakeful hypometabolic physiologic state. *American Journal of Physiology.* September 1 1971;221:795-799. Available at: http://ajplegacy.physiology.org/content/221/3/795. Accessed October 2017.
- Wallace RK, Benson H. The physiology of meditation. *Scientific American.* 1972;226:84-90.
- Wikipedia. List of Systems of the Human Body. Available at: https://en.wikipedia.org/wiki/List_of_systems_of_the_human_body. Accessed October 2017.

CHAPTER 9

THE POWER OF CONNECTION

"To be kept in solitude is to be kept in pain."

—E.O. Wilson, PhD
Retired Harvard Professor
Two-Time Pulitzer Prize Winner

❏ Chapter Goals:

- Develop an understanding of the concept of social connection.
- Review the connection between being socially connected and health.
- Examine the barriers to connecting with others.
- Explore the premise of loneliness.
- Discuss the notion of social isolation.
- Understand what steps can be undertaken to develop enhanced social connections.

❏ Learning Objectives:

- To understand the impact of being socially connected on a person's health
- To review the factors that contribute to social connection
- To grasp the obstacles to being socially connected
- To become familiar with the differences between loneliness and social isolation

❏ Guiding Questions:

- What is social connection?
- What is the impact of a strong social connection on health?
- What factors affect how connected a person is to others?
- What barriers exist to social connection?
- What is social isolation?
- Why does social isolation occur?
- What are the perils of social isolation?
- How can social connection be developed?

Lifestyle Medicine Handbook

❑ Important Terms:

- *Loneliness:* Feelings of being disconnected from others
- *Social connection:* The relationship that people have with the individuals around them
- *Social isolation:* The lack of available and quality relationships
- *Social network:* A social structure that is made up of elements (individuals or organizations) that socially interact with one or more parts of the structure

A growing body of research shows that people need people. People who care about them as individuals. People on whom they can count when they are faced with the challenges inherent in life. People who will provide emotional support if a need arises. People with whom they have mutually satisfying and beneficial relationships. People to whom they feel a sense of connection. As Abraham Maslow's Hierarchy of Needs (Figure 9-1) reveals, a sense of belonging is one of our most important human needs. The only needs more important are physiological needs and safety needs.

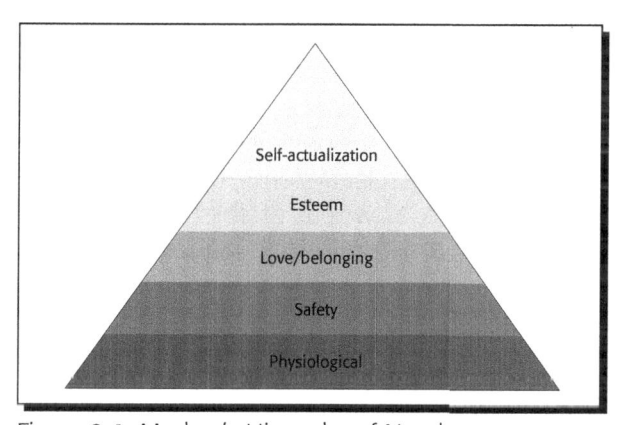

Figure 9-1. Maslow's Hierarchy of Needs

In addition, for people to have continued motivation, they need three things. According to Ryan Deci and Richard Ryan's self-determination theory, these three elements are competence, autonomy, and relatedness (a sense of connection). To make lifestyle changes stick, people often need a connection to others (e.g., a physician, nurse, nutrition expert, fitness professional, health coach or other healthcare professional), who are working to empower them to adopt and sustain healthy habits. This connection could also be a loved one or friend who is supporting the person in the pursuit of health and wellness.

From an evolutionary perspective, people are hardwired to seek human connection. Not only are individuals profoundly influenced by their social environment, they suffer when their social bonds are threatened or severed. The evolutionary impulse to connect is evidenced by the physical pain people feel when cut out from a social circle, rejected from a sports team, or suffering a romantic breakup. These types of situations feel like a threat to their very existence.

During the era of hunting and gathering, individuals existed in tribes, which provided a logistic advantage for procurement of food and separation of labor, a sense of comfort and pride, defense in a dangerous and disorienting environment, and social meaning in a chaotic world. Evolutionary biologists, such as Edward Wilson, describe the human condition as "eusocial," which adds the elements of group selection into natural selection. Group selection favors altruism and cooperation that enables the advanced level of social behavior among humans, which in turn, enables the flourishing of the human species.

What, then, does social connection entail? A number of possible explanations have been advanced. One of the most direct and easy-to-understand definitions of social connection was suggested by best-selling author Brene Brown. "Connection is the energy that exists between people when they feel seen, heard, and valued; when they can give and receive without judgment; and when they derive sustenance and strength from the relationship."

THE POSITIVE HEALTH BENEFITS OF SOCIAL CONNECTION

Social connections are as important to a person's survival and vitality as food, shelter, and safety. Having a sense of social connectedness tends to generate an ongoing positive loop of social, emotional, and physical well-being. While biological explanations are still being investigated, it seems that social ties benefit functioning of the immune system, the endocrine system, and the cardiovascular system. Social circles can also influence health behaviors by providing information, as well as establishing norms and values. Amazingly, research reported in a *Scientific American* article indicates that a strong sense of social connection can increase the duration of a person's lifetime by as much as 50 percent.

THE BIOLOGY OF SOCIAL CONNECTION

People were born to connect. Oxytocin helped individuals form their first social bond with our mothers. Oxytocin, colloquially known as "the love hormone," is produced in the hypothalamus and released by the pituitary gland in the brain. Prosocial activities, such as making love, hugging, cuddling, and holding hands, promote the production and release of oxytocin into the bloodstream. Known best for its direct action to stimulate uterine contractions during pregnancy and subsequent milk letdown postpartum, oxytocin may also play a larger role in social bonding than previously thought.

While still under investigation, the exact mechanism of oxytocin's action on human behavior is thought to reflect release from centrally projecting oxytocin neurons, with synaptic connections to neurons throughout the brain and spinal cord. Various studies suggest that oxytocin works in concert with other neurotransmitters, including GABA, serotonin, and dopamine. Research from Stanford University suggests that social interaction may act as a reward for the brain, as mediated through the effects of oxytocin. Oxytocin acts as a neurotransmitter in the nucleus accumbens, part of the brain's reward circuitry.

Conversely, when the oxytocin receptors are blocked, mice show decreased socializing activity. Oxytocin's prosocial effects are evidenced by its suggested role in increasing trust, reducing fear, improving emotional recognition, increasing eye gazing, and increasing the ability to read emotions behind facial expressions. This factor is supported by a study on children with autism spectrum disorders, which showed that a single inhaled dose of oxytocin increased brain function in regions known to process social information. Oxytocin seems to facilitate social attunement, activating more for social stimuli (human faces) rather than non-social stimuli (cars). Currently, oxytocin is being studied as a possible treatment in patients with PTSD, who have difficulties with emotional and cognitive empathy.

In addition to human to human connections, oxytocin appears to have a role across a variety of species. One study found that the level of oxytocin in both dogs and humans increased substantially after a petting session, which perhaps suggests its role in the emotional bond between humans and dogs. When oxytocin is given intranasally to a dog, the dog displays a higher social orientation and affiliation toward their owner and toward fellow dog partners. It appears that researchers have only scraped the surface of oxytocin's power to promote empathy and social relatedness in mammalian species.

Interestingly, there is not just one location in the brain that controls the ability to socialize. The social brain (Figure 9-2) is complex and calls upon different areas to coordinate and create a social interaction. Being in touch with the other person is key to communication. The amygdala lies deep in the reptilian brain and works to understand emotions. This area needs to communicate with the fusiform face area so that facial expressions can be properly understood. Then, to better understand the person with whom you are speaking, you need to appreciate their mood, since that will help dictate how you speak to them. The medial prefrontal cortex and the superior temporal sulcus help with this factor. These areas of the brain connect with the visual cortex in the posterior of the brain and the auditory cortex on the sides of the brain in the temporal area. Compassionate communication requires a coordination of multiple areas of the brain, as well as concentration on the other person.

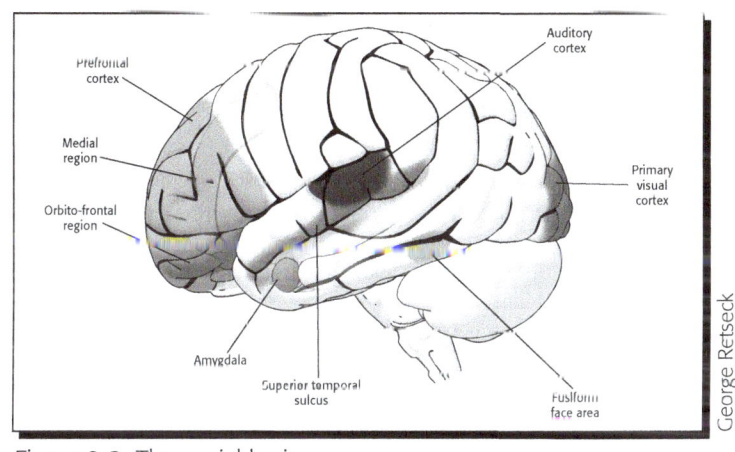

Figure 9-2. The social brain

Neuroscientists have recently discovered the so-called "default network" of the brain, which comes on every time someone is resting (i.e., not actively engaged in a task). Interestingly, the default mode looks very similar to the brain network used for social thinking, such as conjecturing about other people's thoughts, feelings, and goals. This evidence suggests that the default impetus of individuals is to reach out and connect with others—an adaptive evolutionary trait that has promoted the survival and advancement of the human species.

CONNECTIONS THAT KEEP PEOPLE REALLY ALIVE AND THRIVING

Connections to other human beings are not the only important connections. In his book *Connect: 12 Vital Ties That Open Your Heart, Lengthen Your Life, and Deepen Your Soul*, psychiatrist Dr. Edward Hallowell goes into detail about the following 12 vital ties:

- Family of origin
- Immediate family
- Friends and community
- Work, mission, activity
- Beauty
- The past
- Nature and special places
- Pets and other animals
- Ideas and information
- Institutions and organizations
- Whatever is beyond knowledge
- Yourself

Each of these 12 connections serves to energize people. Previously, the power of connecting with people (family and friends) and pets was discussed earlier in this chapter. Connecting with work, projects, and current activities often provides a sense of purpose that has been shown to add almost seven years to life expectancy, according to the work of Blue Zones, with Dan Buettner and his group. Having individuals acknowledge the beauty around them and within them is another piece of the health and wellness puzzle. What we appreciate, appreciates. Thus, when people stop to connect with the beauty, awe-inspiring images, or actions that occur in their lives, they awaken their heart and soul.

Nature and special places that individuals have visited can also have a profound impact on them. Research reveals that living in places with green spaces reduces morbidity, as well as the chances of developing medical conditions and diseases. In fact, just looking at photos of nature with greenery can reduce stress. Connecting with beauty and nature allows people to be fully alive and aware. It takes mindfulness to accomplish this, using all of individuals' senses to enjoy their present moments.

That said, connecting to their past, making sense of their previous experiences, and learning from past mishaps helps people to move forward with confidence. Individuals don't need to dwell in the past; they just need to work to make sense of it with a growth mindset. Connecting with ideas and information, while continuing to learn, is important. Being a lifelong learner, feeding their childlike sense of curiosity and wonder also helps to keep people young. Having a sense of connection to organizations (a person's place of work, volunteer programs) and institutions (college, graduate school, community centers) helps people to feel part of something larger than self.

As such, there is a connection to "Whatever is beyond knowledge," as Dr. Hallowell says. This factor could be a religious or spiritual connection. For some people, this connection plays a large role in their lives and for others, it becomes more important, when illness strikes.

Finally, there is a connection with self. This connection, which is important, is not often emphasized. Feeling like you know yourself—your strengths and weaknesses, is important for health, happiness, and productivity. If a person knows what helps them to create joy, then they are more likely to seek it and enjoy it, literally. Self-love, self-respect, and self-care are all important parts of a healthy lifestyle. Accordingly, connecting with themselves is a key connection for an individual to work on. It takes time, but it is worth it. The journey of self-discovery is part of the lifestyle medicine journey. In fact, the connections to people, pets, places, nature, beauty, the past, work, ideas, organizations, whatever is beyond knowledge, and ourselves all play a role in a person's health and happiness.

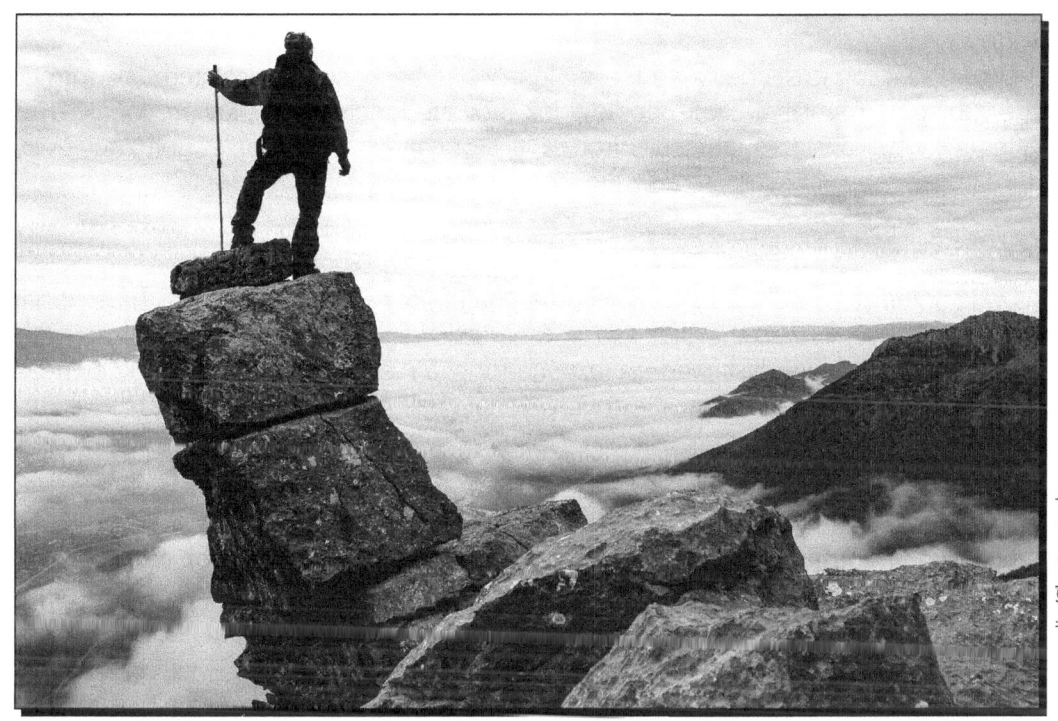

The journey of self-discovery is part of the lifestyle medicine journey.

BARRIERS TO SOCIAL CONNECTION

Despite its obvious relevance for health, research indicates that human-to-human connections are waning at an alarming rate in the United States. This decline could help explain the concomitant rise that has been reported in various emotional responses, such as loneliness, isolation, and alienation.

Why has the level of social connection dwindled so significantly? Among the barriers that can affect a person's ability to build positive relationships include the following:
- Technology (e.g., smartphones and social media)
- Lack of self-confidence (e.g., low self-esteem)
- Lack of interpersonal skills (e.g., invisible wall between people)
- Reluctance to interact with others (e.g., avoid social situations)
- Poor communication skills (e.g., inability to listen to others and to express themselves)
- Fear of change (e.g., resist taking action)
- Their surroundings (e.g., minimal number of actual opportunities for connection)

THE DIFFERENCE BETWEEN LONELINESS AND SOCIAL ISOLATION

A clear distinction exists between feeling lonely and being socially isolated. The former is a subjective mental state. If people think they are lonely, then they are lonely. The latter is a physical state that results from a lack of contact with people. Both, however, have negative health-related consequences, such as:

❑ Loneliness

As was noted previously, it is part of human nature for people to need to have social connection. People who are deficient in their ability to connect or communicate with other individuals are described as experiencing an emotional response known as loneliness. The causes of loneliness vary. Emotional, physical, and social factors can contribute to feelings of loneliness.

❑ Social Isolation

Whereas loneliness is essentially an emotional (mental) state, social isolation is a physical state (i.e., the voluntary or involuntary absence of having contact with other individuals). If individuals are alone, but enjoying it, they are experiencing solitude. On the other hand, if they are alone, but not enjoying it, they are experiencing social isolation. Accordingly, social isolation is considered undesirable.

THE ADVERSE HEALTH EFFECTS OF SOCIAL ISOLATION

Just as social connection is health-promoting, social isolation can have negative implications for a person's mental and physical health. It can exacerbate an individual's feelings of low self-worth, shame, and depression. It can also lead to a fear of interacting with others, as well as a sense of disconnectedness from society as a whole.

In a landmark study conducted in 1979, Lisa F. Berkman and S. Leonard Syme were the first researchers to elucidate the relationship between social and community ties and mortality. Using the 1965 Human Population Laboratory survey of a random sample of 6928 adults in Alameda County, they conclusively found that people who lacked social and community ties were more likely—2.3 more likely for men and 2.8 more likely for women—to die in the follow-up period than those with more extensive contacts.

It is known that individuals who are socially isolated have disrupted sleep patterns, depressed immune function, and higher levels of stress hormones. Individuals who do not feel socially connected also tend to be at a higher risk for certain health-related conditions, such as high blood pressure and an increased level of inflammation. With regard to a person's body systems, it appears that social isolation can negatively impact everything from their cardiac function to skin health, hormone regulation, and even their cognitive faculties.

Social isolation is associated with an increased risk of coronary heart disease. In fact, social isolation rivals hypertension as a cardiovascular risk factor. A study published in the *American Journal of Public Health* used the Social Network Index to measure isolation in 16,849 adults in NHANES III. Low Social Network Index scores were associated with a risk of mortality, similar to that of smoking. Social isolation was also an important predictor of mortality among women along with smoking and high blood pressure.

In another study that looked at the connection between social interactions and health, socially isolated patients had 2.4 times the risk of cardiac death, compared to their more socially connected peers. A low quantity and quality of social ties was linked with development and progression of cardiovascular disease, recurrent heart attack, atherosclerosis, high blood pressure, cancer, delayed cancer recovery, slow wound healing, inflammatory markers, and impaired immune function. Another recently conducted study found that social isolation increases the risk of heart disease by 29 percent and the risk of stroke by 32 percent.

Furthermore, people who have a low amount of social connection tend to be more vulnerable to mental health conditions, such as anxiety, depression, and antisocial behavior. Social interaction promotes general cognitive function, given that participating in a discussion requires listening, practicing empathy to understand the viewpoints of others, memorizing data, updating information, and inhibiting inappropriate responses—all executive functions. Those individuals who have frequent engagement in mental, social, and productive activities have a lower risk of dementia. In contrast, being single, being widowed, or living alone with a limited social network increases the risk of dementia. In fact, loneliness can accelerate cognitive decline in older adults.

While social isolation is most common in elderly individuals, younger adults can also be affected by this condition (as well as by loneliness). Longitudinal findings on subjects, followed from childhood to adulthood, show that social isolation has persistent and cumulative effects on long-term health. Perhaps, the most convincing evidence that social isolation is truly killing people comes from a meta-analysis of 70 studies and 3.4 million people that found that socially isolated individuals have a 30-percent higher risk of dying in the next seven years.

THE IMPACT OF SOCIAL NETWORKS ON HEALTH

Research by Nicholas Christakis shows that health behaviors are spread among network members who are not only geographically close, but socially close. Studies by Christakis and his colleague, James H. Fowler, suggested that a variety of what are normally considered individuals or personal attributes—obesity, smoking status, and happiness—also arise, due to contagion mechanisms that transmit these behaviors within social networks. Thankfully, the same factor applies to happiness, which also spreads through social networks. Conveying presence, being genuine, communicating affirmations, and using effective listening with supportive communication can help develop resilient and positive social networks—one relationship at a time.

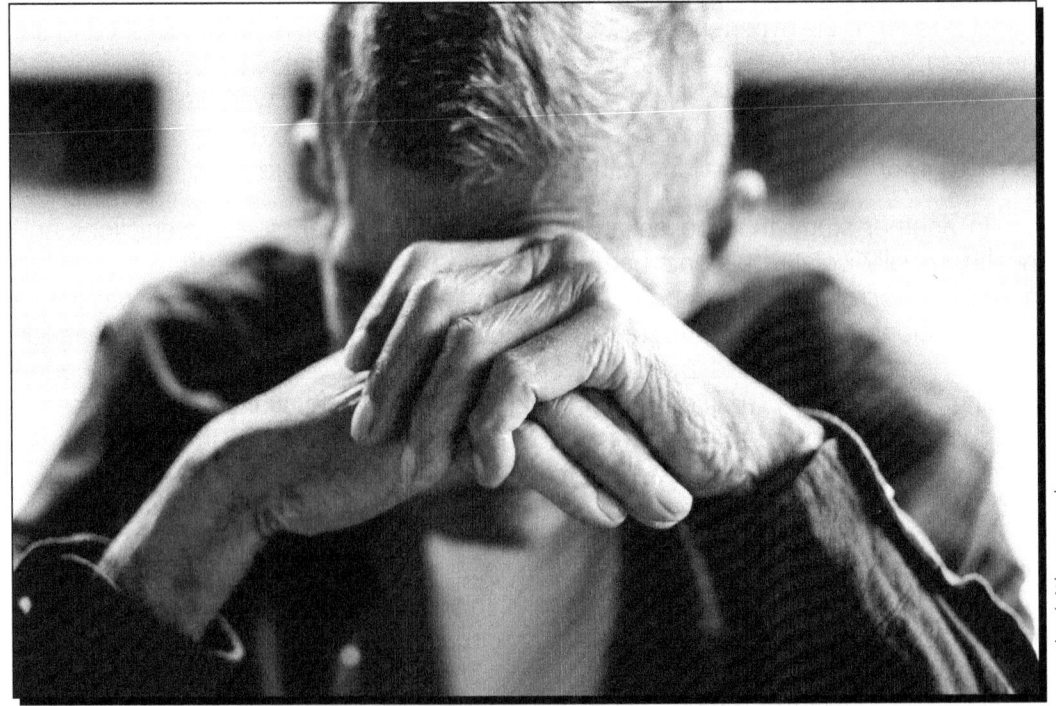

Social isolation has persistent and cumulative effects on long-term health.

STEPS TO ENHANCE A PERSON'S LEVEL OF SOCIAL CONNECTION AND DECREASE LONELINESS

Fortunately, loneliness can be circumvented, although it requires a conscious effort on the lonely person's part to make a change. Ideally, as a society, people will work to combat social isolation, using the Social Ecological Model of Change, with the understanding that the individual's experience is influenced on multiple levels from interpersonal ties, to community norms and networks, to institutional values and culture, and all the way up to policies and laws. Among the more immediate, actionable steps that can help people prevent or overcome loneliness are the following:

- Accept other individuals as they are. Try to build trust with them gradually.
- Have an uplifting attitude and be confident. Most people prefer to associate with positive individuals.
- If they live alone, consider getting a roommate or a pet.
- Be aware that loneliness is a signal that something needs to change.
- Consider volunteering for community service or another activity that they enjoy.
- Focus on developing quality relationships with people who share similar attitudes, interests, and values with them.
- Expect the best from themselves, as well as in others.
- On occasion, think of something that makes them happy or provides them with a sense of enjoyment.
- Identify the reasons why they feel lonely.

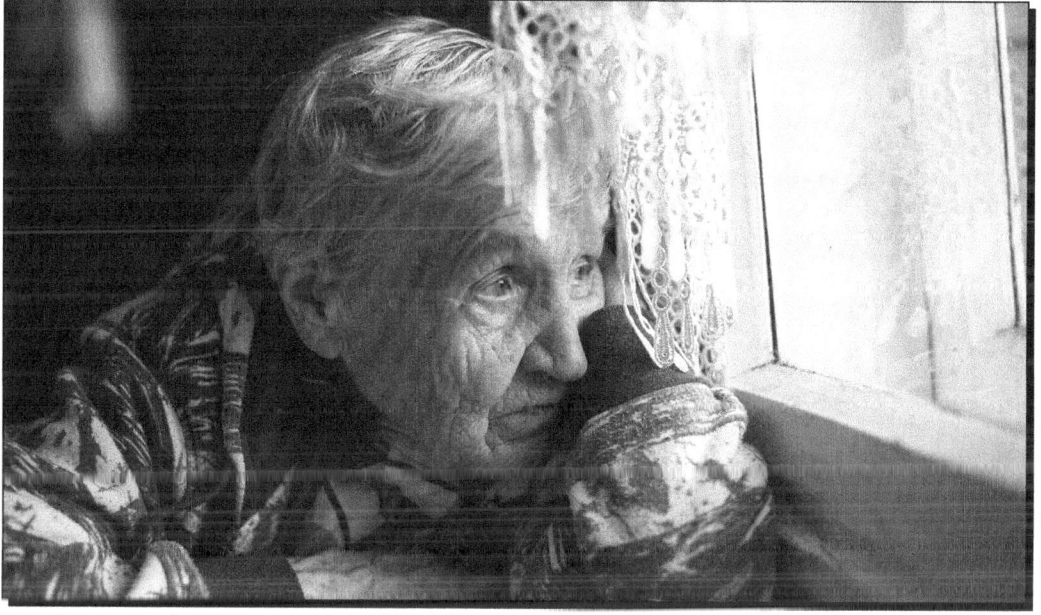

Loneliness can be circumvented, although it requires a conscious effort on the lonely person's part to make a change.

- Start a journal to track their thoughts and feelings.
- Realize that they are not alone—feeling a sense of loneliness is part of human nature.
- Challenge themselves to take the initiative in developing social relationships.
- Understand the effects that loneliness can have on their lives—both mentally and physically.

TAKING SOCIAL CONNECTIONS ONE STEP FURTHER— CREATING HIGH QUALITY CONNECTIONS

Dr. Jane Dutton has done extensive work in creating high quality connections. Her definition of connection is "A connection is the dynamic, living tissue that exists between two people, when there is some contact between them involving mutual awareness and social interaction." To describe a high quality connection, Dr. Dutton uses a medical analogy, "Like a healthy blood vessel that connects parts of our body, a high-quality connection between two people allows the transfer of vital nutrients; it is flexible, strong, and resilient." In contrast, Dr. Dutton describes low quality connections as follows, "A tie exists (people communicate, they interact, and they may even be involved in interdependent work), but the connective tissue is damaged. With low-quality connection, there is a little death in every interaction." There are three essential ingredients for high quality connection:

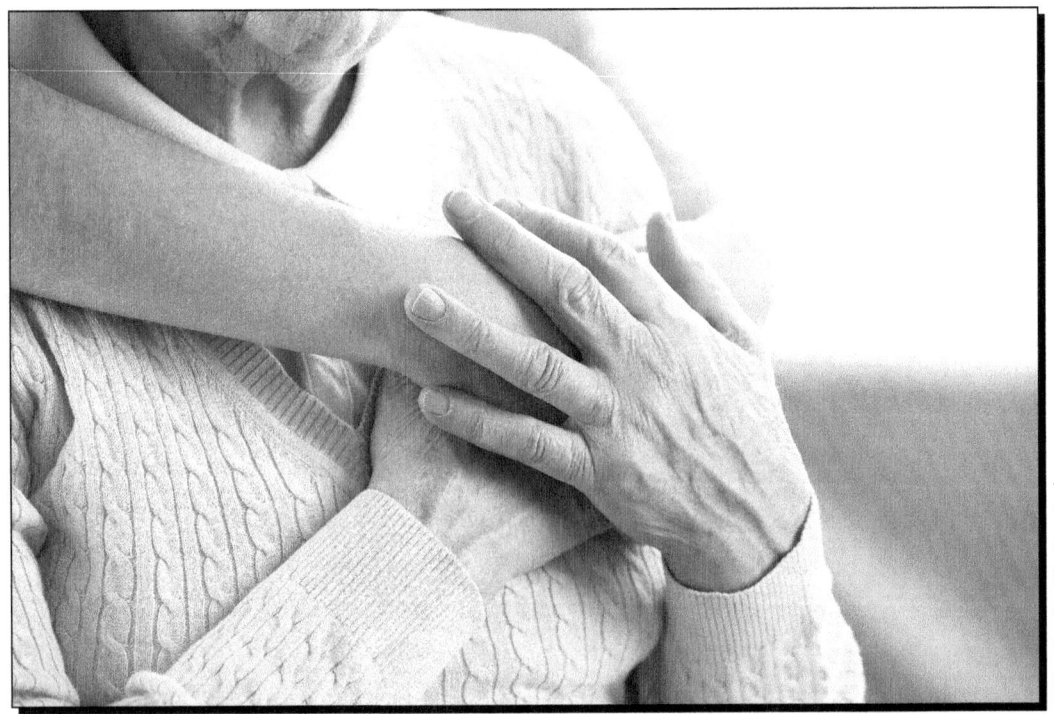

There are three essential ingredients for high quality connection.

- A high emotional carrying capacity (ECC)—the expression of more emotion, both positive and negative, and safety felt in doing so
- The ability to bounce back after setbacks
- Relationship has generativity and openness to new ideas and influence, as well as its ability to deflect behaviors that will shut down generative processes

With high quality connections, people experience:
- Feelings of vitality and aliveness—feeling positive arousal and a heightened sense of positive energy
- Heightened sense of positive regard—a feeling of being known or being loved
- Felt mutuality—Both parties in the connection are engaged and actively participating

Lifestyle medicine practitioners should work to enjoy high quality connections for themselves at work and at home. Knowing these facts and working on it themselves will help them to counsel patients in this area. Most people don't think about the importance of connections or friendships. On the other hand, as lifestyle medicine professionals, it is important that they do. Healthy connections can help people sustain healthy habits.

LIVE AND LEARN WITH DR. BETH FRATES

The power of connections can manifest itself during encounters with patients. The following is an example. I was counseling a woman about her lifestyle, because she was in the overweight category by BMI and wanted to lose weight, mostly because her clothes were so tight that she was on the verge of needing a whole new wardrobe. Since this client was extremely thrifty, she could not bear to buy new clothes. Some of her pants were from 20 years earlier. So, she sought me out to work with me on her diet and exercise.

As it turns out, she had recently changed jobs. The location of her new job prevented her from commuting to work by bicycle. As a result, she had to drive. In addition, at her new job, there was a buffet-style lunch every day. To top it off, because the chef was also an amazing baker, fresh cookies, cakes, and goodies were available after every lunch. The custom at the office was to enjoy a couple of cookies and pack a few more for late afternoon snacks. My patient did just that for four months. By the end of four months, she had put on 15 pounds, due to these lifestyle changes. So, we had some work to do together.

We had weekly walking meetings, in which we discussed nutrition, exercise, sleep, stress resiliency, and social connections. The patient made small changes in all of these areas. Her husband was the cook, and she felt pressure to "show her love" by eating everything on her plate, and they used large plates. As such, working on communicating with her husband and expressing her desire to decrease her portions for health reasons was a goal for her one week. Although they already had a great relationship, they grew even closer.

Subsequently, they started taking evening walks after dinner. In fact, her husband was so supportive, he started adapting his cooking to suit her new whole foods, plant-based eating plan. He also altered her portions to be closer to the recommended sizes. In addition, they moved away from rich desserts to fruits.

In fact, they were having fun, until her husband started to worry that he might have cancer. He noticed a 20-pound weight loss and felt his pants were "falling off." Since he was not trying to lose weight, they were both worried. Thankfully, the husband was able to see his primary care physician quickly, so that their fears could be put to rest. Her husband was told that he was perfectly healthy. He had moved from the overweight BMI category to the normal weight category. They were very relieved, surprised, and thrilled. Together, they have kept the weight off for over five years. Social connections can be a key ingredient in lifestyle changes.

SUGGESTIONS TO PREVENT SOCIAL ISOLATION AND PROMOTE SOCIAL CONNECTION

Physicians and allied healthcare professionals can offer their patients a variety of possible strategies and suggestions to help them prevent social isolation and promote social connection, including the following:
- Be aware that no one-size-fits-all treatment option exists for a disorder, such as social isolation.
- Institute interventions that can help reduce their risk of being socially isolated.
- Pay it forward—participate as a volunteer in activities that they enjoy and that can help enhance their sense of self-worth.
- Treat social isolation as a chronic illness that is a real threat to their health.
- Try to identify and understand the real causes underlying their social isolation and work on addressing them.
- Undertake psychological therapy.

In reality, social connectedness and social networks can take many forms for different people. Geographically, people can be close or far apart. Social network sizes vary from person-to-person, with some networks being large and others being very small.

Regardless of what an individual's social network entails, social connection has more to do with a person's feelings of connection than the number of friends that an individual has. Social connectedness is a byproduct of a person's subjective feelings of being connected. This factor means that individuals can foster, nurture, and build their sense of connection. Engaging in one or more of the following steps can facilitate in this process:
- Actively look for opportunities to socially engage with someone (e.g., go to a movie with a friend).

- Consider participating in a community project (e.g., volunteer for a clean-up campaign).
- Look for new channels of social engagement (e.g., attend church; join a service club, like Kiwanis International; etc.).
- Reach out to someone who may be experiencing difficult times (e.g., death in the family; divorce; etc.).
- Join a chat room on the Internet that provides people with an opportunity to talk online with each other about various topics (e.g., cooking; gardening; movies; favorite sport team, etc.).
- Make a short list of friends, family members, and colleagues who play a supportive and positive role in their life and make a commitment to reach out to them on a regular basis (e.g., face-to-face; telephone; email; etc.).
- Show interest in another person's life (e.g., learn to listen and follow-up accordingly).
- Practice random acts of kindness (e.g., share something; help someone; be unexpectedly nice; etc.).
- Be productive—to a large degree, being connected with others is a choice that individuals can make for themselves (e.g., recognize the value of social connection and do something about it).

FITT PRESCRIPTIONS FOR CONNECTION

F—Frequency: daily, weekly monthly

I—Intensity: quality of interactions (deep or superficial connections; close ties, new connections, etc.)

T—Time: duration of interaction

T—Type: experience/activity (family gathering, volunteer work, meetings, religious services, etc.)

❑ An example FITT prescription for cultivating high quality connections:

F—one day per week
I—deep conversation/connection with friend
T—30 minutes
T—family dinner or meal with a friend

❑ An example FITT prescription for increasing social contact and opening the door for new connections:

F—three days per week
I—superficial/new connection
T—less than five minutes
T—strike up a friendly conversation with someone you don't know well at work, at the store, or at a social event

KEY POINTS/TAKEAWAYS FOR CHAPTER 9

❏ Chapter Review:

- Overall goal: Review the factors that impact a person's level of social connection and ways to enhance social connection.
- Application goal: Understand the connection between social connection, loneliness, and social isolation and an individual's health.

❏ Discussion Questions:

- What are the basic differences between social connection, loneliness, and social isolation?
- What are the barriers to connecting with other individuals?
- What steps can be undertaken to develop social connection?
- What advice should physicians and allied healthcare professionals provide to their patients who are lonely?
- What are the negative health consequences of having a subpar level of social connection?

	TITLE	AUTHORS	JOURNAL	YEAR	KEY FINDINGS
1	Cardiovascular reactivity and the presence of pets, friends, and spouses: the truth about cats and dogs	Allen K, Blascovich J, Mendes WB	*Psychosomatic Medicine*	2002	A study of 240 married couples that sought to examine the effects of the presence of friends, spouses, and pets on cardiovascular reactivity to psychological and physical stress. "Relative to people without pets, people with pets had significantly lower heart rate and blood pressure levels during a resting baseline, significantly smaller increases from baseline levels during the mental arithmetic and cold pressor, and faster recovery."
2	Physiological effects of human/ companion animal bonding	Baun MM, et al.	*Nursing Research*	1984	A small study that recorded blood pressure, heart rate, and respiratory rate of 24 subjects either petting a known or unknown dog, or sitting quietly. They found significant physiologic effects of petting a dog with whom a person has a companion bond. Specifically, they found a decrease in blood pressure, similar to when reading a book, as well as a "greeting response" to entry of a known dog in which blood pressure goes up.

Figure 9-3. The connection prescription evidence

	TITLE	AUTHORS	JOURNAL	YEAR	KEY FINDINGS
3	Social networks, host resistance, and mortality: a nine-year follow-up study of Alameda County residents	Berkman LF, Syme SL	American Journal of Epidemiology	1979	This nine-year follow-up survey of 6,928 adults in Alameda County, California, found that men and women who lacked social and community ties were 2.3 and 2.8 times more likely to die in the follow-up period than those with more extensive contacts, respectively. This was found to be independent of self-reported physical health status, year of death, socioeconomic status, health practices, and utilization of preventive health services.
4	Socially isolated children 20 years later: risk of cardiovascular disease	Caspi A, et al	Archives of Pediatrics & Adolescent Medicine	2006	Longitudinal prospective cohort study of 1,037 children followed from birth to age 26 years that measured social isolation in childhood, adolescence, and adulthood and its relation to heart disease. It found that "socially isolated children were at significant risk of poor adult health compared with nonisolated children (risk ratio, 1.37; 95% confidence interval, 1.17-1.61). This association was independent of other well-established childhood risk factors for poor adult health…"
5	Social reward requires coordinated activity of nucleus accumbens oxytocin and serotonin	Dölen G, et al.	Nature	2013	A mice study that demonstrated how oxytocin acts as a social reinforcement signal within the nucleus accumbens. It also "demonstrates that the rewarding properties of social interaction in mice require the coordinated activity of oxytocin and serotonin (5-HT) in the nucleus accumbens."
6	Loneliness, depression and cognitive function in older U.S. adults	Donovan NJ, et al.	International Journal of Geriatric Psychiatry	2017	This study used longitudinal data from the US Health and Retirement Study (1998-2010) and found that "loneliness and depressive symptoms appear to be related risk factors for worsening cognition but low cognitive function does not lead to worsening loneliness over time."
7	An active and socially integrated lifestyle in late life might protect against dementia	Fratiglioni L, Paillard-Borg S, Winblad B	Lancet Neurology	2004	Systematic review that explores the effect of social network, physical leisure, and non-physical activity on cognition and dementia. The researchers conclude that "an active and socially integrated lifestyle in late life protects against dementia and Alzheimer's disease."
8	Mediterranean lifestyle and cardiovascular disease prevention	Georgousopoulou EN, et al.	Cardiovascular Diagnosis and Therapy	2017	A large study of 2,749 older adults (65-100 years) from the Mediterranean and Greece that showed a strong association between lifestyle parameters (e.g., social life, midday sleep, residential environment) and the presence of cardiovascular disease risk factors in the elderly.

Figure 9-3. The connection prescription evidence (cont.)

	TITLE	AUTHORS	JOURNAL	YEAR	KEY FINDINGS
9	Oxytocin enhances brain function in children with autism	Gordon I, et al.	*Proceedings of the National Academy of Sciences of the United States of America*	2013	In this randomized, double-blind, crossover functional MRI study, the researchers evaluated the impact of a single intranasal administration of oxytocin on brain activity in 17 children and adolescents with autism spectrum disorder. Researchers found enhanced emotion recognition in subjects who received oxytocin. These results suggested that oxytocin may facilitate a social attunement, activating more for social stimuli (i.e., faces) and activating less for non-social stimuli (i.e., cars).
10	Loneliness and social isolation as risk factors for mortality: a meta-analytic review	Holt-Lunstad J, et al.	*Perspectives on Psychology Science*	2015	The authors of this meta-analytic review sought to establish the overall and relative magnitude of social isolation and loneliness and to examine possible moderators. They found increased odds of mortality for social isolation (OR=1.29), loneliness (OR=1.26), and living alone (OR=1.32).
11	Social engagement and cognitive function in old age	Krueger KR, et al.	*Experimental Aging Research*	2009	A study of 838 healthy ~80-year-olds that found that "social activity and social support were related to better cognitive function, whereas social network size was not strongly related to global cognition."
12	The connection prescription: using the power of social interactions and the deep desire for connectedness to empower health and wellness	Martino J, Pegg J, Frates EP	*American Journal of Lifestyle Medicine*	2015	A state-of-the-art review on social connection that found significant evidence that "social support and feeling connected can help people maintain a healthy body mass index, control blood sugars, improve cancer survival, decrease cardiovascular mortality, decrease depressive symptoms, mitigate posttraumatic stress disorder symptoms, and improve overall mental health." It discusses how counseling patients, inquiring about social connection, and prescribing connection can increase the health and well-being of patients.
13	Social isolation: a predictor of mortality comparable to traditional clinical risk factors	Pantell M, et al.	*American Journal of Public Health*	2013	This study analyzed 16,849 adults in the NHANES III database and found that Social Index Scores were predictive of mortality among men, and the risk of mortality was similar to that of smoking. Social isolation was also an important predictor of mortality among women, along with smoking and high blood pressure.

Figure 9-3. The connection prescription evidence (cont.)

	TITLE	AUTHORS	JOURNAL	YEAR	KEY FINDINGS
14	Relationship quality and virtuousness: emotional carrying capacity as a source of individual and team resilience	Stephens JP, et al.	*Journal of Applied Behavioral Science*	2013	In two small studies, researchers "focus on emotional carrying capacity—wherein relationship partners express more of their emotions, express both positive and negative emotions, and do so constructively, as a source of resilience in individuals and teams." They found that emotional carrying capacity is positively related to team resilience and mediates the connection between trust and team resilience.
15	Social support, unstable angina, and stroke as predictors of depression in patients with coronary heart disease	*Su SF, Chang MY, He CP*	*Journal of Cardiovascular Nursing*	2017	A cross-sectional sample of 105 Taiwanese patients from cardiology units that found social support, unstable angina, and stroke may be important predictors of depression in patients with coronary heart disease. Social support was significantly ($r=-0.481$, $p<0.01$) and adversely correlated with depression.
16	Impact of peer health coaching on glycemic control in low-income patients with diabetes: a randomized controlled trial	Thom DH, et al.	*Annals of Family Medicine*	2013	This randomized controlled trial of 249 patients with diabetes utilized 23 controlled diabetics to serve as peer coaches. At six months, the coached group had decreased their hemoglobin A1c by 1.07% as compared to 0.3% in the usual care group ($p=0.01$), and 22.0% of coached vs. 14.9% of usual care patients had hemoglobin A1c levels less than 7.5% ($p=0.04$).
17	Social relationships and health: a flashpoint for health policy	Umberson D, Montez JK	*Journal of Health and Social Behavior*	2010	A discussion of how social relationships affect mental health, health behavior, physical health, and mortality risk. Specifically, "scientific evidence supports the following premises...1) social ties affect mental health, physical health, health behaviors, and mortality risk, 2) social ties are a potential resource that can be harnessed to promote population health, 3) social ties are a resource that should be protected as well as promoted, 4) social ties can benefit health beyond the target individuals by influencing the health of others throughout social networks, 5) social ties have both immediate and long-term cumulative effects on health, and thus represent opportunities for short- and long-term investment in population health... 6) social ties—overburdened, strained, conflicted, abusive—can undermine health, and 7) the costs and benefits of social ties are not distributed equally in the population."

Figure 9-3. The connection prescription evidence (cont.)

	TITLE	AUTHORS	JOURNAL	YEAR	KEY FINDINGS
18	Loneliness and social isolation as risk factors for coronary heart disease and stroke: systematic review and meta-analysis of longitudinal observational studies	Valtorta NK, et al	*Heart*	2016	This systematic review and meta-analysis included 19 studies on coronary heart disease and stroke and found that poor social relationships were associated with a 29% increase in risk of incident coronary heart disease and a 32% increase in risk of stroke.

References

1. Allen K, Blascovich J, Mendes WB. Cardiovascular reactivity and the presence of pets, friends, and spouses: the truth about cats and dogs. *Psychosomatic Medicine*. 2002;64(5):727-739.
2. Baun MM, Bergstrom N, Langston NF, et al. Physiological effects of human/companion animal bonding. *Nursing Research*. 1984;33:126-129. doi:10.1097/00006199-198405000-0000.
3. Berkman LF, Syme SL. Social networks, host resistance, and mortality: a nine-year follow-up study of Alameda County residents. *American Journal of Epidemiology*. 1979;109(2):186-204.
4. Caspi A, Harrington H, Moffitt TE, et al. Socially isolated children 20 years later: risk of cardiovascular disease. *Archives of Pediatrics & Adolescent Medicine*. August 2006;160(8):805-811.
5. Dölen G, Darvishzadeh A, Huang KW, et al. Social reward requires coordinated activity of nucleus accumbens oxytocin and serotonin. *Nature*. 2013;501(7466):179-184. doi:10.1038/nature12518.
6. Donovan NJ, Wu Q, Rentz DM, et al. Loneliness, depression and cognitive function in older U.S. adults. *International Journal of Geriatric Psychiatry*. 2017;32(5):564-573.
7. Fratiglioni L, Paillard-Borg S, Winblad B. An active and socially integrated lifestyle in late life might protect against dementia. *Lancet Neurology*. 2004;3(6):343-353.
8. Georgousopoulou EN, Mellor DD, Naumovski N, et al. Mediterranean lifestyle and cardiovascular disease prevention. *Cardiovascular Diagnosis and Therapy*. 2017;7(Suppl 1):S39-S47. doi:10.21037/cdt.2017.03.11.
9. Gordon I, Vander Wyk BC, Bennett RH, et al. Oxytocin enhances brain function in children with autism. *Proceedings of the National Academy of Sciences of the United States of America*. 2013;110(52):20953-20958. doi:10.1073/pnas.1312857110.
10. Holt-Lunstad J, Smith TB, Baker M, et al. Loneliness and social isolation as risk factors for mortality: a meta-analytic review. *Perspectives on Psychology Science*. 2015;10(2):227-237.
11. Krueger KR, Wilson RS, Kamenetsky JM, et al. Social engagement and cognitive function in old age. *Experimental Aging Research*. 2009;35(1):45-60. doi:10.1080/03610730802545028.
12. Martino J, Pegg J, Frates EP. The connection prescription: using the power of social interactions and the deep desire for connectedness to empower health and wellness. *American Journal of Lifestyle Medicine*. 2015. doi.org/10.1177/1559827615608788.
13. Pantell M, Rehkopf D, Jutte D, et al. Social isolation: a predictor of mortality comparable to traditional clinical risk factors. *American Journal of Public Health*. 2013;103(11):2056-2062. doi:10.2105/AJPH.2013.301261.
14. Stephens JP, Heaphy ED, Carmeli A, et al. Relationship quality and virtuousness: emotional carrying capacity as a source of individual and team resilience. *Journal of Applied Behavioral Science*. 2013;49:13.
15. Su SF, Chang MY, He CP. Social support, unstable angina, and stroke as predictors of depression in patients with coronary heart disease. *Journal of Cardiovascular Nursing*. May 9 2017. doi:10.1097/JCN.0000000000000419.
16. Thom DH, Ghorob A, Hessler D, et al. Impact of peer health coaching on glycemic control in low-income patients with diabetes: a randomized controlled trial. *Annals of Family Medicine*. 2013;11:137-144.
17. Umberson D, Montez JK. Social relationships and health: a flashpoint for health policy. *Journal of Health and Social Behavior*. 2010;51(Suppl):S54-S66.
18. Valtorta NK, Kanaan M, Gilbody S, et al. Loneliness and social isolation as risk factors for coronary heart disease and stroke: systematic review and meta-analysis of longitudinal observational studies. *Heart*. 2016;102(13):1009-1016.

Figure 9-3. The connection prescription evidence (cont.)

REFERENCES

- AARP Foundation. Framework for Isolation in Adults Over 50. Available at: https://www.aarp.org/content/dam/aarp/aarp_foundation/2012_PDFs/AARP-Foundation-Isolation-Framework-Report.pdf. Accessed August 2018.
- Berkman LF, Syme SL. Social networks, host resistance, and mortality: a nine-year follow-up study of Alameda County residents. *American Journal of Epidemiology*. 1979;109(2):186-204.

- Brown B. Quotes: Quotable Quote. Goodreads. Available at: https://www.goodreads.com/quotes/417390-i-define-connection-as-the-energy-that-exists-between-people. Accessed July 2018.
- Caspi A, Harrington H, Moffitt TE, et al. Socially isolated children 20 years later: risk of cardiovascular disease. *Archives of Pediatrics & Adolescent Medicine.* August 2006;160(8):805-811.
- Christakis N. The Hidden Influence of Social Networks. TED. Available at: http://www.ted.com/talks/nicholas_christakis_the_hidden_influence_of_social_networks. Accessed October 2017.
- Christakis NA, Fowler JH. *Connected: The Surprising Power of Our Social Networks and How They Shape Our Lives—How Your Friends' Friends' Friends Affect Everything You Feel, Think, and Do.* New York: Little, Brown and Company; 2009.
- Cornwell EY, Waite LJ. Social disconnectedness, perceived isolation, and health among older adults. *Journal of Health and Social Behavior.* March 2009; 50(1): 31-48.
- Dolen G, Darvishadeh A, Huang KW, et al. Social reward coordinated activity of nucleus accumbens oxytocin and serotonin. *Nature.* September 12 2013;501(7466):179-184.
- Donovan NJ, Wu Q, Rentz DM, et al. Loneliness, depression and cognitive function in older U.S. adults. *International Journal of Geriatric Psychiatry.* May 2017;32(5):564-573.
- Dutton JE, Heaphy ED. The power of high-quality connections. In: Cameron KS, Dutton JE, Quinn RE, eds. *Positive Organizational Scholarship: Foundations of a New Discipline.* San Francisco: Berrett-Koehler; 2003.
- Dutton JE. *Energize Your Workplace: How to Create and Sustain High-Quality Connections at Work.* San Francisco: Jossey-Bass; 2003.
- Fratiglioni L, Paillard-Borg S, Winblad B. An active and socially integrated lifestyle in late life might protect against dementia. *Lancet Neurology.* June 2004;3(6):343-353.
- Georgousopoulou EN, Mellor DD, Naumovski N, et al. Mediterranean lifestyle and cardiovascular disease prevention. *Cardiovascular Diagnosis and Therapy.* 2017;7(Suppl 1):S39-S47. doi:10.21037/cdt.2017.03.11.
- Gordon I, Vander Wyk BC, Bennett RH, et al. Oxytocin enhances brain function in children with autism. *Proceedings of the National Academy of Sciences of the United States of America.* 2013;110(52):20953-20958. doi:10.1073/pnas.1312857110.
- Hakulinen C, Pulkki-Råback L, Virtanen M, et al. Social isolation and loneliness as risk factors for myocardial infarction, stroke and mortality: UKBiobank cohort study of 479 054 men and women. *Heart.* March 27 2018.
- Hallowell EM, Ratey JJ. *Driven to Distraction: Recognizing and Coping With Attention Deficit Disorder From Childhood Through Adulthood.* Revised edition. New York: Anchor Books; 2011.

- Hallowell EM. *Connect: 12 Vital Ties That Open Your Heart, Lengthen Your Life, and Deepen Your Soul.* New York: Pocket Books; 1999.
- Hallowell EM. *The Childhood Roots of Adult Happiness: Five Steps to Help Kids Create and Sustain Lifelong Joy.* New York: The Ballantine Publishing Group; 2002.
- Holt-Lunstad J, Smith TB, Baker M, et al. Loneliness and social isolation as risk factors for mortality: a meta-analytic review. *Perspectives on Psychology Science.* March 2015;10(2):227-237.
- Hung LW, Neuner S, Polepalli JS, et al. Gating of social reward by oxytocin in the ventral tegmental area. *Science.* September 29 2017;357(6358):1406-1411.
- Landiero F, et al. Reducing social isolation and loneliness in older people: a systematic review protocol. *BMJ Open.* 2017;7(5):e013778.
- Leiberman MD. *Social: Why Our Brains Are Wired to Connect.* New York: Random House; 2013.
- Maas J, Verheij RA, de Vries S, Spreeuwenberg P, et al. Morbidity is related to a green living environment. *Journal of Epidemiology and Community Health.* December 2009;63(12):967-973. doi: 10.1136/jech.2008.079038. Epub 2009 Oct 15.
- Martino J, Pegg J, Frates EP. The connection prescription: using the power of social interactions and the deep desire for connectedness to empower health and wellness. *American Journal of Lifestyle Medicine.* 2016. doi.org/10.1177/1559827615608788.
- Neumann ID. Oxytocin: the neuropeptide of love reveals some of its secrets. *Cell Metabolism.* April 2007;5(4):231-233.
- Odendaal JS, Meintjes RA. Neurophysiological correlates of affiliative behaviour between humans and dogs. *Veterinary Journal (London, England: 1997).* 2003;165(3):296-301.
- Olff M. Bonding after trauma: on the role of social support and the oxytocin system in traumatic stress. *European Journal of Psychotraumatology.* 2012;3:1. doi:10.3402/ejpt.v3i0.18597.
- Owen SF, Tuncdemir SN, Bader PL, et al. Oxytocin enhances hippocampal spike transmission by modulating fast-spiking interneurons. *Nature.* August 22 2013;500(7463):458-462. doi:10.1038/nature12330.
- Palgi S. Klein E, Shamay-Tsoory SG. Oxytocin improves compassion toward women among patients with PTSD. *Psychoneuroendocrinology.* 2016;64:143. doi:10.1016/j.psyneuen.2015.11.008.
- Pantell M, Rehkopf D, Jutte D, et al. Social isolation: a predictor of mortality comparable to traditional clinical risk factors. *American Journal of Public Health.* November 2013;103(11):2056-2062.
- Rafnsson SB, Orrell M, d'Orsi E, et al. Loneliness, social integration, and incident dementia over 6 years: prospective findings from the English Longitudinal Study of Ageing. *Journals of Gerontology: Series B.* June 27 2017;gbx087. https://doi.org/10.1093/geronb/gbx087.

- Romero T, Nagasawa M, Mogi K, et al. Oxytocin promotes social bonding in dogs. *Proceedings of the National Academy of Sciences of the United States of America.* June 24 2014;111(25):9085-9090.
- Scheele D, Wille A, Kendrick KM, et al. Oxytocin enhances brain reward system responses in men viewing the face of their female partner. *Proceedings of the National Academy of Sciences of the United States of America.* 2013;110(50):20308-20313. doi:10.1073/pnas.1314190110.
- Stephens JP, Heaphy ED, Carmeli A, et al. Relationship quality and virtuousness: emotional carrying capacity as a source of individual and team resilience. *Journal of Applied Behavioral Science.* 2013;49:13.
- Su SF, Chang MY, He CP. Social support, unstable angina, and stroke as predictors of depression in patients with coronary heart disease. *Journal of Cardiovascular Nursing.* 2017 May 9. doi: 10.1097/JCN.0000000000000419.
- Thom DH, Ghorob A, Hessler D, et al. Impact of peer health coaching on glycemic control in low-income patients with diabetes: a randomized controlled trial. *Annals of Family Medicine.* 2013;11:137-144.
- Turkle S. *Alone Together: Why We Expect More From Technology and Less From Each Other.* New York: Basic Books; 2011.
- Turkle S. *Reclaiming Conversation: The Power of Talk in a Digital Age.* New York: Penguin Books; 2015.
- Umberson D, Montez JK. Social relationships and health: a flashpoint for health policy. *Journal of Health and Social Behavior.* 2010;51(Suppl):S54-S66.
- Valtorta NK, Kanaan M, Gilbody S, et al. Loneliness and social isolation as risk factors for coronary heart disease and stroke: systematic review and meta-analysis of longitudinal observational studies. *Heart.* July 1 2016;102(13):1009-1016.
- Van den Berg MMHE, Maas J, Muller R, et al. Autonomic nervous system responses to viewing green and built settings: differentiating between sympathetic and parasympathetic activity. *International Journal of Environmental Research and Public Health.* 2015;12(12):15860-15874. doi:10.3390/ijerph121215026.
- Wilson EO. *The Social Conquest of Earth.* New York: Liveright Publishing; 2012.

CHAPTER 10

POSITIVELY POSITIVE

"I have decided to be happy, because it's good for my health."

—Voltaire
French Historian, Enlightenment
Writer, and Philosopher

❏ Chapter Goals:

- Develop an understanding of positivity.
- Explore the connection between having a positive attitude and health.
- Review the concept of happiness.
- Discuss the role that gratitude can play in life.
- Learn about the underlying elements of laughter.
- Consider the differences between appropriate and inappropriate humor.
- Examine the key factors attendant to joy.

❏ Learning Objectives:

- To understand the basic forms of positivity
- To be aware of evidence-based information on laughter
- To recognize the benefits of having an attitude of gratitude
- To be cognizant of the attributes of happy people
- To develop a sense of the barriers to feeling joy

❏ Guiding Questions:

- What is positive psychology?
- Why is it important that people develop a more positive attitude toward life?
- What are appropriate ways to cultivate an attitude of gratitude?
- What are the obstacles to being happy?
- How can people find more joy in their lives?
- How can laughter have a positive impact on health?

Lifestyle Medicine Handbook   351

❏ Important Terms:

- *Attitude:* a way of thinking or feeling about something
- *Gratitude:* the quality of being thankful; a readiness to show appreciation for and to return kindness
- *Happiness:* a mental or emotional state of well-being, which can be defined by, among others, positive or pleasant emotions
- *Hope:* a feeling of expectation and desire for a certain thing to occur
- *Humor:* the stimulus (e.g., a joke) that evokes a response
- *Joy:* a feeling of great pleasure and happiness
- *Laughter:* physical reaction characterized by a distinct repetitive vocal sound, certain facial expressions, and contraction of various muscle groups
- *Optimism:* hopefulness and confidence about the future or the successful outcome of something
- *Positive psychology:* the scientific study of optimal human functioning
- *Positivity:* the practice of being or the tendency to be positive or optimistic in attitude
- *Well-being:* the state of being comfortable, healthy, or happy

People have a lot of choices in their lives—what to do, what to wear, what to eat, what to spend their money on, who to spend time with, what to read, when to go to bed, etc. On occasion, the choices that individuals have in life may be limited by their circumstances. One choice that certainly is not constrained by happenstance is a person's attitude. By purposefully choosing a positive attitude and looking for the positive in themselves, as well as the people and places around them, people are setting themselves up for success and joy. While people cannot necessarily choose the situation in which they find themselves, individuals do have a choice of whether and how they embrace positivity as a fundamental tenet of their lives.

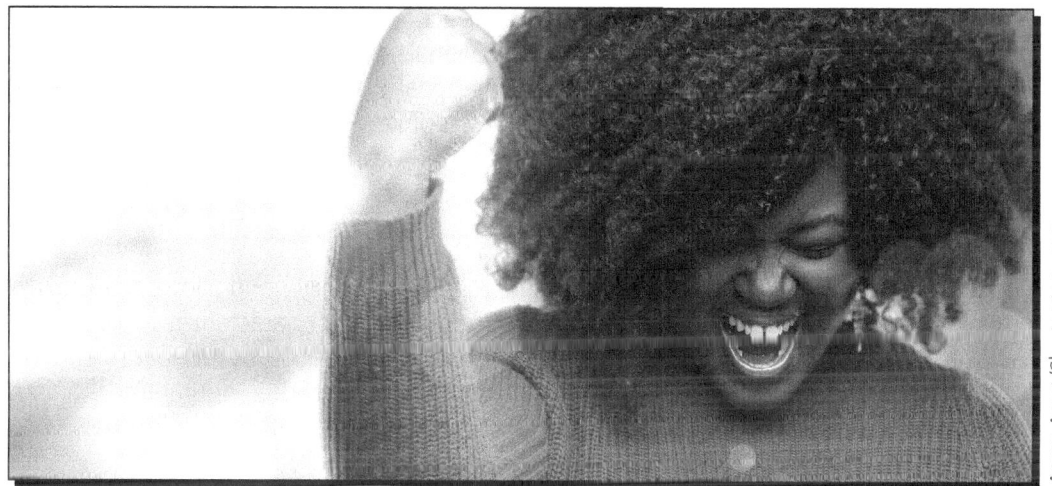

By purposefully choosing a positive attitude and looking for the positive in themselves, as well as the people and places around them, people are setting themselves up for success and joy.

One definite reason to pursue a positive attitude is simply for individuals to consider the adverse impact that negative psychological conditions—depressive symptoms, anger, hostility, anxiety, and hopelessness—have on their health and well-being. This factor has been well documented in the literature for some time. Large numbers of studies reveal the association between negative psychological conditions and higher risks of cardiovascular disease incidence and mortality.

On the other hand, rather than avoiding negative states to prevent disease, individuals can actually promote health and happier lives by cultivating positive emotions. Considerable research has found that optimistic people are, in general, more psychologically and physiologically healthier than those with a pessimistic attitude. Individuals with a positive attitude tend to be happier and more resilient. They have an enhanced ability to cope with stress, as well as difficult situations. They may have stronger immune systems. They often have better relationships with other people. In addition, having a positive attitude can make a person more creative. This creativity may lead a person to make better decisions throughout the day or brainstorming multiple solutions to problems. The benefits of having a positive attitude extend to health as well. According to the Mayo Clinic, optimistic individuals have a reduced risk of death from cardiovascular disease-related issues, a lower likelihood of suffering from depression, and an increased lifespan.

Psychologist Toshiaki Shirai and colleagues looked at the association between perceived level of life enjoyment and the risk of cardiovascular disease incidence and mortality in nearly 90,000 Japanese men and women over the course of 12 years. The findings in Japanese men suggest a protective role of positive psychological conditions on cardiovascular disease. In other words, people who are enjoying their lives also tend to live longer with better health.

Enjoying life takes active effort. Cultivation of positive emotions increases life satisfaction and creates a happy state. Researchers investigated whether people of differing psychological profiles regarding happiness, depression, and life satisfaction tended use happiness promoting strategies. Self-fulfilling individuals, those with high positive and low negative emotions, tended to utilize instrumental goal pursuit, connection, community, social affiliation, and spirituality, when pursuing happiness. These people take an active role in smiling to get themselves in a happy mood, improving their social skills, and working on their self-control. Naturally, this factor begs the question of whether our moods interact with our physiology and our cognitive processing.

Positive mood, in fact, leads to enhanced cognitive flexibility and allows the human brain to think more creatively. Following from Carol Dweck's characterization of growth mindset—the concept that a person's intelligence is malleable by adaptive learning from mistakes and failure—Moser and colleagues postulated a neural mechanism underpinning this psychology. Cognitive testing showed that those individuals who believed that they could learn from their mistakes did indeed perform better after making a mistake. Based on electrical potentials measured from scalp electrodes, the region of the anterior cingulate cortex in those individuals with growth mindset created a larger second signal by electrical activity recording, noting the mistake and telling the brain to pay more attention.

Inevitably, everyone makes mistakes. On the other hand, the research and anecdotal evidence indicate that those persons with high levels of optimism, growth mindset, and positive thinking have increased resilience. Dr. Ruby Nadler and her colleagues showed that positive mood allow for increased cognitive flexibility. The researches brought people into their laboratory and asked them to watch funny or depressing videos to put them in particular mood states. They then had the subjects perform a categorization task.

The researchers found that positive mood enhanced performance, but only on the task where flexibly testing one hypothesis after another produces the best performance. This finding suggests that positive thinking and optimism may improve tasks that demand prefrontal executive functions, like working memory. Optimism has also been linked to improved physiological recovery and psychosocial adjustment to coronary artery bypass surgery, bone marrow transplantation, postpartum depression, traumatic brain injury, lung cancer, breast cancer, failed in vitro fertilization, and even chronic pain.

To gain a deeper appreciation for what positive thinking is and how to cultivate it, it is necessary to first understand what it isn't. It doesn't mean viewing life through rose-colored glasses and ignoring the less pleasant situations in life. Rather, it is based on anticipating the best in a given circumstance—not the worst. It involves making the most of every situation, however challenging it may be. It entails adopting a "can-do," as opposed to a "make-do," attitude toward life.

The individual can self-assist by cultivating a "growth mindset." Furthermore, everyone can assist each other by providing encouragement and complements. Research shows that when individuals receive a compliment, this feedback activates the striatum, and they perform better on a motor task. Compliments are a free and effective strategy to employ in coaching, motivational interviewing, and teaching for healthier behavior change.

As previously mentioned, having a positive attitude is not necessarily automatic; it requires effort and work. It entails a commitment to create and maintain positivity. Among the relatively simple steps that can help a person embrace such an attitude are the following:
- Remember what individuals appreciate, appreciates. If people strive to start a conversation with a positive statement, then the rest of the conversation often follows suit. Appreciative inquiry, which is a coaching tool discussed in Chapter 3, focuses on what is going well and builds on that. When people look for the positive in their friends, colleagues, and family, they often have positive interactions that are productive and enjoyable.
- Identifying the positive in yourself is a great way for you to embrace a positive attitude for the day. Knowing, appreciating, and using your strengths throughout the day brings great joy.

- Find joy in the small pleasures in life (e.g., walking barefoot in the grass, enjoying a meal, etc.). All too often, the big pleasures in life come too infrequently. View life as a blissful mosaic that is often best addressed one piece at a time. This factor will require mindfulness and being present for all the distinct moments in life.
- Be responsible for your own attitude. Attitude is not a byproduct of what happens to a person, but rather how that individual interprets what happens to them. People cannot control everything that happens to them in a day, but they can control their reactions to the events of the day.
- Surround yourself with positive people. Try to avoid being around individuals who cast a negative pall on life (e.g., whiners and complainers). Some people are like "leeches"—they drain the energy out of other individuals. Meanwhile, other people are like "lilies"—they add joy and happiness to the day.
- Upload positivity to the brain. Read books with a positive message. Watch movies with an inspiring theme. Listen to music with uplifting lyrics. Inundate the brain with positive thinking.
- Smile. Release the feel-good hormones (endorphins and serotonin) that are conducive to well-being by smiling.
- Employ a more positive vocabulary. Avoid using negative phrases or emotionally loaded words. Substitute neutral or positive words instead. Help program the brain to think positively by utilizing positive language.
- Maintain a gratitude journal. Write down five things every day in your journal that makes you happy.

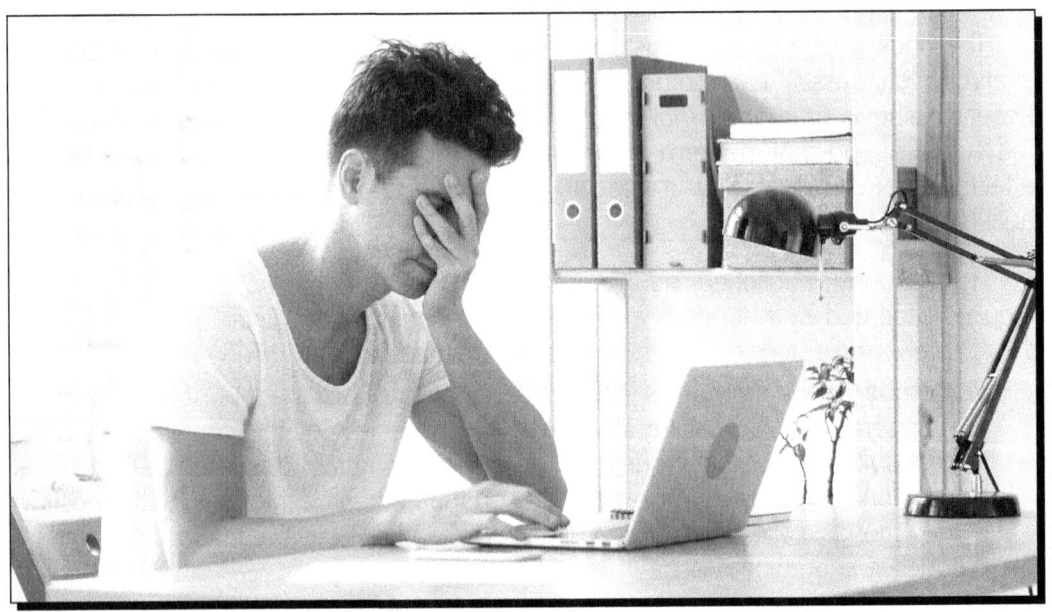

People cannot control everything that happens to them in a day, but they can control their reactions to the events of the day.

- View life's challenges as opportunities, not insurmountable obstacles. Don't expect life to be easy. On occasion, life can be tough. Invest time and energy to figure out the optimal way to manage and deal with the challenges.
- Focus on the good—in yourself, in your life, and in others. Negative thoughts lead to a negative attitude and vice-versa.
- Have a zest for life. Be enthusiastic. Be passionate about life. Approach life with an ardor for joy and happiness. People who have a sense of purpose and feel part of something greater than themselves often feel this zest and passion.
- Don't feel entitled. Don't demand that things be handed to you Realize that it's up to you to get the things you want.
- Be proactive. Decide how you are going to feel, regardless of your circumstances. Choose to be positive and maintain that positivity.
- Adopt a growth mindset. With this mindset described by Carol Dweck, PhD, in her book, *Mindset: The New Psychology of Success*, people look at mistakes and failure as opportunities to grow and learn. This type of outlook on life allows people to take risks, to go outside their comfort zones, and to learn.
- Utilize the power of humor. Be capable of laughing at yourself and life's absurdities. Be aware that humor is a powerful tool that can be used to lift a person's mood and enhance their emotional state.
- Be curious. Using a child-like curiosity each day allows people to live in the moment and be fully present, enjoying each moment as it unfolds. When people feel like they are in learning mode, open and receptive to new ideas, they are less stressed. When people are closed off and in protecting mode, protecting their opinions and ideas, they are often stressed, uncomfortable, and combative. Approach every situation with an attitude of being open to what can be learned from it.
- Find positivity in the ordinary. Be able to put a positive spin on every situation, even negative events. Struggles often make people stronger. Health setbacks can lead to big lifestyle changes.
- Tame your inner critic. Avoid thinking negatively about yourself. Worry less about what others may be thinking.
- Take time for yourself. Do things you enjoy. Think about moments of satisfaction or joy.
- Master the mind. Be open to change and making adjustments in how you think and act, if appropriate. Remember that almost every worthwhile human endeavor, including having a positive attitude, takes focused effort.

One of the most acclaimed and prolific researchers in the world on emotional positivity is Dr. Barbara Fredrickson. Fredrickson's research suggests that positive emotions lead to novel, exploratory, and creative behaviors, which, over time, solidify to long-term resources, such as expanded cognition, psychological resilience, and social relationships. In fact, positive emotions have a unique ability to downregulate lingering negative emotions and the accompanying psychologic and physiologic stress. According to Dr. Fredrickson, positivity can manifest itself in a variety of forms, (i.e., be expressed in a number of ways), including the following 10:

- Joy. Experienced when a person is in a safe and familiar surrounding; things are going their way or even exceed their expectations
- Gratitude. Experienced when an individual receives kindness from another person
- Serenity. Experienced when a person feels contentment when their surroundings are safe and familiar
- Interest. Experienced when a person learns a new skill, meets a new person, or is in a new place—drawing their attention, leading to a sense of fascination and curiosity that makes them want to explore more
- Hope. Experienced when an individual is confronted by unfavorable circumstances, but believes that things can change and improve, which motivates them to tap into their own capabilities and resourcefulness to turn things around
- Pride. Experienced when someone has worked diligently, invested their time and resources, and has succeeded, leading to an achievement for which they can take credit
- Amusement. Experienced when a person is exposed to incongruities that result in unexpected things or behaviors that give them an irrepressible urge to laugh
- Inspiration. Experienced when an individual witnesses or encounters human excellence that rivets their attention, warms their heart, and draws them in to a point that moves them into action to do their best
- Awe. Experienced when a person encounters goodness on a grand scale, making them feel that they are part of something larger than themselves, which results in a transcendent emotion, like gratitude and inspiration
- Love. Experienced when a person stirs good feelings in the heart within a safe and close relationship

3-1 RATIO

In addition to understanding the factors that are affected by, and contribute to, having a positive attitude and embracing emotional positivity, it is also essential to be aware of what positive psychology entails. Collectively, it explores the factors that help an individual lead a full and meaningful life. It also involves efforts to ascertain the purpose of positive emotions that a person has, as well as the different contexts in which they prove to be valuable.

Dr. Martin Seligman, who is considered the forefather of the field of positive psychology, has written several books, including *Learned Optimism, Authentic Happiness*, and *Flourish,* which explore the power of positive thinking and living. Dr. Seligman also focuses on finding people's strengths. A great question for patients is "What are your strengths?" This question is often tough to answer, but it is worth the effort. Everyone has strengths, gifts, and talents. When people talk about their strengths, they often gain confidence. Dr. Seligman has a VIA Institute of Character and an online questionnaire (https://www.viacharacter.org/www/) that approximately five million people have filled out. This questionnaire, which can be filled out by patients in their homes, reveals their top character strengths, like creativity, curiosity, humility, forgiveness, and more. Taking the test can be eye-opening and can open up a new world of possibility for using strengths that were hidden or not appreciated.

In addition, positive psychology is interested in helping people manage negative emotions, thereby allowing individuals to flourish in their lives. Like it or not, human beings are going to experience all kinds of emotions, including negative ones. The key for people is to recognize that negative emotions are a part of living—be willing to accept and experience them, acknowledge them, absorb them, and integrate them into their lives and learn from them. People often refer to surfing the waves of negative and positive emotions. Both come and go. The joy of a home run hit in baseball does not last forever, nor does the sting of a strike out. In that regard, Acceptance Commitment Therapy developed by Steven Hayes, PhD, in 1982, encourages people to:

- Accept their emotions and be present with them, knowing they will only last a short period of time.
- Choose a valued direction by finding a way forward that is in alignment with their priorities and values.
- Take action. Figure out how to make the next concrete step forward in a productive way.

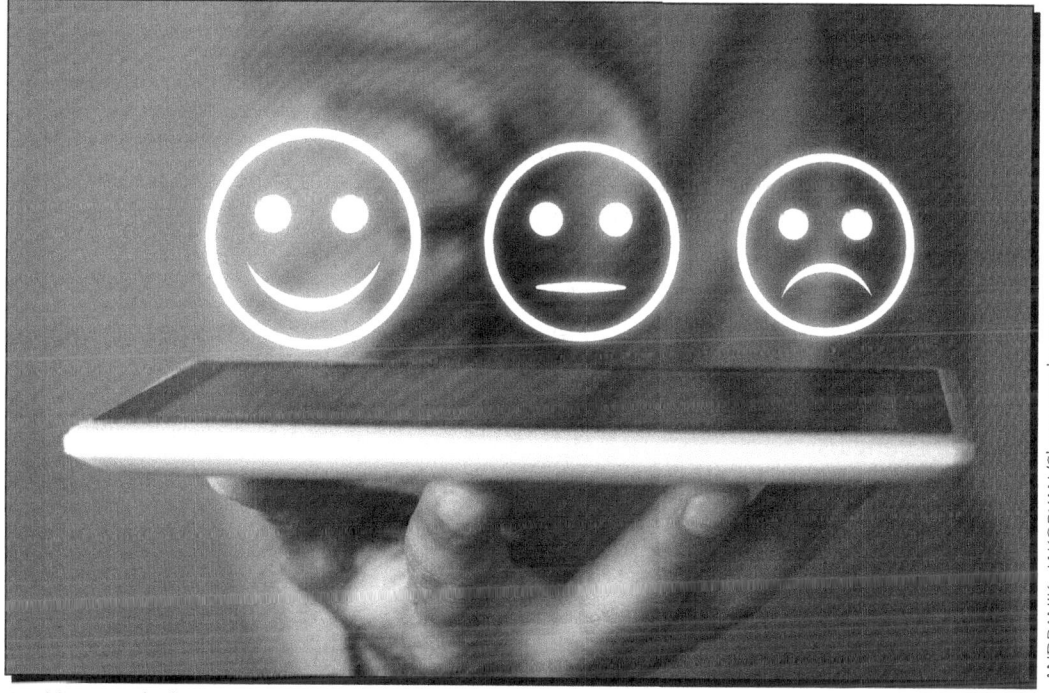

Positive psychology is interested in helping people manage negative emotions, thereby allowing individuals to flourish in their lives.

The positive psychology movement represents a paradigm shift in the focus of traditional psychology research. Rather than focusing predominantly on mental illness, dysfunction, and disease, more studies are being conducted on happiness, optimism, resilience, and positivity. This situation has led to a new discipline—positive psychology—gaining more and more traction with every year. It is an integral part of health and wellness coaching. One practical definition of positive psychology is that it is the scientific study of optimal human functioning. Another definition of positive psychology is "the science of happiness" (also known as subjective well-being).

GRATITUDE

"Gratitude bestows reverence, allowing us to encounter everyday epiphanies, those transcendent moments of awe that change forever how we experience life and the world."

This quote by the 17th century English poet, John Milton, resonates with people. People simply feel better when they feel grateful. Centuries after his statement, there is research to back it up. Gratitude is associated with increased happiness. Not only does it enhance positive emotions, it also helps people deal with adversity, build strong connections and relationships, and even improve their health.

A major contributor to the body of evidence for the value of gratitude in human happiness and health is the aforementioned Dr. Martin Seligman. Over a decade ago, when he was helping spearhead the positive psychology movement, he conducted several research studies on gratitude. In one of them, he compared the effects of five different weekly assignments. One, which was considered a placebo exercise, served as the control. He asked subjects to simply write down early memories, without guiding them in any direction. In this way, they could write about and choose to relive difficult memories, neutral memories or pleasant ones. It was up to the subject. The other assignments were as follows:

- Gratitude visit: write and hand deliver a letter of gratitude.
- Three good things in life: write three things that went well each day, as well as their causes.
- You at your best: write about a time when you were at your best and consider your strengths.
- Using signature strengths in a new way: use one of your top five strengths in a new and different way for one week.

The results of Seligman's study revealed that writing and personally delivering a letter of gratitude to someone, who had never been properly thanked, provided an immediate increase in happiness score, the benefits of which lasted approximately one month. Using signature strengths in a new way and listing three good things also increased happiness. While this study employed a self-report scale and had a small sample size, it revealed that these simple strategies in positive psychology and gratitude can have powerful effects.

Robert Emmons, PhD, from the University of California-Davis, also studied the power of gratitude. In his book, titled, *Thanks: How the New Science of Gratitude Can Make You Happier*, he discusses how gratitude is a chosen attitude and how cultivating an attitude of gratitude can enhance a person's sense of well-being.

The question may be asked, how do people study gratitude? In reality, most of the studies involving gratitude, use self-report scales. For example, Dr. Emmons' gratitude questionnaire, The Gratitude Questionnaire—Six-Item Form (GQ-6), which is a self-report scale on gratitude that employs a Likert system, in which individuals are asked to self-assess how they feel about certain statements, in this instance, the following six assertions:

- I have so much in life to be thankful for.
- If I had to list everything that I felt grateful for, it would be a very long list.
- When I look at the world, I don't see much to be grateful for.
- I am grateful to a wide variety of people.
- As I get older, I find myself more able to appreciate the people, events, and situations that have been part of my life history.
- Long amounts of time can go by before I feel grateful to something or someone.

The Likert scale that Dr. Emmons employed provided respondents with seven possible rankings:

1 = strongly disagree
2 = disagree
3 = slightly disagree
4 = neutral
5 = slightly agree
6 = agree
7 = strongly agree

Dr. Emmons and his colleagues have used this questionnaire and other measures to study the power of gratitude. Their research has found that gratitude increases subjective, emotional well-being. In one of their studies, there were two groups of students. One group listed blessings, while the other was asked to record the hassles or neutral life events that they experienced on a weekly basis, for a two-month period. The subjects who kept gratitude lists were more likely to have made progress in personal goals in the areas of their academics, interpersonal life, or health. Specifically, those individuals who kept a weekly gratitude journal exercised more regularly, reported fewer physical symptoms, felt better about their lives as a whole, and were more optimistic about upcoming week. In another related study conducted by Dr. Emmons and his colleagues, they split the subjects up into three groups:

- #1—a group with a daily gratitude intervention (self-guided exercises)
- #2—a group with a with a focus on things that annoyed them (hassles)
- #3—a group with a focus on social comparison—looking down on others

The subjects in the daily gratitude group showed higher levels of positive states of alertness, enthusiasm, determination, attentiveness, and energy, compared to the other two groups. Furthermore, they were more likely to have helped someone with a personal problem or have offered support to someone. This research revealed that gratitude not only helps people feel happier, it also sets them up to be feel empowered to lend a hand to someone in need. In this way, promoting gratitude helps the person feeling the gratitude, as well as those around that person.

In another study, Dr. Emmons and his colleagues looked at a specific patient population to determine whether gratitude might have important therapeutic effects for certain patients. The subjects were adults with neuromuscular disease. The intervention consisted of a 21-day gratitude exercise, in which the subjects listed their blessings. There was also a control group and the subjects in this group did not do anything different than their usual behavior.

The intervention group reported greater amounts of high-energy positive moods, a greater sense of feeling connected to others, more optimistic ratings of their life, and better sleep. (Sleep was reviewed in detail in Chapter 6. There are other research studies that indicate that gratitude journals, lists, and other interventions can help people improve their sleep. Not only can gratitude influence the mental state of individuals, it can also set them up for healthy habits. This point is an important factor for lifestyle medicine practitioners to consider, when counseling patients.

Dr. Emmons and his colleagues summarized the differences between people who scored high on self-reported gratitude measures versus those individuals who scored low in an article in *The Journal of Personality and Social Psychology*. They report that people with higher gratitude scores have higher positive emotions, life satisfaction, vitality, and optimism, as well as lower levels of depression and stress. In fact, gratitude seems to enhance good feelings better than it decreases unpleasant emotions.

Of note, their research also suggests that grateful people do not deny or ignore negative emotions, feelings, or events. Accordingly, the benefits of feeling grateful don't come from a denial process. Rather, the gratitude helps to empower people to better handle the negative situations that might arise. Other characteristics of people who score high on gratitude include increased capacity to be empathic and to adopt the perspective of others. They were also rated as more generous and more helpful by people in their social networks. Interestingly, they were more likely to acknowledge a belief in the interconnectedness of all life, as well as a commitment and responsibility to others.

Furthermore, their research suggested that people who regularly attend religious services of any kind and those individuals who engage in religious activities of any kind, including simple prayers and reading religious materials, were more likely to be grateful. Moving from religion to the material world, people who score high on gratitude place less emphasis on material items. They were less likely to judge their own success and the success of others based on material possessions, were less envious of wealthy people, and were more likely to share their own material possessions with others.

Of note, Dr. Emmons makes a clear distinction between feeling grateful and feeling indebted. Feeling indebted does not come with all of these otherwise wonderful benefits. In fact, feeling indebted is associated with higher levels of anger, lower levels of appreciation, lower levels of happiness and lower levels of love. As such, lifestyle medicine practitioners can help their patients greatly by enabling them to see the value of gratitude and encouraging them to practice gratitude on a regular basis.

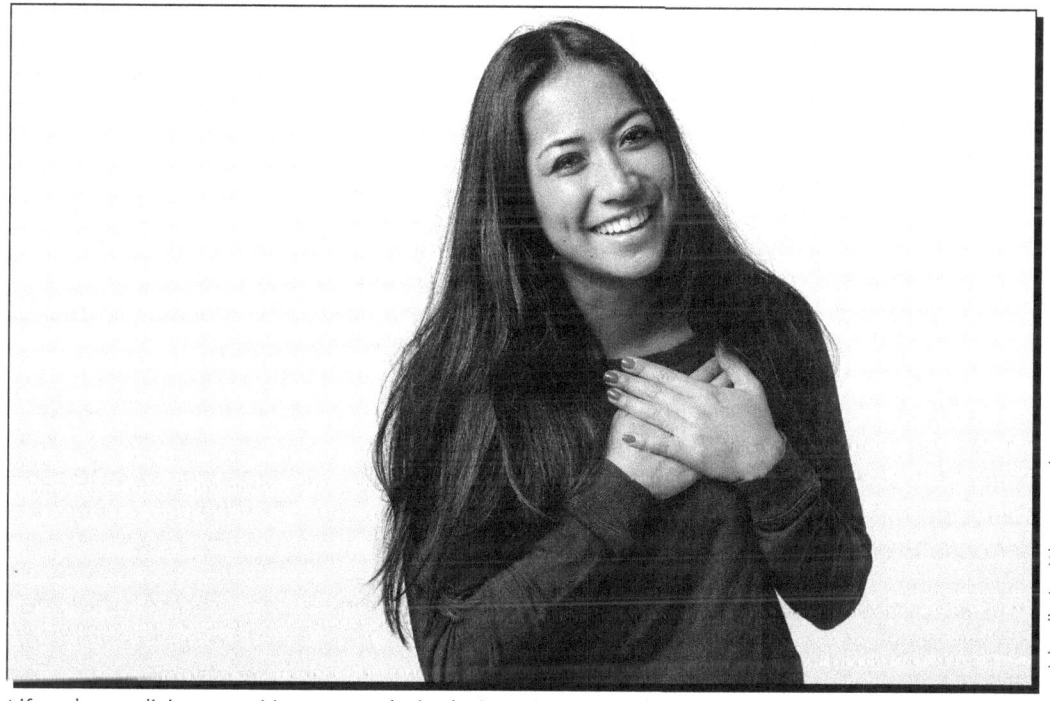

Lifestyle medicine practitioners can help their patients greatly by enabling them to see the value of gratitude and encouraging them to practice gratitude on a regular basis.

LIVE AND LEARN WITH DR. BETH FRATES

I often invite my patients to think about gratitude. Sometimes, I will ask them, "What are you grateful for today?" Other times, I will ask if they want to know about gratitude research and how it might impact their life. Most people are very interested in the research, and can readily list two to three things for which they are grateful.

Over the years, I have had good results with using a gratitude journal. For example, with a client who was a lawyer, a gratitude journal worked in my absence. I had completed 12 weekly sessions with this client, and we focused on increasing movement, increasing vegetable consumption, and increasing the quality of her social connections. The client was very happy with her progress by the end.

Six months later, she contacted me and wanted to work together again for a few booster sessions. She reported that she was feeling down. Of note, when someone has signs of clinical depression, I refer them to my colleagues in my local area, given that lifestyle medicine counseling is not psychological counseling. At any rate, this client felt that a few walking sessions with me to discuss her lifestyle habits would be useful to her.

Unfortunately, I was leaving vacation and was booked solid with appointments the week after I returned. As a result, we needed to look two to three weeks out for an appointment. We had a brief email exchange, during which I reminded her about the value of a gratitude journal for an improved sense of well-being. We had discussed this topic at length, during one of our previous sessions months prior. This client latched onto that suggestion, and for two weeks, she used a gratitude journal at night, in which she listed two to three things for which she was grateful.

Subsequently, when I returned from vacation, I reached out to this client to check on her, and she reported feeling markedly better. In fact, she was feeling so much better, that she did not feel a huge rush to see me, as she had experienced, when she contacted me two weeks earlier. The gratitude journal, alone, had helped to improve her outlook and mindset.

Like everything else in lifestyle medicine, if practitioners can practice what they preach, they will be more motivating and compelling. Thus, this Live and Learn is an invitation to all the readers of this handbook to try a gratitude journal for 30 days. See how it goes. By trying something for themselves, practitioners have the ability to speak about personal experiences, as well as be more capable of guiding patients in more productive ways, as they will have experienced the pros and cons of adopting the new habit. Not only do they know the challenges, they also know first-hand the benefits of keeping a gratitude journal.

HAPPINESS

What is happiness, anyway? Does it mean the accumulation of wealth, a person meeting their soulmate, or having the perfect body? Perhaps it's about the attainment of the perfect job or about having particularly high status in the community. Would an individual be happier if they had the home of their dreams, owned a sports car, or could take a luxurious vacation? Most Americans have been exposed to an array of cultural messages that claim that these things are the key to happiness.

If this were in fact the case, then people with wealth, perfect bodies, or fabulous homes would all be happy. This situation is not the case. In fact, ironically, many of these people may actually be relatively unhappy. Research shows a poor correlation between happiness and external possessions. This situation exists because happiness comes from within. Happiness is actually a choice. Accordingly, a feasible working definition of happiness is having a sense of joy, contentment, or positive well-being, combined with the feeling that life is good, meaningful, and worthwhile. According to Aristotle, happiness is "the whole aim and end of human existence."

Yet, happiness is not something individuals can simply procure, but rather it's a byproduct of leveraging their strengths, promoting goodness in the world, and pursuing a life of meaning. Viktor Frankl, Austrian psychiatrist and Holocaust survivor, reminds people that despair is suffering without meaning. In reality, the capacity to turn tragedy into triumph is in each person.

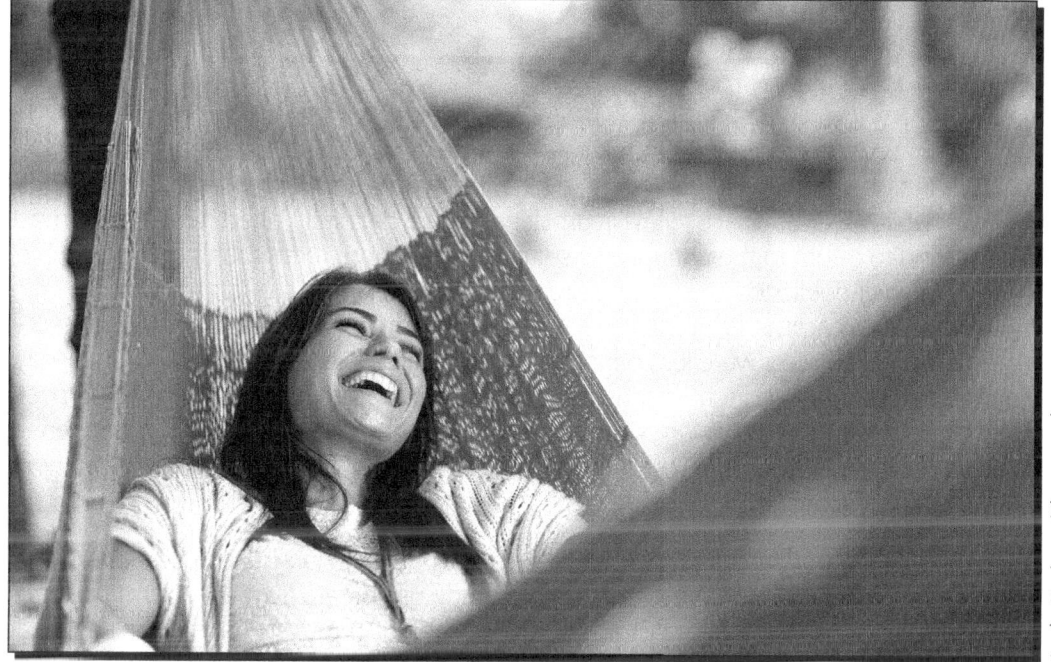

Happiness is having a sense of joy, contentment, or positive well-being, combined with the feeling that life is good, meaningful, and worthwhile.

Researchers have found that happiness seems to be made up of the following three components: genetic set point (50 percent), life circumstances (10 percent), and intentional activity (40 percent). In other words, hereditary tendencies can lead a person to be melancholy or cheerful, pessimistic or optimistic—but that's only half the story. Surprisingly, life circumstances, such as where they live, what type of job they have, how old they are, and whether or not they have a an expensive car only account for 10 percent of the happiness pie (Figure 10-1). That means an astonishing 40 percent of whether or not an individual is happy is up to them—how they choose to spend their time and, especially, how they choose to think. Attitude is key, and, fortunately, attitudes can be changed with awareness and practice.

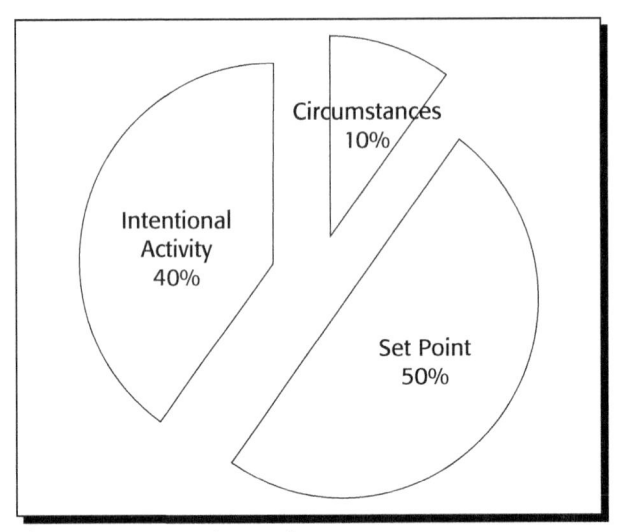

Figure 10-1. Happiness pie

The set point theory of happiness states that there's a genetic baseline for happiness to which individuals are bound to return, even after major catastrophes or major triumphs. While the ups and downs of life circumstances can definitely affect well-being, most people tend to return to their happiness set point after about three months. For example, in 1978, a well-publicized study compared the happiness levels of lottery winners with those of accident victims. After the initial euphoria of winning a large sum of money wore off, most lottery winners were less happy than might otherwise be suspected. Conversely, life satisfaction of the accident victims before they were disabled robustly predicted post-disability satisfaction in paraplegics. In general, major traumas or events that happened three or more months ago generally do not significantly affect an individual's happiness level. Eventually, they are likely to return to their genetic set point.

People are able to increase their happiness set point by upregulating the "intentional activity" factor of the happiness equation. In a study using data from the German Socio-Economic Panel Survey, the largest and longest series of observations of happiness that exists to date, the personal trait most closely associated with life satisfaction is altruism. The more individuals practice compassion and seek to help others, the happier they are in life.

There is also data from work by Sonja Lyubomirsky and colleagues to suggest that pursuing altruistic goals actually causes happiness. When she had college students perform five acts of kindness over a week, the students reported a significant boost in their happiness, compared to subjects in the control group. This data and anecdotal experience suggest that part of the antidote for unhappiness may be counterintuitive—individuals looking beyond themselves putting their energy into others. In happiness, just as in health, a person's genes are not their destiny.

THE HAPPINESS-HEALTH CONNECTION

Hundreds of evidence-based studies verify the benefits of happiness on almost all aspects of life. When compared to their less happy peers, happy people are more sociable, charitable, and cooperative, likely to get married and stay married, and likely to have a richer network of friends and social support. These individuals tend to be better leaders, earn higher incomes, live longer, and be more resilient in the face of hardship.

Happiness has also been linked to physical health. While researchers are somewhat unsure if good health leads to happiness or vice versa, happiness has been associated with good health in at least four ways:
- Protects the heart.
- Strengthens the immune system.
- Reduces stress and anxiety.
- Diminishes the number of aches and pains.

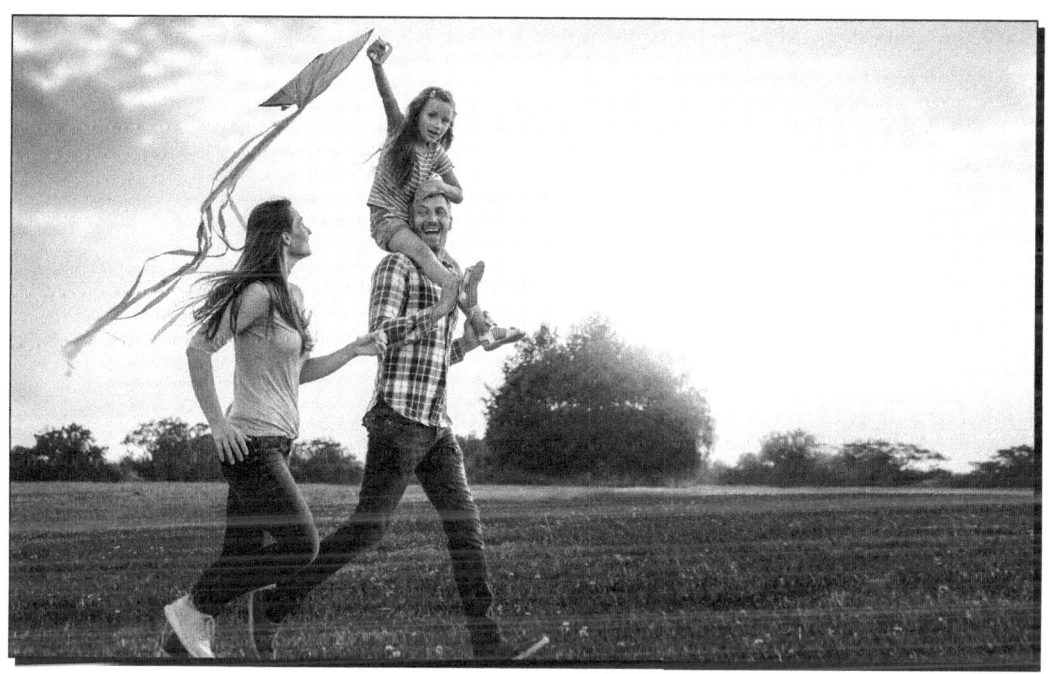

In happiness, just as in health, a person's genes are not their destiny.

❑ Obstacles to Happiness

Unfortunately, not everyone is as happy as they could be. Achieving happiness is not always easy. Frequently, it involves recognizing obstacles that stand in the way of one's happiness and then working to break those barriers down. Among the common obstacles that can limit a person's happiness are the following:
- Fearing failure
- Feeling that they are not worthy of happiness
- Being too sensitive to criticism
- Trying to be what others want them to be, instead of being true to themselves
- Living in the past
- Having unrealistic expectations
- Not having occasional moments of solitude
- Avoiding new things and challenges
- Experiencing negative feelings (e.g., guilt, greed, resentment, self-doubt, anger, etc.)

❑ Strategies for Overcoming Barriers to Happiness

Whether they want to or not, people are going to encounter obstacles in their lives, including barriers to their being happy. One of the major keys to happiness is overcoming those obstacles. Some of those barriers may be beyond the control of the individual. Others can be overcome. In that regard, the following tips can be helpful for individuals:
- To the degree possible, do what you like to do.
- Focus on achieving dreams and goals—not on money and possessions.
- Take advantage of every opportunity.
- Take charge of your life.
- Ignore (avoid, if possible) negative people in your life.
- Get into and remain in a flow state when doing things.
- Don't allow fear to rule your life.
- Adopt a growth mindset.
- Adopt an attitude of gratitude to increase energy, optimism, and empathy.
- Engage life—with joy, passion, and exuberance.

LAUGHTER

It seems as if it would go without saying that happy people have more fun, right? In fact, people who choose to be happy and exemplify positivity often look for more opportunities to laugh. It's been written (though never documented) that the average four-year-old laughs 300 times per day, but the average 40-year-old only laughs four times per day. The importance of such an observation is reinforced by the oft-cited quote, "You don't stop laughing because you grow old. You grow old because you stop laughing."

❑ What Is Laughter?

Humor is the stimulus, such as a joke, that evokes a response. Laughter, often the response to humor, is a physical reaction in humans, typically consisting of rhythmical, often audible, contractions of the diaphragm and other parts of the respiratory system. Laughter is part of human behavior regulated by the brain, helping individuals clarify their intentions in social interaction situations, as well as providing an emotional context to their circumstances.

Laughter can be either spontaneous or simulated. If it is spontaneous, its basis is genuine. In contrast, if it is simulated, its roots are forced.

There are more than 100 theories concerning why people laugh. Five of the more commonly held theories are as follows:
- Superiority theory—humor springs out of feelings of superiority; an individual increases their own sense of self-esteem at the expense of someone else.
- Incongruity theory—humor occurs when an incongruity exists between what a person expects and what actually happens.
- Benign violation theory—laughter occurs when something is violated (e.g., morals, social codes, linguistic norms, or personal dignity), but the violation isn't threatening.
- Release theory—humor results from the physical manifestation of repressed desires (i.e., the release of sexual or aggressive tension).
- Relief theory—humor helps individuals cope with stressful situations (i.e., tension is released during emotional moments).

There are many ways to laugh, from giggles to guffaws and chuckles to cackles. The type of laughter depends on a variety of factors, including the setting, the circumstances, and the individuals themselves. Among the types of laughter are the following:
- Etiquette laughter
- Contagious laughter
- Nervous laughter
- Belly laughter
- Silent laughter
- Stress-relieving laughter
- Pigeon laughter (i.e., not opening the mouth when laughing)
- Snorting laughter
- Canned laughter
- Cruel laughter

There are also a number of reasons that people laugh; some of the reasons are obvious (e.g., in response to jokes or humor), others not so much. Surprisingly, most laughter is not in response to comedy. For example, some individuals laugh to show that they like people and that they agree with them, understand them, and are part of the same group as them. In fact, research indicates that individuals are approximately 30 times more likely to laugh when they are with someone else than by themselves. Other people laugh simply because someone else is laughing or because they want to share their laughter. Regardless of the rationale behind laughing, it allows people to share meaning with others, make themselves feel better, reinforce existing relationships, and fostering the development of new relationships.

❏ Laughter Is Medicine

While laughter makes people feel better in the moment, there appear to be long-term health (both mental and physical) benefits of laughter as well.

The Mental Health Benefits of Spontaneous Laughter:

- Improves affect.
- Improves depression.
- Improves anxiety.
- Decreases stress.
- Decreases agitation (in dementia patients).

The Physical Health Benefits of Spontaneous Laughter:

- Increases the release of epinephrine and norepinephrine.
- Decreases cortisol levels.
- Increases systolic blood pressure (similar to exercising).
- Increases stroke volume.
- Increases cardiac output.
- Releases endorphin.
- Increases pain tolerance.
- Increases natural killer cell activity.
- Decreases total peripheral resistance.
- Dilates the blood vessels and improves *circulation*.

❏ Is Laughter Appropriate in a Medical Setting?

Depending upon the circumstances, humor and laughter can be valuable tools in a lifestyle medicine professional's toolbox. Employed properly, humor can help improve communication between patients and their physicians or allied healthcare professionals by building an emotional connection between everyone involved. It can also help ease a patient's pain, as well as show the patient the human side of the team of lifestyle medicine practitioners. In addition to helping everyone cope, laughter can also help lighten the mood of the situation.

It is important to remember that insensitive humor (i.e., cynical, derogatory, dark, and negative) should be strictly off-limits. Furthermore, some patients will simply not be open to the use of humor and laughter. Humor and laughter require a certain measure of trust and understanding between the patient and the healthcare provider, following the lead of the patient is the best (and most appropriate) strategy. When employed appropriately in the proper setting, laughter is, indeed, one of the best medicines.

FITT PRESCRIPTION FOR LAUGHTER

F—Frequency: daily or weekly
I—Intensity: spontaneous, tickling, belly laughing
T—Time: duration of laughter episode
T—Type: environment/entertainment (laughter yoga, comedy club, favorite sitcom, etc.)

❏ An example FITT prescription for laughter:

F—once per week
I—belly laughing
T—30 minutes
T—laughter yoga class

KEY POINTS/TAKEAWAYS FOR CHAPTER 10

❏ Chapter Review:

- Overall goal: Understand the impact having a positive attitude has on a patient's health.
- Application goal: Be aware of how to incorporate positivity in a patient's life.

❏ Discussion Questions:

- What are the key components of happiness?
- What can individuals do to embrace a positive attitude?
- What are the ways in which positivity manifests itself?
- How is happiness associated with good health?
- What are the common barriers to happiness?
- What can individuals do to overcome obstacles to happiness?
- What are common theories concerning why people laugh?
- What are the mental and physical health benefits associated with laughter?

	TITLE	AUTHORS	JOURNAL	YEAR	KEY FINDINGS
1	Heart health when life is satisfying: evidence from the Whitehall II cohort study	Boehm JK, et al.	European Heart Journal	2011	A study of 7,956 originally healthy subjects from the Whitehall II cohort that investigated satisfaction in seven life domains as possible predictors of incident coronary heart disease. Subjects that scored higher than average in all categories had up to 13% less risk of heart disease, heart attacks, and angina. Associations for lower incidence of coronary heart disease were evident for increased satisfaction in four life domains (job, family, sex life, feelings about yourself as a person).
2	Counting blessings versus burdens: an experimental investigation of gratitude and subjective well-being in daily life	Emmons RA, McCullough ME	Journal of Personality & Social Psychology	2003	A two-month study where subjects were divided into three groups that either listed blessings, hassles, or neutral life events each week or daily in a journal. It found that the subjects who kept gratitude lists were more likely to have made progress in personal goals (academic, interpersonal, or health-based), exercise more regularly, report fewer physical symptoms, and feel better about their lives, and were more optimistic about the upcoming week.
3	Optimism and the experience of pain: benefits of seeing the glass as half full	Goodin BR, Bulls HW	Current Pain and Headache Reports	2013	This review article explores the health-promoting effects of having an optimistic outlook. It finds that optimism is linked to "enhanced physiological recovery and psychosocial adjustment to coronary artery bypass surgery, bone marrow transplantation, postpartum depression, traumatic brain injury, Alzheimer's disease, lung cancer, breast cancer, and failed in vitro fertilization." Furthermore, "optimism seems to benefit the pain experience and its course of treatment."
4	The laughter prescription: a tool for lifestyle medicine	Louie D, Brooks K, Frates E	American Journal of Lifestyle Medicine	2014	A review of laughter and its physiologic effects, as well as recommendations for how physicians can harness the power of laughter for their patients.
5	The grateful disposition: a conceptual and empirical topography	McCullough ME, Emmons RA, Tsang JA	Journal of Personality and Social Psychology	2002	A collection of four studies that examined the correlates of the disposition toward gratitude. It revealed that scoring high on the Gratitude Questionnaire (6-7) was correlated with higher positive emotions, life satisfaction, vitality, and optimism, and lower depression and stress. It also found evidence suggesting that gratitude was negatively associated with envy and materialistic attitudes. Furthermore, the associations persisted after controlling for extraversion/positive affectivity, neuroticism/negative affectivity, and agreeableness.

Figure 10-2. Positive emotions: laughter, optimism, and gratitude evidence

	TITLE	AUTHORS	JOURNAL	YEAR	KEY FINDINGS
6	Better mood and better performance: learning rule-described categories is enhanced by positive mood	Nadler RT, Rabi R, Minda JP	*Psychological Science*	2010	A study of 87 university students exposed to music and video clips to create affective states (positive, negative, or neutral). Volunteers who listened to the positive music and watched the positive video were better at learning a rule to classify sets of complex pictures. There was no difference in affective states for non-category learning or non-rule-described learning.
7	Lifestyle medicine for depression	Sarris J, et al.	*BMC Psychiatry*	2014	Reviews the role of various lifestyle factors in the pathogenesis of depression. It finds that many individual elements considered to be lifestyle medicine are modifiers of overall mental health and depression, but stresses that more rigorous research needs to be done to "address the long-term application of Lifestyle Medicine for depression prevention and management."
8	The affective profiles in the USA: happiness, depression, life satisfaction, and happiness-increasing strategies	Schütz E, et al.	*PeerJournal*	2013	Two studies in Sweden of 900 and 500 participants that evaluated affect profiles and how they were related to happiness, life satisfaction, and overall emotional well-being. They found that "promoting positive emotions can positively influence a depressive-to-happy state as well as increasing life satisfaction. Moreover, the present study shows that pursuing happiness through strategies guided by agency, communion, and spirituality is related to a self-fulfilling experience."
9	Positive psychology progress: empirical validations of interventions	Seligman ME, et al.	*American Psychologist*	2005	A study of 411 subjects that compared the effects of five weekly interventions. They found that using signature strengths in a new way or writing down three good things that happened each day increased happiness and decreased depressive symptoms for six months. It also found that writing and personally delivering a letter of gratitude to someone who had never been properly thanked resulted in an immediate increase in happiness score that lasted one month.
10	Optimism, well-being, depressive symptoms, and perceived physical health: a study among stroke survivors	Shifren K, Anzaldi K	*Psychology, Health & Medicine*	2017	Examined the relationship between optimism, well-being, depressive symptoms, and perceived physical health among stroke survivors.

Figure 10-2. Positive emotions: laughter, optimism, and gratitude evidence (cont.)

	TITLE	AUTHORS	JOURNAL	YEAR	KEY FINDINGS
11	Perceived level of life enjoyment and risks of cardiovascular disease incidence and mortality: the Japan public health center-based study	Shirai K, et al.	*Circulation*	2009	A ~12-year prospective cohort study of 88,175 Japanese men and women 40 to 69 years of age that examined the effects of perceived level of enjoyment on cardiovascular disease incidence and mortality. They found that Japanese men who had a low level of perceived life enjoyment showed an increased risk for stroke and coronary heart disease, incidence, and mortality. However, for women, perceived level of life enjoyment was not associated with risks of cardiovascular disease incidence or mortality.
12	Relationship quality and virtuousness: emotional carrying capacity as a source of individual and team resilience	Stephens JP, et al.	*Journal of Applied Behavioral Science*	2013	In two small studies, researchers "focus on emotional carrying capacity—wherein relationship partners express more of their emotions, express both positive and negative emotions, and do so constructively, as a source of resilience in individuals and teams." They found that emotional carrying capacity is positively related to team resilience and mediates the connection between trust and team resilience.
13	Social rewards enhance offline improvements in motor skill	Sugawara SK, et al.	*PLOS ONE*	2012	Forty-eight healthy participants were trained to perform a specific keyboard sequence task and then either received praise for their own training performance, watched an evaluator praise another participant's performance, or experienced no praise. The next day the participants who received a compliment directly from the evaluator performed better than other participants.
14	The effect of laughter Yoga on general health among nursing students	Yazdani M, et al.	*Iranian Journal of Nursing and Midwifery Research*	2014	A small study done on 38 nursing students that consisted of eight one-hour sessions of laughter yoga as compared to a control group. At the end of the one-month study, they found a significant difference in the mean scores of general health between the two groups. Specifically, the laughter yoga group had improved the signs of physical and sleep disorders, lowered anxiety and depression, and promoted their social functioning.

Figure 10-2. Positive emotions: laughter, optimism, and gratitude evidence (cont.)

References

1. Boehm JK, Peterson C, Kivimaki M, et al. Heart health when life is satisfying: evidence from the Whitehall II cohort study. *European Heart Journal.* 2011;32(21):2672-2677. doi:10.1093/eurheartj/ehr203.
2. Emmons RA, McCullough ME. Counting blessings versus burdens: an experimental investigation of gratitude and subjective well-being in daily life. *Journal of Personality & Social Psychology.* 2003;84(2):377-389. doi:10.1037//0022-3514.84.2.377.
3. Goodin BR, Bulls HW. Optimism and the experience of pain: benefits of seeing the glass as half full. *Current Pain and Headache Reports.* 2013;17(5):329-338. Available at: http://www.ncbi.nlm.nih.gov/pmc/articles/PMC3935764/.
4. Louie D, Brooks K, Frates E. The laughter prescription: a tool for lifestyle medicine. *American Journal of Lifestyle Medicine.* 2014.
5. McCullough ME, Emmons RA, Tsang JA. The grateful disposition: a conceptual and empirical topography. *Journal of Personality and Social Psychology.* 2002;82(1):112-127.
6. Nadler RT, Rabi R, Minda JP. Better mood and better performance: learning rule-described categories is enhanced by positive mood. *Psychological Science.* 2010;21:1770-1776.
7. Sarris J, O'Neil A, Coulson CE, et al. Lifestyle medicine for depression. *BMC Psychiatry.* 2014;14:107. doi:10.1186/1471-244X-14-107.
8. Schütz E, Sailer U, Al Nima A, et al. The affective profiles in the USA: happiness, depression, life satisfaction, and happiness-increasing strategies. *PeerJournal.* 2013;1:e156. doi:10.7717/peerj.156.
9. Seligman ME, Steen TA, Park N, et al. Positive psychology progress: empirical validations of interventions. *American Psychologist.* 2005;60(5):410-421.
10. Shifren K, Anzaldi K. Optimism, well-being, depressive symptoms, and perceived physical health: a study among Stroke survivors. *Psychology, Health & Medicine.* May 5 2017:1-12. doi:10.1080/13548506.2017.1325505. Epub ahead of print.
11. Shirai K, Iso H, Ohira T, et al. Perceived level of life enjoyment and risks of cardiovascular disease incidence and mortality: the Japan public health center-based study. *Circulation.* 2009;120:956-963.
12. Stephens JP, Heaphy ED, Carmeli A, et al. Relationship quality and virtuousness: emotional carrying capacity as a source of individual and team resilience. *Journal of Applied Behavioral Science.* 2013;49:13.
13. Sugawara SK, Tanaka S, Okazaki S, et al. Social rewards enhance offline improvements in motor skill. *PLOS ONE.* 2012;7(11):e48174. https://doi.org/10.1371/journal.pone.0048174.
14. Yazdani M, Esmaeilzadeh M, Pahlavanzadeh S, et al. The effect of laughter Yoga on general health among nursing students. *Iranian Journal of Nursing and Midwifery Research.* 2014;19(1):36-40. Available at: http://www.ncbi.nlm.nih.gov/pmc/articles/PMC3917183/.

Figure 10-2. Positive emotions: laughter, optimism, and gratitude evidence (cont.)

REFERENCES

- 8 Things Happy People Do Differently [Video]. Available at: https://www.youtube.com/watch?v=3OQDI-BZdnI. Accessed October 2017.
- Baby Laughing Hysterically at Ripping Paper (Original) [Video]. Available at: http://www.youtube.com/watch?v=RP4abiHdQpc. Accessed October 2017.
- Ben-Shahar T. *Happier: Learn the Secrets to Daily Joy and Lasting Fulfillment.* New York: McGraw-Hill; 2007.
- Breuning LG. *Habits of a Happy Brain: Retrain Your Brain to Boost Your Serotonin, Dopamine, Oxytocin, & Endorphin Levels.* Avon, MA: Adams Media; 2016.
- Brickman P, Coates D, Janoff-Bulman R. Lottery winners and accident victims: is happiness relative? *Journal of Personality and Social Psychology.* 1978;36(8):917.
- Cooper JM. Aristotle on the goods of fortune. *Philosophical Review.* May 1 1985;94(2):173-196.
- Dhar AK, Barton DA. Depression and the link with cardiovascular disease. *Frontiers in Psychiatry.* 2016;7:33. doi:10.3389/fpsyt.2016.00033.
- Dweck I. *Mindset: The New Psychology of Success—How We Can Learn to Fulfill Our Potential.* Updated edition. New York: Ballantine Books; 2016.
- Easterlin RA. Income and happiness: toward a unified theory. *Economic Journal.* July 2001;111(473):465-484.
- Egger G, Binns A, Rossner S. Chapter 16. In: Egger G, Binns A, Rossner S, eds. *Lifestyle Medicine: Managing Diseases of Lifestyle in the 21st Century.* 2nd ed. North Ryde, N.S.W.: McGraw-Hill; 2010.

- Emmons RA, McCullough ME. Counting blessings versus burdens: an experimental investigation of gratitude and subjective well-being in daily life. *Journal of Personality & Social Psychology.* 2003;84(2):377-389. doi:10.1037//0022-3514.84.2.377.
- Emmons RA. Gratitude Scale. Available at: http://www.psy.miami.edu/faculty/mmccullough/gratitude/2-Page%20Blurb%20on%20the%20Gratitude%20Questionnaire.pdf. Accessed July 2018.
- Emmons RA. *Thanks: How the New Science of Gratitude Can Make You Happier.* New York: Houghton Mifflin; 2007.
- Frankl VE. *Man's Search for Meaning.* Boston, MA: Beacon Press; 1959.
- Frederickson BL. *Positivity: Top Notch Research Reveals the 3-to-1 Ratio That Will Change Your Life.* New York: Three Rivers Press; 2009.
- Fredrickson B. *Love 2.0.* New York: Hudson Street Press; 2013.
- Fredrickson BL. Positive emotions broaden and build. Pages 1-53. In: Plant EA, Devine PG, eds. *Advances on Experimental Social Psychology, 47.* Burlington: Academic Press; 2013.
- Goodin BR, Bulls HW. Optimism and the experience of pain: benefits of seeing the glass as half full. *Current Pain and Headache Reports.* 2013;17(5):329-338. Available at: http://www.ncbi.nlm.nih.gov/pmc/articles/PMC3935764/. Accessed October 2017.
- Hayes SC, Luoma JB, Bond FW, et al. Acceptance and commitment therapy: model, processes and outcomes. *Behaviour Research and Therapy.* 2006;44(1):1-25.
- Hayes SC, Strosahl KD, Wilson KG. *Acceptance and Commitment Therapy: The Process and Practice of Mindful Change.* New York: Guilford Press; 2012.
- Headey B. The set point theory of well-being has serious flaws: on the eve of a scientific revolution. *Social Indicators Research.* 2010;97:7-21.
- Lane RD. Neural correlates of conscious emotional experience. Pages 345-370. In: Lane RD, Nadel L, eds. *Series in Affective Science: Cognitive Neuroscience of Emotion.* New York: Oxford University Press; 2000.
- Laughter Yoga on Discovery Channel [Video]. Available at: http://www.youtube.com/watch?v=ahhN3Ryw4O4. Accessed October 2017.
- Layous K, Chancellor J, Lyubomirsky S. Positive activities as protective factors against mental health conditions. *Journal of Abnormal Psychology.* February 2014;123(1):3-12.
- Layous K, Sweeny K, Armenta C. The proximal experience of gratitude. *PLOS ONE.* July 7 2017;12(7):e0179123.
- Louie D, Brook K, Frates E. The laughter prescription: a tool for lifestyle medicine. *American Journal of Lifestyle Medicine.* July 1 2016;10(4):262-267.
- Lyubomirsky S, Sheldon KM, Schkade D. Pursuing happiness: the architecture of sustainable change. *Review of General Psychology.* 2005;9(2):111-131. Available at: https://escholarship.org/uc/item/4v03h9gv. Accessed August 2018.

- Lyubomirsky S, Tkach C, Sheldon KM. Pursuing sustained happiness through random acts of kindness and counting one's blessings: tests of two six-week interventions. Unpublished raw data. 2004. doi:10.1037/1089-2680.9.2.111.
- Lyubomirsky S. *The How of Happiness: A Scientific Approach to Getting the Life You Want.* New York: Penguin Books; 2008.
- Maruta T, Colligan RC, Malinchoc M, et al. Optimists vs pessimists: survival rate among medical patients over a 30-year period. *Mayo Clinic Proceedings.* 2000;75:140-143.
- Mayo Clinic Staff. Positive Thinking: Stop Negative Self-Talk to Reduce Stress. Mayo Clinic. Available at: https://www.mayoclinic.org/healthy-lifestyle/stress-management/in-depth/positive-thinking/art-20043950. Accessed July 2018.
- McCullough ME, Emmons RA, Tsang JA. The grateful disposition: a conceptual and empirical topography. *Journal of Personality and Social Psychology.* 2002;82:112. 10.1037/0022-3514.82.1.112.
- Moser JS, Schroder HS, Heeter C, et al. Mind your errors: evidence for a neural mechanism linking growth mind-set to adaptive posterror adjustments. *Psychological Science.* 2011;22(12):1484-1489.
- Nadler RT, Rabi R, Minda JP. Better mood and better performance: learning rule-described categories is enhanced by positive mood. *Psychological Science.* 2010;21:1770-1776.
- Ng MY, Wong WS. The differential effects of gratitude and sleep on psychological distress in patients with chronic pain. *Journal of Health Psychology.* 2013;18(2):263-271.
- Provine RR, Fischer KR. Laughing, smiling and talking: relation to sleeping and social context in humans. *Ethology.* 1989;83:295-305.
- Provine RR. Laughing, tickling, and the evolution of speech and self. *Current Directions in Psychological Science.* 2004;13(6):215-218.
- Ruberton PM, Huynh HP, Miller TA. The relationship between physician humility, physician-patient communication, and patient health. *Patient Education and Counseling.* July 2016;99(7):1138-1145.
- Schütz E, Sailer U, Al Nima A, et al. The affective profiles in the USA: happiness, depression, life satisfaction, and happiness-increasing strategies. *PeerJournal.* 2013;1:e156. doi:10.7717/peerj.156.
- Seligman ME. *Flourish: A Visionary New Understanding of Happiness and Well-being.* New York: Free Press; 2011.
- Seligman MEP, Steen TA, Park N, et al. Positive psychology progress: empirical validation of interventions. *American Psychologist.* 2005;60(5):410-421. http://dx.doi.org/10.1037/0003-066X.60.5.410.
- Seligman MEP. *Authentic Happiness: Using the New Positive Psychology to Realize Your Potential for Lasting Fulfillment.* New York: Atria Paperback; 2002.

- Seligman MEP. Optimism, pessimism, and mortality. *Mayo Clinic Proceedings.* 2000;75(2):133-134.
- Shifren K, Anzaldi K. Optimism, well-being, depressive symptoms, and perceived physical health: a study among stroke survivors. *Psychology, Health & Medicine.* May 5 2017:1-12. doi: 10.1080/13548506.2017.1325505. [Epub ahead of print]
- Shirai K, Iso H, Ohira T, et al. Perceived level of life enjoyment and risks of cardiovascular disease incidence and mortality: the Japan public health center-based study. *Circulation.* September 15 2009;120(11):956-963.
- Sugawara SK, Tanaka S, Okazaki S, et al. Social rewards enhanced offline improvements in motor skill. *PLOS ONE.* 2012;7(11):e48174.
- Yazdani M, Esmaeilzadeh M, Pahlavanzadeh S, Khaledi F. The effect of laughter yoga on general health among nursing students. *Iranian Journal of Nursing and Midwifery Research.* 2014;19(1):36-40. Available at: http://www.ncbi.nlm.nih.gov/pmc/articles/PMC3917183/. Accessed October 2017.

CHAPTER 11

SUBSTANCE ABUSE

"What is addiction, really? It is a sign, a signal, a symptom of distress. It is a language that tells us about a plight that must be understood."

—Alice Miller, PhD
Swiss Psychologist and
Psychoanalyst
Author

❏ Chapter Goals:

- Understand the key factors involved in substance abuse.
- Recognize why people abuse substances.
- Become aware of the symptoms and signs of various kinds of substance abuse.
- Discern the connection between health and substance abuse.
- Learn basic counseling for individuals who are abusing substances.

❏ Learning Objectives:

- To comprehend what substance abuse details
- To be cognizant of why substance abuse is important
- To understand the impact of substance abuse on health
- To learn treatment options for various forms of substance abuse
- To consider possible lifestyle interventions for substance abuse

❏ Guiding Questions:

- What is substance abuse?
- What are the signs and symptoms of substance abuse?
- What is the impact of substance abuse on society?
- What is the impact of substance abuse on health?
- What are common ways of treating substance abuse?
- What are barriers to treating substance abuse?
- What techniques can lifestyle medicine practitioners use when dealing with patients who abuse substances?

❏ Important Terms:

- *Addiction:* A compulsive use of a habit-forming substance despite negative consequences, characterized by tolerance and by well-defined physiological symptoms upon withdrawal
- *Dependence:* The body's physical need for a specific substance (agent) as evidenced by withdrawal or tolerance
- *Overdose:* When the body receives a level of drugs that it cannot tolerate
- *Tolerance:* The body's diminished response to the same amount of a substance that is the result of repeated use of markedly increased amounts of the given substance to achieve the desired effect.
- *Withdrawal:* Specific signs and symptoms occurring after discontinuing the given substance

Addiction is complex chronic disease, often arising from individual and environmental factors. The scientific understanding of addiction is constantly evolving and by no means is this text meant to be exhaustive in its description of addiction. On the other hand, an understanding of the basic biology, common addictive substances, and the expanding conception of addiction is helpful for effectively counseling people suffering with addiction.

According to the American Society of Addiction Medicine (ASAM) website:

> "Addiction is a primary, chronic disease of brain reward, motivation, memory, and related circuitry. Dysfunction in these circuits leads to characteristic biological, psychological, social and spiritual manifestations. This is reflected in an individual pathologically pursuing reward and/or relief by substance use and other behaviors.
>
> "Addiction is characterized by inability to consistently abstain, impairment in behavioral control, craving, diminished recognition of significant problems with one's behaviors and interpersonal relationships, and a dysfunctional emotional response. Like other chronic diseases, addiction often involves cycles of relapse and remission. Without treatment or engagement in recovery activities, addiction is progressive and can result in disability or premature death."

It is widely accepted that nearly half of addiction has a genetic etiology and is also influenced by age, gender, ethnicity, and co-morbid mental illness. Environmental factors include, but are not limited to, the availability of addictive substances, peer pressure, and a history of abuse and violence. From a developmental perspective, the earlier a person begins using addictive substances, the more likely that addiction will take hold. Adolescent brains, especially the prefrontal cortex, are still developing, a factor that influences decision-making and judgement.

Addiction has neurobiological underpinnings rooted in the more primitive reward circuitry of the brain. Pleasure generates a reinforcing reward stimulus for the brain. This factor is communicated by the neurotransmitter dopamine and encoded in the nucleus accumbens. The neurons of the ventral tegmental area (VTA) contain dopamine, which is released to the nucleus accumbens and registers as a jolt of pleasure.

In order to reinforce this behavior and make sure it is repeated in the future the nucleus accumbens interacts with area of the brain that control memory and behavior. The amygdala establishes associations between environmental cues and whether or not that particular experience is rewarding or aversive. The hippocampus encodes the pleasurable experience as a memory in order to repeat the behavior in the future. Regions of the prefrontal cortex then provide executive control over choices made regarding whether or not to seek reward.

Under normal conditions, this circuit controls an individual's response to natural rewards, such as food, sex, and social interactions. Addictive drugs, however, also activate the reward pathway, the power of which causes the neurons to ramp up their production of dopamine. Simultaneously, the brain decreases the number of cells that respond to dopamine. This factor enables the phenomenon of tolerance by which the user must increase the amount of a pleasurable substance in order to produce the same "high." Naturally, this situation creates the potential for substance abuse.

Addiction and substance abuse mutually reinforce each other. Addiction is marked by a change in behavior caused by the biochemical changes in the brain, after continued substance abuse. Subsequently, continued substance abuse then reinforces addiction. Addiction is a component of substance use disorder and represents the most severe form of the disorder.

Considering the following ASAM acronym "ABCDE" can help diagnose and clarify the challenges facing a person who suffers from addiction:

- A—an inability to consistently Abstain
- B—an impaired capacity to control Behavior
- C—an increased "Craving" to smoke
- D—a Diminished ability by an individual to recognize significant problems that may be occurring with their behavior and interpersonal relationships.
- E—a dysfunctional Emotional response to their situation

SUBSTANCE USE DISORDER

The *Diagnostic and Statistical Manual of Mental Disorders*, Fifth Edition (DSM-5), no longer uses the terms substance abuse and substance dependence. Rather, it refers to substance use disorders. Substance use disorders occur when the recurrent use of alcohol and/or drugs causes clinically and functionally significant impairment, such as health problems, disability, and failure to meet major responsibilities at work, school, or home. According to the DSM-5, a diagnosis of substance use disorder is based on evidence of impaired control, social impairment, risky use, and pharmacological criteria. The most common substance use disorders in the United States include alcohol use disorder, tobacco use disorder, cannabis use disorder, stimulant use disorder, and opioid use disorder. The health impact of excessive use of these substances is discussed in this chapter.

Substance use disorder is an insidious problem in the United States. The leading causes of death at the beginning of the 21st century in the United States were tobacco (435,000 deaths; 18.1 percent of total US deaths), poor diet and physical inactivity (365,000 deaths, 15.2 percent), and alcohol consumption (85,000 deaths, 3.5 percent). Substance use disorder exacts a tremendous toll on the physical and fiscal health of this nation. Every year, federal, state, and local governments spend an estimated $600 billion on various aspects of substance abuse. On the other hand, for every dollar federal and state governments spend in that regard, only two cents go to prevention and treatment.

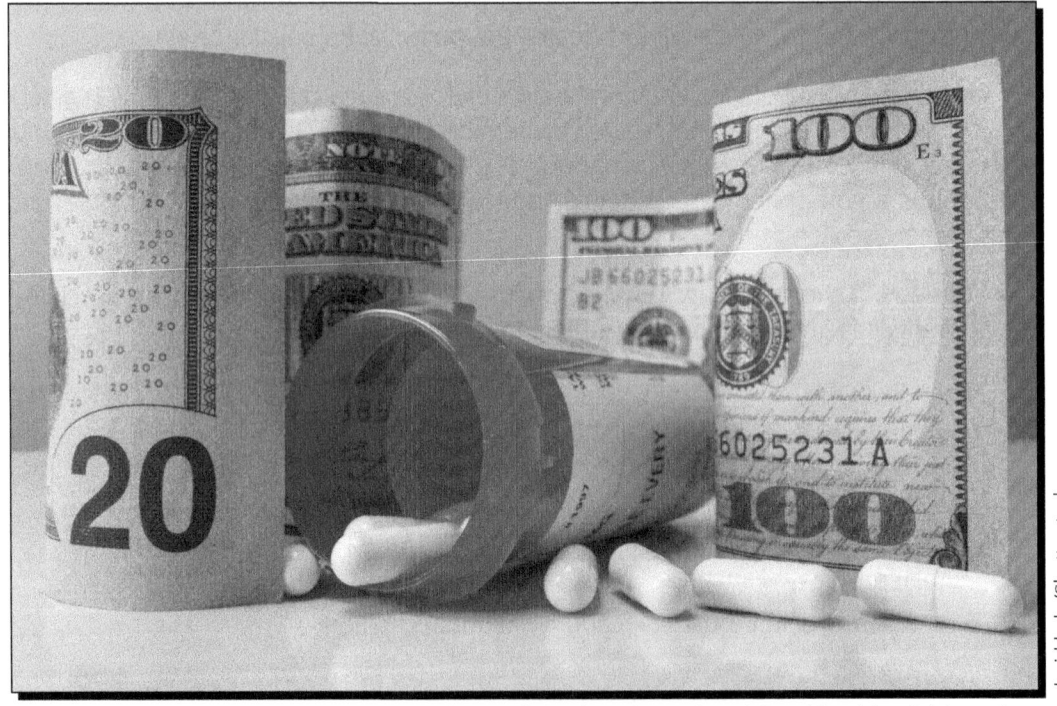

Substance use disorder exacts a tremendous toll on the physical and fiscal health of this nation.

Examples of the impact that substance use disorder can have at an individual and societal level include the following:

- Costs involved in healthcare expenses, diminished level of productivity in the workplace, and secondary crime-related activities
- Broken families, child abuse, death due to negligence or accident, destroyed careers, domestic violence, and physical abuse
- Changes in a person's brain chemistry
- Diminished personal health

A number of individuals don't understand why or how other people use substances in excess. They often mistakenly believe that these individuals lack the moral fortitude or willpower to stop their substance abuse. In reality, substance use disorder is a complex issue that, more often than not, can require more than good intentions or a strong will to quit.

In fact, education, outreach, and empathy are key to helping people understand the possible risks of substance use disorder and getting them to change their untoward behavior. In that regard, lifestyle medicine practitioners have a crucial role in tailoring an appropriate treatment approach to each patient's substance use pattern and personal circumstances.

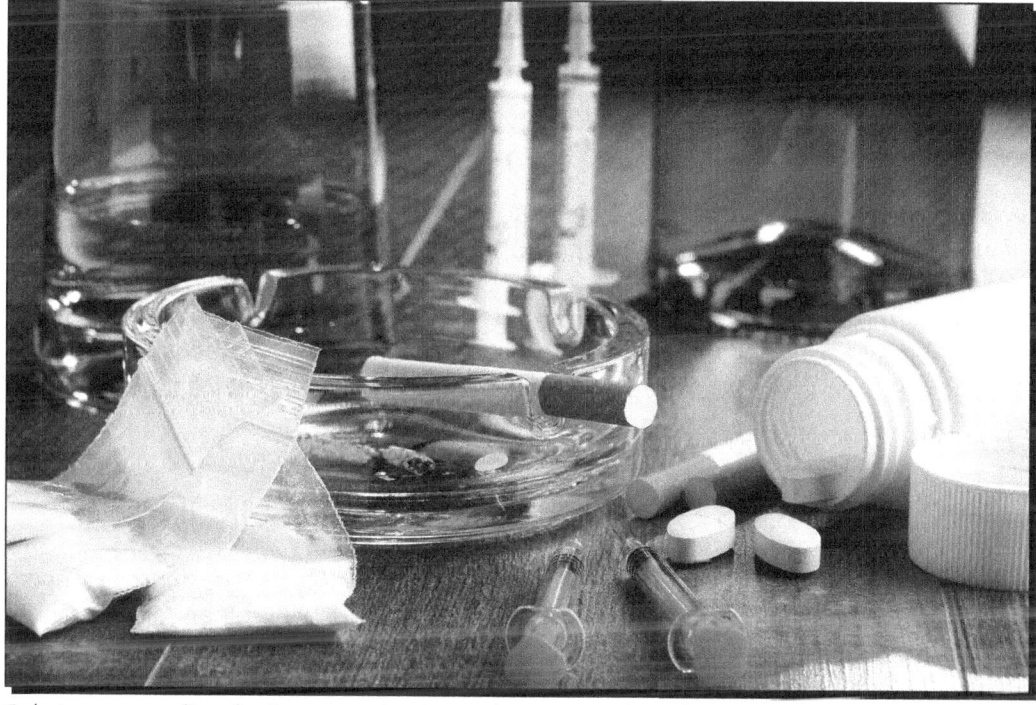

Substance use disorder is a complex issue that, more often than not, can require more than good intentions or a strong will to quit.

LIVE AND LEARN WITH DR. BETH FRATES

There's nothing like the emergency room to learn about medicine. During my internship, I had an experience that I can still remember like it was yesterday. A 35-year-old man came in by ambulance with chest pain. He had significant EKG changes and was admitted to the hospital for careful monitoring, after his myocardial infarction (heart attack).

The usual suspects for heart disease were not there. He did not have a family history of heart disease. He did not smoke. He did not have diabetes, high blood pressure, or high cholesterol. He was not overweight. He was not sedentary. He was a young, fairly fit man. His case was a mystery.

Because I was the intern on his case, I spent a great deal of time with him, explaining our rationale for ordering different tests and then sharing the results. He was going to be discharged for follow-up with his primary care physician. I remember sitting with him, hands on my head, staring at the floor, saying, "This must be so frustrating for you. We can't figure out what happened here. I imagine you might be afraid this could happen again since we don't know the etiology—the cause—of your heart attack. I want to make sure we have examined every possibility here."

Then, he said, "Cocaine. I did cocaine." I looked up slowly and quietly. Feeling surprised, I said softly, "Oh. I thought I asked you about drugs when you were first admitted." He responded, "Yes. You did. I lied. I was scared. I was not sure if I would be arrested or what would happen, if I told you. But, you and your team are working so hard to figure this out, and I can tell you care a lot about this. I want to help you help me. So, I need to come clean here."

Well, I was again surprised, but I was so grateful that he told the truth. With that information, we had an explanation and a plan to help him prevent another heart attack. This interaction taught me the power of Theodore Roosevelt's words, "No one cares how much you know, until they know how much you care." It was not until this patient was convinced that we cared deeply about him as a person that he was comfortable sharing his true story with us. Empathy is key when working with people struggling with substance use disorders.

THE SUBSTANCES OF SUBSTANCE USE DISORDER

Individuals use, and are prone to overusing, a wide variety of substances, ranging from chocolate to drugs. Some of these substances are lawful, others are illegal. All are potentially harmful. Five of the most common, as well as the most likely to be destructive, of these substances are alcohol, cannabis, tobacco, stimulants, and opioids. Each of these substances is discussed in detail in the following sections.

ALCOHOL

Statistics indicate that alcohol (from a numbers standpoint) is the most widely used substance in the United States. A number of Americans drink more than the recommended level of alcohol consumption, based on the American Heart Association's guidelines of up to one drink per day for women and two drinks per day for men. It should be noted that this guideline refers to the amount consumed on any single day, as opposed to as an average over several days.

In fact, over 86 percent of people of ages 18 or older state that, at some point in their lives, they have drunk alcohol. Almost that many individuals (70 percent) report consuming alcohol in the past year. The problem that has arisen over time is that a number of people drink to excess.

A 2017 study in the *Journal of the American Medical Association (JAMA)*, found that one in eight American adults is a heavy drinker, i.e., for men that is more than four drinks on any given day or more than 14 drinks per week; for women that is more than three drinks on any day or more than seven drinks per week. Binge drinking, for a typical adult, is defined as consuming five or more drinks in about two hours for men or four or more drinks for women in the same timeframe. The more drinks on any day, as well as the heavier drinking days over time, the greater the risk not only for alcohol abuse, as well as for other health and personal problems. At-risk drinking is characterized as four drinks on any day or more than 14 per week for men, and more than three drinks on any day or more than seven per week for women. This delineation might surprise some readers and some patients. In fact, many, many people drink to excess and fall into the category of at risk drinking.

If a person's problem-drinking becomes severe, that individual is given the medical diagnosis of alcohol use disorder (AUD). AUD is a chronic relapsing brain disease characterized by compulsive alcohol use, loss of control over alcohol intake, and a negative emotional state when not using. An estimated 16 million people in the United States have AUD. To be diagnosed with AUD, individuals must meet certain criteria outlined in the *Diagnostic and Statistical Manual of Mental Disorders* (DSM). The severity of AUD—mild, moderate, or severe—is based on the number of the following criteria occurring within a 12-month period:

- Alcohol is often taken in larger amounts or over a longer period than was intended.
- There is a persistent desire or unsuccessful efforts to cut down or control alcohol use.
- A great deal of time is spent in activities necessary to obtain alcohol, use alcohol, or recover from its effects.
- Craving, or a strong desire or urge for alcohol, exists.
- Recurrent alcohol use occurs, resulting in a failure to fulfill significant role obligations at work, school, or home.

- Alcohol use continues, despite having persistent or recurrent social or interpersonal problems, caused or exacerbated by the effects of alcohol.
- Important social, occupational, or recreational activities are given up or reduced because of alcohol use.
- Recurrent alcohol use occurs in situations in which it is physically hazardous.
- Alcohol use continues, despite knowledge of having a persistent or recurrent physical or psychological problem that is likely to have been caused or exacerbated by alcohol.
- A need exists for markedly increased amounts of alcohol to achieve intoxication or the desired effect; or a markedly diminished effect occurs with the continued consumption of the same amount of alcohol.
- When the effects of alcohol are wearing off, withdrawal symptoms (e.g., trouble sleeping, shakiness, irritability, anxiety, depression, restlessness, nausea, sweating, etc.) are experienced; or more alcohol (or a closely related substance, such as benzodiazepine) is taken to relieve or avoid the symptoms of withdrawal.

Mild alcohol use is defined by the presence of two to three of these symptoms. Moderate alcohol use refers to the presence of four to five of the symptoms. As such, six or more of the symptoms constitutes severe alcohol use.

One potential side effect of drinking too much alcohol is alcohol intoxication, a physical state that is also commonly referred to as drunkenness. A physiological condition that may result in psychological alterations of consciousness, drunkenness is induced by consuming alcohol, which enters the bloodstream faster than it can be metabolized by the body. During metabolism, ethanol (alcohol) is broken down into non-intoxicating by-products.

When individuals suffer from alcohol intoxication, they experience clinically significant problematic behavior or psychological changes (e.g., inappropriate sexual or aggressive behavior, mood (ability, impaired judgment) that developed during or shortly after alcohol was consumed. Among the signs or symptoms that may arise from excessive alcohol use are the following:
- Slurred speech
- Lack of coordination
- Unsteady gait
- Nystagmus (side-to-side movements of the eyes)
- Impairment in attention or memory
- Stupor or coma
- Signs or symptoms that are not attributable to another medical condition and are not better explained by another medical disorder, including intoxication with another substance

THE IMPACT OF ALCOHOL ON HEALTH

Drinking to excess over an extended time or consuming too much alcohol on a single occasion can damage the body, including the following problems:

❏ Heart:

- Cardiomyopathy—stretching and drooping of the heart muscle
- Arrhythmias—irregular heart beat
- Stroke
- High blood pressure

❏ Liver:

- Steatosis, or fatty liver
- Alcoholic hepatitis
- Fibrosis
- Cirrhosis

❏ Pancreas:

- Pancreatitis—a dangerous inflammation and swelling of the blood vessels in the pancreas that prevents proper digestion

❏ Immune System:

- Weakens the immune system, making the body a much easier target for disease.
- Chronic drinkers are at a heightened risk for pneumonia and tuberculosis, compared to non-drinkers.
- Drinking a lot on a single occasion slows the body's ability to ward off infections, even up to 24 hours after getting drunk.

Drinking a lot on a single occasion slows the body's ability to ward off infections, even up to 24 hours after getting drunk.

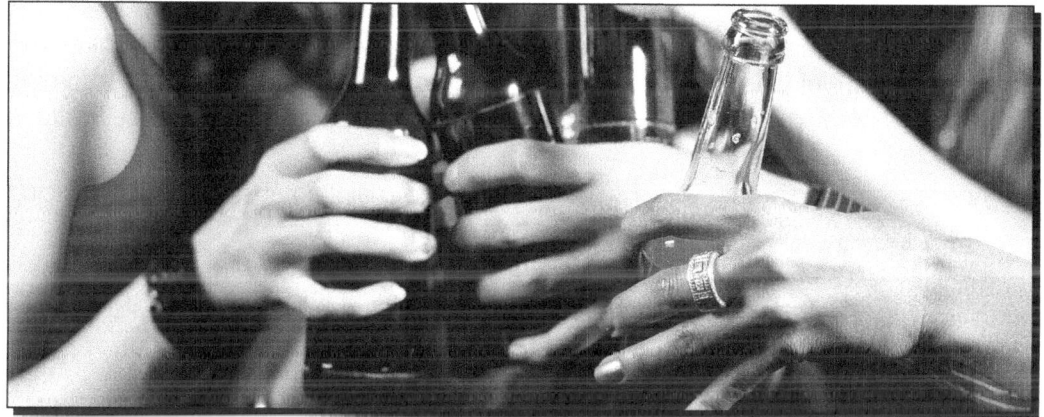

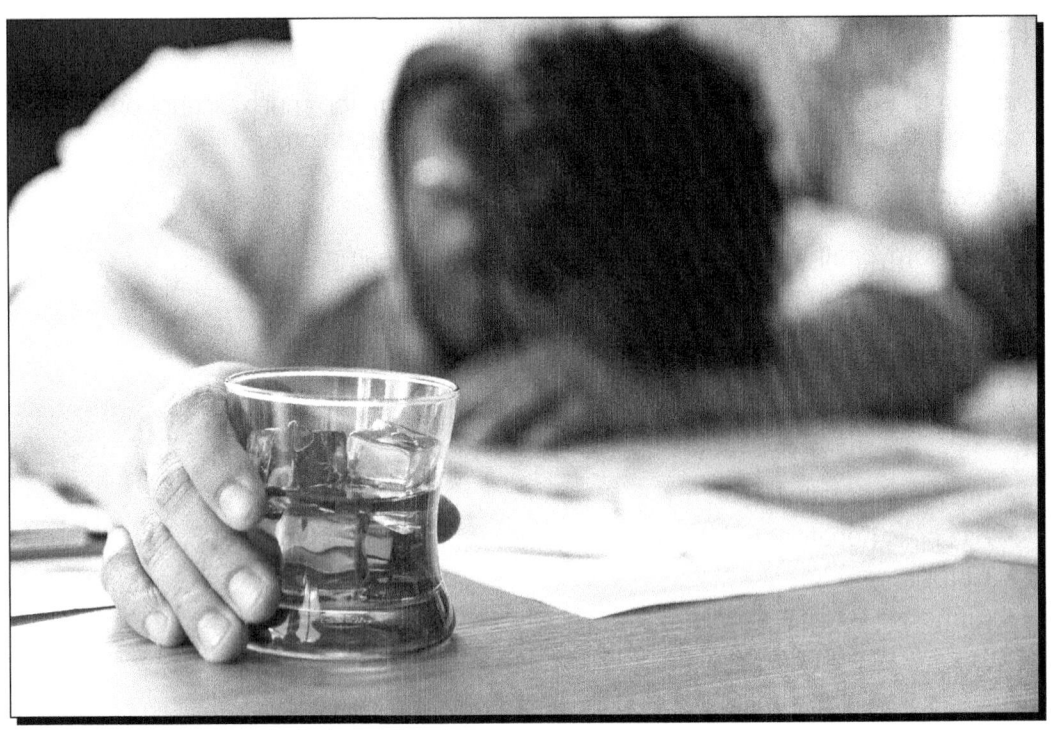

No medicine can cure alcohol use disorder.

Drinking too much alcohol can also increase an individual's risk of developing certain cancers, including cancers of the mouth, esophagus, throat, liver, and breast. In addition, chronic AUD can cause brain damage, in this instance, a neurological disorder referred to as Wernicke-Korsakoff syndrome (WKS). WKS results from a thiamine deficiency. Most researchers believe that Wernicke's encephalopathy occurs as a result of severe acute deficiency of thiamine (vitamin B1), while Korsakoff's psychosis is a chronic neurologic consequence of Wernicke's encephalopathy. WKS leads to various degrees of cognitive impairment, as well as cardiovascular dysfunction. Figure 11-1 details regions of the brain that are vulnerable to alcoholism-related abnormalities.

No medicine can cure AUD. Some medications, however, can make drinking less enjoyable to a point where individuals don't want to drink as much, if at all. According to a *Harvard Medical School Special Health Report*, three FDA-approved medications that help in that regard are:
- Acamprosate (Campral), which makes it easier to maintain abstinence by reducing the unpleasant effects from abstaining from alcohol
- Disulfiram (Antabuse), which makes a person feel sick or throw up if they drink
- Naltrexone (ReVia or Vivitrol), which reduces the pleasurable effects of alcohol and reduces cravings

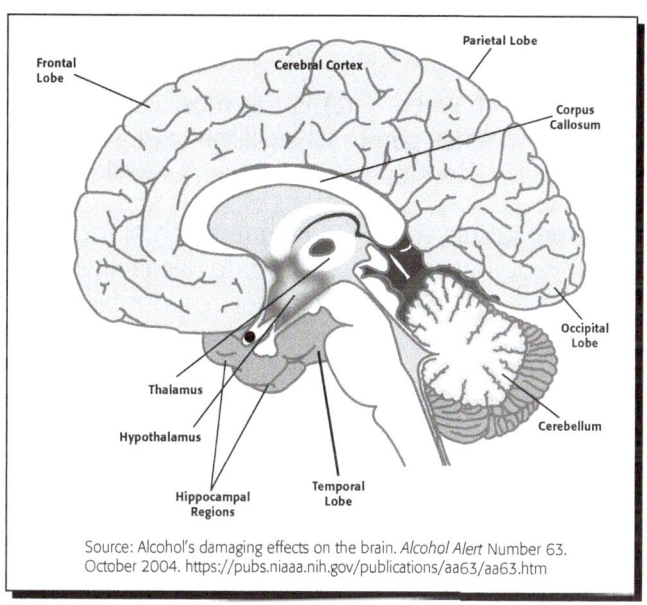

Figure 11-1. Regions of the brain that are vulnerable to alcoholism-related abnormalities

No one-size-fits-all treatment plan exists for alcoholism. In general, individuals have a variety of treatment options, including alcohol detoxification (completed under professional medical care); inpatient rehabilitation (undertaken in a facility that features a structured treatment environment); alcohol counseling (guidance is received from an alcohol counselor who addresses any underlying issues that may be causing a person's drinking problem); and government-issued services and resources (government-funded programs designed to treat alcohol-related problems).

There are also a number of groups in the United States that support people who are struggling with AUD. It is important for individuals who have a drinking problem to know that they're not alone in their situation. There are organizations that offer resources and tools for individuals who are impacted by the harmful effects of alcohol. Among the groups, in that regard, are the following:

- Al-anon and Alateen
- Alcoholics Anonymous
- Secular Organizations for Sobriety
- SMART Recovery
- WhoYouWant2Be.org
- Women for Sobriety

CANNABIS

Cannabis (e.g., marijuana, pot, weed, etc.) is the most commonly used illicit drug in the United States, due in no small part to its legalization in a number of states. Similar to alcohol, cannabis users can develop a use disorder, as well as become intoxicated.

Cannabis use disorder occurs when the recurrent use of the drug leads to clinically and functionally significant impairment (similar to alcohol use), such as physical problems, disability, and a failure to meet major responsibilities at home, work, or school. Its diagnosis is based on evidence of impaired control, social impairment, risky use, and specific pharmacological criteria. Recently conducted research indicates that over four million Americans met the diagnostic criteria for cannabis use disorder.

The primary effects of cannabis are caused by the more than 100 different chemical compounds in the plant. Among the acute effects of using cannabis are euphoria and anxiety. In turn, very high levels of cannabis can lead to auditory and visual hallucinations.

The psychological effects of cannabis, commonly referred to as a "high," are subjective and can vary, based on the circumstances (e.g., the individual, the method of use, and the relative strength of the drug). Cannabis use can also have a number of subjective and highly tangible effects, such as an increased level of enjoyment of food taste and aroma, an enhanced appreciation of music and comedy, and marked distortions concerning the perception of time and space. In some instances, cannabis can result in altered body image, ataxia (loss of full control of bodily movements), and dissociative mental states, such as depersonalization and derealization.

Smoking cannabis appears to entail the same risks as smoking tobacco, given that carcinogens are present in all smoke. On the other hand, medical marijuana has been approved to treat nausea and vomiting associated with chemotherapy and appetite stimulation in illnesses, such as cancer. While it may be helpful in treating chronic pain, neuropathic pain, and spasticity due to multiple sclerosis, more research is needed in this area.

On occasion, cannabis use can result in cannabis intoxication. When that situation occurs, users typically experience one or more of the following side effects: conjunctival injection, increased appetite, dry mouth, and tachycardia. More serious side effects can include panic, paranoia, and acute psychosis. The degree to which individuals are affected by the various side effects varies from person to person, as well as with the amount and strength of the cannabis used.

At some point, some long-term or heavy cannabis users decide to quit using the drug. Going through cannabis withdrawal is not easy. On the other hand, it is not impossible, although long-term or heavy cannabis users often experience more serious side effects than do individuals who didn't use the drug as heavily or for as long a duration of time. As

Lifestyle Medicine Handbook   389

a rule, within a week of discontinuing cannabis use that heretofore has been heavy and prolonged (i.e., daily or almost daily use for a period of at least a few months), individuals will experience three or more of the following signs and symptoms:
- Irritability, anger, or aggression
- Nervousness or anxiety
- Sleep difficulty (e.g., insomnia, disturbing dreams)
- Decreased appetite or weight loss
- Restlessness
- Depressed mood
- At least one of the following physical symptoms, causing significant discomfort: abdominal pain, shakiness/tremors, sweating, fever, chills, or headache

THE IMPACT OF CANNABIS USE ON HEALTH

Cannabis use (e.g., smoking, vaporizing, eating, drinking it as brewed tea, etc.) can have a number of mostly negative effects on a person, with a few arguably positive, including the following:

❑ Effects of Cannabis on Physical Aspects of Health:

- Speed up heart rate.
- Increased risk of heart attack, particularly in older people and in individuals with heart problems.
- Relax and enlarge breathing passages.
- Expand the blood vessels in the eyes (making the eyes look bloodshot).
- In some instances, raise blood pressure, as well as heart rate, thereby reducing the blood's capacity to carry oxygen.
- Possibly cause orthostatic hypotension (head rush or dizziness upon standing).
- Possible increased risk of an aggressive form of testicular cancer that predominantly affects young adult males.
- Long-term and short-term effects on the brain
- Breathing problems (e.g., irritated lungs, daily coughing and phlegm, more frequent incidence of lung illness, a higher risk of lung infections)
- Problems with child development during and after pregnancy (e.g., lower birth weight)

❑ Effects of Cannabis on Mental Aspects of Health:

- Altered senses (e.g., seeing brighter colors)
- Altered sense of time
- Anxiety
- Changes in mood
- Depression

- Difficulty with thinking and problem-solving
- Impaired body movement
- Impaired memory
- Reduced life satisfaction
- Suicidal thoughts among teenagers
- Worsening symptoms in individuals with schizophrenia
- Delusions (when taken in high doses)
- Hallucinations (when taken in high doses)
- Psychosis (when taken in high doses)

TOBACCO

Despite the fact that smoking harms nearly every organ of the body, leads to a number of diseases, and diminishes the health of individuals in general, an estimated 36.5 million adults in the United States currently smoke. Even though the percentage of U.S. adults who smoke cigarettes has generally declined every year since 1965, cigarette smoking remains the leading preventable cause of death in the United States, causing more than 480,000 deaths annually (approximately one in five deaths).

In fact, smoking causes more deaths than the following causes combined: alcohol use, firearm-related incidents, human immunodeficiency virus, illegal drug use, and motor vehicle accidents. Another startling statistic is the fact that more than 10 times as many U.S. citizens have died prematurely from cigarette smoking than have died in all the wars fought by the United States.

Who starts smoking and why? While a variety of individuals who are likely to begin exists, three of the more probable groups are people with parents or friends who smoke, individuals who just "wanted to try it," and people who thought it was "cool" to smoke. In reality, teenagers are the group of people who are most predisposed to smoking. Approximately 90 percent of smokers start smoking before they reach the age of 19—a statistic made even more compelling by the fact that the younger someone is when they start smoking, the more likely they are to become addicted to the practice.

The nicotine in cigarettes, which quickly enters the bloodstream, is addictive, which makes it difficult to stop smoking. Within a few seconds of entering your body, the nicotine reaches your brain, causing it to release adrenaline, which, in turn, creates a burst of pleasure and energy. The buzz doesn't last for too long, however. As a result, the smoker feels tired and a little down, wanting to experience the buzz again. This scenario is what makes an individual light up their next cigarette.

Over time, the body is able to build up a high tolerance to nicotine. As a result, the individual will need to smoke more and more cigarettes to experience the pleasure effects of the nicotine and prevent withdrawal symptoms. Eventually, this up-and-down cycle, repeated over and over, leads to addiction.

Addiction keeps people smoking, even when they want to quit. Overcoming addiction is more difficult for some people than others. More often than not, a person may need to make more than one attempt to quit. Like many chronic diseases, nicotine addiction can involve cycles of relapse and remission. Without treatment or engagement in targeted recovery activities, however, addiction can be progressive and can have dire health-related consequences.

Tobacco use disorder is a condition characterized by the harmful consequences of repeated tobacco use, a pattern of compulsive tobacco use, and (on occasion) physiological dependence on tobacco (i.e., tolerance and/or withdrawal). This disorder is only diagnosed when tobacco use becomes persistent and causes significant occupational, social or medical impairment.

❑ Tobacco Withdrawal

Over time, a person's body and brain get used to having nicotine in them. When a person quits smoking, the body begins to adjust to normal levels of chemicals. In reaction, the smoker may feel different withdrawal symptoms, including irritability, anxiety, difficulty concentrating, increased appetite, restlessness, depressed mood, and insomnia. Experiencing these signs and symptoms, which can begin to appear relatively soon after the last cigarette, can cause clinically significant distress or impairment in social, occupational, or other key areas of functioning.

Withdrawal can be uncomfortable. The feelings associated with withdrawal usually are the strongest in the first week after a person quits. Many people don't like or can't tolerate the experience. As a result, they start smoking again to feel better. The key for them is to develop a viable strategy to stay smoke-free. In that regard, lifestyle medicine practitioners can provide counsel, comfort, and compassion to their patients who are smokers.

❑ The Impact of Smoking on Health

Smoking cigarettes can have a negative impact on nearly every organ and system of the body. A review of the various systems of the body and how each is adversely impacted by smoking is warranted, as the following indicates:

Circulatory System

Smoking is the most consequential single risk factor in heart disease, including coronary artery disease, sudden cardiac death, ischemic stroke, aortic aneurysm formation, peripheral vascular disease, and Buerger's disease. In fact, individuals who smoke are also two to four times more likely to develop coronary heart disease. Even smoking one cigarette a day puts you at increased risk for signs of early cardiovascular disease. This occurs due to increased inflammation and subsequent damage to the blood vessels. The blood vessels are lined with a thin layer of endothelial cells which keep the blood circulating fluidly throughout the body. The toxins from cigarette smoke causes an inflammatory reaction of in this fragile endothelial lining, leading to the formation of atherosclerotic plaque in the blood vessel wall. These plaques are composed of various white blood cells and particles of oxidized LDL. As more smoke causes more inflammation, the plaque enlarges with a larger risk of rupture. Rupture of the plaque can then cause the artery to clog, cutting of circulation to the heart muscle and leading to rapid death of heart cells (or "myocytes"). This is called a myocardial infarction, or more commonly a heart attack.

Damage to blood vessels is not just confined to the arteries of the heart, however. Nicotine causes blood vessels all over the body to tighten, which restricts the flow of blood and increases blood pressure. Over time, the ongoing narrowing, along with inflammatory damage to the vessels can cause peripheral artery disease. Damage to the blood vessels can also decrease their strength and elasticity, which increases the risk for abdominal aortic aneurysms.

Digestive System

Smoking causes destruction to the teeth and gums which can cause tooth loss. Just as cigarette smoke gets into the lungs, the toxins also seep into the gastrointestinal tract. Therefore, smoking increases the risk of mouth, throat, larynx, and esophageal cancer. Smokers have a higher risk of pancreatic cancer.

Endocrine System

Studies have also shown that smoking increases the risk of developing insulin resistance and type 2 diabetes. In fact, the risk of developing diabetes is 30 to 40 percent higher for active smokers than nonsmokers.

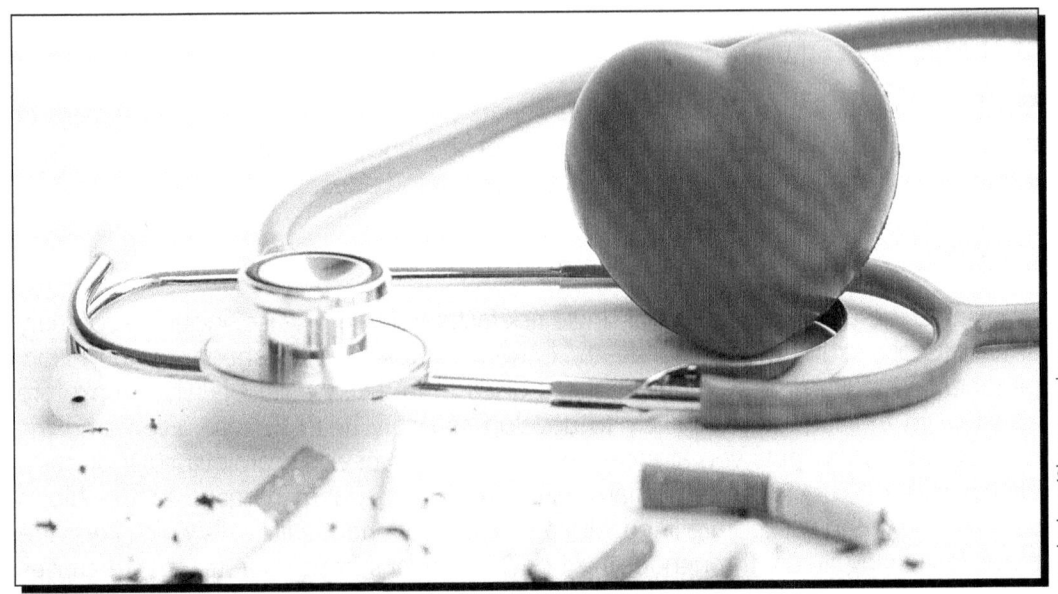

Individuals who smoke are also two to four times more likely to develop coronary heart disease.

Lifestyle Medicine Handbook 393

Immune System

The chemicals in cigarette smoke cause ongoing damage to cells throughout the body. As such, the immune system must continually work to fight off this damage. This situation clearly weakens the immune system to the point that it makes the patient predisposed to infections. It may also limit the immune system's ability to target and destroy cancer cells once they arise.

Dermatologic System

Tobacco smoke changes the structure and color of the skin. It ruins the elasticity in the skin, causes bags under the eyes, results in a toughening of the skin, leads to wrinkles, and gives rise to stretch marks. It also predisposes a patient to fungal nail infections. Furthermore, nicotine increases hair loss, balding, and graying. In addition, it confers an elevated risk for skin cancers, warts, psoriasis, and poor wound healing.

Muscular System

Tobacco smoke reduces muscular strength and flexibility. Diminished blood flow due to damage in the circulatory system decreases the ability of a person to exercise the muscles. Lower levels of oxygen hinder muscle growth. As lung capacity and oxygen supply decrease, muscles are starved for the oxygen that they need to grow and develop.

Nervous System

Nicotine, one of the core ingredients of tobacco, is a mood-altering drug that provides an initial boost of energy. Once this boost wears off, however, cravings mount. Physical withdrawal from nicotine can impair cognitive functioning and cause feelings of anxiety, irritation, and depression. Smoking also confers a two to fourfold increased risk of stroke. Just like the arteries that the supply the heart are vulnerable to plaque rupture, thrombosis, and subsequent ischemia, so too are the arteries that supply the brain. Smoking can also increase the risk for cataracts (clouding of the eye's lens that makes it hard to see). Furthermore, it can cause age-related macular degeneration (AMD), which is damage to the small spot near the eye's center needed for central vision.

Reproductive System

Recall that nicotine reduces blood flow causing peripheral artery disease. A few of these affected arteries are those that supply the reproductive organs. Therefore, smoking can compromise sexual performance in men by making it more difficult to achieve erection. Smoking can also reduce male sperm count, which can reduce fertility, as well as increase risks for birth defects and miscarriage.

Women can have diminished sexual satisfaction due to decreased lubrication and decreased ability to achieve orgasm. For those women trying to become pregnant, smoking makes it more difficult. It can also affect the baby's health before and after birth by increasing the risk of preterm delivery, stillbirth, low birth weight, sudden infant death syndrome, ectopic pregnancy, and orofacial cleft.

Respiratory System

Smoking has a very deleterious impact on the respiratory system. For example, smoking causes lung cancer, increasing the risk of lung cancer by 25 times that of a nonsmoker. For more details, please refer to the following section "A Note on How Smoking Causes Lung and Other Cancers." In addition to cancer, smoking damages the airways and the alveoli in the lungs, thereby impairing gas exchange. Over time, this situation can lead to chronic obstructive pulmonary disease (COPD)—either emphysema or chronic bronchitis. Smoking can also trigger and exacerbate asthma. Given the lung damage, these patients are also at increased risk for infections such as pneumonia and influenza.

Skeletal System

Nicotine results in weaker bones in post-menopausal women, and increases risk for broken bones.

Renal/Urinary System

Given that the toxic chemicals from tobacco are excreted by the kidneys into the urine, these chemicals come in contact with the kidneys, the ureter, and the bladder. One of the biggest risk factors for the development of bladder cancer is smoking. Fifty percent of all cases of bladder cancer are found in smokers. Patients who smoke are at higher risk of kidney dysfunction and failure than those who do not.

❏ A Note on How Smoking Causes Lung and Other Cancers

Researchers believe that smoking causes lung cancer by damaging the cells that line the lungs. When cigarette smoke is inhaled, which is full of carcinogens (cancer-causing substances), changes in the lung tissue begin almost immediately. Initially, the body may be able to repair the damage. In time, however, with each repeated exposure to these carcinogens, the lungs become increasingly damaged. Eventually, cancer develops.

Cigarette smoke contains over 4,000 chemicals, including 43 known cancer-causing compounds, as well as 400 other toxins. Figure 11-2 illustrates several of the more common ingredients that are present in cigarettes that can have serious health-related consequences. Of those elements, nicotine is one of the most damaging to a person's health. According to the American Lung Association, cigarettes contain a variety of seemingly implausible substances, including the following:

- Acetone—found in nail polish remover
- Acetic acid—an ingredient in hair dye
- Ammonia—a common household cleaner
- Arsenic—used in rat poison
- Benzene—found in rubber cement
- Butane—used in lighter fluid
- Cadmium—active component in battery acid
- Carbon monoxide—released in car exhaust fumes
- Formaldehyde—embalming fluid
- Hexamine—found in barbecue lighter fluid
- Lead—used in batteries
- Methanol—a main component in rocket fuel
- Naphthalene—an ingredient in moth balls
- Nicotine—used as insecticide
- Tar—material for paving roads
- Toluene—used to manufacture paint

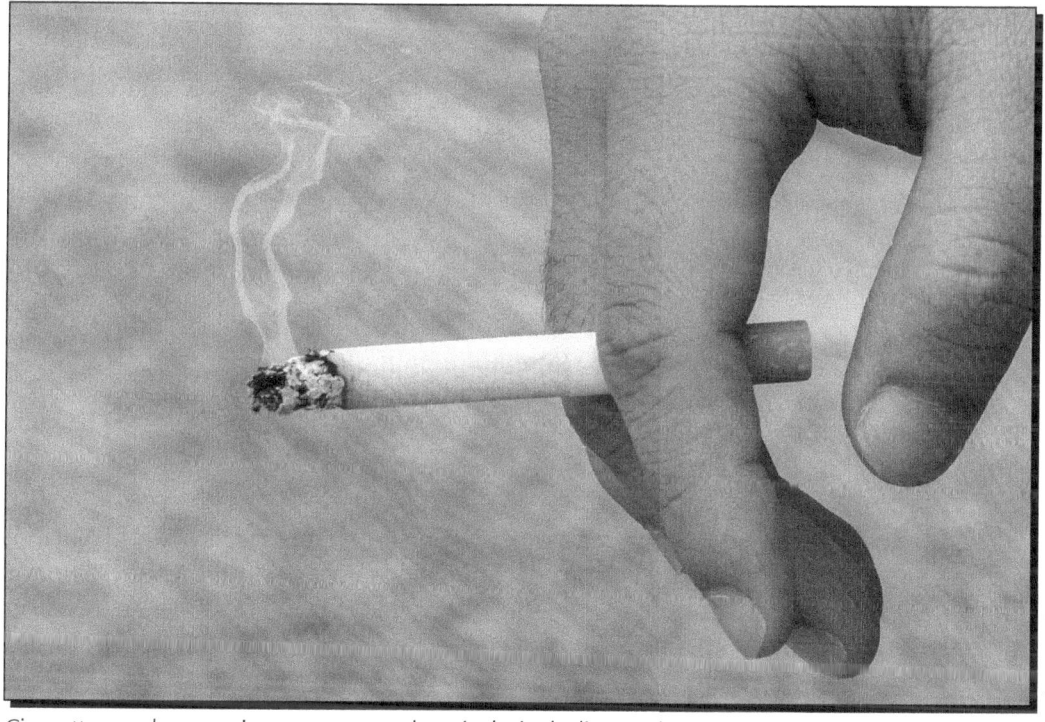

Cigarette smoke contains over 4,000 chemicals, including 43 known cancer-causing compounds, as well as 400 other toxins.

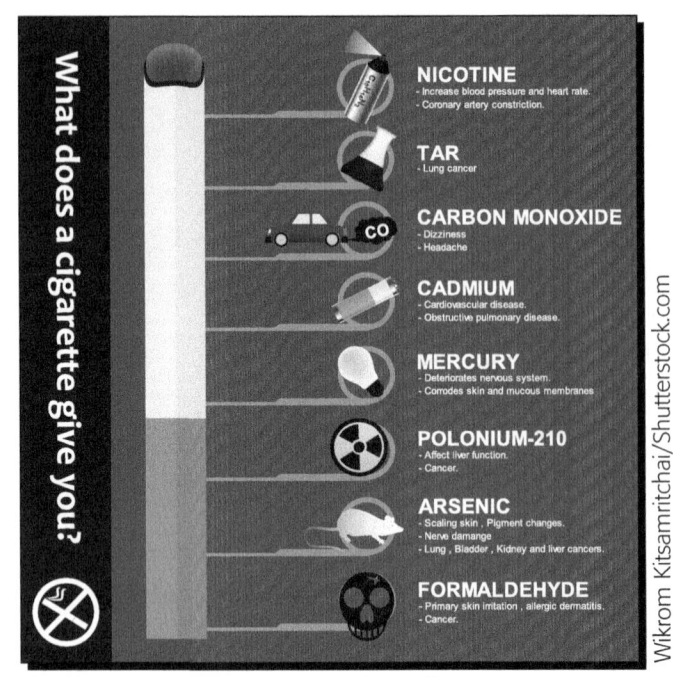

Figure 11-2. Common cigarette ingredients

These ingredients are toxic to every part of the body with which they have contact. This factor is why cigarette smoke is tremendously carcinogenic and confers a heightened cancer risk for nearly every organ in the body including:

- Bladder
- Blood (acute myeloid leukemia)
- Cervix
- Colon and rectum (colorectal)
- Esophagus
- Kidney and ureter
- Larynx
- Liver
- Oropharynx (includes parts of the throat, tongue, soft palate, and the tonsils)
- Pancreas
- Stomach
- Trachea, bronchus, and lung

❏ The Benefits of Quitting Smoking

Quitting smoking can have positive consequences on a person's health. Not only can it preclude new damage to the body from occurring, it can also help repair any damage that has already been done. Furthermore, quitting smoking is the best way to lower an individual's risk of getting cancer. The following examples illustrate four health-related outcomes of quitting smoking:

- Heart attack risk decreases substantially one year after quitting smoking
- The risk of stroke drops to that of a non-smoker within two to five years of quitting smoking.

- The risk of developing cancers of the mouth, throat, esophagus, and bladder decrease by 50 percent five years after quitting smoking.
- The risk of developing lung cancer drops by 50 percent 10 years after quitting smoking.

Treatment options for nicotine addiction span the spectrum, from behavior support to pharmacologic treatment. Often, a patient will need to try and experiment with different modalities before finding the right approach. Numerous behavioral approaches exist and are offered for free. A few of the pharmacologic approaches are discussed here in greater detail.

❑ Nicotine Replacement Strategies

Nicotine replacement (e.g., gum, inhalers, lozenges, patches, and sprays) is recognized as a relatively safe, as well as effective, aid to smoking cessation. Not only does it help smokers reduce their feelings of withdrawal and their cravings to smoke, it also doubles a person's chances of quitting smoking for good.

While nicotine replacement therapy (NRT) can induce a variety of mild-to-moderate side effects, it can be an integral part of almost every smoker's strategy to quit smoking. Among the more common and the less common side effects of NRT are the following:

More Common Side Effects of NRT:

- Acid or sour stomach
- Belching
- Coughing
- Heartburn
- Indigestion
- Mouth and throat irritation

Less Common Side Effects of NRT:

- Anxiety
- Back pain
- Change in taste
- Diarrhea
- Dizziness
- Feeling of burning, numbness, tightness, tingling, warmth, or heat
- Feelings of drug dependence
- Flu-like symptoms
- General pain
- Hiccups

- Mental depression
- Pain in the jaw and neck
- Pain in the muscles
- Passing gas
- Problems with teeth
- Trouble with sleeping
- Unusual tiredness or weakness

❏ Assistive Medications

On occasion, patients who want to quit smoking can be given medication that will augment their efforts. In that regard, two FDA-approved medications that can assist patients in quitting smoking are Chantix and Zyban:

- Chantix:
    ✓ An oral drug (varenicline)
    ✓ It competes with the nicotine in cigarettes from binding to nicotine receptors in the brain.
    ✓ It blocks the stronger stimulation by nicotine.
    ✓ Smokers do not experience the full effect of smoking while taking varenicline.
- Zyban:
    ✓ Bupropion (brand name Wellbutrin)
    ✓ It is used as an anti-depressant.
    ✓ Bupropion is a pill taken to reduce a person's craving for tobacco.
    ✓ It does not contain nicotine.
    ✓ It decreases cravings, we well as withdrawal symptoms.

STIMULANTS

Stimulants increase alertness, attention, and energy, as well as elevate blood pressure, heart rate and respiration. They include a wide range of drugs, including amphetamines, methamphetamine, and cocaine. Symptoms of stimulant use disorders include cravings for stimulants, failure to control use when attempted, continued use despite interference with major obligations or social functioning, use of larger amounts over time, development of an increased level of tolerance, spending a great deal of time to obtain and use stimulants, and withdrawal symptoms that occur after stopping or reducing use, including fatigue, vivid and unpleasant dreams, sleep problems, increased appetite, or irregular problems in controlling movement.

Perhaps, the most common stimulant used daily by over 80 percent of the U.S. population is caffeine, with roughly 400 million cups of coffee consumed daily. Caffeine is a stimulant to the central nervous system that works by blocking receptors for adenosine, a byproduct of cellular activity that normally produces feelings of tiredness and the need to sleep. Regular use of caffeine causes mild physical dependence. Daily doses of caffeine found in about one cup of coffee (approximately 100 mg), which can lead to physical dependence, can lead to withdrawal symptoms upon cessation. These symptoms could include headaches, depressed mood, muscle pains, lethargy, and irritability. The 5th edition of the DSM now includes caffeine withdrawal as an official diagnosis for the first time. Thankfully, compared to many other drugs, the effects of caffeine are relatively short-term, with symptoms beginning 12 to 24 hours after the last dose and abating within two to nine days.

OPIOIDS

Opioid use disorder, which has recently been spotlighted as an epidemic in the United States, is a medical condition characterized by a problematic pattern of opioid use that causes clinically significant impairment and distress. Every day, 116 people die from opioid-related drug overdoses. Opioid use disorders are evidenced by individuals having an intense desire to consume them, an inability to control their use, persistent use despite negative social consequences and not meeting major obligations, increased tolerance and use over time, and the appearance of withdrawal symptoms upon cessation or reduction of their use. Characteristic withdrawal symptoms include agitation, anxiety, nausea and vomiting, muscle aches, diarrhea, sweating, and insomnia.

Opioids include substances such as morphine, heroin, fentanyl, codeine, and oxycodone. While these substances reduce the perception of pain, they can also produce drowsiness, mental confusion, euphoria, nausea, constipation, and respiratory depression. The euphoric response to opioid medications is highly addictive. The drugs are potent triggers of the brain's reward pathway. People who become addicted and start misusing opioids often try to intensify their experience by snorting or injecting them, which increases the risk of overdosing.

Since 1999, opiate overdose deaths have increased 265 percent among men and 400 percent among women. In 2016 alone, in the U.S., there were over 64,600 opiate-related drug overdose deaths. Alarmingly, this factor contributed to the decrease in life expectancy in the U.S. for the second year in a row.

Given that opioid use disorder has become a public health crisis, numerous efforts are underway to prevent opioid use disorder and manage those individuals who are already using opioids and addicted. Naloxone (trade name Narcan), which is an antagonist of the opioid receptors, is used in the emergency treatment of an overdose. Long-term treatment and care focuses on reducing the physical and psychological condition of the addicted person. Opioid substitution or maintenance therapy, using drugs like methadone and buprenorphine, which are longer-acting and lead to less euphoric formulations of opioids, is used to reduce cravings and withdrawal symptoms.

Often, these medications are combined with detox programs, behavior therapy like CBT, and social support services. Like all forms of addiction therapy, treatment for opioid addiction requires a multidisciplinary and multimodal approach.

OTHER ADDICTIONS

Both behavioral and neuroscience research is rapidly accumulating to show that addiction is not limited to what have been traditionally thought of as "addictive substances," like tobacco and alcohol. Indeed, functional MRI brain imaging confirms that substances in foods, like sugar, salt, and fat, trigger the brain's reward pathway. This factor is also true for various forms of technology, which provide an instant "hit" of gratification from a new email, a Facebook like, or an Instagram heart. For those individuals interested in learning more about the addictive nature of these modern phenomena and abundant ingredients, refer to the references section at the end of this chapter. It is crucial for the lifestyle medicine practitioner to understand that the scope of what constitutes addiction is expanding, as more and more insight is gained into the neural pathways and cognitive processes that underpin addictive behaviors.

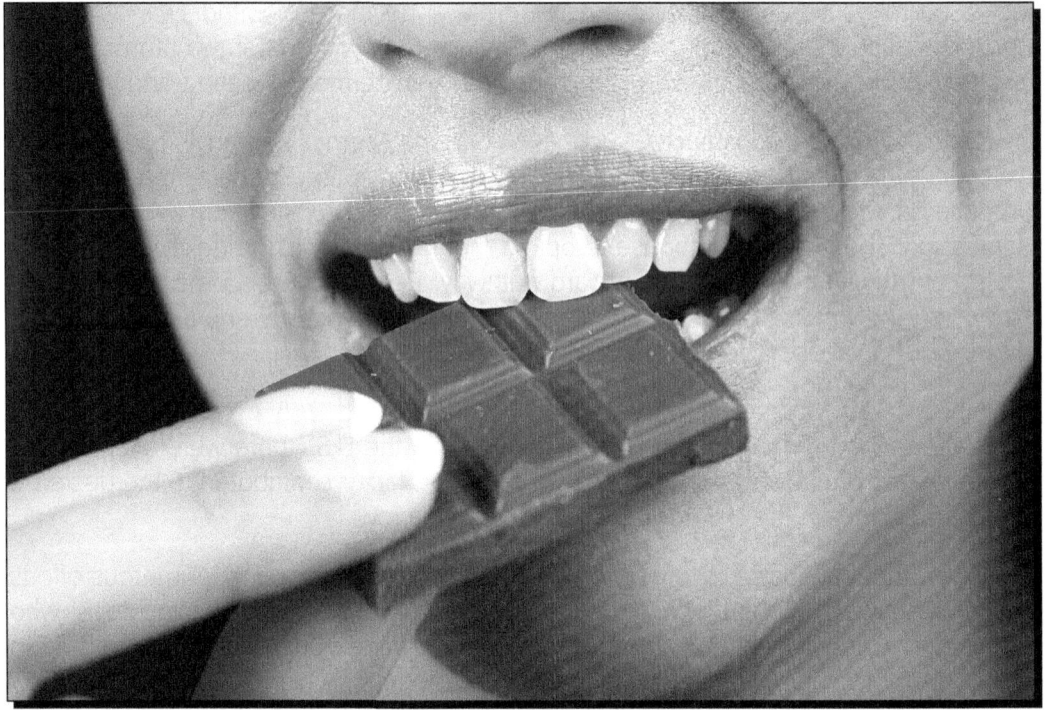

Functional MRI brain imaging confirms that substances in foods, like sugar, salt, and fat, trigger the brain's reward pathway.

COUNSELING PATIENTS WITH ADDICTION

Education and counseling are at the core of how physicians and allied healthcare professionals can help their patients who suffer from substance abuse. While many individuals who abuse substances believe that they can stop on their own, they often cannot. They need help—the exact kind of assistance provided by lifestyle medicine practitioners. In that regard, physicians and allied healthcare professionals have a variety of tools and techniques in their toolbox that they can employ with their patients who are addicted to substances, including:

- Utilizing the Transtheoretical Model of Change
- Using motivational interviewing
- Listening
- Connecting
- Asking questions—showing curiosity
- Being non-judgmental
- Being appreciative to be sitting together and learning
- Showing compassion—empathy
- Exhibiting honesty
- Applying the Frates COACH Approach (curiosity, open, appreciative, compassionate, honest)

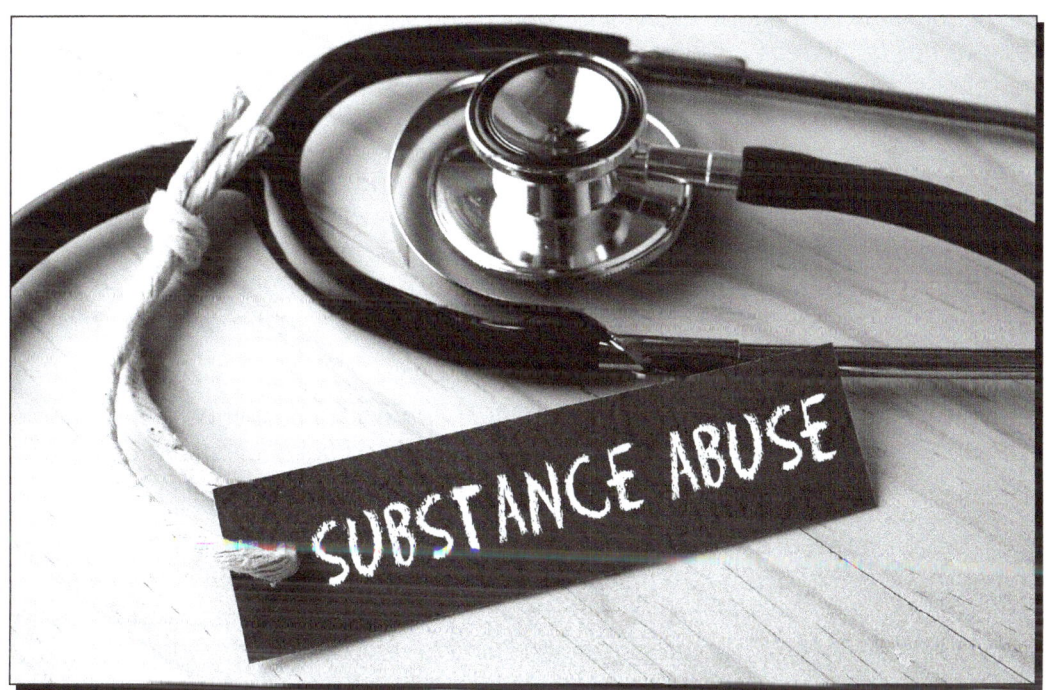

While many individuals who abuse substances believe that they can stop on their own, they often cannot.

Among the questions that physicians and allied healthcare professionals could ask their patients during an intervention for substance use are the following:
- What is happening in your life right now?
- How would your life be different without this substance?
- What is good about using this substance?
- What is bad about using this substance?
- What would it take for you to stop using this substance?

LIVE AND LEARN WITH DR. BETH FRATES

Utilizing the Frates COACH Approach can really help, when counseling patients with substance use disorders. In that regard, lifestyle medicine practitioners should employ compassion, openness, appreciation, compassion, and honesty at all times. When I was running my pilot wellness group for stroke survivors and caregivers, I experienced a very challenging situation. On the very first day, the patients and caregivers were strolling in and last to arrive was a gentleman wheeling his wife into the room. He looked very stressed and frustrated.

After situating her at the table, he headed for the door. Quickly I said, "Oh excuse me. You don't have to leave. We would be delighted if you would join us. It is up to you. You are welcome to participate in the discussion. Rolling his eyes, he replied "Okay."

At the time, I thought everything was going along pretty smoothly. We had reviewed all of the reasons why people have strokes, and everyone shared their own personal stories. Then, we went over risk factors for stroke. Each person shared the risk factors that they knew they had. Even the caregivers shared this information.

Everything went well, until we got to Mr. Escape (the gentleman who tried to run off after getting his wife situated). Mr. Escape, paused when it was his turn. Basically, he squinted his eyes, looked straight at me, and slammed his hand on the table and then announced, in a low, loud voice, "I smoke, and I'm not quitting!" It was a belligerent response. Thankfully, I have studied behavior change and was already using health coaching methods in my interactions.

This scenario was ripe for the Frates COACH Approach. I remember feeling angry when he seemed to be angry at me. This scenario could have fallen into a negative vicious cycle. I also remember thinking, "Take deep breaths. Pause. Think."

I knew I needed a break, so I reached into my purse pretending to look for something special. While rummaging around in my purse, I was taking time to pause and collect my thoughts. I knew that everyone in the group was watching me, wondering how I would respond. I was searching for empathy, and I found it.

With the Frates COACH Approach, I needed to focus on curiosity. What was making him so angry, and why does he want to keep smoking? I figured he had tried to quit many times previously without success, and, was likely frustrated. Probably, everyone has tried to wrestle him down to make him quit smoking. I needed to be open. Although I may not be successful at helping to empower him to quit today, he might not be ready. I must be open to however the conversation flows. In addition, I must be appreciative that he is talking to me and that he chose to stay in the room to participate in the group instead of racing out the door.

Mostly, I knew I needed to express compassion and thus, I was searching for my empathy, while rummaging through my purse. Lastly, I needed to be honest. He said he was not going to quit, but I still needed to find a way to empower him to consider quitting at a later date and to tell him that one of the best things he could do for himself is to quit smoking.

After rummaging in my purse for a minute or two, I pulled out one of my business cards. Then, I used motivational interviewing. I used a reflection. "I hear you. You are smoking, and you are not going to quit." Then, I asked permission to share some information, "May I say something?" To date, no one has answered no to this question.

After giving me permission to say something, I proceeded with "I know you are not ready to consider quitting smoking now. However, it is one of the best things you could do for your health. The smoke has a negative impact on you and the second-hand smoke has a negative impact on your wife. So, when you are ready to quit, please give me a call. I would be delighted to help you, when you are ready."

After that, I handed my card to him. He was silent and looked a bit confused. For the next couple of weeks, I did not ask Mr. Escape about his smoking. The rest of the group was staring in complete silence.

During the subsequent sessions, I did discuss the risks of smoking and the impact of second-hand smoke, which is part of the curriculum in the stroke prevention wellness group. I did not look at Mr. Escape or do anything that I felt might make him uncomfortable. Four weeks later, Mr. Escape entered the wellness group stating, "I have an announcement to make. I cut down on my cigarettes. I have a plan to quit in a month."

The whole room started clapping. I keep my facial expression and body language pretty steady and solid. In contrast, all of the members of the stroke group cheered and then clapped. They all wanted what was best for him and his wife. I asked him one question, "How does that feel?" He answered, "Great!" My lesson was that when someone is in a pre-contemplative state to change a behavior, empathy is one of the best possible therapeutic tools.

KEY POINTS/TAKEAWAYS FOR CHAPTER 11

❑ Chapter Review:

- Overall goal: Understand the underlying factors associated with substance abuse.
- Application goal: Be aware of how to effectively address substance abuse in a patient.

❑ Discussion Questions:

- What is substance abuse?
- What are the signs and symptoms of addiction?
- How can individuals safely withdraw from abusing substances?
- What is the impact of three of the more common forms of substance abuse (alcohol, cannabis, smoking) on a person's health?
- How does alcohol abuse affect a person's well-being?
- What tools can lifestyle medicine practitioners use to deal with substance abuse in their patients?

	TITLE	AUTHORS	JOURNAL	YEAR	KEY FINDINGS
1	Hatching the behavioral addiction egg: Reward Deficiency Solution System (RDSS) as a function of dopaminergic neurogenetics and brain functional connectivity linking all addictions under a common rubric	Blum K, et al.	Journal of Behavioral Addictions	2014	This selective literature review of psychiatry and behavioral addiction literature and neurogenetics identified the importance of dopaminergic pathways and resting-state, functional connectivity of brain reward circuits.
2	Managing problem drinking: screening tools and brief interventions for primary care physicians	Dwyer-Clonts M, Frates E, Suzuki J	American Journal of Lifestyle Medicine	2016	"This article draws on randomized controlled trials and literature on screening techniques, motivational interviewing, the trasntheoretical model of behavior change, and medication-assisted treatments" to enhance brief intervention methodologies aimed to help primary care doctors reduce alcohol consumption among patients who were screened as problem drinkers.

Figure 11-3. Smoking, alcohol, and addiction evidence

	TITLE	AUTHORS	JOURNAL	YEAR	KEY FINDINGS
3	Detecting alcoholism: the CAGE questionnaire	Ewing JA	*JAMA*	1984	Identified four key questions, using the pneumonic "CAGE," that could be used to help make a diagnosis of alcoholism. "The questions focus on Cutting down, Annoyance by criticism, Guilty feeling, and Eye-openers."
4	Carrot addiction	Kaplan R	*Australian and New Zealand Journal of Psychiatry*	1996	A case report on carrot addiction and a literature review and discussion on the role of beta carotene in addiction behavior.
5	In search of how people change: applications to addictive behaviors	Prochaska JO, Diclemente CC, Norcross JC	*American Psychologist*	1992	Summarizes key transtheoretical constructs of stages and processes of change and how they pertain to addiction.

References

1. Blum K, Febo M, McLaughlin T, et al. Hatching the behavioral addiction egg: Reward Deficiency Solution System (RDSS) as a function of dopaminergic neurogenetics and brain functional connectivity linking all addictions under a common rubric. *Journal of Behavioral Addictions.* 2014;3(3):149-156.
2. Dwyer-Clonts M, Frates E, Suzuki J. Managing problem drinking: screening tools and brief interventions for primary care physicians. *American Journal of Lifestyle Medicine.* 2016. Available at: http://journals.sagepub.com/doi/full/10.1177/1559827616629929. Accessed October 2017.
3. Ewing JA. Detecting alcoholism: the CAGE questionnaire. *JAMA.* 1984;252(14):1905-1907.
4. Kaplan R. Carrot addiction. *Australian and New Zealand Journal of Psychiatry.* 1996;30(5):698-700. Available at: https://www.ncbi.nlm.nih.gov/pubmed/8902181. Accessed October 2017.
5. Prochaska JO, Diclemente CC, Norcross JC. In search of how people change: applications to addictive behaviors. *American Psychologist.* September 1992;27(9):1102-1114.

Figure 11-3. Smoking, alcohol, and addiction evidence (cont.)

REFERENCES

- ABC News. Quiz: Do You Have an Unhealthy Food Addiction? September 7, 2011. Available at: http://abcnews.go.com/Health/quiz-addicted-food/story?id=14406763. Accessed October 2017.
- American Lung Association. What's in a Cigarette? Available at: http://www.lung.org/stop-smoking/smoking-facts/whats-in-a-cigarette.html. Accessed July 2018.
- American Psychiatric Association. *Diagnostic and Statistical Manual of Mental Disorders.* 5th ed. Arlington, VA: American Psychiatric Publishing; 2013.
- American Society of Addiction Medicine. Definition of Addiction. Available at: https://www.asam.org/resources/definition-of-addiction. Accessed May 2018.
- Blum K, et al. Hatching the behavioral addiction egg: Reward Deficiency Solution System (RDSS) as a function of dopaminergic neurogenetics and brain functional connectivity linking all addictions under a common rubric. *Journal of Behavioral Addictions.* 2014;3(3):149-156.
- Center on Addiction. Addiction by the Numbers. Available at: https://www.centeronaddiction.org/. Accessed July 2018.

- Centers for Disease Control and Prevention (CDC). Health Effects of Cigarette Smoking Fact Sheet. Available at: https://www.cdc.gov/tobacco/data_statistics/fact_sheets/health_effects/effects_cig_smoking/index.htm. Accessed July 2018.
- Centers for Disease Control and Prevention (CDC). Prescription Painkiller Overdoses. Available at: https://www.cdc.gov/vitalsigns/prescriptionpainkilleroverdoses/index.html. Accessed July 2018.
- Centers for Disease Control and Prevention (CDC). Trends in Current Cigarette Smoking Among High School Students and Adults, United States, 1965–2014. Available at: https://www.cdc.gov/tobacco/data_statistics/tables/trends/cig_smoking/index.htm. Accessed July 2018.
- Centers for Disease Control and Prevention (CDC). Youth and Tobacco Use Fact Sheet. Available at: https://www.cdc.gov/tobacco/data_statistics/fact_sheets/youth_data/tobacco_use/index.htm. Accessed July 2018.
- Ciccolo JT, Jennings EG, Busch AM. Behavioral approaches to enhancing smoking cessation. In: Rippe JM, ed. *Lifestyle Medicine*. 2nd ed. Boca Raton, FL: CRC Press; 2013:245-254.
- Daly JW, Holmen J, Fredholm BB. Is caffeine addictive? The most widely used psychoactive substance in the world affects same parts of the brain as cocaine. *Lakartidningen*. 1998;95:5878-5883.
- Dennis M, Babor TF, Roebuck C, et al. Changing the focus: the case for recognizing and treating cannabis use disorders. *Addiction*. 2002;97:(s1):4-15.
- Drugs.com. Nicorette Side Effects. Available at: https://www.drugs.com/sfx/nicorette-side-effects.html. Accessed July 2018.
- Dwyer-Clonts M, Frates E, Suzuki J. Managing problem drinking: screening tools and brief interventions for primary care physicians. *American Journal of Lifestyle Medicine*. 2016. Available at: http://journals.sagepub.com/doi/full/10.1177/1559827616629929. Accessed October 2017.
- Egger G, Binns A, Rossner S. Chapter 17. In: Egger G, Binns A, Rossner S. *Lifestyle Medicine: Managing Diseases of Lifestyle in the 21st Century*. 2nd ed. North Ryde, N.S.W.: McGraw-Hill; 2010.
- Enoch MA, Goldman D. The genetics of alcoholism and alcohol abuse. *Current Psychiatry Reports*. 2001;3(2):144-151.
- Evans SM, Griffiths RR. Low-dose caffeine physical dependence in normal subjects: dose-related effects. In: Harris L, ed. Problems of Drug Dependence 1990: Proceedings of the 52nd Annual Scientific Meeting, the Committee on Problems of Drug Dependence, Inc. NIDA Research Monograph 105. Washington, D.C.: Government Printing Office; 1991.
- Fagerstrom K, Heatherton T, Kozlowski L. Nicotine addiction and its assessment. *Ear, Nose, and Throat Journal*. 1990;69(11):763-765.
- Film Bilder. Nuggets [Video]. Available at: https://www.youtube.com/watch?v=HUngLgGRJpo. Accessed October 2017.

- Foote J, Wilkens C, Kosanke N, Higgs S. *Beyond Addiction: How Science and Kindness Help People Change.* New York: Simon & Schuster; 2014.
- Freedman ND, Silverman DT, Hollenbeck AR, et al. Association between smoking and risk of bladder cancer among men and women. *JAMA.* 2011;306(7):737-745. doi:10.1001/jama.2011.1142.
- Gearhardt A, Corbin W, Brownell KD. Preliminary validation of the Yale Food Addiction Scale. *Appetite.* 2009;52(2):430-436.
- Global Addiction Association. Addiction Scales and Assessment. Available at: http://www.globaladdiction.org/scales.php. Accessed October 2017.
- Grant BF, Chou SP, Saha TD, et al. Prevalence of 12-month alcohol use, high-risk drinking, and DSM-IV alcohol use disorder in the United States, 2001-2002 to 2012-2013: results from the National Epidemiologic Survey on Alcohol and Related Conditions. *JAMA Psychiatry.* 2017;74(9):911-923. doi:10.1001/jamapsychiatry.2017.2161.
- Griffiths MD. Grasp a Carrot: A Brief Look at Compulsive Carrot Eating. Psychology Today. Available at: https://www.psychologytoday.com/blog/in-excess/201307/grasp-carrot. Accessed October 2017.
- Hackshaw A, Morris JK, Boniface S, et al. Low cigarette consumption and risk of coronary heart disease and stroke: meta-analysis of 141 cohort studies in 55 study reports. *BMJ.* 2018;360:j5855.
- Hari J. Everything You Think You Know About Addiction Is Wrong. TED. Available at: https://www.ted.com/talks/johann_hari_everything_you_think_you_know_about_addiction_is_wrong?language=en. Accessed October 2017.
- Harvard Medical School. Alcohol Use and Abuse: A Harvard Medical School Special Report. Available at: http://hrccatalog.hrh.ca/InmagicGenie/DocumentFolder/alcohol%20use%20and%20abuse.pdf. Accessed July 2018.
- Hedegaard H, Warner M, Minino AM. Drug overdose deaths in the United States, 1999–2016. NCHS Data Brief, no 294. Hyattsville, MD: National Center for Health Statistics; 2017. Available at: https://www.cdc.gov/nchs/data/databriefs/db294.pdf. Accessed July 2017.
- Hill KP. Medical marijuana for treatment of chronic pain and other medical and psychiatric problems: a clinical review. *JAMA.* 2015;313(24):2474-2483. doi:10.1001/jama.2015.6199.
- Jamal A, King BA, Neff LJ, et al. Current cigarette smoking among adults—United States, 2005–2015. *Morbidity and Mortality Weekly Report.* 2016;65:1205-1211. doi: http://dx.doi.org/10.15585/mmwr.mm6544a2.
- Juliano LM, Griffiths RR. A critical review of caffeine withdrawal: empirical validation of symptoms and signs, incidence, severity, and associated features. *Psychopharmacology.* 2004;176:1-29.
- Kaplan R. Carrot addiction. *Australian and New Zealand Journal of Psychiatry.* 1996;30(5):698-700. Available at: https://www.ncbi.nlm.nih.gov/pubmed/8902181. Accessed October 2017.

- Kessler DA. *The End of Overeating: Taking Control of the Insatiable American Appetite.* New York: Rodale; 2009.
- Kitchen Daily. America's Coffee Obsession: Fun Facts That Prove We're Hooked. Huffington Post. Available at: https://www.huffingtonpost.com/2011/09/29/americas-coffee-obsession_n_987885.html. Accessed July 2018.
- Kochanek KD, Murphy SL, Xu JQ, et al. Mortality in the United States, 2016. NCHS Data Brief, no 293. Hyattsville, MD: National Center for Health Statistics; 2017.
- Lustig RH. *The Hacking of the American Mind: The Science Behind the Corporate Takeover of Our Bodies and Brains.* New York: Penguin Random House; 2017.
- Merriam-Webster. Addiction. Available at: http://www.merriam-webster.com/dictionary/addiction. Accessed July 2018.
- Moir D, Rickert WS, Levasseur G, et al. A comparison of mainstream and sidestream marijuana and tobacco cigarette smoke produced under two machine smoking conditions. *Chemical Research in Toxicology.* 2008;21(2):494-502. doi:10.1021/tx700275p.
- Mokdad AH, Marks JS, Stroup DF, et al. Actual causes of death in the United States, 2000. *JAMA.* March 10 2004;291(10):1238-1245.
- National Institute on Alcohol Abuse and Alcoholism. *Alcohol Alert.* Available at: https://pubs.niaaa.nih.gov/publications/aa63/aa63.htm. Accessed July 2018.
- National Institute on Alcohol Abuse and Alcoholism. Alcohol Facts and Statistics. Available at: https://www.niaaa.nih.gov/alcohol-health/overview-alcohol-consumption/alcohol-facts-and-statistics. June, 2017. Accessed July 2018.
- National Institute on Alcohol Abuse and Alcoholism. Alcohol's Effect on the Body. Available at: https://www.niaaa.nih.gov/alcohol-health/alcohols-effects-body. Accessed July 2018.
- National Institute on Alcohol Abuse and Alcoholism. Screening Tests. Available at: http://pubs.niaaa.nih.gov/publications/arh28-2/78-79.htm. Accessed October 2017.
- National Institute on Drug Abuse. Cigarettes and Other Tobacco Products. Available at: https://www.drugabuse.gov/publications/drugfacts/cigarettes-other-tobacco-products. Accessed July 2018.
- National Institute on Drug Abuse. Heroin. Available at: https://www.drugabuse.gov/publications/research-reports/heroin. Accessed July 2018.
- National Institute on Drug Abuse. Marijuana. Available at: https://www.drugabuse.gov/publications/drugfacts/marijuana. Accessed July 2018.
- National Institute on Drug Abuse. Nationwide Trends. Available at: https://www.drugabuse.gov/publications/drugfacts/nationwide-trends. Accessed July 2018.
- National Institute on Drug Abuse. Principles of Adolescent Substance Use Disorder Treatment: A Research-Based Guide. Available at: https://www.drugabuse.gov/publications/principles-adolescent-substance-use-disorder-treatment-research-based-guide. Accessed July 2018.

- National Institute on Drug Abuse. Principles of Drug Addiction Treatment: A Research-Based Guide. 3rd ed. Available at: https://www.drugabuse.gov/publications/principles-drug-addiction-treatment-research-based-guide-third-edition. Accessed July 2018.
- National Institute on Drug Abuse. What Science Tells Us About Opioid Abuse and Addiction. Available at: https://www.drugabuse.gov/about-nida/legislative-activities/testimony-to-congress/2016/what-science-tells-us-about-opioid-abuse-addiction. Accessed July 2018.
- Pharmacotherapies for Alcohol and Substance Abuse Consortium. About Substance Abuse. Available at: https://pasa.rti.org/About/Substance-Abuse. Accessed July 2018.
- Prescott CA, Kendler KS. Genetic and environmental contributions to alcohol abuse and dependence in a population-based sample of male twins. *American Journal of Psychiatry.* 1999;156(1):34-40.
- Prochaska JO, Norcross J, DiClemente C. *Changing for Good: A Revolutionary Six-Stage Program for Overcoming Bad Habits and Moving Your Life Positively Forward.* New York; HarperCollins, 1994.
- Ries RK, Fiellin DA, Miller SC, et al. *The ASAM Principles of Addiction Medicine.* 5th ed. Philadelphia: Lippincott Williams & Wilkins; 2014.
- Silverman K, Evans SM, Strain EC, et al. *New England Journal of Medicine.* October 15 1992;327(16):1109-1114.
- Stein J, Silver JK, Frates EP. *Life After Stroke: The Guide to Recovering Your Health and Preventing Another Stroke.* Baltimore, MD: Johns Hopkins University Press; 2006.
- Striley CLW, Griffiths RR, Cottler LB. Evaluating dependence criteria for caffeine. *Journal of Caffeine Research.* 2011;1(4):219-225. doi:10.1089/jcr.2011.0029.
- Studeville G. Caffeine addiction is a mental disorder, doctors say. *National Geographic.* Jan. 19, 2005.
- Substance Abuse and Mental Health Services Administration. Substance Use Disorders. Available at: https://www.samhsa.gov/disorders/substance-use. Accessed July 2018.
- Suckling J, Nestor LJ. The neurobiology of addiction: the perspective from magnetic resonance imaging present and future. *Addiction.* 2017;112(2):360-369. doi:10.1111/add.13474.
- Tashkin DP. Effects of marijuana smoking on the lung. *Annals of the American Thoracic Society.* 2013;10(3):239-247.
- Trüeb RM. Association between smoking and hair loss: another opportunity for health education against smoking? *Dermatology.* 2003;206:189-191.
- U.S. Department of Health and Human Services, Office of the Surgeon General. *Facing Addiction in America: The Surgeon General's Report on Alcohol, Drugs, and Health.* Washington, DC. HHS; 2016. Available at: https://addiction.surgeongeneral.gov/surgeon-generals-report.pdf. Accessed October 2017.

- U.S. Department of Health and Human Services, Office of the Surgeon General. Executive Summary. *Facing Addiction in America: The Surgeon General's Report on Alcohol, Drugs, and Health.* Washington, DC: HHS; 2016. Available at: https://addiction.surgeongeneral.gov/executive-summary.pdf. Accessed October 2017.
- U.S. Department of Health and Human Services. The Opioid Epidemic by the Numbers in 2016. Available at: https://www.hhs.gov/opioids/sites/default/files/2018-01/opioids-infographic.pdf. Accessed July 2018.
- U.S. National Library of Medicine: MedlinePlus. Opiate and Opioid Withdrawal. Available at: https://medlineplus.gov/ency/article/000949.htm. Accessed July 2018.
- Volkow ND, Boyle M. Neuroscience of addiction: relevance to prevention and treatment. *American Journal of Psychiatry*. Epub April 25 2018.
- Volkow ND, Koob GF, McLellan AT. Neurobiologic advances from the brain disease model of addiction. *New England Journal of Medicine.* January 28 2016;374(4):363-371.
- Zilverstand A, Huang AS, Alia-Klein N, et al. Neuroimaging impaired response inhibition and salience attribution in human drug addiction: a systematic review. *Neuron.* June 6 2018;98(5):886-903.

CHAPTER 12

STAYING THE COURSE

"Act as if what you do makes a difference. It does."

—William James, M.D.
American Philosopher and
Psychologist
Harvard University
1842 – 1910

❑ Chapter Goals:

- Understand what lifestyle medicine practitioners need to do to "stay the course" professionally, during both good and bad times.
- Examine the fundamental components of self-care.
- Recognize signs that might indicate a need for greater attention to self-care.
- Review the importance of lifelong learning.
- Understand that being "busy" is a decision and that our priorities dictate what we choose to do

❑ Learning Objectives:

- To recognize the need for self-care
- To be able to recognize the signs and symptoms of burnout
- To grasp the essential steps involved in self-care
- To learn how to make a difference in the life of a patient
- To understand the connection between the four "always" and the role of a lifestyle medicine practitioner
- To accept the premise that professional competence is an ongoing journey, rather than a static point in life

❑ Guiding Questions:

- What steps should physicians and allied healthcare professionals take concerning their own personal self-care?
- What can lifestyle medicine practitioners do to avoid burning out professionally?
- What does lifelong learning entail?
- What can physicians and allied healthcare professionals do to continue to thrive and be passionate about the impact that they have on others?

❏ Important Terms:

- *Burnout:* Physical or mental collapse resulting from overwork or stress
- *Caring:* Displaying kindness and concern for others
- *Commitment:* The quality of being dedicated to a cause, activity, etc.
- *Compassion:* Empathy; concern for another person
- *Competence:* The ability to do something effectively and efficiently
- *Lifelong learning:* The ongoing development and acquisition of the knowledge and skills needed to perform a job or a task
- *Self-care:* Any activity deliberately undertaken by a person to take care of their mental, emotional, spiritual, and physical health

On occasion, physicians and allied healthcare professionals forget that they are people and patients too. They don't take care of themselves. They don't continue to grow professionally. They lose sight of their goal to be a difference-maker in the lives of their patients. They lose their determination to be caring, compassionate, and competent, as well as committed to being the best at what they do. In short, they're no longer on the professional journey that they originally started on.

Why and to what degree lifestyle medical practitioners may veer off their professional path that they have followed tends to vary from individual to individual. What is known, however, is that physicians and allied healthcare professionals who want to stay the course in lifestyle medicine can enhance the likelihood of that occurring by adhering to the four "always":
- *Always* practice what they preach
- *Always* be learning
- *Always* be values-oriented
- *Always* be a difference-maker

ALWAYS PRACTICE WHAT THEY PREACH

A number of reasons can be advanced concerning why lifestyle medicine practitioners should always practice what they preach. For one, by their actions, they need to set an unspoken standard for their patients concerning what is appropriate behavior and what is not. For another, they need to lead their patients by example. When they advise one thing, but do another, they can erode the trust that their patients have in their advice. In this instance, leading by example can entail a variety of factors, including saying what they mean, meaning what they say, and taking care of themselves (i.e., self-care).

As people, physicians and allied healthcare professionals are not immune to health-related problems. More simply stated, they're not invincible. They need to engage in self-care. They need to do for themselves what they advocate that their patients do (i.e., establish and maintain their health, as well as prevent and deal with illness/disease). In essence, self-care is a broad concept, encompassing the following factors:

- Hygiene (general and personal)
- Nutritional (type, quality, and quantity of food consumed)
- Lifestyle (exercise; leisure-time activities; not smoking, etc.)
- Environmental (living conditions, workplace setting, etc.)
- Socioeconomic (income level, education, occupation, etc.)
- Self-medication (over-the-counter drugs and products)

Each of the aforementioned aspects of self-care can entail a variety of steps, for example:

❑ Good hygiene, including:

- Washing hands
- Brushing teeth on a regular basis
- Washing food

❑ Healthy eating, including:

- Consuming a nutritious balanced diet, with appropriate levels of calorie intake
- Avoiding "empty" calories

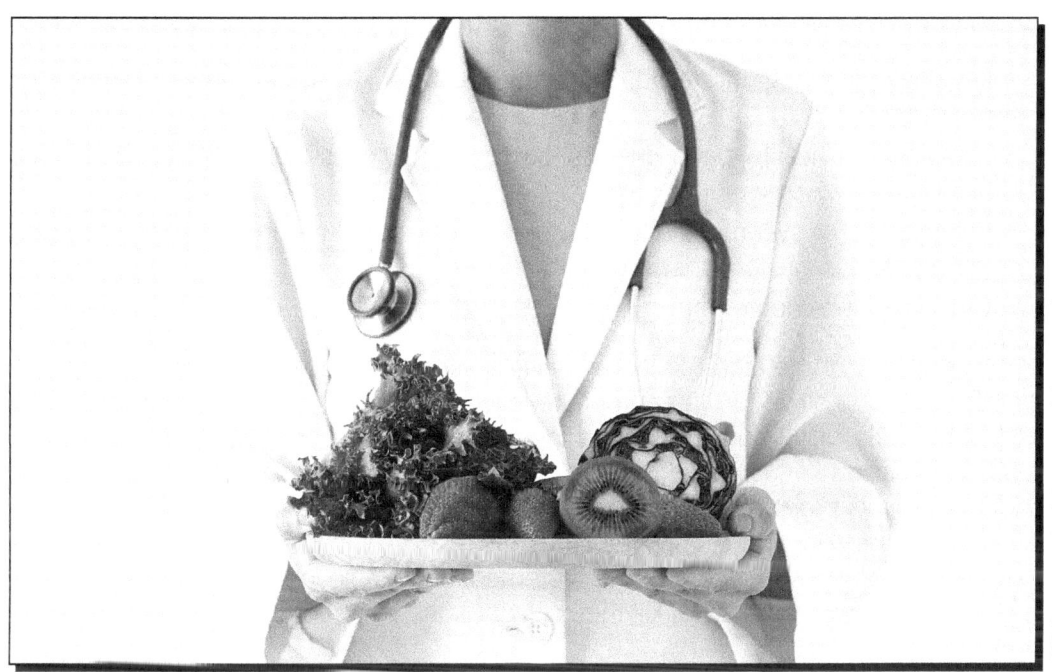

Lifestyle medicine practitioners should always practice what they preach.

❏ Suitable lifestyle, including:

- Engaging in an appropriate level of physical activity, such as walking and cycling
- Quitting smoking
- Limiting alcohol use
- Getting recommended vaccinations
- Practicing safe sex
- Using sunscreen

❏ Acceptable environment, including:

- Avoiding physical exposure to air pollution, toxins, etc.
- Ideally, having access to healthy food
- Living in an environment that is conducive to being physically active
- Residing in an area that is convenient for being socially connected

❏ Healthy socioeconomic circumstances, including:

- Being literate about health-related matters
- Having the capacity to obtain, process, and understand basic health information and services
- Having a job that does not expose the individual to unsafe or unhealthy conditions

❏ Self-awareness of and being proactive toward physical and mental health, including:

- Regularly engaging in health screenings, as well as other proven, diagnostic measures
- Knowing key health-related indices, such as body mass index, cholesterol level, blood pressure, etc.
- Being aware of over-the-counter drugs, medicines, and products that can be used to help treat or prevent specific health-related issues
- Using over-the-counter drugs, medicines, and products in a responsible manner

As a review of the aforementioned factors suggests, the key for lifestyle medicine practitioners is to strive for an appropriate level of balance in all aspects of their lives, including work, play, family, relationships, and rest. Self-neglect in this regard can lead to tragic consequences. Physicians and allied healthcare professionals are not immune to the problems that other people face, particularly those individuals who are workaholics and perfectionists, such as depression, substance abuse, divorce, and suicide. Alarmingly, with regard to the aforementioned, research shows that physicians are more than twice as likely to kill themselves as the general population.

On a more positive note, research also indicates that physicians who exhibit an appropriate level of self-care are also more likely to advocate such behavior in their patients. For example, physicians who exercise on a regular basis are more inclined to encourage their patients to be physically active. In fact, the same basic predisposition holds true for physicians, with regard to all of the pillars of lifestyle medicine.

Conversely, individuals who are not active in practicing self-care tend to experience certain triggers (i.e., red flags) that signal that all may not be well with regard to their health, including:

❑ Physical reactions:

- Fatigue
- Sleep disturbances
- Appetite changes
- Headaches
- Upset stomach
- Chronic muscle tension
- Sexual dysfunction

❑ Emotional reactions:

- Feeling overwhelmed/emotionally spent
- Feeling helpless
- Feeling inadequate
- Sense of vulnerability
- Increased mood swings
- Irritability
- Crying more easily or frequently
- Suicidal/violent thoughts or urges

❑ Behavioral reactions:

- Sense of isolation/withdrawal
- Restlessness
- Changes in alcohol or drug consumption
- Changes in relationships with other individuals (personally and professionally)

❑ Cognitive reactions:

- Disbelief
- A sense of numbness
- Replaying events in the mind (over and over)
- Decreased level of concentration
- Confusion; an impaired level of memory
- Difficulty making decisions or solving problems
- Distressing dreams/fantasies/nightmares

ALWAYS BE LEARNING

Abraham Lincoln, once remarked, "I don't think much of a man who is not wiser today than he was yesterday." President Lincoln's observation could just as well refer to lifestyle medicine practitioners. Physicians and allied healthcare professionals who want to remain on top of their craft must be lifelong learners.

Lifestyle medicine practitioners who understand the need for, as well as the benefits of, lifelong learning have an unquenchable thirst for knowledge, a steadfast desire to learn, and an indefatigable willingness to be teachable. They are aware that the ever-evolving body of knowledge is an invaluable asset that should be inculcated, processed, and utilized.

Physicians and allied healthcare professionals have a number of opportunities to continue their process of learning. For example, they could attend professional meetings (e.g., ACLM annual conference). Not only do the scheduled sessions provide a somewhat structured venue for learning, the subsequent interaction with their colleagues (between the presentations, at the end of the day, over lunchtime, etc.) is also a learning-rich window. The networking and connections that can take place at a professional gathering can inspire, motivate, and reinvigorate one's sense of passion and love of a particular field.

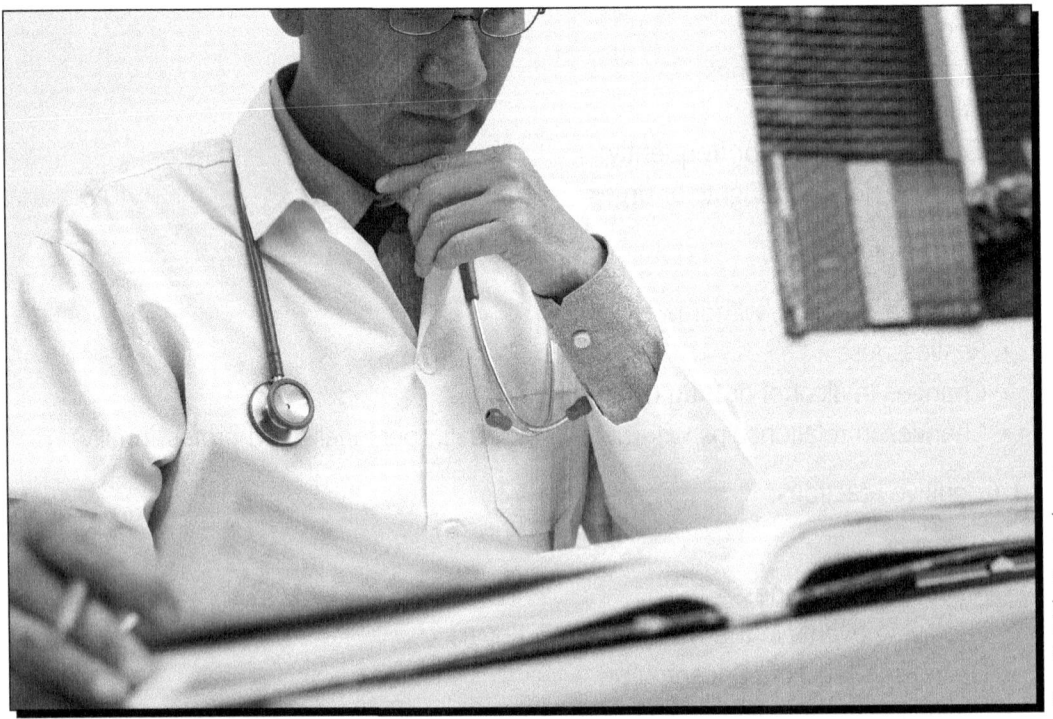

Physicians and allied healthcare professionals who want to remain on top of their craft must be lifelong learners.

Lifestyle medicine practitioners who want to be consummate professionals tend to be insatiable readers. Not only are they aware of the plethora of medical-related websites that exists, they frequently utilize them to access up-to-date information that can aid them in doing their job.

The bottom line is that those who are committed to lifelong learning are fully aware of the fact that learning involves more than "book smarts." Rather, it also entails "life smarts"—the ability to appropriately apply assimilated information to address the needs and interests of their patients.

❏ What Is Learning?

Literally dozens of possible definitions of learning exist. One of the best definitions of learning is achieving a new state of understanding of a particular factor in life, which enables the individual to make sense of it. Such understanding is acquired in two primary ways—education and experience.

It is important to note that education entails more than simply the systematic formal education that a lifestyle medicine practitioner receives while in school. Not surprisingly, a person's experiences often have a more meaningful impact on that individual's level of knowledge than their structured, formal education. "Experience" encompasses what they learn collectively—intellectually and emotionally—from the information-gathering opportunities to which they are exposed. Furthermore, a person's experiences not only affect their level of knowledge, they also heighten their ability to process and apply information.

❏ Why Is Learning Important?

The importance of learning extends to all professions in life, including lifestyle medicine. Learning leads to an enhanced level of competence and provides credibility—both of which are critical attributes for physicians and allied healthcare professionals. All other factors being equal, while knowledge is not the only attribute that a lifestyle medicine practitioner needs to be an effective clinician, an increased understanding of lifestyle medicine and treatment options can improve the quality of the care being delivered.

Furthermore, credibility is an important attribute to possess, as it often creates respect and inspires in the clinician. If patients believe and experience an effective clinician handling the diverse demands of their craft, they may be more likely to respond positively to that provider's recommendations.

The potential benefits of learning are not confined to providing a boost to a person's level of competence and credibility. Learning has also been found to help make people happier, healthier, and live longer (not to mention wealthier). It can also help people improve their ability to adapt to an ever-changing world, to manage their lives effectively, and to undertake yet unidentified opportunities for personal/professional growth.

❑ Tips for Effective Learning

Being an effective learner is a basic requirement for success in any field, and requires commitment and dedication. Because information and knowledge on almost everything is increasing rapidly, it can be argued that many physicians and allied healthcare professionals need to expand their level of knowledge simply to remain current. In that regard, the first step in becoming an effective learner is making a resolute commitment to do so.

Effective learning entails several components. Not only do individuals need to be able to accurately absorb the information they learn, they also need to be able to recall it at a later date, and to utilize it appropriately in a wide variety of situations. Subsequently, the more confident people are in their ability and efforts to learn, the more likely they will be to try new things, develop their understanding and skills, and pursue their interests.

The key issue is understanding what can lifestyle medicine practitioners do to become better learners? Like most things in life, effective learning does not occur by accident. It also does not happen overnight. It takes both attention and practice. The following tips (which by no means is an exhaustive list) can be helpful to people who want to become better learners:

- Be engaged.
- Be persistent.
- Be a voracious reader.
- Challenge themselves.
- Plan their learning.
- Be open to new ideas.
- Be prepared to learn.
- Be a critical thinker.
- Be a problem-solver.
- Brainstorm.
- Use mnemonic techniques.
- Map their task flow.
- Be self-motivated.

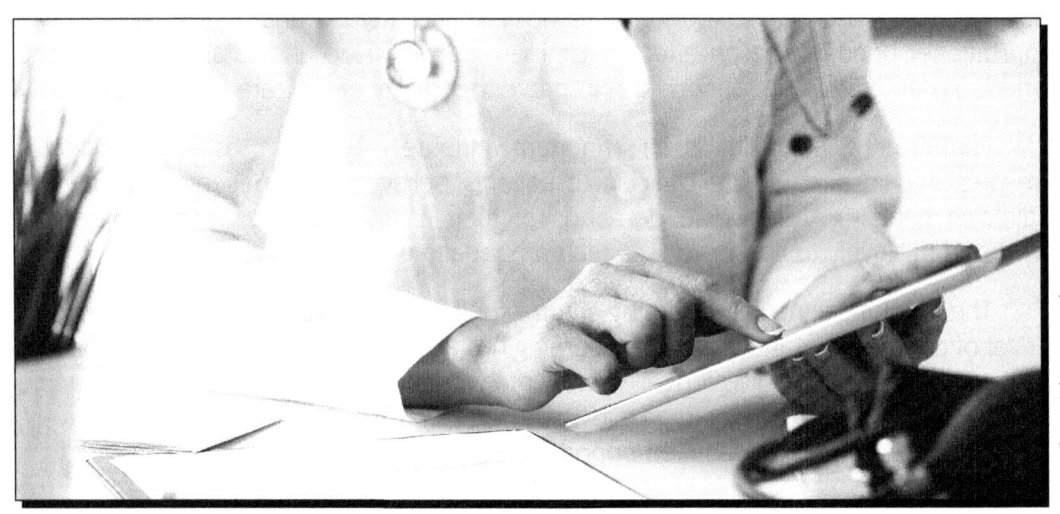

The first step in becoming an effective learner is making a resolute commitment to do so.

ALWAYS BE VALUES-ORIENTED

Values exist, whether individuals recognize their existence or not. When professionals acknowledge their values, and live a life that is consistent with those values, their life and their job become more meaningful and fulfilled.

Values are priorities that serve as a person's filter concerning how they will act and react to the circumstances that they are confronted with in life. In essence, values tell individuals how to spend their time—right here, right now. There are hundreds of specific examples of values, and people perceive the importance of certain values differently. Two particularly relevant values to lifestyle medicine are caring (concern with the needs and interests of another person) and compassion (a deep awareness of the suffering of another individual, coupled with a desire to help relieve it).

An individual's values allow them to create priorities, which are important in the lives of lifestyle medicine practitioners for two reasons. First, they enable people to focus on spending their time appropriately. Time is the single most valuable commodity a person has (other than health). It is the one thing that a person cannot buy or buyback. It is a finite resource. Once a moment has passed, it's gone forever. Second, values help individuals stick to a clear and consistent course of action in their lives. They serve as a compass that helps keep people on the proper path in life.

Values provide the moral authority for who an individual is as a person. The presence of ethically grounded principles can help instill a sense of legitimacy (i.e., a moral bearing) in a professional for a number of reasons, including reinforcement as to why that individual's opinions and efforts matter. In general, a values-centered lifestyle medicine practitioner is more capable of inspiring confidence and rallying others to achieve a specific purpose.

A variety of terms (e.g., values, morals, principles, ethics, virtues, etc.) can be used to express what an individual feels is important in life with regard to personal conduct. Although some distinction exists between each word, they often are often considered synonyms for each other. They key point is that each descriptor is a relative parameter of a person's behavior.

Importantly, values are like fingerprints—unique and personal. Individuals impart them all over everything they do. The words and actions of a professional that are grounded in values-driven principles can leave a profound positive impression. Alternatively, behavior that is not rooted in a strong moral code is much less likely to be perceived by others in a favorable light.

❏ Why Do Values Matter?

Research indicates that positive people will be more effective in what they do than negative individuals. Given the consequential impact that values can have on a person's professional destiny, it can be argued that individuals should make a concerted effort to keep their values positive. This step means that having a positive attitude may predispose lifestyle medicine practitioners to achieving their professional goals, with the converse being true as well.

Values also play a critical role in making decisions. Every decision can present its own unique and inherent challenges. Having well-established and defined values generally makes it easier to reach a decision and address whatever problematic issues might exist in arriving at a particular course of action when dealing with their patients.

❑ Values—A Bucket List for the Soul

Leading a values-based life is a choice. Although the core principles and values that guide a person's behaviors can be impacted by a myriad of factors (e.g., upbringing, peer influences, culture, etc.), individuals have the capacity to determine what values they hold dear. A person can also determine if there are any governing principles that may be lacking in their life. Identifying deficient areas can lead an individual to appropriately reevaluate and recalibrate their core values.

If physicians and allied healthcare professionals don't stick to their values when they're being challenged or tested, they're not values—they're illusions of convenience. A willingness to overlook an occasional detour in their values means that a person's principles weren't grounded in the first place. Challenging circumstances are part of every person's life, on occasion. Far too often, however, many people view difficult times in an entirely negative perspective. This mindset does not have to be the case. It is often within these tough situations that an individual can find a perfect chance to learn and grow from the experience. Arguably, life's ups and downs can provide windows of opportunity for professionals to engage their values, particularly in the context of addressing problematic matters concerning their patients.

If individuals feel like they have to start compromising who they are as people and what is most important to them as a human being because of others, it is probably time for them to change the people around them. While striking a balance between one set of circumstances and another possible option can be a suitable course of action, depending on the situation, it is never appropriate for a person to make compromise on their values.

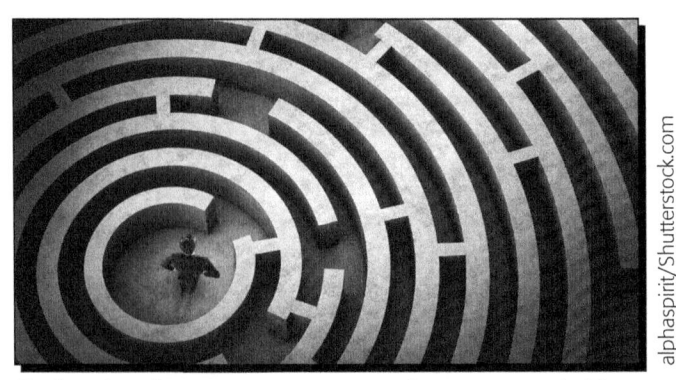

Challenging circumstances are part of every person's life.

ALWAYS BE A DIFFERENCE-MAKER

While anyone can be a difference-maker, not everyone has the passion, work ethic, mindset, and commitment to excel at what they do. Five attributes that commonly characterize a difference-maker include:

- They are able to ask the right questions (e.g., refer to the Frates COACH Approach).
- They are able to understand the situation from the patient's point of view.
- They are able to think outside the box, including being able to interact with professionals outside of their immediate network of associates and colleagues.
- They're always looking for better ways to do things. For them, "good enough" is never good enough.
- They take ownership of their actions. First and foremost, they're concerned about the welfare of their patients. When it comes to their patients, they never say (or think) that "it's not my job."

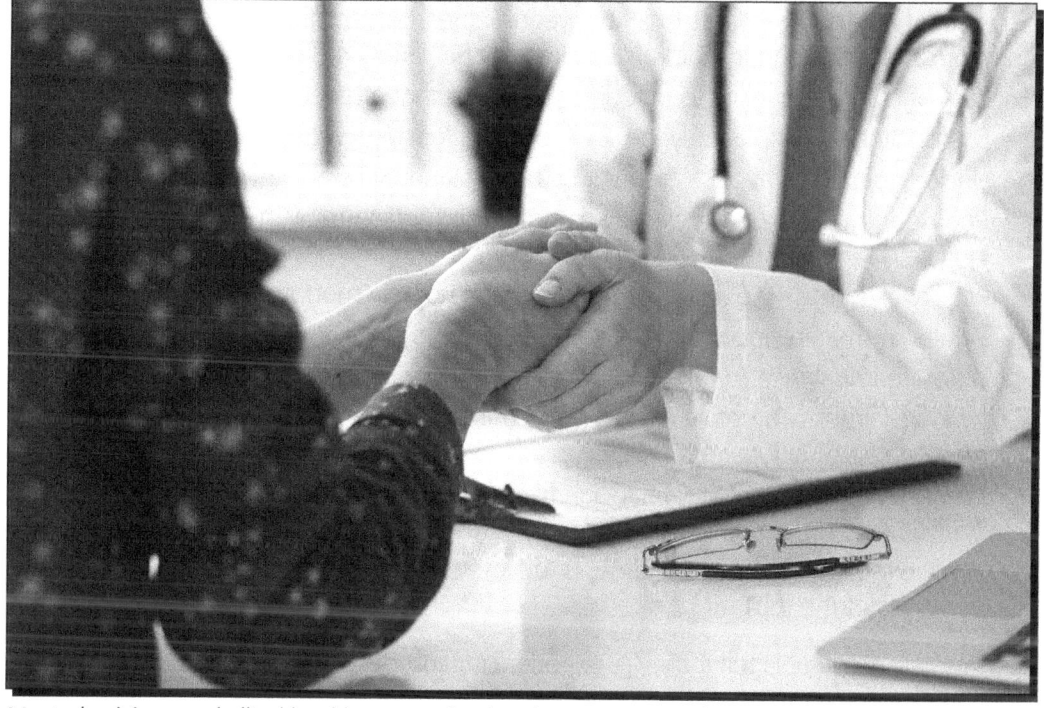

Most physicians and allied healthcare professionals are aware of the fact that they are difference-makers ... improving the lives of their patients, one step at a time ... impacting the realm of healthcare, one piece of sound advice at a time ... using their skills to make the world a better place, one patient at a time.

Most physicians and allied healthcare professionals are aware of the fact that they are difference-makers ... improving the lives of their patients, one step at a time ... impacting the realm of healthcare, one piece of sound advice at a time ... using their skills to make the world a better place, one patient at a time.

BURNOUT

Many physicians and allied healthcare professionals are busier than ever. They often feel rushed. They feel physically and emotionally drained. They have a reduced sense of accomplishment toward what they do. They tend to become somewhat callous or indifferent to what they do. They are probably exhausted and overwhelmed. On occasion, their job-related performance is compromised. Taken together, they are suffering from job burnout, resulting from being exposed to multiple chronic stressors over an extended period of time.

The matter of job burnout appears to be of particular concern for physicians. Research indicates that U.S. physicians suffer more burnout than other American workers. In fact, a recent Medscape Lifestyle Report disclosed that the current level of physician burnout is almost 50 percent.

With regard to job burnout, at least three critical issues need to be addressed: what causes job burnout, how can individuals tell if they're experiencing job burnout, and what should individuals do if they're feeling overly stressed at work?

❏ What causes job burnout?

Professional burnout can be more than simply working long hours. Frequently, it occurs because of mismatches that exist between values, expectations, and resources. Job burnout can transpire in individuals as a result of a variety of factors, including:
- Lack of control (inability to influence decisions that affect them)
- Dysfunctional workplace dynamics (poor relationships with coworkers)
- Unclear job expectations (ambiguous understanding of what the job entails)
- Poor job fit (mismatch regarding the skills and interests of the job holder and the job itself)
- Activity extremes (the job is either too chaotic or too monotonous)
- Values mismatch (incompatible goals and values)
- Work-life imbalance (work does not leave enough time or energy for other things)
- Lack of fairness (a sense of inequity concerning key factors, e.g., workload, pay, employee evaluations, etc.)
- Insufficient rewards (the financial [pay and benefits], social [recognition], and intrinsic [feeling of doing a good job] rewards are not sufficiently satisfying)
- Work overload (insufficient time is devoted to resting and recovering from the demands of the job)

❏ How can individuals tell if they're experiencing job burnout?

If individuals answer in the affirmative to any of the following questions, they may be experiencing job burnout:

- Do they no longer have the energy they once had to a point where their productivity is less than it once was?
- Do they have trouble motivating themselves to put in the (often high) effort that is needed to perform the work that is required of them?
- Do they have trouble getting out of bed to face another day of the same?
- Do they feel impatient, moody, or frustrated more easily than they normally would?
- Do they consistently have trouble sleeping?
- Do they find it more difficult to get excited about life or to look on the bright side, in general?
- Do they use food, drugs, or alcohol as a bridge to "feel better"?
- Do they withdraw from interpersonal relationships at work?
- Do they lack a feeling of being satisfied with their job-related accomplishments?

❑ What should individuals do if they're feeling overly stressed at work?

Lifestyle medicine practitioners need to be proactive in their efforts not only to deal with the potential signs and symptoms of workplace burnout, should they arise, but also to help prevent its occurrence in the first place. A fundamental strategy for dealing with the issue of job burnout can encompass a number of viable steps for individuals, including the following:

- Engage in self-care (treat their body right)
- Socially connect with others (establish strong social relationships)
- Expand the envelope (have a life outside of work)
- Make relaxing a part of their routine (take at least a 15-minute break every day)
- Communicate with their supervisor (have an ongoing dialogue with their boss)
- Be clear about their job responsibilities (know what the job entails and what others expect of them)
- Learn to say "no" (set and adhere to reasonable limits about what they can do at work)
- Don't accept boredom as an irrefutable characteristic of the job (ask for a change in duties)
- Learn to delegate (be aware that time is an irreplaceable asset)
- Realize that they can't change everything (change what they can, accept what they can't)
- Be introspective (try to ascertain the source of their discontent and then address it)
- Don't do anything rash (be cool—haste makes waste)
- Work with a purpose (understand and accept the fact that they are difference-makers because of what they do—they make life better for their patients)

SELF-CARE

Self-care often seems intuitive to many healthcare professionals, but it can be surprisingly difficult to "practice what you preach." Many health professionals are inherently caring, giving, and used to putting the health of patients and loved ones first. These attributes are admirable, and allow providers to take exceptional care of others. Often, these same characteristics can lead people to neglect their own health. Such a situation leads to a deficit in being able to take care of themselves, which is not only important to avoid burnout, but it is also fundamental to practicing lifestyle medicine.

Healthcare providers are typically highly motivated, driven individuals. Society rewards these types for the extraordinary number of hours they work. It is often easy to justify the hours worked by convincing themselves that it is for the good of the patients, or it is something that needs to be done to forward a career. While there are inevitably periods of time when long hours or engaging in unsustainable work behaviors can be beneficial and necessary (e.g., a big project deadline/presentation, etc.), these practices are not sustainable long term.

WHAT MAKES SELF-CARE SO CHALLENGING?

Most individuals know the guidelines recommend: getting seven to eight hours of sleep, exercising for 150 minutes each week, eating a healthy diet, etc. What prevents people from translating knowledge into action? One of the most common barriers cited is the lack of time. After an 8- to 12-hour workday, commuting to and from work, making dinner, spending time with loved ones, answering emails, and additional work or household needs, it is difficult to find yet another 30 minutes to exercise. It seems that life is already full of responsibilities, obligations, and tasks. How do people find the time to perform self-care activities?

The simple answer is that people rarely find time—instead, they make time. Perhaps the most critical concept to understand regarding self-care is that being busy is a decision. Another way to imagine the phrase "I am too busy" is to replace it with "It is not a high enough priority for me right now." There is nothing wrong with this. In fact, there are many things in life that are not truly important right now—watching a television show, cleaning out the garage, organizing the cupboards, etc. Sometimes meetings or conference calls may fall into this category. A more difficult situation arises when decisions involve more personal issues.

As an example, a colleague asks if you want to get lunch together. However, you typically work through your lunch break. It is easy to respond to this colleague with "I am busy." The reality is the additional time spent working during your lunch hour ensures you leave on time. This approach may be absolutely fine in that situation, but what if the dynamics of that situation are changed slightly?

Instead of it being a work colleague, let's say that your best friend is passing through town and only had time to meet during lunch. Chances are high that the work would get put off until later, and lunch with your friend would take precedence. This situation demonstrates two important concepts; prioritization and opportunity cost. In the first situation, despite the colleague being a friend, getting out of work on time to be home with loved ones is more important relative to the alternative choices that day. The opportunity cost of going to lunch means having to delay work later in the day resulting in getting home later. By choosing to do one activity, it precludes doing another in its place. However, if this situation were a rare chance to see a best friend that may not be available later, this opportunity becomes more important than getting out of work on time because you will not be able to have lunch with a friend later that day, week, month, or year. This scenario may seem like an obvious example, but this prioritization of daily choices is frequently done unconsciously for every decision that is made each day.

The same rationale applies to self-care. Reflecting on whether or not 30 minutes of exercise were accumulated in a day can essentially be thought of as "exercise was or was not a high enough priority today." Some days, exercising may not be a high enough priority. That is okay. Exercise may or may not take priority relative to other activities that day.

The important concept is not being critical of yourself for not exercising, but understanding that you dictate what your priorities are every day. You get to make those choices. There is an opportunity cost to every choice you make—choosing one activity, often negates your ability to perform another activity. If there are facets of life that "should" be improved, or if you are unhappy with how the activities of a day unfold, the person ultimately responsible for making these changes is you.

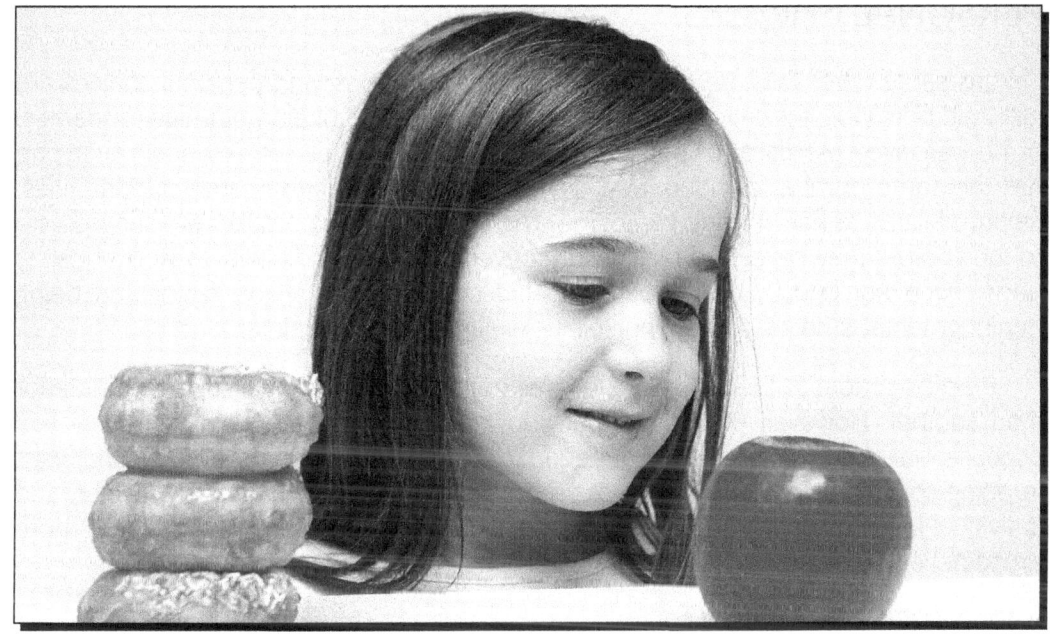

There is an opportunity cost to every choice you make.

TIME IS INVALUABLE

As previously discussed, time is the one commodity that you cannot buy more of or buy back. Everyone is given the same 24 hours each day. Each individual gets to decide how every minute of that time is spent. Although health is commonly viewed as the most valuable asset you have, its value is predicated on having time to enjoy it. People have also argued that it takes too much time to engage in all of the lifestyle behaviors to keep an individual healthy. Why spend so much time exercising, in exchange for a similar amount of time extended in your life? You are spending all of your "extra" time exercising! The problem with that notion is that it does not take into account the quality of your life. Lifestyle medicine doesn't just extend life, it makes it better throughout. Rather than think you don't have time to practice self-care, the case could be made that you don't have the time to *not* practice good self-care habits. Recognizing that there is only a finite amount of time in your life, wouldn't you want to have the most fulfilling, wonderful existence possible?

Clearly, there are things that are more important than exercising for 30 minutes—e.g., going to work in order to provide for a family, spending time with children, enjoying dinner with a spouse. Whether you consciously or unconsciously recognize this, these choices are made every day. Work will ask for increased productivity, colleagues will ask for help with projects/tasks, organizations will ask for volunteer efforts, and loved ones will ask for favors. The fact is, if you do not choose how to spend your time, someone else will choose for you. Taking control of your health is a personal decision that only an individual can make.

PERSONAL CHOICES

On this same note, self-care choices are intimate decisions, and personal choices are just that: *personal*. It is critical that lifestyle medicine practitioners not judge, disparage, or be perceived as critical of personal decisions made by others. Although everyone has the same number of hours in a day, not everyone has the same opportunities, responsibilities, or hardships to overcome. The choices a person makes are subordinate to the choices they have. The reality is that everyone's life and ability to make healthy decisions is *not* equal. Life is not fair. Being conscientious of this factor and being nonjudgmental is necessary for yourself, as well as for the people around you.

Practicing more or "better" self-care does not make an individual superior or inferior than another. However, practicing what you preach not only exemplifies ideals you espouse, but also provides real-world feedback about the inherent challenges that exist in doing so. Understanding the complex interaction between work, family, career, and individual interests on a personal level enables lifestyle medicine providers to be more empathetic to the struggles others may be facing.

If self-care were easy, everyone would do it. Much like working out, self-care takes time, effort, and perseverance. Although it is a life-long commitment that is filled with challenges, self-care ultimately boils down to the personal decisions that are made every day. These decisions may seem difficult at times, but the choices that are made typically reflect the priorities a person holds. The key to continued success is appreciating the true value that lifestyle behaviors bring to life. Once this is done, prioritizing self-care becomes much easier.

LIVE AND LEARN WITH DR. BETH FRATES

No one is perfect. Everyone struggles. People who love exercise sometimes stop exercising. Why? Usually because life happens. Things come up. Competing interests arise. For me, this happened after I had my two boys. I felt like I should be spending every minute with them while I was home. When I was teaching at the medical school, I would race home to see them. In fact, my first ticket I received for speeding was coming home around 5:30 p.m., racing to catch every minute before my son's bedtime at 7 p.m.

When I had my second son, things got more difficult. I felt like they needed me. I felt like it would be selfish if I were to go and jog, while they were awake. I really wanted to spend every waking moment with them, if I were not working. I could feel that my body was moving differently, my mood was not quite as chipper, and my energy was not as high as it usually was. My husband kept telling me to take the time to exercise, but I refused.

Then, one day we discovered that both boys were big enough and old enough to sit in a baby jogger. So, we purchased a double-baby jogger. This way, while I was jogging, I could still be talking with them and connecting with them. It was great. We watched the leaves fall in October, and in the spring, we had the opportunity to smell the flowers after they bloomed. Including my boys in the exercise plan was what I needed to get moving again. It felt great. And, by the time my youngest son was a teenager, he was asking to run with me.

That was not the only time that I fell off of my exercise routine. When the boys were in elementary school, I co-authored a book about life after stroke. It was a lot of work. But, I was passionate about the material, as my father suffered a stroke when I was 18, and I really wanted people to avoid this health setback. At any rate, the mix of working, writing, being a mom, being a wife, and being a daughter were all taking a toll on me.

I felt like I had no time. I was always under the gun with deadlines for the book. So, every free minute I had, I would sit and write. Well, that led me to the same place I had been six years earlier. I was sedentary, noticing my pants fitting more tightly on my bottom, feeling stressed, feeling less energy, and feeling overall unfit. I could not devote time to myself, because I thought that was selfish. Imagine that. I believed that self-care was selfish.

One day while looking up information about dogs, because my husband and boys wanted to adopt a puppy, I had a eureka moment. I searched on pub med (a public portal for medical research articles) and found research that indicated that dogs could help people exercise more regularly. Then, I read an article about dogs reducing stress and more. I was sold. It was clear from the articles, that the people who adopted the dog needed to provide the dog with adequate exercise for the health of the dog and for the sake of the furniture, shoes, and socks in the house, as the dog would go on chewing sprees if they were not fatigued by some exercise.

This justification was just the excuse I needed to get me to run again. I knew that I would run if it meant that another being (human or animal) would benefit. I also did not want a dog chewing everything in sight and wreaking havoc on the house. So, we did get a dog, and I did run and walk the dog religiously. We both benefited from that.

It is good to know yourself and know what will make you make the time to exercise. It all starts with self-awareness and honestly with yourself. In fact, it's important to use the Frates COACH Approach with yourself. Be curious about your own motives and actions. Be open about possible solutions to the problem and consider going outside the box. Be appreciative for all that you have and all that has happened to you to help inform you about the best path forward. Be compassionate with yourself. Understand that everyone is human. Thus, stumbling and falling off an exercise routine just means that you will learn and grow from the experience which will make you even stronger than you were previously. Lastly, be honest with yourself. Telling yourself that it is no big deal if you are spending the majority of the day sitting and your gaining five pounds a year is not a big deal. This mentality will not help you. This way of thinking is hiding from the truth—not speaking the truth. Being honest with yourself means looking in the mirror, seeing your flaws, acknowledging them, making a plan to address them and still feeling awesome anyway.

This approach is called, "flawsome." When you realize you are not perfect, and no one else is, it frees you to improve. When you do experience setbacks and lapses in healthy living, remember that your story of recovery and re-engaging with exercise will be an inspirational one to friends, colleagues, and patients alike.

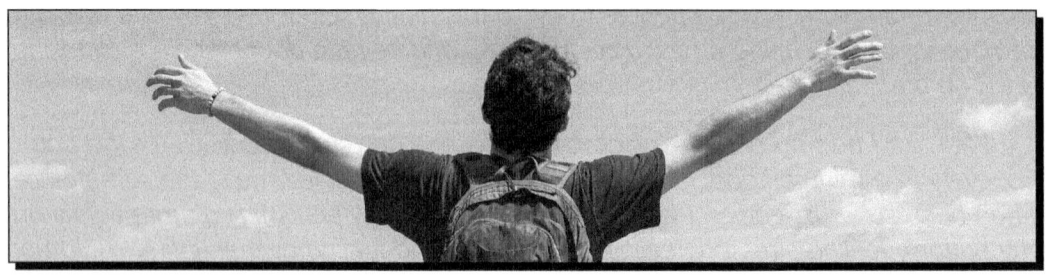

When you realize you are not perfect, and no one else is, it frees you to improve.

WHERE TO START?

The weekly lifestyle medicine schedule in Appendix A provides a snapshot of many of the lifestyle behaviors associated with positive health benefits. It provides a rudimentary summary of what might be reasonable goals for which you should strive. It is in no way comprehensive, and additional efforts beyond what is listed can provide further health benefits. The schedule addresses the six major pillars of lifestyle medicine (i.e., physical activity, diet, sleep, stress management, relationships, and toxin avoidance).

A simple way to evaluate your self-care is to think about the previous week and identify how many of these boxes you could check. The unchecked boxes represent potential areas for improvement. If there is a specific domain that you are lacking in, the sample calendar offers possible ways to schedule these activities into daily life.

Scheduling can help people fit more health-promoting behaviors into their busy lives, since most individuals tend to prioritize things that are scheduled, whether it is a meeting, conference call, work, or a personal training session. Essentially, committing to a block of time in a calendar provides a predetermined space to engage in activities that matter. Why shouldn't exercise or sleep take a similar priority to a conference call or meeting?

Importantly, these behaviors do not need to be done in isolation. It is arguably easier and valuable to combine healthy habits together. Exercising with a friend facilitates a social connection, in addition to the physical activity. Leveraging the daily commute to bike or walk to work can further increase efficiency. Similarly, using the stairs, instead of the elevator at the office, is a great way to incorporate additional physical activity into the day. Rather than sitting around a conference table or at a desk, walking meetings represent another great substitution to build physical activity into a typical day.

In terms of nutrition, money and time can be saved by planning ahead. This effort necessitates prioritizing grocery shopping and food preparation, but this small investment pays dividends throughout the week. The majority of meals are already made, ready to eat. No need to drive to a restaurant, wait to be served, and then come home. It is easy to grab-n-go with healthy, portioned meals that are ready to eat.

Regarding sleep, there is no shortcut in this instance. It means planning ahead and holding yourself accountable for going to bed at the same time each night. With all of the distractions that exist (e.g., computers, cell phones, email, television, etc.), it helps to have a bedtime routine that is free from electronics and allows time to transition to sleep.

BEYOND THE BASICS

While the schedule provides a tangible goal to work toward, the quantities of the aforementioned behaviors should be viewed as a floor, rather than a ceiling. If you are already getting more physical activity weekly than 150 minutes, there is no need to cut back. Benefits from exercise continue to accrue with increasing durations, but there are diminishing returns. In other words, the relative increase in health benefits is less, with increasingly higher levels of activity.

The guidelines for many of the lifestyle medicine domains (i.e., physical activity, diet, sleep, and smoking) were created as a means to balance efficiency and provide realistic public health targets for people to work toward. They are constructed from multiple large studies that analyze mortality or morbidity, with respect to a specific disease entity, such as cardiovascular disease or diabetes, as the outcome. This approach aids in helping prevent certain health problems, as well as slowing disease progression, should a particular medical condition occur.

Instead of focusing on disease avoidance, however, what if there was a focus on cultivating wellness? Using osteoporosis as an example, individuals are encouraged to perform resistance training to help improve their bone density. Instead of motivating people with a threat of worsening bone density, perhaps, the point could be emphasized how resistance training will improve strength, increase confidence, make their activities of daily living easier, and make their quality of life better. This subtle shift changes the entire dynamic of behavior change from engaging in activity to avoid a "punishment" to pursuing a "reward."

The major lifestyle medicine domains, with the exception of smoking, can be considered on a continuous scale. As such, an opportunity exists to achieve more or less within a single domain, such as exercising fewer or more minutes or eating fewer or more vegetables, etc. Despite the potential health implications that varying doses might have, the focus is typically on getting individuals to this average threshold, the recommended guidelines, that theoretically provides the highest return on investment, with regard to disease avoidance. While these numbers are excellent as population targets, there is reason to believe that significant variability exists between individuals.

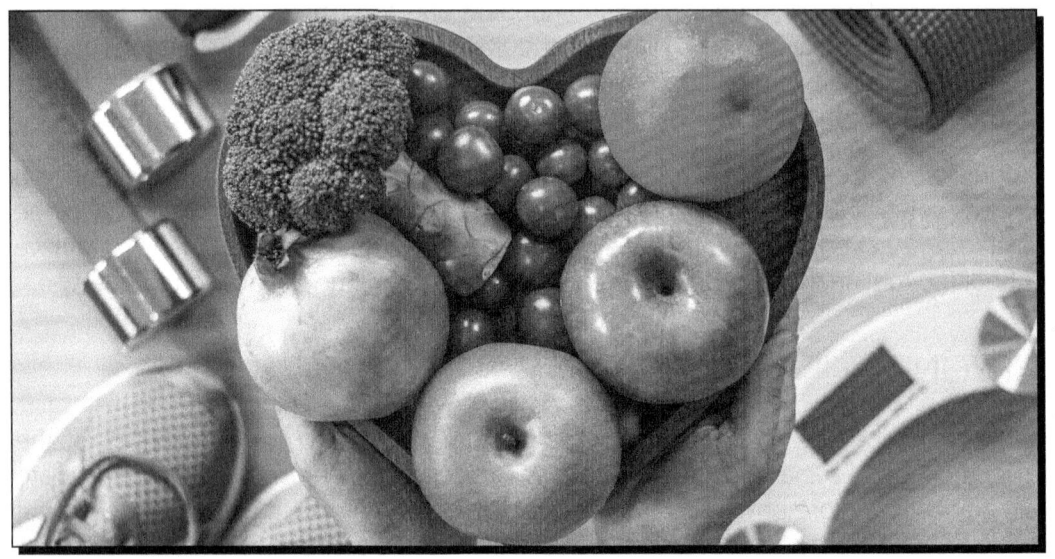

Instead of focusing on disease avoidance, what if there was a focus on cultivating wellness?

This concept can be illustrated by some people needing nine hours of sleep to feel refreshed, whereas others might only require six hours. To force a person who needs six hours of sleep to sleep an additional one to two hours, so that they meet the recommended guidelines doesn't make much sense. Furthermore, restricting the nine-hour person to seven to eight hours would almost certainly worsen their functioning, health, and quality of life. Higher, and potentially lower, levels of lifestyle medicine may be necessary to reap the ultimate reward—vitality and optimal functioning. That begs the question, if lifestyle is the medicine, what is the ideal dose?

THE HEALTH CONTINUUM

To answer the aforementioned question, consider the concept of health. What is health? Often, health is viewed as a lack of disease, but it is more than a binary entity. Similar to most of the lifestyle medicine domains, health represents a continuum, with disease and death being toward one extreme and wellness and optimal functioning representing the other (see Figure 12-1). This concept was first introduced by Dr. John Travis in his Illness-Wellness Continuum. While traditional medicine has focused almost exclusively on slowing the progression of disease and death, lifestyle medicine is relatively unique in that it can reverse this trajectory and move people toward wellness and optimal functioning.

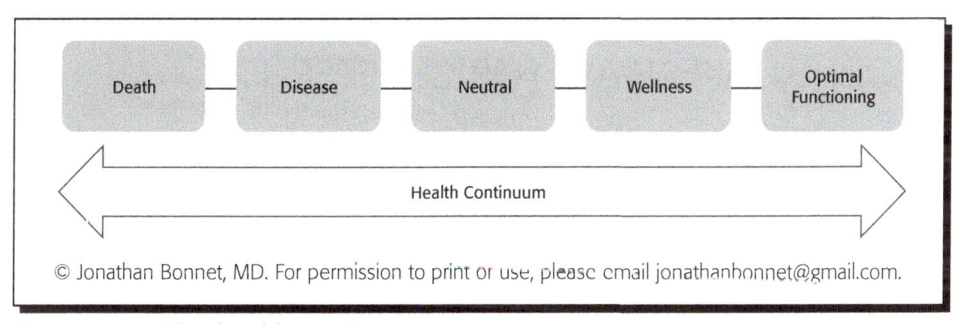

Figure 12-1. The health continuum

The optimal dose of lifestyle medicine on an individual level varies from person to person and changes with time. For example, the recommended duration and intensity of physical activity differs for children, as compared to adults. As individuals age, resistance training increases in importance to help combat the 35 to 40 percent loss of muscle mass that occurs between 20 and 80 years of age. Sleep recommendations are also vastly different across the lifespan, with the National Sleep Foundation recommending 14-17 hours for newborns, compared with seven to eight hours for those 65 years or older.

These may seem like relatively obvious examples of personalizing the lifestyle medicine dose. Given the known *intra*variability that exists across the lifespan, it seems likely that *inter*variability exists among similar aged individuals as well. Combining this notion of a tailored prescription, with a focus on the improved functioning and quality of life that lifestyle medicine provides, leads an individual to health optimization.

LIFESTYLE MEDICINE 2.0—HEALTH OPTIMIZATION

Optimization is defined as "an act, process, or methodology of making something (such as a design, system, or decision) as fully perfect, functional, or effective as possible." Health optimization seeks to maximize an individual's well-being, functioning, and quality of life. The concept of optimal functioning is not a purely physical or mental state; rather, it is a representation of human potential. Although it is different for everyone, it can be illustrated with the following assignment: "Think of a time when you felt or performed your best. What did that look like? How did that feel?"

The answer to these queries provides a glimpse of the potential an individual has. While it may not be the pinnacle of functioning, it is likely beyond where a person is at currently. While there is no known lifestyle medicine dose to optimize functioning for everyone at a population level, there certainly is a prescription that optimizes health on an individual level. The challenge is figuring out what it is. Although discerning what these lifestyle medicine parameters are for each individual is beyond the scope of this book, the previous chapters provide information on how to craft an individualized lifestyle medicine prescription.

Lifestyle medicine is the wave of the future for healthcare and for health optimization. Everyone can use a dose of it. One day, lifestyle medicine will be mainstream.

KEY POINTS/TAKEAWAYS FOR CHAPTER 12

❑ Chapter Review:

- Overall goal: Review the factors that can support lifestyle medicine practitioners on their professional journey, and also help define them as difference-makers.
- Application goal: Understand what lifestyle medicine practitioners need to do to take care of themselves and maintain their professional edge in their craft.

❑ Discussion Questions:

- What are four of the core attributes that lifestyle medicine practitioners who want to stay the course must have?
- Why should physicians and allied healthcare professionals practice what they preach?
- What factors does self-care encompass?
- Why is lifelong learning important?
- How does a person's values-orientation affect their life?
- What traits commonly characterize someone who is a difference-maker?
- What are common triggers that signal a person's health may not be what it should be?
- Why does a person do what they do each day?
- Who is responsible for self-care? What barriers exist?

- What does being busy mean?
- What areas of my personal self-care are not optimized? Do I want to change that?

	TITLE	AUTHORS	JOURNAL	YEAR	KEY FINDINGS
1	Personal exercise habits and counseling practices of primary care physicians: a national survey	Abramson S, et al.	Clinical Journal of Sport Medicine	2000	The authors demonstrated that physicians who exercise were more likely to counsel their patients to exercise. Physicians that do aerobic training counsel on aerobic training, and those that do strength training counsel on strength training. The main barriers that physicians faced preventing them from counseling on exercise were: inadequate time, lack of knowledge/experience with exercise counseling.
2	Physician disclosure of healthy personal behaviors improves credibility and ability to motivate	Frank E, Breyan J, Elon L	Archives of Family Medicine	2000	This study compared the effect that two different educational videos had on physicians' abilities to motivate patients to adopt healthy habits. It found that subjects viewed the video in which the physician discussed their own personal health habits with subtle supporting cues (i.e., apple on the desk, bike helmet in view) to be more believable and motivating regarding exercise and diet.
3	A model for predicting the counseling practices of physicians	Lewis CE, Wells KB, Ware J	Journal of General Internal Medicine	1986	A random sample survey of 151 physicians that found significant associations between the counseling practices reported and physicians' personal health habits, attitudes, and specialties. "In general, physicians who had poor health habits did not fully counsel patients about those habits; however, physicians attempting to improve poor habits counseled patients significantly more often than physicians who were not trying to change their own behavior." They ultimately concluded that "health maintenance efforts among physicians may have a multiplier effect."
4	Emotional distress and occupational burnout in health care professionals serving HIV-infected patients: a comparison with oncology and internal medicine services	Lopez-Castillo J, et al.	Psychotherapy and Psychosomatics	1999	A cross-sectional survey of 196 healthcare professionals at four hospitals that found that 38% of healthcare professionals reported diagnostic levels of psychological distress, including depression, anxiety, and impaired functioning at a rate comparable to their patients.

Figure 12-2. Self-care evidence

	TITLE	AUTHORS	JOURNAL	YEAR	KEY FINDINGS
5	The painful truth: physicians are not invincible	Miller NM, McGowen RK	Southern Medical Journal	2000	A review of some of the psychosocial problems physicians face, including depression, suicide, marital problems, and other stress-related concerns. "Discusses possible factors related to the development of these problems and suggests a variety of solutions to improve physician self-care."
6	Physicians' health practices strongly influence patient health practices	Oberg EB, Frank E	Journal of the Royal College of Physicians of Edinburgh	2009	"Physicians can positively influence patients' health habits by counselling them about prevention and health-promoting behaviors. Physical counselling is strongly related to one's own health practices, so addressing providers' own health behaviors is key to substantially increasing health promotion counselling in general practice."
7	Caring for oneself to care for others: physicians and their self-care	Sanchez-Reilly S, et al.	Journal of Supportive Oncology	2013	"Discusses validated methods to increase self-care, enhance self-awareness, and improve patient care." They recommend regularly appraising and regulating six areas of work life: workload, control, reward, community, fairness, and values. Other suggestions include, but are not limited to, performing reflective exercises, prioritizing relationships, adopting healthy lifestyles, and working to improve empathy.
8	Personal health practices and patient counseling of German physicians in private practice	Voltmer E, Frank E, Spahn C	International Scholarly Research Notices: Epidemiology	2013	A study of 414 physicians in private practice in Germany that found doctors who had better personal exercise ($p=0.007$), fruit and vegetable consumption ($p=0.001$), smoking ($p=0.012$), and alcohol ($p=0.047$) behaviors counseled their patients significantly more often on related topics.

References

1. Abramson S, Stein J, Schaufele M, et al. Personal exercise habits and counseling practices of primary care physicians: a national survey. *Clinical Journal of Sport Medicine*. 2000;10(1):40-48.
2. Frank E, Breyan J, Elon L. Physician disclosure of healthy personal behaviors improves credibility and ability to motivate. *Archives of Family Medicine*. 2000;9(3):287-290.
3. Lewis CE, Wells KB, Ware J. A model for predicting the counseling practices of physicians. *Journal of General Internal Medicine*. 1986;1(1):14-19.
4. Lopez-Castillo J, Gurpegui M, Ayuso-Mateos JL, et al. Emotional distress and occupational burnout in health care professionals serving HIV-infected patients: a comparison with oncology and internal medicine services. *Psychotherapy and Psychosomatics*. 1999;68:348-356.
5. Miller NM, McGowen RK. The painful truth: physicians are not invincible. *Southern Medical Journal*. 2000;93:966-973.
6. Oberg EB, Frank E. Physicians' health practices strongly influence patient health practices. *Journal of the Royal College of Physicians of Edinburgh*. 2009;39(4):290-291. Available at: https://www.ncbi.nlm.nih.gov/pmc/articles/PMC3058599/. Accessed October 2017.
7. Sanchez-Reilly S, Morrison LJ, Carey E, et al. Caring for oneself to care for others: physicians and their self-care. *Journal of Supportive Oncology*. 2013;11(2):75-81.
8. Voltmer E, Frank E, Spahn C. Personal health practices and patient counseling of German physicians in private practice. *International Scholarly Research Notices: Epidemiology*. 2013. Available at: https://www.hindawi.com/journals/isrn/2013/176020/abs/. Accessed October 2017.

Figure 12-2. Self-care evidence (cont.)

REFERENCES

- Abramson S, Stein J, Schaufele M, Frates E, Rogan S. Personal exercise habits and counseling practices of primary care physicians: a national survey. *Clinical Journal of Sport Medicine*. 2000;10(1):40-48.
- Action FCTO. Physical activity and public health—a recommendation from the Centers for Disease Control and Prevention and the American College of Sports Medicine. *JAMA*. 1995;273:402-407.
- Bass K, McGeeney K. US Physicians Set Good Health Example. Gallup News. October 3, 2012. Available at: http://www.gallup.com/poll/157859/physicians-set-good-health-example.aspx. Accessed October 2017.
- Cho J. Healing the Healer: Why Physicians and Medical Professionals Must Practice Self-Care. Forbes. March 30, 2016. Available at: https://www.forbes.com/sites/jeenacho/2016/03/30/healing-the-healer-why-physicians-and-medical-professionals-must-practice-self-care/#353efe43797a. Accessed May 2017.
- Church TS, Earnest CP, Skinner JS, et al. Effects of different doses of physical activity on cardiorespiratory fitness among sedentary, overweight or obese postmenopausal women with elevated blood pressure: a randomized controlled trial. *JAMA*. May 16 2007;297(19):2081-2091.
- Frank E, Breyan J, Elon L. Physician disclosure of healthy personal behaviors improves credibility and ability to motivate. *Archives of Family Medicine*. 2000;9(3):287-290.
- Fung B. Is Your Doctor Healthier Than You? The Atlantic. August 6, 2012. Available at: http://www.theatlantic.com/health/archive/2012/08/is-your-doctor-healthier-than-you/260706/. Accessed October 2017.
- Hirshkowitz M, Whiton K, Albert SM, et al. The National Sleep Foundation's sleep time duration recommendations: methodology and results summary. *Sleep Health*. 2015;1(1):40-43.
- Lewis CE, Wells KB, Ware J. A model for predicting the counseling practices of physicians. *Journal of General Internal Medicine*. 1986;1(1):14-19.
- López-Castillo J, Gurpegui M, Ayuso-Mateos JL, et al. Emotional distress and occupational burnout in health care professionals serving HIV-infected patients: a comparison with oncology and internal medicine services. *Psychotherapy and Psychosomatics*. 1999;68(6):348-356.
- Merriam-Webster. Optimization. Available at: https://www.merriam-webster.com/dictionary/optimization. Accessed May 2018.
- Miller MN, Mcgowen KR, Quillen JH. The painful truth: physicians are not invincible. *Southern Medical Journal*. 2000;93(10).
- Oberg EB, Frank E. Physicians' health practices strongly influence patient health practices. *Journal of the Royal College of Physicians of Edinburgh*. 2009;39(4):290-291. Available at: https://www.ncbi.nlm.nih.gov/pmc/articles/PMC3058599/. Accessed October 2017.

- Parks T. Report Reveals Severity of Burnout by Specialty. AMA Wire. January 31, 2017. Available at https://wire.ama-assn.org/life-career/report-reveals-severity-burnout-specialty. Accessed May 2017.
- Peckham C. Medscape Lifestyle Report 2017: Race and Ethnicity, Bias and Burnout. Available at: https://www.medscape.com/features/slideshow/lifestyle/2017/overview#page=1. Accessed October 2017.
- Pollock ML, Franklin BA, Balady GJ, et al. AHA Science Advisory. Resistance exercise in individuals with and without cardiovascular disease: benefits, rationale, safety, and prescription: an advisory from the Committee on Exercise, Rehabilitation, and Prevention, Council on Clinical Cardiology, American Heart Association. Position paper endorsed by the American College of Sports Medicine. *Circulation.* February 22 2000;101(7):828.
- Proctor DN, Balagopal P, Nair KS. Age-related sarcopenia in humans is associated with reduced synthetic rates of specific muscle proteins. *Journal of Nutrition.* 1998;128:351S-355S.
- Sanchez-Reilly S, Morrison LJ, Carey E, et al. Caring for oneself to care for others: physicians and their self-care. *Journal of Supportive Oncology.* 2013;11(2):75-81.
- The Wellspring. Key Concept #1: The Illness-Wellness Continuum. Available at: http://www.thewellspring.com/wellspring/introduction-to-wellness/357/key-concept-1-the-illnesswellness-continuum.cfm. Accessed May 2018.
- Travis J, Ryan RS. *The Wellness Workbook: How to Achieve Enduring Health and Vitality.* 3rd ed. New York: Random House; 1981.
- U.S. Department of Health and Human Services. 2008 Physical Activity Guidelines for Americans. Available at: www.health.gov/paguidelines. Accessed November 2008.
- Voltmer E, Frank E, Spahn C. Personal health practices and patient counseling of German physicians in private practice. *International Scholarly Research Notices: Epidemiology.* 2013. Available at: https://www.hindawi.com/journals/isrn/2013/176020/abs/. Accessed October 2017.
- Webber D, Guo Z, Mann S. Self-care in health: we can define it, but should we also measure it? *SelfCare.* 2013;4(5):101-106.
- WHO. The Role of the Pharmacist in Self-Care and Self-Medication. Report of the 4th WHO Consultative Group on the Role of the Pharmacist 1998. Available at: http://apps.who.int/medicinedocs/en/d/Jwhozip32e/. Accessed June 2018.
- Winett RA, Carpinelli RN. Potential health-related benefits of resistance training. *Preventive Medicine.* November 1 2001;33(5):503-513.

APPENDIX A

A Weekly Health Prescription

Health is one of the most precious and important commodities an individual has. While health is not a destination, it is the currency which allows a person to live the type of fulfilled life that they desire. Lifestyle-related behaviors (e.g., physical inactivity, poor diet, smoking, etc.) are the primary actual causes of death in the United States, as well as significant contributors to a decreased quality of life. This factor has been known for decades. The challenge has been, and will continue to be, translating what we know into what we routinely do.

For many people, scheduled events take priority. A schedule that includes healthy events will allow us to appropriately prioritize healthy activities. Figure A-1 illustrates a series of evidence-based lifestyle medicine practices laid out in a suggested weekly schedule. It is designed specifically for a normal 40-hour work week and attempts to take into account what days/nights tend to be more stressful or time-pressed (e.g., Monday). It addresses the primary domains of lifestyle medicine, including physical activity, diet, sleep, stress, and love. Smoking is the only domain not specifically targeted. Getting 7-8 hours of sleep and eating at least five fruits or vegetables are recommended every day.

Figure A-1 is merely an example schedule. A person can easily swap the items included to any day of the week. For individuals with alternate work schedules or with different responsibilities on particular days of the week, the entire checklist of items is included. Readers should feel free to create their own healthy week so that it is personalized to them. Once they have a schedule set, they can enter it as a recurring event in their phone with daily reminders.

Sunday	Monday	Tuesday	Wednesday	Thursday	Friday	Saturday
☐ Sleep 7-8 hrs	☐ Sleep 7-8 hrs	☐ Sleep 7-8 hrs	☐ Sleep 7-8 hrs	☐ Sleep 7-8 hrs	☐ Sleep 7-8 hrs	☐ Sleep 7-8 hrs
☐ Walk/jog/run 45 mins	☐ Relaxation activity for 15 mins	☐ Relaxation activity for 15 mins	☐ Lunchtime walk (15 mins)	☐ Walk/jog/run 45 mins	☐ Meet up with friend for 30 mins; optional alcoholic drink***	☐ Walk/jog/run 45 mins
☐ Religious/spiritual practice 15-60 mins	☐ Make to-do list/schedule for the week	☐ Family activity for 30 mins**	☐ Family dinner or meal w/ friend	☐ Muscle strengthening	☐ Family activity for 30 mins**	☐ Muscle strengthening
☐ Call or visit parents or children 15 mins	☐ Three good things*			☐ Three good things*	☐ Three good things*	☐ Family dinner or meal w/ friend
# Fruits/Veggies ☐☐☐☐☐	# Fruits/Veggies ☐☐☐☐☐	# Fruits/Veggies ☐☐☐☐☐	# Fruits/Veggies ☐☐☐☐☐	# Fruits/Veggies ☐☐☐☐☐	# Fruits/Veggies ☐☐☐☐☐	# Fruits/Veggies ☐☐☐☐☐

*Before you go to bed, write down three good things that happened to you today.
**Family activity can be anything and with anyone whom you consider family (parents, children, significant other, relatives, pets, etc.). For example, play a board game, participate in a card game, go for a walk, play outside, sit and talk, share dinner together, read a book, etc. Keep in mind that doing something with your pet also counts!
***If you do not drink, there is no recommendation to start. However, there may be some cardiovascular benefits from consuming alcohol. If you are a male you can enjoy up to two drinks per day. If you are a female, you can enjoy up to one drink per day.

© Jonathan Bonnet, MD; for permission to print or use, please email jonathanbonnet@gmail.com

Figure A-1. Suggested weekly schedule

CHECKLIST

PHYSICAL ACTIVITY

❑ Walk/jog/run 45 minutes x 3 days

❑ Lunchtime walk (15 minutes) x 1 day

❑ Muscle strengthening x 2 days

DIET

❑ At least five fruits/veggies a day x 7 days

SMOKING

❑ Don't smoke! Try to quit if you do.

SLEEP

❑ Sleep 7-8 hours x 7 days

STRESS

❑ Three good things* x 3 days

❑ Relaxation activity for 15 minutes x 2 days

❑ Make to-do list/schedule for the week x 1 day

❑ Meet up with friend for 30 minutes; optional alcoholic drink*** x 1 day

LOVE AND CONNECTION

❑ Family activity for 30 minutes** x 2 days

❑ Family dinner or meal w/ friend x 2 days

❑ Religious/spiritual practice 15-60 minutes x 1 day

❑ Meet up with friend for 30 minutes; optional alcoholic drink*** x 1 day

❑ Call or visit parents/children 15 minutes x 1 day

---

*Before you go to bed, write down three good things that happened to you today.

**Family activity can be anything and with anyone whom you consider family (parents, children, significant other, relatives, pets, etc.). For example, play a board game, participate in a card game, go for a walk, play outside, sit and talk, share dinner together, read a book, etc. Keep in mind that doing something with your pet also counts!

***If you do not drink, there is no recommendation to start. However, there may be some cardiovascular benefits from consuming alcohol. If you are a male you can enjoy up to two drinks per day. If you are a female, you can enjoy up to one drink per day.

ABOUT THE AUTHORS

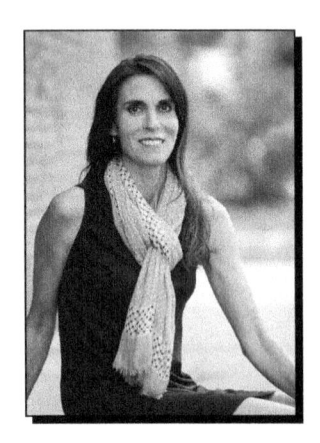

Beth Frates, MD is trained as a physiatrist and a health and wellness coach. Her expertise is in lifestyle medicine, and she works to empower patients to reach their optimal level of wellness by adopting healthy habits. A member of the Board of Directors of the American College of Lifestyle Medicine, Dr. Frates is helping to shape the scope of this new specialty. She is an award-winning teacher at Harvard Medical School, where she is an assistant clinical professor, and she developed and taught a college lifestyle medicine curriculum at the Harvard Extension School, which is one of the most popular courses offered at the school. She shared a lifestyle medicine syllabus, which can be downloaded through the ACLM website, in hopes that her work can serve as a template for other instructors and professors hoping to teach a course in lifestyle medicine. As the Director of Wellness Programming at the Stroke Institute for Research and Recovery at Spaulding Rehabilitation Hospital, Dr. Frates has created and implemented a 12-month wellness program for stroke survivors and their caregivers. She is co-author of the book *Life After Stroke: The Guide to Recovering Your Health and Preventing Another Stroke* and co-author of three chapters on behavior change in different medical textbooks.

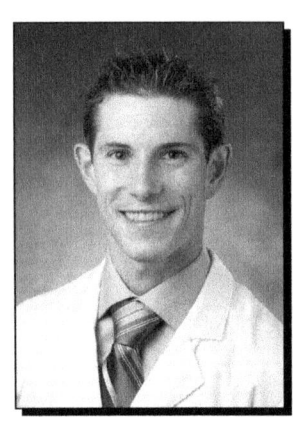

Jonathan P. Bonnet, MD is a board-certified family, sports, and obesity medicine physician. He has a background in exercise physiology and is also a certified personal trainer. He has been a teaching assistant for the Introduction to Lifestyle Medicine course at the Harvard University Extension School and was elected to the board of the American College of Lifestyle Medicine from 2014-2016. Jonathan has published research in sleep medicine, nutrition, sports and exercise, obesity, and behavior change and is on the editorial board of the American Journal of Lifestyle Medicine.

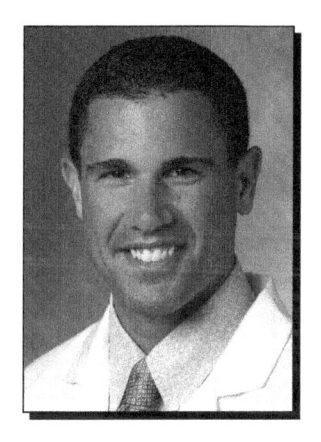

Richard Joseph, MD is currently a senior resident physician in the HVMA Primary Care Residency Program at Brigham & Women's Hospital (BWH). This program is a collaboration between BWH, Harvard Vanguard Medical Associates (HVMA), the Department of Population Medicine at Harvard Medical School, and the Harvard Pilgrim Health Care Institute. Prior to his clinical training, Rich earned his joint MD/MBA from Stanford University. While at Stanford, Rich helped develop the lifestyle medicine seminar, "an interdisciplinary course for Stanford clinicians, medical students, and graduate students that encourages physicians to facilitate behavioral change and promote a culture of health and wellness in patients." The course has enjoyed great success as measured by ongoing growth in enrollment. After residency, Rich plans to design care delivery models that provide a unique combination of primary care, lifestyle medicine interests, and health and fitness.

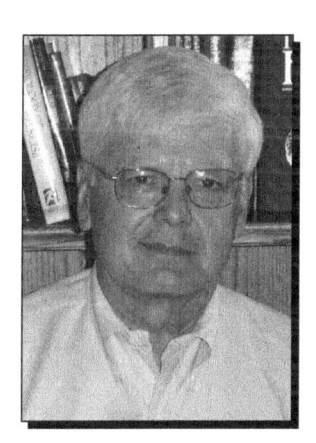

James A. Peterson, PhD is a sports medicine consultant who resides in Monterey, CA. A fellow of ACSM, he has written over 100 books, as well as over 100 published articles. Previously, he served as the director of sports medicine for StairMaster Sports/Medical Products (1990-1995). Before that, he was a member of the faculty at the United States Military Academy at West Point (1971-1990).